Biomarkers in Oncology

Heinz-Josef Lenz
Editor

Biomarkers in Oncology

Prediction and Prognosis

Springer

Editor
Heinz-Josef Lenz, M.D., F.A.C.P.
Division of Medical Oncology
Norris Comprehensive Cancer Center
Keck School of Medicine
University of Southern California
Los Angeles, CA, USA

ISBN 978-1-4419-9754-8 ISBN 978-1-4419-9755-5 (eBook)
DOI 10.1007/978-1-4419-9755-5
Springer New York Heidelberg Dordrecht London

Library of Congress Control Number: 2012944172

Printed on acid-free paper

Springer is part of Springer Science+Business Media (www.springer.com)

This book is dedicated to all patients with cancer and their families, and to my parents, who always encouraged me to pursue my dream and taught me compassion and care.

Preface

This book attempts to address the complexity of biomarker identification, development, and clinical relevance in solid tumors and hematological malignancies. It provides an overview on validated biomarkers, which already impact treatment, decisions, and shed some light onto the future development of new biomarkers. We also address the challenges and limitations of biomarker validation and diagnostic test development. We include novel and cutting-edge technologies, which in the future will be increasingly utilized, such as circulating tumor cells. This book gives hematologists, oncologists, basic scientists, and physician scientists an overview on the status of biomarker integration into the clinical practices. We are fortunate to have benefited from the expertise of the internationally renowned authors and experts with clinical and basic science background who contributed to this book. Our hope is that this book can stimulate innovative translational research collaborations by providing insights into how biomarkers in different diseases using different technologies were identified and validated.

Los Angeles, CA, USA Heinz-Josef Lenz, M.D., F.A.C.P.

Acknowledgements

I would like to thank all of my coauthors, who worked diligently on their contributions to the book. Many of them reviewed and provided invaluable feedback regarding chapters in the book.

My editor, Michael D. Sova, deserves a special thank you for his essential and calm guidance throughout the process of preparing this book.

Finally, I would like to acknowledge my wife, Maria, and my children, Felicitas, Cosima, Annika, and Daria for their support and understanding throughout the process of writing this book, which all too frequently necessitated my absence from family activities.

Contents

Contributors

Nazish Ahmad, B.A., D.O. Department of Medicine, University of Southern California, Los Angeles, CA, USA

Al B. Benson III, M.D., F.A.C.O. Department of Hematology and Oncology, Department of Medicine, Feinberg School of Medicine, Robert H. Lurie Comprehensive Cancer Center, Northwestern Memorial Hospital, Chicago, IL, USA

Charles D. Blanke, M.D. Division of Medical Oncology, British Columbia Cancer Agency, Vancouver, BC, Canada

Helene Blons, M.D., Ph.D. Department of Biology, Hôpital Europ*é*en Georges-Pompidou, Paris, France

Valerie Boige, M.D., Ph.D. Department of Medicine, Institut Gustave Roussy, Villejuif, France

Jon Burrows, Ph.D. OncoPlex Diagnostics, Rockville, MD, USA

Janine M. Davies, M.D., B.N., M.Sc. Division of Hematology/Oncology, Lineberger Comprehensive Cancer Center, University of North Carolina at Chapel Hill, Chapel Hill, NC, USA

Casimir P. Eitner, B.Sc. OncoPlex Diagnostics, Rockville, MS, USA

Gregory A. Endress NeoDiagnostix, Inc., Rockville, MD, USA

Agustin A. Garcia, M.D. Division of Medical Oncology, University of Southern California, Los Angeles, CA, USA

Armin Gerger, M.D. Division of Medical Oncology, Norris Comprehensive Cancer Center, Keck School of Medicine, University of Southern California, Los Angeles, CA, USA

Barbara J. Gitlitz, M.D. Division of Medical Oncology, Department of Internal Medicine, Norris Comprehensive Cancer Center, Keck School of Medicine, University of Southern California, Los Angeles, CA, USA

Amir Goldkorn, M.D. Division of Medical Oncology, Department of Internal Medicine, Norris Comprehensive Cancer Center, Keck School of Medicine, University of Southern California, Los Angeles, CA, USA

Steffen Heeg, M.D. Department of Hematology and Oncology, University of Freiburg Medical Center, Freiburg, Germany

Ilia Ichetovkin, Ph.D. Head of Oncology, Vela Diagnostics, Fairfield, NJ, USA

David H. Ilson, M.D., Ph.D. Department of Medical Oncology Solid Tumor GI, Memorial Sloan-Kettering Cancer Center, New York, NY, USA

Daniel J. Knauer, Ph.D. Manager, Oncology R&D, Vela Diagnostics, Fairfield, NJ, USA

Melissa J. LaBonte, Ph.D. Division of Medical Oncology, Norris Comprehensive Cancer Center, Keck School of Medicine, University of Southern California, Los Angeles, CA, USA

Pierre Laurent-Puig, M.D., Ph.D. Department of Biochemistry, Hôpital Européen Georges-Pompidou, Paris, France

Thierry Lecomte, M.D., Ph.D. Department of Hepato-Gastroenterology, CHRU of Tours, CHU Trousseau, Chambray-lès-Tours, France

Heinz-Josef Lenz, M.D., F.A.C.P. Division of Medical Oncology, Norris Comprehensive Cancer Center, Keck School of Medicine, University of Southern California, Los Angeles, CA, USA

Howard J. Lim, M.D., Ph.D., F.R.C.P.C. Department of Medical Oncology, British Columbia Cancer Agency, Vancouver, BC, Canada

Edwin Y. Lin, M.D. Department of Medical Oncology, Norris Comprehensive Cancer Center, Keck School of Medicine, University of Southern California, Los Angeles, CA, USA

Stephen V. Liu, M.D. Division of Medical Oncology, Department of Internal Medicine, Norris Comprehensive Cancer Center, Keck School of Medicine, University of Southern California, Los Angeles, CA, USA

Marie-Anne Loriot, M.D., Ph.D. Department of Biology, Hôpital Européen Georges-Pompidou, Paris, France

Stan Louie, Ph.D. Clinical Pharmacy and Pharmaceutical Economics and Policies, University of Southern California, Los Angeles, CA, USA

Sumithra J. Mandrekar, Ph.D. Department of Health Sciences Research, Mayo Clinic, Rochester, MN, USA

Ben Markman, M.B.B.S., F.R.A.C.P. Monash Institute of Medical Research, Monash University, Victoria, Australia

Howard L. McLeod, Pharm.D. Department of Pharmacy, Eshelman School of Pharmacy, University of North Carolina at Chapel Hill, Chapel Hill, NC, USA

Bud Mishra, Ph.D. Department of Computer Science and Mathematics, Courant Institute of Mathematical Sciences, New York University, New York, NY, USA

Daniel P. Petrylak, M.D. Signal Transduction Program, Cedar Street, New Haven, CT, USA

Courtney K. Phillips, M.D. Department of Urology, Mount Sinai School of Medicine, New York, NY, USA

Richard M. Pinnola, B.S. NeoDiagnostix, Inc., Rockville, MD, USA

Vladimir Poponin, Ph.D. Nant Holdings, LLC, Costa Mesa, CA, USA

Derek G. Power, M.D. Department of Medicine, Gastrointestinal Oncology Service, Memorial Sloan Kettering Cancer Center, New York, NY, USA

David Ian Quinn, M.B.B.S.(Hons), Ph.D., F.R.A.C.P., F.A.C.P. Department of Oncology, Norris Comprehensive Cancer Center, Keck School of Medicine, University of Southern California, Los Angeles, CA, USA

Ravin Rupani, M.D. Department of Hematology and Oncology, Norris Comprehensive Cancer Center, University of South California, Los Angeles, CA, USA

Jared Russell, B.S. Pharmacology and Pharmaceutical Sciences, University of Southern California, Los Angeles, CA, USA

Daniel J. Sargent, Ph.D. Department of Health Sciences Research, Mayo Clinic, Rochester, MN, USA

Patrick Soon-Shiong, M.D. Departments of Microbiology, Immunology, and Molecular Genetics, Bioengineering, University of California, Los Angeles, Los Angeles, CA, USA

Gregory P. Swanson, M.D. Department of Radiation Oncology, Radiology and Urology, University of Texas Health Science Center at San Antonio, San Antonio, TX, USA

Josep Tabernero, M.D. Department of Medical Oncology Service, Vall d'Hebron University Hospital, Barcelona, Spain

Thomas Wray Tombler Jr., Ph.D. ADD Biosensors, Somerset, NJ, USA

Lex H.T. Van der Ploeg, Ph.D. Rhythm Pharmaceuticals, Managing Director VDP, LLC, Rhythm, Boston, MA, USA

Maxwell T. Vergo, B.S., M.D. Division of Hematology and Oncology, Department of Medicine, Feinberg School of Medicine, Robert H. Lurie Comprehensive Cancer Center, Northwestern Memorial Hospital, Chicago, IL, USA

Eduardo Vilar, M.D., Ph.D. Department of Internal Medicine, University of Michigan Comprehensive Cancer Center, Ann Arbor, MI, USA

Cornelius F. Waller, M.D. Department of Hematology and Oncology, University of Freiburg Medical Center, Freiburg, Germany

Tong Xu, Ph.D. Division of Medical Oncology, Department of Internal Medicine, Norris Comprehensive Cancer Center, Keck School of Medicine, University of Southern California, Los Angeles, CA, USA

Chapter 1
Predictive Markers in Colon Cancer

Armin Gerger, Melissa J. LaBonte, and Heinz-Josef Lenz

Introduction

Over the past several decades, significant progress has been made towards improving survival outcome of patients with colorectal cancer (CRC), which is due in part to the approval and incorporation of multiple new chemotherapeutic agents including irinotecan, oxaliplatin, and the biologically targeted agents, bevacizumab, cetuximab, and panitumumab [1]. However, the prognosis for patients with metastatic colorectal cancer (mCRC) remains poor, with a 5-year survival rate of about 8% and >50% of CRC patients demonstrating recurrent or metastatic disease regardless of curative operations [2]. The antimetabolite 5-fluorouracil (5-FU) and the oral 5-FU pro-drug, capecitabine, remain the backbone in CRC treatment regimens. The single agent response rates (RR) of 5-FU had been shown to range from 20 to 25% in patients with mCRC [3]. In addition, it has further been demonstrated that 5-FU can be safely substituted for capecitabine when combined with oxaliplatin without any loss of efficacy [4]. Combining 5-FU with DNA-damaging agents, oxaliplatin or irinotecan, increases tumor RR to 40–50% and prolongs overall survival (OS) [5, 6]. In recent years, the biologically targeted agents such as bevacizumab, a recombinant monoclonal antibody (mAb) against the pro-angiogenic vascular endothelial growth factor (VEGF), cetuximab, a chimeric mAb against the epidermal growth factor receptor (EGFR), and panitumumab, a fully humanized EGFR mAb have emerged as key components in mCRC management demonstrating additional clinical benefit [7].

While there have been many advances in new drug development for CRC, several key questions remain: Why is the benefit from therapeutic agents seen only

A. Gerger, M.D. • M.J. LaBonte, Ph.D. • H.-J. Lenz, M.D., F.A.C.P. (✉)
Division of Medical Oncology, Norris Comprehensive Cancer Center, Keck School of Medicine, University of Southern California, 1441 Eastlake Avenue, Los Angeles, CA 90033, USA
e-mail: lenz@usc.edu

H.-J. Lenz (ed.), *Biomarkers in Oncology: Prediction and Prognosis*,
DOI 10.1007/978-1-4419-9755-5_1, © Springer Science+Business Media New York 2013

in selected patient populations? Why do some patients develop severe toxicities from these drugs? How can we individualize cancer treatment by preselecting patients for the most appropriate treatment strategies? Currently, a lack of validated predictive biomarkers for almost all therapeutic agents and patient screening restricts our ability to tailor specific drugs to specific patient cohorts, and may be viewed as one of the largest barriers and challenges to the success of individualized CRC therapy. The "one size fits all" approach to CRC therapy has been replaced with the realization that treatment strategies need to be tailored on an individual patient-specific basis due to the multitude of factors that have been shown to contribute to the outcome of therapy [8]. With the knowledge of both the molecular biology of the patient and the cancer expanding at an exponential rate, the significant heterogeneity within both has become more apparent. In recent years, major efforts have been made on the identification of predictive biomarkers in CRC, which in turn would allow the identification of the patients who will benefit from therapy, while sparing others of needless toxicity and the financial burden of a treatment that will fail to demonstrate any benefit [9]. Biomarkers are defined as measurable molecular, cellular, or functional parameters indicative of a particular genetic, epigenetic, or functional status of a biological system. Effective biomarkers are reproducible, repeatable, and measurable through a minimally invasive procedure, can be prognostic when they are indicative of the natural course and outcome of the disease, regardless of the treatment, and become predictive when they can be significantly correlated with the clinical response to a particular treatment regimen [10].

Despite extensive research into biomarkers in CRC, progress to date on the identification, validation, and integration of predictive biomarkers into routine clinical practice has been slow and unsatisfactory, resulting in the need to address several critical questions: can single markers sufficiently describe the impact of a given treatment on a predefined subset of CRC patients? Would a more comprehensive pathway approach to categorize CRC patients for treatment benefit yield more promising results? At least, in part, these questions are currently being addressed with the introduction of tumoral *KRAS* status as a predictive biomarker for the anti-EGFR mAbs, cetuximab and panitumumab [11]. Recent evidence suggests that the benefit of cetuximab is limited to mCRC patients carrying a *KRAS* wild-type tumor status. Results from several clinical trials demonstrated RR of up to 60% with cetuximab plus chemotherapy in the *KRAS* wild-type patient populations, indicating a valuable and robust biomarker predicting increased response to a given regimen [12]. However, it has further been shown that the presence of a *KRAS* wild-type tumor does not exclusively dictate that EGFR-targeting mAbs will be effective. This is evidenced in the reported RR, which indicates that 40% of *KRAS* wild-type patients also do not benefit from EGFR mAb-targeted treatment. The 40% of mCRC patients with *KRAS* mutant tumors simply failed to respond to treatment. Within the patients harboring *KRAS* mutant tumors additional factors, such as mutation of *BRAF*, *NRAS*, and loss of PTEN or *PIK3CA* activation, might contribute to the resistance to EGFR-targeting mAbs and need to undergo further testing [13]. While *KRAS* mutational status represents a significant step forward in the concept of individualized treatment in mCRC, this success ultimately poses further challenges.

It is now widely recognized that even patients with similar clinicopathological characteristics can demonstrate significant variability in their treatment responses and clinical outcome. It is becoming increasingly apparent that disease progression is not a linear chain of events, but largely driven by a multitude of signaling networks and the analysis of a single marker may fail to predict treatment efficacy with a high degree of accuracy and reproducibility. Therefore, it is critical to adopt and implement a more global pathway-based approach whereby analysis of multiple components within the molecular networks being targeted can be evaluated. Moreover, it is now well characterized that many of the pathways that are currently the focus of novel therapeutic development are highly complex with multiple downstream effectors, which can determine drug efficacy. The goal of treatment on an individualized basis should finally involve a simultaneous patient-specific analysis of clinical and pathologic characteristics and analysis of a patient's germline genetic and tumor biomarker profile.

Predictive Markers and Anti-EGFR Therapy

Anti-EGFR mAbs represent an important treatment option in the management of mCRC. Two FDA-approved anti-EGFR mAbs, cetuximab and panitumumab, function through blockade of ligand-induced EGFR tyrosine-kinase activation and prevent activation of downstream intracellular signaling pathways including the phosphatidylinositol 3-kinase (PI3K)/AKT, mitogen-activated protein kinase (MAPK), and signal transducer and activator of transcription 3 (STAT3) pathways [14]. This inhibition ultimately results in a decrease in cellular proliferation and induction of apoptosis. It has been shown that 50–70% of CRCs exhibit EGFR expression. A subset of tumor cells develop dependence or addiction to continuous EGFR signaling that drives their proliferation and survival, and subsequent inhibition of EGFR and therefore rapid withdrawal of pro-survival signaling can lead to catastrophic events within the cell that result in cell-cycle arrest and programmed cell death. It has therefore been hypothesized that increased EGFR dependency might be associated with the increased efficacy of anti-EGFR mAbs. However, EGFR expression, primarily measured by immunohistochemistry (IHC), has failed to provide any definitive correlation with response to cetuximab [8]. In contrast, increased *EGFR* copy number has been associated with tumor responses to anti-EGFR mAbs and the level of sensitivity to cetuximab was proportional to the level of mRNA expression of two EGFR ligands: epiregulin and amphiregulin [15–17].

Not surprisingly given that EGFR is strongly expressed in skin cells, patients treated with anti-EGFR mAbs experience skin reactions with various degrees of severity. This raised the question whether skin toxicity could be used as a surrogate marker for anti-EGFR therapies. In the NCIC CTG CO.17 clinical trial that investigated single-agent cetuximab efficacy in heavily pretreated mCRC patients, a rash of grade 2 or higher was strongly associated with improved OS (hazard ratio (HR) for death 0.33; 95% confidence interval (CI) 0.22–0.50; $P<0.001$) [18]. Preliminary data from the Evaluation of Various Erbitux REgimens by means of Skin and Tumour biopsies (EVEREST) trial suggests that in patients with tumors expressing wild-type *KRAS* who had no or mild skin reactions, dose escalation of cetuximab in combination with irinotecan may improve RR compared with standard-dose cetuximab, although this result did not reach statistical significance. Similar to what is observed with bevacizumab-induced hypertension, the utility of skin toxicity as a predictive marker for anti-EGFR therapy is limited in its use as it cannot be assessed a priori. A larger body of evidence is available for predictive biomarkers to anti-EGFR treatment, with the ability to identify patients that will fail to respond to anti-EGFR treatment. More comprehensive data suggests that oncogenic mutations in genes of the intracellular signaling pathways of the EGFR-signaling cascade are responsible for primary intrinsic resistance to anti-EGFR treatment in mCRC patients.

KRAS

The first identified biomarker for response to anti-EGFR therapies was *KRAS*. *KRAS* is a GTPase protein and an oncogene that has been shown to be mutated in 30–40% of CRC patients [12]. Under normal cellular conditions, wild-type *KRAS* activity is tightly regulated and only transiently activated. However, the activating mutation in *KRAS* renders the RAS/RAF/MEK/MAPK and PI3K/AKT pathways constitutively active, even in the presence of EGFR inhibition. Of the *KRAS*-mutant CRC patients, 85–90% harbor mutations in codon 12 or 13 and 5% in both codons 61 and 146 [19].

A large body of evidence confirmed the preliminary findings by Lievre and colleagues that *KRAS*-mutated tumors in patients with mCRC lacked response to cetuximab treatment [11]. In an updated analysis of the randomized CRYSTAL trial in 540 mCRC patients treated with first-line FOLFIRI ± cetuximab, there was a statistically significant difference in favor of *KRAS* wild-type compared to *KRAS*-mutant tumors for RR, progression-free survival (PFS), and overall survival. The OPUS trial of 233 patients also demonstrated that a benefit from the addition of cetuximab to FOLFOX-4 therapy was restricted to the *KRAS* wild-type population [12]. To date, almost all studies investigating cetuximab and panitumumab efficacy have demonstrated that patients harboring *KRAS*-mutant mCRC fail to benefit from these EGFR-targeted agents.

All patients with mCRC are now tested for seven mutations in *KRAS* codons 12 and 13 before receiving anti-EGFR mAbs. In the majority of the translational *KRAS* studies that have been conducted, codon 12 and 13 mutations have been grouped together, without specific subgroup analyses. However, reports now indicate that not all *KRAS* mutant tumors respond equally to EGFR-targeted treatment, with a small subset of patients with *KRAS*-mutated tumors responding to anti-EGFR therapy. In these tumors, codon 13 mutations were overrepresented when compared with the overall *KRAS*-mutated tumor population. In vitro data support this finding with *KRAS* codon 13 mutations exhibiting weaker transforming activity than *KRAS* codon 12 mutations [20]. Based on these observations, De Roock and colleagues conducted a large exploratory retrospective pooled analysis of chemotherapy-refractory mCRC patients treated with cetuximab and chemotherapy investigating the association of *KRAS* G13D mutation in relation to outcome. The authors found an association between longer PFS and OS among patients with *KRAS* G13D-mutated tumors compared to other *KRAS*-mutated tumor types. However, these preliminary data need to be further validated in prospective randomized trials before drawing any conclusions about treating *KRAS* G13D-mutated tumors with anti-EGFR therapy [21].

Further evidence supports that not all *KRAS* mutations respond equally to treatment and need to be evaluated on an individual basis. A retrospective European consortium study showed that *KRAS* codon 61 mutant tumors have a lower RR than wild-type tumors and, because the mutation incidence is similar to some *KRAS* codon 12 mutations, suggested that *KRAS* codon 61 should be included in the *KRAS* mutation testing. By contrast with a previous report, *KRAS* codon 146 mutations did not affect cetuximab efficacy. The co-occurrence of *KRAS* codon 146 mutations with other *KRAS* mutations is an additional indication that this might not be an important oncogenic codon [19].

Despite the ability to utilize *KRAS* mutational status in determining patient sensitivity to EGFR-mAbs, not all *KRAS* wild-type patients respond to these mAbs. Approximately 40–60% of *KRAS* wild-type patients fail to respond to EGFR targeting mAbs, which may indicate other molecular determinants within the downstream signaling pathways that may mediate sensitivity to this family of targeted agents.

BRAF

BRAF, v-raf murine sarcoma viral oncogene homolog B1, is located immediately downstream of *KRAS* in the signaling cascade. While several mutations in *BRAF* have been identified, the best-described and most prevalent mutation is the activating *V600E* mutation located in exon 15 that results in constitutive activation of the RAF/MEK/ERK pathway. Analysis of both *KRAS* and *BRAF* mutations in the same patient population has demonstrated that mutations in these two genes are mutually exclusive. The mutation frequency for *BRAF* has been shown significantly lower, with its identification in only 5–10% of CRC patients [22]. This frequency has been shown to be dependent on the patient population investigated, since *BRAF* mutations confer poor prognosis. *BRAF* mutations are associated with the CpG island methylator phenotype (CIMP) and microsatellite instability, whereas *KRAS* mutations are more common in CIMP-low and microsatellite-stable tumors [13].

A number of studies to date have reported that the *V600E* mutation in *BRAF* precludes response to anti-EGFR therapy. Di Nicolantonio and colleagues reported that patients with *BRAF* mutations failed to respond to cetuximab therapy [22]. In support of this, a recent study by Loupakis and colleagues reported similar findings with lack of response and shorter PFS and OS in *BRAF*-mutated tumors

[23]. Further evidence in support of these findings comes from two recent studies which noted lower RR and shorter PFS and OS in *BRAF*-mutated tumors [19, 24]. In contrast, pooled analysis of the OPUS and CRYSTAL trials demonstrated that *BRAF* mutation status does not appear to be a strong predictive biomarker for the addition of cetuximab to chemotherapy; however, the sample size of *BRAF*-mutated tumors was too small to draw definitive conclusions [25]. While the clinical data supports the importance of mutations in *BRAF* in association with resistance to anti-EGFR therapies, future trials of large cohorts of *KRAS* wild-type patients treated with anti-EGFR therapies are required to fully explore the predictive role of *BRAF* mutations in determining response.

NRAS

NRAS represents another downstream effector of the EGFR-signaling pathway and mutations in *NRAS* might also have negative effects on response to anti-EGFR therapies. *NRAS* and *KRAS* are very closely related, having 85% amino acid sequence identity. *NRAS* mutations occur in a smaller percentage, approximately 2–5% of CRC, than *KRAS* or *BRAF* mutations and seem to arise at a later stage in the development of CRC, similar to the stage at which mutations in p53 appear to arise [10].

In a recent retrospective European consortium analysis, patients with *NRAS*-mutant mCRC showed a significantly lower RR (7.7% vs. 38.1%, odds ratio (OR) 0.14, 95% CI 0.007–0.70; $P = 0.013$) than did patients with *NRAS* wild-type tumors. There was no significant difference between *NRAS* wild-type vs. mutants in disease control, median PFS, and OS. However, *NRAS* mutations were significantly associated with lower response and disease control rates in a multivariate analysis (including mutation status of *KRAS*, *PIK3CA* exon 20, *PIK3CA* exon 9, *BRAF*, and *NRAS*, and age, sex, number of previous chemotherapy lines, and center as covariates) and retained in the conditional inference trees [19]. *NRAS* status in mCRC therefore represents a promising predictive biomarker and warrants further exploration and validation in prospective trials.

PI3K

PI3Ks belong to a family of heterodimeric lipid kinases. PI3K isoforms have been grouped into three classes based on their structural features and lipid substrate preferences [26]. The PI3K class IA molecules are heterodimers, composed of regulatory (p85) and catalytic (p110) subunits. Activation of class I PI3Ks is initiated by growth factor receptors, such as insulin and insulin-like growth-factor-1 receptors (IGFR1), platelet-derived growth-factor receptors (PDGFRs), and members of the HER-family [13]. It was originally hypothesized that *PIK3CA* mutations could constitutively activate the PI3K/AKT axis and may render the inhibition of the upstream EGFR ineffective to its oncogenic signaling. In CRC, mutations in the p110α (encoded by *PIK3CA*) isoform roughly occur in 15–20% of patients [27]. More than 80% of *PIK3CA* mutations in CRC occur in exon 9 (60–65%; E542K, E545K) or exon 20 (20–25%; H1047R) [13, 19]. In vitro studies have demonstrated that the gain-of-function induced by *PIK3CA* exon 20 mutations (coding for the kinase domain) is independent of RAS binding, whereas the mutations in exon 9 (coding for the helical domain) require the RAS–GTP interaction [28].

Sartore-Bianchi and colleagues demonstrated a lack of response to anti-EGFR therapy in mCRC patients harboring *PIK3CA* mutations [29]. In contrast, in a cohort of 200 patients, Prenen and colleagues reported no strong rationale for the use of *PIK3CA* mutations as a single predictive marker for response to anti-EGFR treatment [30]. One reason for the conflicting data could be the apparent differences between the mutations in exon 9 and exon 20, which ultimately represent different biological subgroups that were not separately analyzed in both studies. In addition, different proportions of exon 9 and exon 20 mutations in the patient cohorts might explain the results, at least in part. Recently, De Roock and colleagues reported for the first time an association between *KRAS* mutations and *PIK3CA* exon 9 (not exon 20) mutations in mCRC. These results are in line with the finding that the gain-of-function induced by *PIK3CA* exon 9 mutations (helical domain) requires the RAS–GTP interaction. Moreover, their data suggest that only *PIK3CA* exon 20 mutations are associated with worse outcome after cetuximab treatment [19]. These data holds promise for further translational investigations and biological studies. However, because of the low number of *PIK3CA* exon 20 mutations, these results should be regarded as both preliminary and explorative.

PTEN

PTEN, phosphatase and tensin homologue, is a tyrosine phosphatase enzyme that functions as negative regulator of the PI3K/AKT pathway, thereby attenuating its downstream signaling. Essentially, PTEN functions to maintain equilibrium in PI3K signaling by dephosphorylating PI3K's product, thereby converting it from an active to inactive state. The COOH-terminal region of the PTEN protein has been shown to be required for its tumor suppressor function. Mutations in *PTEN* produce truncated proteins lacking the COOH-terminal region, which then are rapidly degraded, resulting in loss of PTEN protein expression. While *PTEN* mutations are infrequent in CRC, they may be more common in MSI-High (MSI-H) tumors. Also allelic losses at chromosome 10q23 or hypermethylation of the *PTEN* promoter region can result in loss of PTEN activity. It has been observed that *PTEN* promoter hypermethylation is a frequent occurrence in MSI-H tumors (19.1%) compared to 2.2% of MSI-Low/microsatellite stable tumors [13, 31]. Loss of PTEN, as measured by IHC in mCRC, has been reported to predict lack of benefit from cetuximab treatment [32, 33]. Interestingly, PTEN expression was shown to be inconsistent between the primary tumor and distant metastases site(s). Distant metastases often showed loss of PTEN, whereas the primary tumor retained normal functioning PTEN [33]. Since there are numerous differences in translational PTEN studies, including PTEN

Table 1.1 Predictive biomarkers of monoclonal antibodies in colorectal cancer

Drug	Biomarker	Biological function	Predictive function
Anti-EGFR therapy (cetuximab and panitumumab)	EGFR copy number [15, 16]	EGFR gene amplification	Increased response to anti-EGFR therapy
	Epiregulin and amphiregulin overexpression [17]	EGFR ligands	Increased response to anti-EGFR therapy
	Skin rash (surrogate marker) [18]	NA	Early marker of response to anti-EGFR therapy
	KRAS mutations codon 12, 13, and 61 [13, 19, 21]	Constitutive activation of downstream pathways	Resistance to anti-EGFR therapy (codon 13 mutations lower RR, but no difference in PFS and OS)
	BRAF V600E mutation [13, 19]	Constitutive activation of the RAF/MEK/ERK pathway	Resistance to anti-EGFR therapy
	NRAS mutations [13, 19]	Constitutive activation of downstream pathways	Resistance to anti-EGFR therapy
	PIK3CA mutation in exon 20 [13, 19]	Constitutive activation of PI3K/AKT axis	Resistance to anti-EGFR therapy
	PTEN IHC [23, 32]	Negative regulator of PI3K/AKT signaling	Los of PTEN by IHC predicts resistance to anti-EGFR therapy
Bevacizumab	IL-8 plasma level [43]	VEGF-independent pro-angiogenic factor	Shorter PFS with bevacizumab plus FOLFIRI
	VEGF-1154 G/A polymorphism [46]	GG increased VEGF expression	GG fourfold higher risk of tumor progression with bevacizumab plus FOLFIRI
	VEGF-634 G/C polymorphism [46]	GG lower VEGF expression	GG higher RR with bevacizumab plus FOLFIRI
	Hypertension (surrogate marker) [47]	NA	Early marker of response to bevacizumab

IL interleukin; *VEGF* vascular endothelial growth factor; *PFS* progression-free survival; *OS* overall survival; *RR* response rate; *NA* not applicable; *EGFR* epidermal growth factor receptor; *IHC* immunohistochemistry

antibodies, IHC scoring algorithms, and whether PTEN expression was measured in the primary or metastatic tumor tissue, future studies are needed to determine the role of PTEN as a predictive marker for anti-EGFR therapy (Table 1.1).

Predictive Markers and Bevacizumab

Angiogenesis, the sprouting or intussusception of preexistent blood vessels to form new vessels, is a crucial component for the delivery of oxygen, nutrients, growth factors, and hormones that are essential for tumor growth and disease progression [34]. Several key signaling pathways have been implicated in angiogenesis; however the current understanding and research place greater importance on the VEGF pathway. VEGF is a ligand produced by tumor cells and the associated stroma that stimulates angiogenesis by binding to either one of the two highly related receptor tyrosine kinases (RTKs), VEGF receptor 1 [VEGFR-1, also known as fms-like tyrosine kinase (FLT-1)] and VEGF receptor 2 [VEGFR-2, also known as kinase insert domain receptor (KDR)]. Ligand binding activates multiple downstream signaling pathways including the PI3K/AKT, MAPK, and focal adhesion pathways, which ultimately results in the increased proliferation, migration, and survival of endothelial cells [35]. The hypothesis that tumor progression may be driven in part through increased angiogenesis and therefore be arrested by angiogenesis inhibitors has been confirmed experimentally by a large body of evidence [36]. Bevacizumab, a recombinant humanized anti-VEGF mAb, prevents VEGF-A from binding to its receptors and activating downstream signaling networks. The addition of bevacizumab to standard chemotherapy has proven efficacious in multiple advanced cancers such as mCRC. The approval of bevacizumab for use in mCRC was based on the results of the pivotal phase III AVF2107 trial, which demonstrated improved efficacy in chemotherapy-naive patients with the combination of bolus 5-FU and irinotecan plus bevacizumab in comparison to chemotherapy alone (RR 44.8 vs. 34.8%, $P=0.004$; median PFS 10.6 vs. 6.2 months, HR 0.54, $P<0.001$; median OS 20.3 vs. 15.6 months, HR 0.66, $P<0.001$) [37, 38]. The large phase III trials, NO 16966 and ECOG 3200, provided further support for the benefit of bevacizumab when added to conventional chemotherapeutic regimens in mCRC [38, 39].

While there is a reported benefit of the addition of bevacizumab to chemotherapy in mCRC, the clinical benefit has been limited to a subset of patients resulting in the need for the identification of biomarkers that may be used in determining which patients will benefit from its incorporation into their treatment regimen. Despite the effects of bevacizumab in unselected mCRC patients, the ability to target therapy towards a well-selected subgroup of patients would increase the likelihood of benefit and would improve its cost-effectiveness and therapeutic outcomes. Although several biomarkers associated with angiogenesis measured before treatments have been shown to provide potential prognostic value, there is limited information on biomarkers for clinical response and outcome to bevacizumab treatment in CRC patients. While no one biomarker has been widely agreed upon, several studies have shown promising data. Another challenge is establishing adequate criteria for measurement of response to bevacizumab in CRC. Bevacizumab has been shown to act predominately as a cytostatic agent, thereby increasing the time to show effective benefit, making objective response measurements such as tumor shrinkage less useful for determining its efficacy [40, 41].

VEGF Expression and Circulating Biomarkers

There is a biological rationale to suggest that the level of VEGF expression by a tumor would determine its responsiveness to bevacizumab. However, the examination of VEGF expression in a retrospective analysis of 278 mCRC patients failed to identify a patient subgroup with a differential response to bevacizumab therapy [42]. Intuitively, one would suggest that baseline or dynamic plasma concentration of VEGF would be helpful in predicting response to VEGF inhibitors. Baseline VEGF levels as predictive biomarkers and VEGF modulation after bevacizumab therapy are still a matter of debate with contrasting results and requires further validation. In a recently published study, Kopetz and colleagues found no association between bevacizumab therapy and VEGF modulations in mCRC patients. However, elevated interleukin (IL)-8 levels at baseline were associated with decreased PFS [43]. IL-8 is a member of the chemokine family that has been implicated to play an important role in CRC growth, angiogenesis, and metastasis. This raises the question of whether alternative angiogenic factors are potentially involved in resistance to anti-VEGF treatment, and sustained tumor angiogenesis through VEGF-independent mechanisms occurs.

VEGF Germline Polymorphisms

Angiogenesis is largely a host-mediated event [44]. Will therefore germline genetic variability be the key to predicting angiogenesis inhibitor effects? In a pioneering study, Schneider and colleagues investigated the association of *VEGF* and *VEGFR-2* polymorphisms with efficacy and toxicity in the ECOG 2100 phase III trial (paclitaxel versus paclitaxel plus bevacizumab as first-line therapy in metastatic breast cancer) and found that the *VEGF-2578 AA* and *VEGF-1154 AA* genotypes predicted a superior OS for patients treated with the combination, but not in patients in the control arm, thus supporting its potential use as a predictive (not prognostic) marker. Two additional genotypes, *VEGF-634 CC* and *VEGF-1498 TT*, were associated with a significantly less grade 3 or 4 hypertension in the combination arm when compared with the alternate genotypes combined. All candidate genotypes in the study were compared with primary tumor expression of *VEGF* and *VEGFR-2*, but there was no statistically significant association found [45]. In mCRC, a small study reported an association between the minor allele of *VEGF-1154* and increased PFS and the *VEGF-634* wild-type and higher RR; however no significant influence on OS and toxicity was found by the investigated *VEGF* polymorphisms [46]. Although these data need to be confirmed in larger clinical trials, investigation of host-related germline polymorphisms may assist in the identification of patients who are more sensitive to bevacizumab containing regimens.

Interestingly, hypertension might be a useful surrogate marker of VEGF activity and predicts the efficacy of bevacizumab as VEGF signaling leads to local vasodilatation and reduced blood pressure by upregulating the production of nitric oxide and other vasodilatators. Bevacizumab inhibits VEGF signaling, which leads to a rapid increase in blood pressure. Preliminary data from small, single-arm studies in mCRC have demonstrated that hypertension induced by bevacizumab treatment was associated with increased RR and extended PFS and OS [47]. Although hypertension may represent an early marker of response in some patients treated with bevacizumab, its utility as a predictor of response remains limited as it cannot be used a priori to select patients who may derive benefit.

Predictive biomarker research in angiogenesis inhibitors is an actively growing field. Although current data are promising, it is still uncertain which biomarker can reliably predict bevacizumab efficacy. With increasing numbers of angiogenesis inhibitors being developed, the need for predictive biomarkers is more critical than ever. Such efforts should be diligently pursued due to the early phases of angiogenesis inhibitor drug development, to move from demonstrating small advantages in unselected populations to the use in selection for individualized therapy. In addition, as preliminary biomarkers are developed, their continued development in large, well-designed prospective clinical trials will be imperative to guide their success and direct the efficacy, safety, and cost considerations associated with these agents.

Predictive Markers and Oxaliplatin

Oxaliplatin is a third-generation platinum compound used in combination with 5-FU and leucovorin (LV) in CRC treatment regimens. It functions through generation of platinum-DNA cross-links that inhibits DNA replication and transcription, which ultimately results in DNA damage and cell death [48]. There have been several key phase III trials establishing the efficacy of combination therapy with oxaliplatin in CRC, in both the adjuvant and metastatic settings. Oxaliplatin activity as a single agent in CRC is not reported [49]. The primary toxicity observed following oxaliplatin treatment is neurotoxicity, presenting as acute or chronic sensory neuropathy. Although many patients recover from neuropathy rapidly after drug discontinuation, not all patients recover completely and even worsen after oxaliplatin withdrawal [1].

Oxaliplatin binds irreversibly to erythrocytes and/or forms complexes with albumin and other plasma proteins. The remaining free fraction of oxaliplatin is biotransformed non-enzymatically and subsequently forms complexes with chloride, glutathione, methionine, and cysteine. The cytotoxicity of oxaliplatin is thought to occur through the formation of DNA adducts which ultimately results in DNA damage and apoptosis. Intracellular oxaliplatin is activated by nonenzymatic hydrolysis and displacement of the oxalate group. Extracellular conjugation of oxaliplatin to albumin results in renal excretion of inactive drug species. Removal of the oxaliplatin-induced DNA cross-link formation by the nucleotide excision repair (NER) pathway might impair oxaliplatin efficacy, although there is no evidence that the mismatch repair complex is involved in resistance to oxaliplatin [48]. Excision repair cross-complementing gene (ERCC1) is an excision nuclease within the NER pathway which plays an important role in repairing DNA cross-link formations. ERCC1 forms a heterodimer with xeroderma pigmentosum group F (XPF), which stabilizes this endonuclease. The protein ERCC1 is responsible for the rate-limiting process of NER, with higher expression levels and/or activity resulting in increased DNA repair. Based on the biological function of the NER pathway and the mode of action of oxaliplatin, low ERCC1 level and/or activity may increase oxaliplatin efficacy through induction of apoptosis. Additional components of the NER pathway that have been implicated in mediated response to oxaliplatin include xeroderma pigmentosum group D (XPD) and X-ray repair cross-complementing 1 (XRCC1) [50].

Excision Repair Cross-Complementing Group 1

In mCRC, a small number of published reports have investigated ERCC1 as a predictive biomarker for oxaliplatin. Shirota and colleagues reported an association between low *ERCC1* gene expression and increased OS in mCRC patients treated with oxaliplatin-based chemotherapy [51]. A retrospective analysis of the phase III randomized CAIRO study that included 506 patients investigated several biomarkers with putative predictive and/or prognostic functions and found no association between ERCC1 protein expression and outcome in mCRC patients treated with oxaliplatin plus capecitabine in second- and third-line treatment [52]. The influence of functional germline polymorphisms in drug target genes on outcome was examined in 166 patients with mCRC receiving first-line therapy with FOLFOX-4 using peripheral blood samples for genotyping. In the multivariate model, *ERCC1-118 TT* genotype, *XPD-751 AC* genotype, and *XPD-751 CC* genotype were significantly associated with an increased risk of tumor progression. In combination analyses, the median PFS was 11.2 months for patients without any of the 3 genotypes, 9.8 months for those with 1 of the high-risk genotypes, and 8 months for those with both the *ERCC1-118 TT* and either *XPD-751 AC* or *CC* genotypes (HR=2.84; *P*=0.002) [53]. In experimental models, the *ERCC1-118 T* allele variants showed potential functional consequences with a trend to higher *ERCC1 mRNA* levels than those observed in the presence of the *ERCC1-118 C* allele, which supports the biological mechanism of oxaliplatin resistance.

Glutathione S-Transferase pi 1

Variable chemosensitivity to oxaliplatin may also depend on detoxification pathways, including the glutathione S-transferase (GST) family of isoenzymes. A single nucleotide polymorphism (SNP) in *GSTP1* causing an isoleucine to valine substitution significantly reduces GSTP1 activity. Inherited homozygous deletions in either *GST Theta 1* (*GSTT1*) or *GST Mu 1* (*GSTM1*) lead to the absence of enzymatic activity. In a recent study of FOLFOX-4-treated mCRC patients, neurotoxicity was significantly associated with the *GSTP1-105 A/G* polymorphism. Carriers of the *GSTP1-105 GG* genotype demonstrated a higher probability to develop grade 3 neurotoxicity than carriers of *GSTP1-105 AG* and *GSTP1-105 AA* genotypes [53]. Germline polymorphisms in the genes of NER pathway therefore represent promising predictive biomarkers for oxaliplatin efficacy and toxicity; however, their clinical significance remains to be further established and validated.

Predictive Markers and Irinotecan

Irinotecan is a topoisomerase I (TOPO1) inhibitor. Irinotecan has demonstrated efficacy in patients with mCRC as a single agent, in combination with the mAbs cetuximab and panitumumab in the *KRAS* wild-type population, and in combination with 5-FU and LV [1, 49]. However, no role for irinotecan in the adjuvant setting of CRC has been established yet. In the randomized phase III BICC-C trial comparing the safety and efficacy of three different irinotecan-containing regimens in the first-line treatment of mCRC, irinotecan plus oral capecitabine (CapeIRI) had to be prematurely discontinued because of safety concerns including a remarkable amount of grade 4 toxicities with diarrhea as the most common grade 3 or 4 toxicity [54].

Irinotecan acts as a pro-drug of SN-38 (7-ethyl-10-hydroxycamptothecin), which once inside the cell is 100- to 1,000-fold more cytotoxic [55]. Irinotecan functions through inhibition of TOPO1, which ultimately leads to single- and double-strand DNA breaks, DNA fragmentation, cell-cycle arrest, and cell death. TOPO1 plays a critical role in the uncoiling DNA for replication and transcription. TOPO1 is overexpressed in about 40–50% of CRC patients [56]. Intracellularly, irinotecan is converted to its active metabolite SN-38 by the enzyme carboxylesterase (CES). CES is an enzyme found in serum, liver, and intestine among other tissues. SN-38 is further conjugated to an inactive glucuronide (SN-38G) by uridine diphosphate glucuronosyltransferases (UGT) and excreted in the bile and, to a lesser extent, in the urine. The major isozyme in this conjugation is UGT1A1, but others (e.g., UGT1A 6, 7, and 9) also have been found to be important [57]. Irinotecan inactivation can also be mediated by cytochrome P-450 isoform 3A (CYP3A4) and CYP3A5, although the latter enzyme has shown only weak catalytic activity [58]. Investigations in heritable familial hyperbilirubinemia syndromes (Gilbert's- and Crigler–Najjar syndrome type I and II) led to the findings of genetic variants in UGT1A, associated with enzyme activity [59].

In colon cancer, one report suggested that the enzymatic activity of CES is correlated with an increased toxicity in the form of neutropenia and diarrhea in patients treated with irinotecan-based chemotherapy [60]. It would be biologically plausible that a high expression of CES in tumor tissue may be correlated with a better response to irinotecan; however, to date, there is no data supporting this hypothesis.

Topoisomerase I

In human CRC cell lines, it was shown that increased levels and activity of the target enzyme TOPO1 were correlated with response to irinotecan treatment [61]. The randomized phase III FOCUS trial evaluated the clinical benefit of 5-FU alone versus 5-FU plus oxaliplatin or 5-FU plus irinotecan and attempted to identify biomarkers of efficacy and toxicity to these treatments. Patients with high TOPO1 protein expression benefited from the addition of either drug (HR 0.48–0.70 in all categories; interaction $P=0.005$; overall $P=0.001$ for irinotecan; $P=0.05$ for oxaliplatin). High TOPO1 expression was associated with a major OS benefit with first-line combination chemotherapy (HR 0.60; median benefit 5.3 months); patients with moderate or low TOPO1 did not benefit (HR=0.92 and 1.09, respectively; interaction $P=0.005$). With increasing expression of TOPO1, the outcome with 5-FU alone was worse, but the addition of a second drug became worthwhile, with a major improvement in survival for the highest expressing patients. While the predictive association of TOPO1 with oxaliplatin was interesting, it was unexpected and statistically weaker than with irinotecan, so should be interpreted with caution [62]. Despite the promising results of this large biomarker analysis, the results of an independent validation in 545 patients from the CAIRO clinical trial treated with capecitabine, irinotecan, and oxaliplatin did not corroborate these findings, reporting no associations between TOPO1 and PFS or OS with first-line combination chemotherapy [52].

UDP-Glucuronyltransferase 1A1 Germline Polymorphisms

*UGT1A1*28* is a common allele with seven TA repeats in a TATA box of the promoter of *UGT1A1* compared with the wild-type allele (*UGT1A1*1*), which has six TA repeats. The seven TA repeats are associated with decreased gene transcription and expression of *UGT1A1* and reduced enzymatic activity compared with the six TA repeats. Patients homozygous for *UGT1A1*28* have reduced glucuronidation of SN-38 and an elevated risk of neutropenia compared with patients with one or two wild-type alleles [10]. The US Food and Drug Administration amended the irinotecan label to include *UGT1A1*28* as a risk factor for severe neutropenia in 2005 based on the findings of 4 pharmacogenetic studies. The warning recommended that these patients should receive a reduction in their starting dose of irinotecan. A recent meta-analysis of ten irinotecan pharmacogenetic studies enrolling a total of 825 patients assessed the correlation between irinotecan-induced hematologic toxicities in *UGT1A1*28* patients, irinotecan dose and overall toxicity [63]. The clinical action for the *UGT1A1* genotype status cannot be utilized in a simple as treat or do not treat manner. The association between genotype and hematologic toxicity is influenced by the dose of irinotecan administered. The *UGT1A1*28* genotype seems to be strongly predictive when high doses of irinotecan (>250 mg/m^2) are given, but only moderately or not predictive in intermediate or low doses, respectively. Also, there is a lack of empirical evidence if dosing irinotecan on the basis of genotypes influences the efficacy of the drug [64]. In a recent study, Cecchin and colleagues investigated the contribution of other members of the UGT1A family to irinotecan toxicity in 250 patients with mCRC and found that *UGT1A7*3* is the only marker predicting severe hematologic toxicity after the first cycle of irinotecan-based chemotherapy. A specific haplotype and gender together predicted severe hematologic toxicity during the entire course of therapy. In addition, *UGT1A1*28/*28* was a significant predictor of RR [65]. These data again highlight that a combination of biomarkers, rather than single biomarker, may better predict efficacy and/or toxicity of a given treatment regimen.

Predictive Markers and 5-FU

Although 5-FU has been in clinical use for over 40 years, it remains the backbone of treatment for both early and advanced CRC. The majority of the chemotherapeutic regimens in CRC incorporate 5-FU or its oral pro-drug, capecitabine, in both the adjuvant and palliative setting. 5-FU functions through inhibition of the enzyme thymidylate synthase (TS), resulting in inhibition of the de novo synthesis of thymidylate, an essential component for DNA synthesis, thereby preventing viable thymine nucleosides from being incorporated into DNA and RNA [66]. More than 80% of the administered 5-FU is primarily catabolized in the liver by the enzyme dihydropyrimidine dehydrogenase (DPD), which is a rate-limiting step for 5-FU catabolism [50, 67].

Thymidylate Synthase

Significant effort has been directed at the evaluation of the differences in expression and activity of several key enzymes in the 5-FU pathway that have been suggested to be responsible for resistance to 5-FU, including TS, thymidine phosphorylase (TP), and DPD. Preclinical models showed increased TS gene expression or gain of gene copy number as indicators for 5-FU resistance [68]. Although conflicting results for TS mRNA and protein expression have been reported, several independent trials consistently reported that low levels of intra-tumoral TS expression are a strong predictive marker for response to 5-FU-based regimes in patients with mCRC. A large meta-analysis of over 3,000 patients by Popat and colleagues analyzed 20 independent studies stratifying OS and/or PFS in CRC patients by TS expression status. The authors concluded that tumors expressing high levels of TS appeared to have reduced OS compared with tumors expressing low TS levels [69]. Several genetic determinants for TS expression have been previously described. A variable number tandem repeat polymorphism in the TS promoter–enhancer region (TSER) leads to double (2R) or triple (3R) tandem repeat of a 28 bp sequence. This tandem repeat polymorphism has been demonstrated to alter the transcriptional and/or translational efficacy of the *TS* gene, with a 3.6-fold increase in *TS* mRNA expression of the homozygous 3R variant compared with the 2R allele [70, 71]. As a result, patients with CRC that are homozygous 3R/3R may demonstrate a lower RR to 5-FU-based regimens. However, a substantial proportion of homozygous 3R/3R patients were identified to have low TS expression levels. An SNP resulting in a G>C exchange has been described within the 3R variant of the *TS* gene. Whereas the G allele of this SNP has been linked to increased gene expression and protein levels, the 3RC polymorphism was found to lead to significantly decreased TS expression compared to the 3RG variant. These findings may explain the observation that patients with the 3R/3R polymorphism have low TS gene expression levels and therefore might benefit from 5-FU-based chemotherapy [10, 72]. However, a significant population of patients with low TS gene expression levels fail to respond to 5-FU-based therapy resulting in the critical need to evaluate in prospective studies with consistent methodology the precise predictive value for both intra-tumoral TS expression and germline gene variants before successful clinical implementation. In addition to evaluation of TS, evaluation of other candidate biomarkers involved in 5-FU metabolism must be diligently pursued.

Dihydropyrimidine Dehydrogenase

In CRC, low DPD expression theoretically leads to decreased degradation of 5-FU and thus higher 5-FU availability. Levels of DPD activity can vary widely between individuals: 3–5% of the population is partially deficient and 0.2% completely deficient [73]. A number of polymorphisms in *DPD* can cause enzyme deficiency, leading to severe toxicity after 5-FU treatment [74]. In addition, intra-tumoral *DPD* mRNA expression has been found to influence response to capecitabine, suggesting a predictive role in mCRC [75]. However, translational data do not unequivocally support a predictive effect of DPD on 5-FU response, toxicity, and clinical outcome [52]. Despite extensive investigation, the pharmacogenetic basis of varied DPD activity remains to be fully elucidated and prospective studies are needed to fully explore the role of DPD to predict 5-FU efficacy and toxicity before clinical implementation.

Microsatellite Instability

Microsatellite instability (MSI) corresponds to an alteration in the length of highly repeated DNA sequences termed microsatellites, resulting in a deficient mismatch repair (dMMR) system. A panel of 5–10 microsatellite loci is used to diagnose MSI cases, for which three categories have been defined: MSI-H, MSI-Low (MSI-L), and microsatellite stable (MSS) for cases without MSI. MSI-H can be found in approximately 15% of sporadic CRC, which is largely due to *MLH1*-promoter hypermethylation. MSI rates have been shown to vary between tumor stages, with 22, 12, and 2% reported in stage II, III, and IV colon cancer, respectively [9, 76]. Because of the low MSI frequency in stage IV, most of the translational studies have been performed in the adjuvant setting. MSI represents a strong and well-validated prognostic factor in adjuvant colon cancer. In a meta-analysis including 32 studies it was confirmed that patients with MSI-H tumors have higher survival rates than those with MSS tumors [77]. Supporting in vitro data, MSI-H was also suggested as predictive biomarker for lack of response to adjuvant 5-FU-based chemotherapy. The CALGB-89803 study reported a predictive effect of MSI-H with improved outcome in stage III CRC patients treated with 5-FU, LV, and irinotecan compared with those receiving 5-FU/LV alone [78]. However, the PETACC-3 study, including 1,327 colon cancer patients, failed to confirm these findings. In a recent study, Sargent and colleagues showed that only patients with stage III MSS colon cancer benefit from adjuvant 5-FU chemotherapy (DFS: HR 0.64; $P=0.001$). In contrast, patients with stage II MSI colon cancer showed a trend to decreased DFS (HR 2.30; $P=0.09$) and a significantly lower OS (HR=2.95; $P=0.04$) when given 5-FU [79]. Although the study by Sargent and colleagues provides evidence that colon cancer patients with dMMR do not benefit from 5-FU/LV therapy, the current standard for stage III disease remains FOLFOX. To date, there are no data showing how the MSI-H results would apply to oxaliplatin-based chemotherapy, thus not justifying excluding patients based on MSI tumor status from the FOLFOX regimen. However, in the appropriate clinical setting, it may be reasonable to include MSI tumor status in the clinical decision-making process, in particular in stage II colon cancer based on the good prognosis and a putative detrimental effect of 5-FU in MSI-H tumors (Table 1.2).

Conclusions

Given the growing number of therapeutic options and the complexity of treatment planning for patients with CRC, treatment options and selection have demonstrated incremental improvements. However, there are no clearly defined guidelines on the best method to best incorporate the new active drugs and regimens into the treatment plans for individual patients. Despite a plethora of promising predictive biomarkers developed, *KRAS* status remains the only marker with sufficient evidence to justify routine clinical assessment for selection of anti-EGFR therapy in mCRC patients.

Table 1.2 Predictive biomarkers of chemotherapy agents in colorectal cancer

Drug	Biomarker	Biological function	Predictive function
Oxaliplatin	ERCC1 gene expression [51]	High ERCC1 increases DNA repair	Decreased OS with oxaliplatin-based chemotherapy
	ERCC1-118 C/T polymorphism [53]	T allele higher ERCC1 mRNA levels	Increased risk for tumor progression with oxaliplatin-based chemotherapy
	GSTP1-105 A/G polymorphism [53]	G allele lower enzyme activity (detoxification)	GG higher neurotoxicity
Irinotecan	Carboxylesterase mRNA expression in PBMC [60]	Converts irinotecan to its active metabolite	High expression predictive for increased toxicity (neutropenia, diarrhea)
	Topoisomerase I (TOPO1) [62]	Uncoiling DNA for replication and transcription	High TOPO1 protein expression predictive for irinotecan response
	UGT1A1*28 TA repeat polymorphism [63, 64]	*28 (7) TA repeats associated with reduced glucuronidation of active metabolite	*28/*28 predicts elevated risk of neutropenia
5-FU	TS mRNA and protein expression [69]	De novo synthesis of thymidylate	High TS predicts 5-FU resistance
	TSER 28-bp 2R/3R repeat polymorphism [71]	3R/3R higher TS mRNA expression	3R/3R predicts 5-FU resistance
	TSER 3R G/C [72]	3RC associated with decreased TS expression	3RC predicts higher 5-FU response
	DPD mRNA expression [75]	Catabolizes 5-FU	Low expression predicts higher capecitabine efficacy
	Variety of DPD polymorphisms [74]	DPD enzyme deficiency	Higher risk for toxicity
	MSI-High [79]	Deficient MMR system	MSI-High predicts 5-FU resistance in stage II colon cancer

ERCC1 excision repair cross-complementing rodent repair deficiency, complementation group 1; *OS* overall survival; *GST1* glutathione S-transferase pi 1; *PBMC* peripheral blood mononuclear cells; *TS* thymidylate synthase; *TSER* thymidylate synthase enhancer region; *DPD* dihydropyrimidine dehydrogenase; *MSI* microsatellite instability; *MMR* MSI and mismatch repair; *5-FU* 5-Fluorouracil

Challenges in finding strong and reliable predictive biomarkers include biological issues inherent to the complexity and redundancy of pathways regulating tumor proliferation, progression, survival, and drug metabolism. A more comprehensive profile of biomarkers describing the biological mechanisms than a single marker is suggested to increase the ability to predict the efficacy and toxicity of a given therapy. Many putative predictive biomarkers have been described in small, limited studies; however, there has to be considerably better validation pursued before any can be thought of as being associated with therapy outcome and therefore incorporated into routine clinical testing. Once a biomarker pattern is identified, standardized techniques will be required for measurements to ensure both inter- and intra-observer reliability. An integrated, collaborative effort among laboratory scientists, clinical oncologists, and pharmaceutical companies is critically needed to successfully incorporate mechanism-based predictive biomarkers for CRC therapies into routine practice within the clinical setting.

References

1. Cunningham D, Atkin W, Lenz HJ, et al. Colorectal cancer. Lancet. 2010;375:1030–47.
2. O'Connell JB, Maggard MA, Ko CY. Colon cancer survival rates with the new American joint committee on cancer sixth edition staging. J Natl Cancer Inst. 2004;96:1420–5.
3. Modulation of fluorouracil by leucovorin in patients with advanced colorectal cancer: evidence in terms of response rate. Advanced Colorectal Cancer Meta-Analysis Project. J Clin Oncol. 1992;10:896–903
4. Van Cutsem E, Twelves C, Cassidy J, et al. Oral capecitabine compared with intravenous fluorouracil plus leucovorin in patients with metastatic colorectal cancer: results of a large phase III study. J Clin Oncol. 2001;19:4097–106.
5. Douillard JY, Cunningham D, Roth AD, et al. Irinotecan combined with fluorouracil compared with fluorouracil alone as first-line treatment for metastatic colorectal cancer: a multicentre randomised trial. Lancet. 2000;355:1041–7.
6. Giacchetti S, Perpoint B, Zidani R, et al. Phase III multicenter randomized trial of oxaliplatin added to chronomodulated fluorouracil-leucovorin as first-line treatment of metastatic colorectal cancer. J Clin Oncol. 2000;18:136–47.
7. Eng C. The evolving role of monoclonal antibodies in colorectal cancer: early presumptions and impact on clinical trial development. Oncologist. 2010;15:73–84.
8. Wilson PM, Labonte MJ, Lenz HJ. Molecular markers in the treatment of metastatic colorectal cancer. Cancer J. 2010;16:262–72.
9. Tejpar S, Bertagnolli M, Bosman F, et al. Prognostic and predictive biomarkers in resected colon cancer: current status and future perspectives for integrating genomics into biomarker discovery. Oncologist. 2010;15:390–404.
10. Winder T, Lenz HJ. Molecular predictive and prognostic markers in colon cancer. Cancer Treat Rev. 2010;36:550–6.
11. Lievre A, Bachet JB, Le Corre D, et al. KRAS mutation status is predictive of response to cetuximab therapy in colorectal cancer. Cancer Res. 2006;66:3992–5.
12. Allegra CJ, Jessup JM, Somerfield MR, et al. American society of clinical oncology provisional clinical opinion: testing for KRAS gene mutations in patients with metastatic colorectal carcinoma to predict response to anti-epidermal growth factor receptor monoclonal antibody therapy. J Clin Oncol. 2009;27:2091–6.

13. Roock WD, Vriendt VD, Normanno N, Ciardiello F, Tejpar S. KRAS, BRAF, PIK3CA, and PTEN mutations: implications for targeted therapies in metastatic colorectal cancer. Lancet Oncol. 2010;12(6):594–603.
14. Ciardiello F, Tortora G. EGFR antagonists in cancer treatment. N Engl J Med. 2008;358:1160–74.
15. Personeni N, Fieuws S, Piessevaux H, et al. Clinical usefulness of EGFR gene copy number as a predictive marker in colorectal cancer patients treated with cetuximab: a fluorescent in situ hybridization study. Clin Cancer Res. 2008;14:5869–76.
16. Sartore-Bianchi A, Moroni M, Veronese S, et al. Epidermal growth factor receptor gene copy number and clinical outcome of metastatic colorectal cancer treated with panitumumab. J Clin Oncol. 2007;25:3238–45.
17. Jacobs B, De Roock W, Piessevaux H, et al. Amphiregulin and epiregulin mRNA expression in primary tumors predicts outcome in metastatic colorectal cancer treated with cetuximab. J Clin Oncol. 2009;27:5068–74.
18. Jonker DJ, O'Callaghan CJ, Karapetis CS, et al. Cetuximab for the treatment of colorectal cancer. N Engl J Med. 2007;357:2040–8.
19. De Roock W, Claes B, Bernasconi D, et al. Effects of KRAS, BRAF, NRAS, and PIK3CA mutations on the efficacy of cetuximab plus chemotherapy in chemotherapy-refractory metastatic colorectal cancer: a retrospective consortium analysis. Lancet Oncol. 2010;11:753–62.
20. Guerrero S, Casanova I, Farre L, Mazo A, Capella G, Mangues R. K-ras codon 12 mutation induces higher level of resistance to apoptosis and predisposition to anchorage-independent growth than codon 13 mutation or proto-oncogene overexpression. Cancer Res. 2000;60: 6750–6.
21. De Roock W, Jonker DJ, Di Nicolantonio F, et al. Association of KRAS p.G13D mutation with outcome in patients with chemotherapy-refractory metastatic colorectal cancer treated with cetuximab. JAMA. 2010;304:1812–20.
22. Di Nicolantonio F, Martini M, Molinari F, et al. Wild-type BRAF is required for response to panitumumab or cetuximab in metastatic colorectal cancer. J Clin Oncol. 2008;26:5705–12.
23. Loupakis F, Ruzzo A, Cremolini C, et al. KRAS codon 61, 146 and BRAF mutations predict resistance to cetuximab plus irinotecan in KRAS codon 12 and 13 wild-type metastatic colorectal cancer. Br J Cancer. 2009;101:715–21.
24. Laurent-Puig P, Cayre A, Manceau G, et al. Analysis of PTEN, BRAF, and EGFR status in determining benefit from cetuximab therapy in wild-type KRAS metastatic colon cancer. J Clin Oncol. 2009;27:5924–30.
25. Bokemeyer C, Kohne C, Rougier P, Stroh C. Cetuximab with chemotherapy (CT) as first-line treatment for metastatic colorectal cancer (mCRC): analysis of the CRYSTAL and OPUS studies according to KRAS and BRAF mutation status. J Clin Oncol. 2010;28:15s. ASCO Meeting Abstracts 2010;28: 3506.
26. Markman B, Atzori F, Perez-Garcia J, Tabernero J, Baselga J. Status of PI3K inhibition and biomarker development in cancer therapeutics. Ann Oncol. 2010;21:683–91.
27. Barault L, Veyrie N, Jooste V, et al. Mutations in the RAS-MAPK, PI(3)K (phosphatidylinositol-3-OH kinase) signaling network correlate with poor survival in a population-based series of colon cancers. Int J Cancer. 2008;122:2255–9.
28. Zhao L, Vogt PK. Helical domain and kinase domain mutations in p110alpha of phosphatidylinositol 3-kinase induce gain of function by different mechanisms. Proc Natl Acad Sci USA. 2008;105:2652–7.
29. Sartore-Bianchi A, Martini M, Molinari F, et al. PIK3CA mutations in colorectal cancer are associated with clinical resistance to EGFR-targeted monoclonal antibodies. Cancer Res. 2009;69:1851–7.
30. Prenen H, De Schutter J, Jacobs B, et al. PIK3CA mutations are not a major determinant of resistance to the epidermal growth factor receptor inhibitor cetuximab in metastatic colorectal cancer. Clin Cancer Res. 2009;15:3184–8.
31. Goel A, Arnold CN, Niedzwiecki D, et al. Frequent inactivation of PTEN by promoter hypermethylation in microsatellite instability-high sporadic colorectal cancers. Cancer Res. 2004;64:3014–21.

32. Frattini M, Saletti P, Romagnani E, et al. PTEN loss of expression predicts cetuximab efficacy in metastatic colorectal cancer patients. Br J Cancer. 2007;97:1139–45.
33. Loupakis F, Pollina L, Stasi I, et al. PTEN expression and KRAS mutations on primary tumors and metastases in the prediction of benefit from cetuximab plus irinotecan for patients with metastatic colorectal cancer. J Clin Oncol. 2009;27:2622–9.
34. Carmeliet P, Jain RK. Angiogenesis in cancer and other diseases. Nature. 2000;407:249–57.
35. Ferrara N. Vascular endothelial growth factor: basic science and clinical progress. Endocr Rev. 2004;25:581–611.
36. Folkman J. Tumor angiogenesis: therapeutic implications. N Engl J Med. 1971;285:1182–6.
37. Hurwitz H, Fehrenbacher L, Novotny W, et al. Bevacizumab plus irinotecan, fluorouracil, and leucovorin for metastatic colorectal cancer. N Engl J Med. 2004;350:2335–42.
38. Saltz LB, Clarke S, Diaz-Rubio E, et al. Bevacizumab in combination with oxaliplatin-based chemotherapy as first-line therapy in metastatic colorectal cancer: a randomized phase III study. J Clin Oncol. 2008;26:2013–9.
39. Giantonio BJ, Catalano PJ, Meropol NJ, et al. Bevacizumab in combination with oxaliplatin, fluorouracil, and leucovorin (FOLFOX4) for previously treated metastatic colorectal cancer: results from the eastern cooperative oncology group study E3200. J Clin Oncol. 2007;25:1539–44.
40. Grothey A, Hedrick EE, Mass RD, et al. Response-independent survival benefit in metastatic colorectal cancer: a comparative analysis of N9741 and AVF2107. J Clin Oncol. 2008;26:183–9.
41. Brower V. Evidence of efficacy: researchers investigating markers for angiogenesis inhibitors. J Natl Cancer Inst. 2003;95:1425–7.
42. Jubb AM, Hurwitz HI, Bai W, et al. Impact of vascular endothelial growth factor-A expression, thrombospondin-2 expression, and microvessel density on the treatment effect of bevacizumab in metastatic colorectal cancer. J Clin Oncol. 2006;24:217–27.
43. Kopetz S, Hoff PM, Morris JS, et al. Phase II trial of infusional fluorouracil, irinotecan, and bevacizumab for metastatic colorectal cancer: efficacy and circulating angiogenic biomarkers associated with therapeutic resistance. J Clin Oncol. 2010;28:453–9.
44. Ferrara N. Role of vascular endothelial growth factor in regulation of physiological angiogenesis. Am J Physiol Cell Physiol. 2001;280:C1358–66.
45. Schneider BP, Wang M, Radovich M, et al. Association of vascular endothelial growth factor and vascular endothelial growth factor receptor-2 genetic polymorphisms with outcome in a trial of paclitaxel compared with paclitaxel plus bevacizumab in advanced breast cancer: ECOG 2100. J Clin Oncol. 2008;26:4672–8.
46. Formica V, Palmirotta R, Del Monte G, et al. Predictive value of VEGF gene polymorphisms for metastatic colorectal cancer patients receiving first-line treatment including fluorouracil, irinotecan, and bevacizumab. Int J Colorectal Dis. 2011;26:143–51.
47. Jubb AM, Harris AL. Biomarkers to predict the clinical efficacy of bevacizumab in cancer. Lancet Oncol. 2010;11:1172–83.
48. Kweekel DM, Gelderblom H, Guchelaar HJ. Pharmacology of oxaliplatin and the use of pharmacogenomics to individualize therapy. Cancer Treat Rev. 2005;31:90–105.
49. Raftery L, Goldberg RM. Optimal delivery of cytotoxic chemotherapy for colon cancer. Cancer J. 2010;16:214–9.
50. Koopman M, Venderbosch S, Nagtegaal ID, van Krieken JH, Punt CJ. A review on the use of molecular markers of cytotoxic therapy for colorectal cancer, what have we learned? Eur J Cancer. 2009;45:1935–49.
51. Shirota Y, Stoehlmacher J, Brabender J, et al. ERCC1 and thymidylate synthase mRNA levels predict survival for colorectal cancer patients receiving combination oxaliplatin and fluorouracil chemotherapy. J Clin Oncol. 2001;19:4298–304.
52. Koopman M, Venderbosch S, van Tinteren H, et al. Predictive and prognostic markers for the outcome of chemotherapy in advanced colorectal cancer, a retrospective analysis of the phase III randomised CAIRO study. Eur J Cancer. 2009;45:1999–2006.
53. Ruzzo A, Graziano F, Loupakis F, et al. Pharmacogenetic profiling in patients with advanced colorectal cancer treated with first-line FOLFOX-4 chemotherapy. J Clin Oncol. 2007;25:1247–54.

54. Fuchs CS, Marshall J, Mitchell E, et al. Randomized, controlled trial of irinotecan plus infusional, bolus, or oral fluoropyrimidines in first-line treatment of metastatic colorectal cancer: results from the BICC-C Study. J Clin Oncol. 2007;25:4779–86.
55. Rivory LP, Robert J. Molecular, cellular, and clinical aspects of the pharmacology of 20(S) camptothecin and its derivatives. Pharmacol Ther. 1995;68:269–96.
56. Boonsong A, Curran S, McKay JA, Cassidy J, Murray GI, McLeod HL. Topoisomerase I protein expression in primary colorectal cancer and lymph node metastases. Hum Pathol. 2002;33:1114–9.
57. Gagne JF, Montminy V, Belanger P, Journault K, Gaucher G, Guillemette C. Common human UGT1A polymorphisms and the altered metabolism of irinotecan active metabolite 7-ethyl-10-hydroxycamptothecin (SN-38). Mol Pharmacol. 2002;62:608–17.
58. Santos A, Zanetta S, Cresteil T, et al. Metabolism of irinotecan (CPT-11) by CYP3A4 and CYP3A5 in humans. Clin Cancer Res. 2000;6:2012–20.
59. Bosma PJ, Chowdhury JR, Bakker C, et al. The genetic basis of the reduced expression of bilirubin UDP-glucuronosyltransferase 1 in Gilbert's syndrome. N Engl J Med. 1995;333:1171–5.
60. Cecchin E, Corona G, Masier S, et al. Carboxylesterase isoform 2 mRNA expression in peripheral blood mononuclear cells is a predictive marker of the irinotecan to SN38 activation step in colorectal cancer patients. Clin Cancer Res. 2005;11:6901–7.
61. Jansen WJ, Zwart B, Hulscher ST, Giaccone G, Pinedo HM, Boven E. CPT-11 in human colon-cancer cell lines and xenografts: characterization of cellular sensitivity determinants. Int J Cancer. 1997;70:335–40.
62. Braun MS, Richman SD, Quirke P, et al. Predictive biomarkers of chemotherapy efficacy in colorectal cancer: results from the UK MRC FOCUS trial. J Clin Oncol. 2008;26:2690–8.
63. Hoskins JM, Goldberg RM, Qu P, Ibrahim JG, McLeod HL. UGT1A1*28 genotype and irinotecan-induced neutropenia: dose matters. J Natl Cancer Inst. 2007;99:1290–5.
64. Hoskins JM, McLeod HL. UGT1A and irinotecan toxicity: keeping it in the family. J Clin Oncol. 2009;27:2419–21.
65. Cecchin E, Innocenti F, D'Andrea M, et al. Predictive role of the UGT1A1, UGT1A7, and UGT1A9 genetic variants and their haplotypes on the outcome of metastatic colorectal cancer patients treated with fluorouracil, leucovorin, and irinotecan. J Clin Oncol. 2009;27:2457–65.
66. Longley DB, Harkin DP, Johnston PG. 5-fluorouracil: mechanisms of action and clinical strategies. Nat Rev Cancer. 2003;3:330–8.
67. Rich TA, Shepard RC, Mosley ST. Four decades of continuing innovation with fluorouracil: current and future approaches to fluorouracil chemoradiation therapy. J Clin Oncol. 2004; 22:2214–32.
68. Berger SH, Jenh CH, Johnson LF, Berger FG. Thymidylate synthase overproduction and gene amplification in fluorodeoxyuridine-resistant human cells. Mol Pharmacol. 1985;28:461–7.
69. Popat S, Matakidou A, Houlston RS. Thymidylate synthase expression and prognosis in colorectal cancer: a systematic review and meta-analysis. J Clin Oncol. 2004;22:529–36.
70. Morganti M, Ciantelli M, Giglioni B, et al. Relationships between promoter polymorphisms in the thymidylate synthase gene and mRNA levels in colorectal cancers. Eur J Cancer. 2005;41:2176–83.
71. Pullarkat ST, Stoehlmacher J, Ghaderi V, et al. Thymidylate synthase gene polymorphism determines response and toxicity of 5-FU chemotherapy. Pharmacogenomics J. 2001;1:65–70.
72. Mandola MV, Stoehlmacher J, Muller-Weeks S, et al. A novel single nucleotide polymorphism within the 5′ tandem repeat polymorphism of the thymidylate synthase gene abolishes USF-1 binding and alters transcriptional activity. Cancer Res. 2003;63:2898–904.
73. Walther A, Johnstone E, Swanton C, Midgley R, Tomlinson I, Kerr D. Genetic prognostic and predictive markers in colorectal cancer. Nat Rev Cancer. 2009;9:489–99.
74. Diasio RB, Johnson MR. The role of pharmacogenetics and pharmacogenomics in cancer chemotherapy with 5-fluorouracil. Pharmacology. 2000;61:199–203.
75. Vallbohmer D, Yang DY, Kuramochi H, et al. DPD is a molecular determinant of capecitabine efficacy in colorectal cancer. Int J Oncol. 2007;31:413–8.

76. Koopman M, Kortman GA, Mekenkamp L, et al. Deficient mismatch repair system in patients with sporadic advanced colorectal cancer. Br J Cancer. 2009;100:266–73.
77. Popat S, Hubner R, Houlston RS. Systematic review of microsatellite instability and colorectal cancer prognosis. J Clin Oncol. 2005;23:609–18.
78. Bertagnolli MM, Niedzwiecki D, Compton CC, et al. Microsatellite instability predicts improved response to adjuvant therapy with irinotecan, fluorouracil, and leucovorin in stage III colon cancer: Cancer and Leukemia Group B Protocol 89803. J Clin Oncol. 2009;27:1814–21.
79. Sargent DJ, Marsoni S, Monges G, et al. Defective mismatch repair as a predictive marker for lack of efficacy of fluorouracil-based adjuvant therapy in colon cancer. J Clin Oncol. 2010;28:3219–26.

Chapter 2
Prognostic Markers in Breast Cancer

Agustin A. Garcia and Nazish Ahmad

Introduction

Selection and identification of appropriate therapy for breast cancer patients require the use of validated and clinically relevant prognostic and predictive factors. A prognostic indicator may be defined as any factor that provides information on clinical outcome independent of treatment and separates poor from favorable groups [1]. Prognostic factors are associated with expression of biologic characteristic, which is involved in either the metastatic and or growth rate potential of the primary tumor [1, 2]. A useful prognostic factor has the following characteristics [3].

1. It has significant and independent value, validated by clinical testing.
2. Its determination must be feasible, reproducible, and widely available with quality control.
3. It must be readily interpretable by the clinician and have therapeutic implications.

Prognostic factors can help better quantify the risk of recurrence in breast cancer. Their value lies in defining patients at low risk, for whom adjuvant therapy is not indicated, and identifying high risk groups who would most benefit from treatment [4]. The availability of intensive chemotherapy for the worst prognostic groups as well as efficacious, low-toxicity adjuvant chemotherapy and hormonotherapy has made prognostication mandatory [5].

A.A. Garcia, M.D. (✉)
Division of Medical Oncology, University of Southern California, 1441 Eastlake Av, Rm 3449, Los Angeles, CA 90033, USA
e-mail: aagarcia@usc.edu

N. Ahmad, B.A., D.O.
Department of Medicine, University of Southern California, Los Angeles, CA, USA

H.-J. Lenz (ed.), *Biomarkers in Oncology: Prediction and Prognosis*,
DOI 10.1007/978-1-4419-9755-5_2,

A predictive factor, on the other hand, is able to provide information on the likelihood of response to a given therapy [1, 2]. In the case of a pure predictive factor, patient outcomes in the absence of the specific treatment are the same regardless of whether marker results are "positive" or "negative" [2]. In clinical practice many of the factors used frequently have both prognostic and predictive values.

Pathologic Evaluation

The most important prognostic indicators that should be determined for every breast cancer are size, histologic type, histologic grade, and lymph node status [4–6]. Tumor size is the simplest to measure and is the most reliable and clinically useful tool for assessing short-term and long-term prognosis in node negative breast cancer. Histologic grade of tumor is assigned according to size and shape of nuclei and the number of mitoses seen [4]. Histologic type defined as tubular, papillary, medullary, mucinous, cribiform, ductal, or lobular is a valuable marker as they predict the probability of recurrence and survival [4, 5]. Tubular, mucinous, and, to a lesser extent, medullary tumors, are associated with a better prognosis. Histologic grade has also strong prognostic value [6]. The histologic involvement and number of axillary lymph node metastases is the strongest single prognostic factor in breast cancer [1, 7, 8].

Estrogen and Progesterone Receptors

Estrogen and progesterone receptor positivity offer a favorable prognosis and also predict good response to endocrine therapy in both adjuvant and metastatic settings [9, 10]. Estrogen mediates its functions through two specific intracellular receptors, the ER alpha and ER beta, which act as hormonal dependent transcriptional regulators [11, 12]. Overexpression of the PR serves as a functional assay because it indicates that the ER pathway is intact, even if the tumor is reported ER negative [13]. The ER and PR status can be measured using immunohistochemistry (IHC). About 50–85 % of breast cancers contain measurable amount of ER with concentrations of at least 10 fmol/mg of cytosol protein. The presence of ER implies that normal cellular mechanisms for processing estrogen have been maintained despite malignant change, particularly if PR is present. The clinical importance of ER relates principally to the fact that its presence identifies hormone-sensitive tumors. Roughly 50–60 % of patients with significant amount of ER in their tumors respond favorably to hormone or endocrine therapy [10]. Patients with ER positive tumors have prolonged disease free survival after primary treatment, superior overall survival, and longer survival after recurrence compared with patients with ER negative tumors, and this advantage is independent of axillary node status [14]. ER and PgR should be evaluated on every primary invasive breast cancer and metastatic lesions if the results would influence treatment [15].

Ductal carcinoma in situ (DCIS) constitutes a spectrum of noninvasive proliferative epithelial lesions with a predilection for the terminal duct- lobular units of the breast and represents up to one fourth of the breast cancer diagnoses [16]. ER and PR do not represent strong prognostic factors in patients with DCIS.

Markers of Proliferation

In general, markers of an elevated proliferative rate correlate with a worse prognosis in untreated patients [17]. One of the markers of proliferative rate in breast tumor specimens is DNA flow cytometry by S-phase. Many studies suggest that high proliferative rate as determined by S phase analysis is an independent predictor of prognosis. In many studies S phase was significant in univariate but not multivariate analyses [18–26]. The implementation of DNA flow cytometry as a marker for proliferative rate is complicated by variations in method of tissue preparations and difference in instrumentations and method for converting information on to the histograms to the S phase estimate. In addition, interpretation of individual studies is complicated by the fact that many are too small to have statistical power, cut offs have not been prospectively defined, and study populations have not been controlled for adjuvant systemic treatments [27].

Immunohistochemical staining is used to measure prognostic and predictive value of proliferation markers like Ki 67, TK, Cyclin E, Cyclin D, cyclin inhibitors p27 and p21, and topoisomerase II [27]. 160,000 patients with invasive breast carcinoma in 132 studies were analyzed to determine the prognostic and predictive role of each marker. The authors concluded that prognostic and predictive value remains undefined because the majority of the studies on these markers had level of evidence III or IV and literature reviewed is not standardized in terms of reagents, procedure, and scoring [17].

The routine use of these markers of cell proliferation is not justified based on the available published data.

HER2

The HER2/neu oncogene is a member of the erb-like oncogene family and is related to epidermal growth factor receptor. The gene has been shown to be amplified in 15–30 % of breast cancers and is associated with more aggressive behavior [28]. In most studies, the overexpression of HER2 in primary tumor tissue is associated with worse survival [28, 29]. Other studies conclude that overexpression is associated with other factors such as negative hormone status, high grade, and young age [30]. HER2 amplification in tumor tissue of both node positive and node negative disease has been shown to be a poor prognostic marker in some studies [31, 32]. Trastuzumab is a humanized monoclonal antibody that binds to the extracellular domain of HER2 [33].

Like many other studies, one clinical trial demonstrated that trastuzumab was associated with a longer time to disease progression, a higher rate and longer duration of response, a lower rate of death, and longer survival [34]. Her2 expression and/or amplification should be evaluated in every primary invasive breast cancer either at time of diagnosis or at recurrence to guide selection of trastuzumab in adjuvant and or metastatic setting.

There is considerable interest in biologic markers able to predict response of cancer patients to therapy. Studies have shown that both groups (HER2 positive and negative) of patients benefit from CMF based regimens. However, the use of anthracycline based regimens appears to be beneficial only for HER2 positive patients [35–37]. This may be related to coexpression or coamplification of topoisomerase II in the presence of HER2 [38].

Whether taxane based therapy is of any use in patient with HER2 positive tumor is controversial [27]. In one study of 474 women with advanced stage breast cancer, three different doses of paclitaxel monotherapy were given and there was no association of HER2 status with response rate, disease free survival, or overall survival [39]. Yet in another study of 297 patients with metastatic breast cancer, HER2 positive patients benefited from paclitaxel and doxorubicin as supposed to cyclophosphamide and doxorubicin [40]. Therefore, Her2 status should not be used as the sole criteria to administer a taxane in the adjuvant setting.

Complex interactions exist between HER2 and ER pathways and HER2 overexpression promotes estrogen-independent growth and is associated with resistance to tamoxifen in vitro and in animal models [27]. Multiple studies have shown that overexpression of HER2 in early stage breast cancer or metastatic cancer is associated with lack of efficacy of adjuvant tamoxifen [41, 42]. The interaction of HER2 with endocrine therapy may vary depending on the type of hormonal agent in question. In a trial of 324 primary breast cancer patients not eligible for surgery received either letrozole or tamoxifen. The study concluded that HER2 positive and ER positive patients were more likely to respond to letrozole than tamoxifen [43]. In contrast, another trial comparing anastrazole vs. tamoxifen vs. the combination of the two failed to show befits from Aromatase inhibitors for HER2 positive tumors [44, 45]. HER2 status should not be used to withhold endocrine therapy for a patient with hormone-receptor positive breast cancer, nor should it be used to select one specific type of endocrine therapy over another.

Tumor Markers

CA 15-3, CA 27.29 and CEA

CA 15-3 and CA 27.29 are well-characterized assays that allow the detection of circulating MUC-I antigen in peripheral blood. Several studies support the relevance of this circulating marker in early stage breast cancer [46–48]. In one study of 1,046 women with breast cancer without metastases at time of diagnosis, elevated preoperative serum marker of cancer antigen 15-3 was correlated with worse prognosis [46]. In another study of 362 node negative patients, prognostic contribution of CA 15-3 was highly significant and its relationship with prognosis is continuous with the risk of relapse increasing progressively from approximately 10 U/ml [47]. However, the use of MUC I antigen in peripheral blood to make treatment decisions on early breast cancer is unclear. Therefore, routine measurement of CA 15-3 and 27.29 at diagnosis or for monitoring patient is not recommended [27, 49, 50].

On the other hand, these tumor markers may be used for monitoring patients with metastatic disease during active therapy, along with history, physical, and diagnostic imaging. The markers alone are not recommended for monitoring response to treatment but may be used to indicate treatment failure in the absence of readily measurable disease.

The routine use of carcinoembryonic antigen (CEA) for screening, diagnosing, staging, routine surveillance of breast cancer patients after primary therapy is not recommended [27]. However, in absence of readily measurable disease, an increasing CEA may be used to indicate treatment failure.

uPA/PAI-1

Urokinase plasminogen activator and plasminogen activator inhibitor are part of the plasminogen activating system, which plays an important role in invasion, angiogenesis, and metastasis [51]. High levels of both uPA and PAI-1 are associated with poor prognosis and therefore the data provided by the European Organization for Research and Treatment of Cancer-Receptor and Biomaker Group (EORTC) was analyzed to confirm prognostic value of the markers. The dataset included 8,377 breast cancer patients followed for 79 months and the authors concluded that apart from lymph node status, high levels of uPA and PAI-1 were the strongest predictors of relapse and survival [52]. A prospective trial of 556 patients in a follow-up of 32 months confirmed strong and independent prognostic importance of uPA and PAI-1 for patients with node-negative breast cancer [53]. The authors concluded that patients with low tumor levels had statistically significantly lower risk of disease recurrence and adjuvant chemotherapy can be avoided as supposed to patients with high tumor levels whom benefited from adjuvant chemotherapy (Fig. 2.1).

p53 Expression

High tissue p53 protein expression appears to be univariate predictor of poor outcome in many studies [54–57]. Yet, other studies have failed to find an association between p53 and clinical outcomes [58, 59]. In addition, IHC for p53 detects both mutated p53 and stabilized wild type p53 but misses p53 deletions. Therefore, in

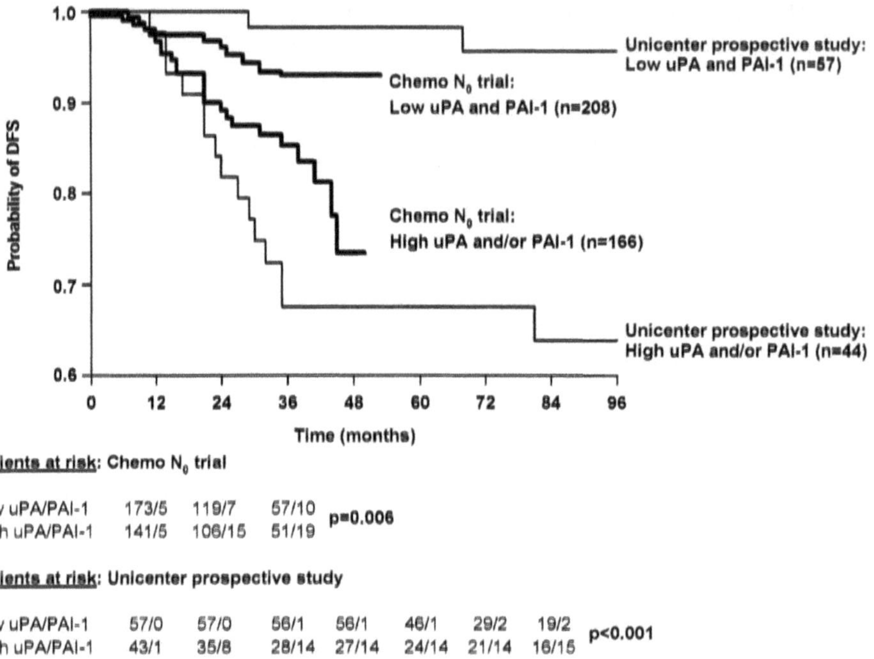

Fig. 2.1 Kaplan–Meier curves showing the impact of tumor levels of urokinase-type plasminogen activator (uPA) and plasminogen activator inhibitor type 1 (PAI-1) on the probability of disease-free survival (DFS) (reprinted from [53], with permission from Oxford University Press)

order for p53 to be used as a prognostic factor or a predictor of benefit from systemic therapies, genetic abnormalities in p53 need to be more clearly defined. The routine use of p53 as prognostic marker is not recommended since most studies analyzing p53 have not taken therapy into consideration and the results may be strongly biased in one direction or another.

Cathepsin D

Cathepsin D is a lysosomal aspartyl protease expressed in all tissues and involved in protein catabolism and tissue remodeling. In the literature, there is controversy regarding the prognostic role of cathepsin D in primary breast cancer. In one study of 2,810 patients with follow-up of 88 months, cytosolic extracts from primary breast tumors were analyzed for cathepsin D. The authors concluded that high levels of Cathepsin D are strongly associated with poor prognosis in patients with primary breast cancer. In addition, there is a weak relationship with no clinical significance between cathepsin D and classical prognostic factors such as older age, postmenopausal status, tumor size, lymph node status and hormone receptor positivity [60]. In general, the studies on cathepsin D are variable with no assay standardization and inconsistent associations with outcome and with little regard to confounding effects of systemic therapy. Therefore, the routine use of cathepsin D measurements for management of patients with breast cancer is not recommended [27].

Cyclin E

Cycling E is a 50-kDa protein expressed in the late G1 phase of the cell cycle. Cyclin E/CDK complex promotes transition of cells to the S phase promoting DNA synthesis. The complex activity is inhibited by p21 and p27 proteins [61]. Amplification of cyclin E gene leads to cleaving of cyclin E protein to low molecular weight (LMW) fragments which is seen in breast cancer [62]. LMW fragments have greater affinity for CDK2 hence more effective in inducing cell cycle progression and resisting inhibition by p21 and p27 [63]. Due to methodological differences in the assays, conflicting results and lack of high level studies, the routine measurements of cycling E for management of patients with breast cancer is not recommended [27, 64–67].

Multiparameter Gene Expression Analysis

The use of multiparameter gene expression analysis represents the most exciting recent development in developing prognostic and predictive markers in breast cancer [68]. Research indicates that gene expression profiling may provide information about tumor behavior and that it can be used as a prognostic marker in a subset of patients that have received uniform therapy (Figs. 2.2 and 2.3). Several technologies have been developed to generate molecular signatures, including cDNA and oligonucleotide arrays and multiplex PCR technologies. Few assays have been subjected to rigorous assay quality control and clinical validation. These include Onco*type* DX, MammaPrint test, the Breast Cancer Gene Expression Ratio and the Rotterdam Signature. The first three are commercially available.

Oncotype DX

Onco*type* DX is an RT-PCR assay that measures the expression of 21 genes in RNA extracted from FFPE tissue [69]. The 21 gene panel includes gene involved in tumor cell proliferation and hormonal response, characteristics that have been reported to be associated with chemotherapy response in general [70]. The 21 genes in Onco*type* DX were selected from a much larger set of genes following the analysis of retrospective test sets of clinical material from several sources, including specimens from a cooperative group trial in which patients with ER positive, node negative breast cancer received tamoxifen vs. tamoxifen plus chemotherapy (NSABP B-20). After the prognostic algorithm was developed, the assay was validated by the analysis of

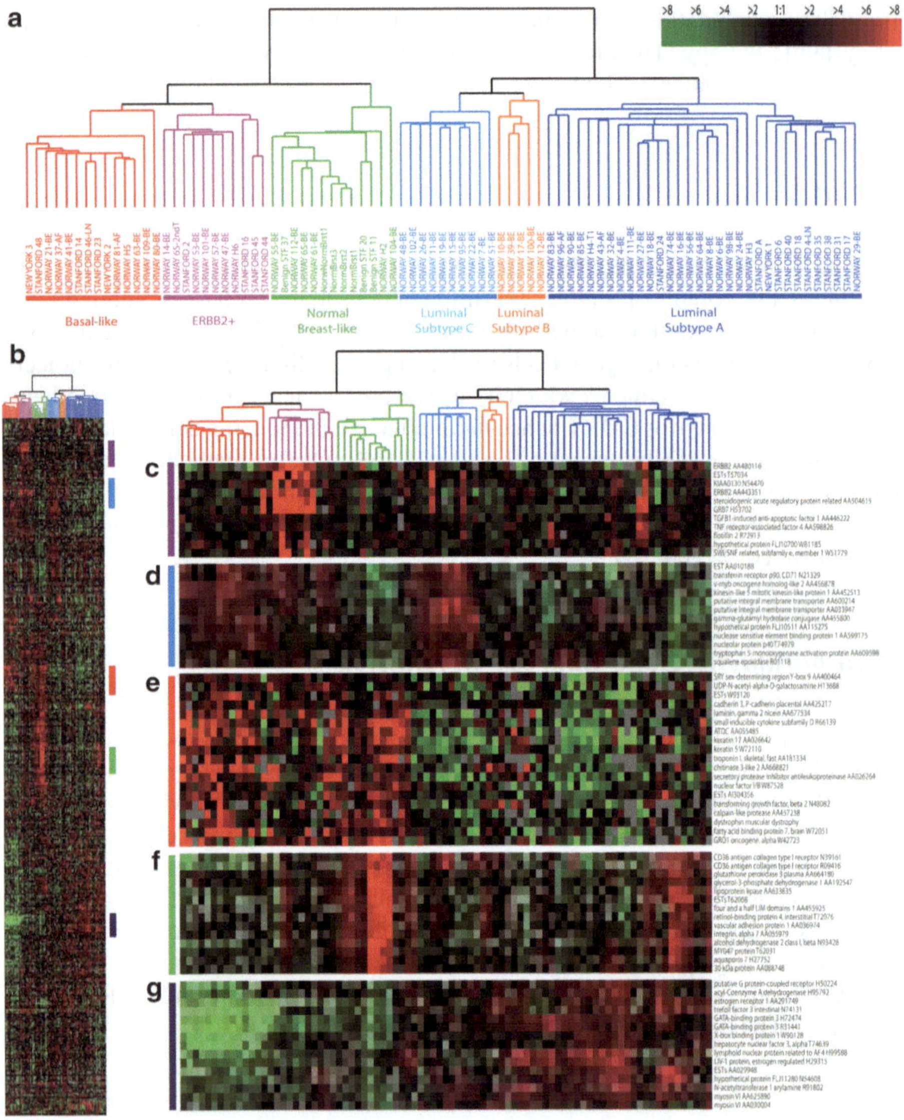

Fig. 2.2 Gene expression patters of breast cancer dividing tumors into subtypes based on differences in gene expression (reprinted from [68], ©2001 National Academy of Sciences, USA)

specimens and data from a second set of patients with node negative, ER positive breast cancer treated only with tamoxifen, who were enrolled in the NSABP clinical trial B14 [9]. Patient are assigned to either low, intermediate, or high risk group depending on an empirically derived, prospectively defined mathematical formula from the levels of expression of the 21 genes [69] (Figs. 2.4 and 2.5). An analysis of data collected from NSABP trial B20 reported that patients with high recurrence score assay had a large benefit from chemotherapy as supposed to patients with low

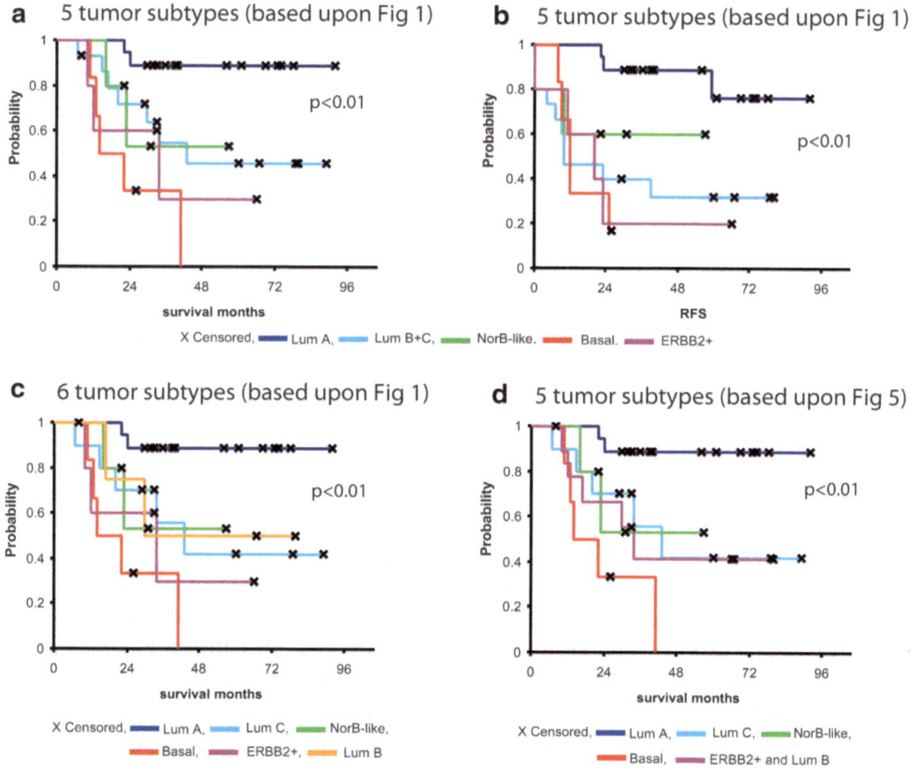

Fig. 2.3 Overall and relapse-free survival analysis based on different gene expression (reprinted from [68], ©2001 National Academy of Sciences, USA)

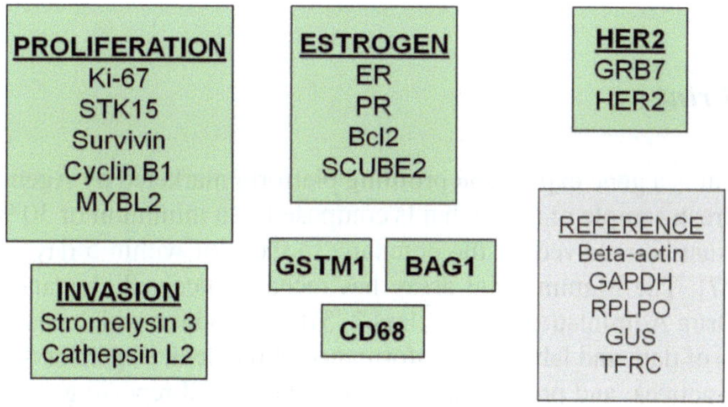

Fig. 2.4 Panel of 21 genes and the recurrence-score algorithm (reprinted from [69] with permission from the Massachusetts Medical Society)

recurrence score [70]. The NSABP 14 trial reproduced the results and concluded that the test is a significant predictor of recurrence independent of age and tumor size and a significant predictor of overall survival [71]. A cost utility analysis applying a

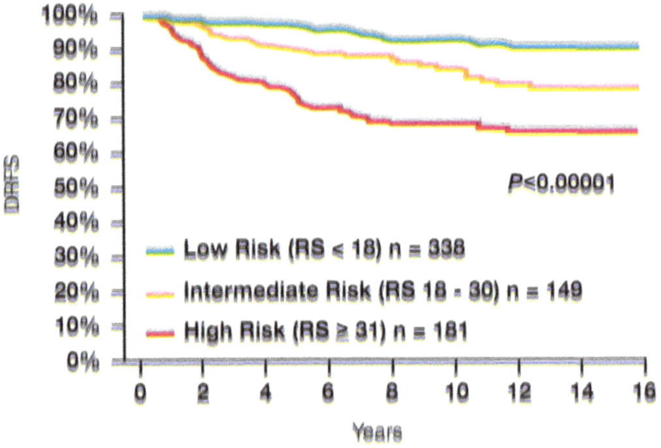

Fig. 2.5 Likelihood of distant recurrence, according to recurrence-score categories (reprinted from [69] with permission from the Massachusetts Medical Society)

Markov decision analytic model concluded that Onco*type* DX would result in an average increase in quality adjusted survival of 8.6 years and a reduction in overall costs of $202,828 [72]. Therefore, the American Society of Clinical Oncology recommends the use on Onco*type* DX to identify patients who are predicted to obtain the most therapeutic benefit from adjuvant tamoxifen and may not require adjuvant chemotherapy. In addition, patients with high recurrence scores appear to obtain marked benefit from adjuvant chemotherapy possibly even higher than that from tamoxifen [27]. Emerging data suggests that this assay may provide also prognostic information in patients with lymph node involvement [73].

MammaPrint

MammaPrint is a gene expression profiling platform marketed by Agendia. The test requires a fresh sample of tissue that is composed of a minimum of 30 % malignant cells and must be received by the company in their kit within 5 days of obtaining material [27]. The MammaPrint assay has recently received clearance by the US Food and Drug Administration as a class 2, 510(k) product, which ensures independent review of data and labeling, conformance of the device sponsor to good manufacturing practices, and post marketing surveillance and reporting to US Food and Drug Administration [27]. A number of studies were conducted in order to validate this assay. Initially, 78 patients with node negative breast cancer were analyzed on oligonucleotide microarrays. The data collected from these patients was then subjected to supervised classification to establish a 70 gene RNA expression profile that correlated with a relatively short interval to distant metastases [74]. The signature was then tested on 295 patients with stage I or II primary breast cancer younger than 53 years of age in both node positive and node negative patients [75]. The authors

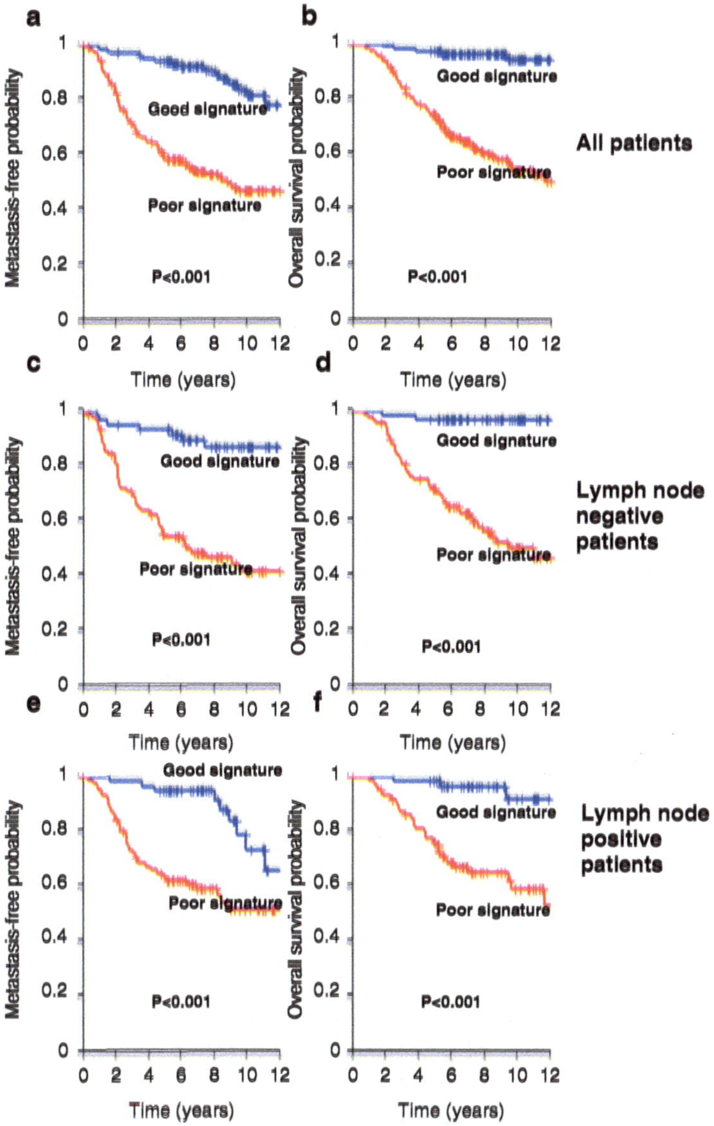

Fig. 2.6 Kaplan–Meier Analysis of the Probability of patients remaining free of Distant Metastases According to Whether They Had a Good-Prognosis or a Poor-Prognosis Signature (reprinted from van de Vijver MJ, He YD, van't Veer LJ et al. A gene expression signature as a predictor of survival in breast cancer. N Eng J Med 2002; 347(25):1999–2009 with permission from the Massachusetts Medical Society)

concluded that gene expression profile studied is a more powerful predictor of the outcome of disease in young patients with breast cancer than standard systems (Fig. 2.6). Another validation trial was completed by TRANSBIG research network and confirmed that the 70 gene signature added independent prognostic information to conventional clinical and histological risk factors [76]. Therefore, Mammaprint profiling appears to identify groups of patients with very good or very poor prognosis but it is difficult to assess whether these results are affected by therapy or not. Furthermore, the tissue handling requirements as stated above make it challenging in current clinical practice [27].

Breast Cancer Gene Expression Ratio Assay

Breast cancer gene expression ratio assay looks at 2 genes and their association between tumor recurrences. In initial study, the authors identified 3 genes, HOXBOX13 (a homeodomain-containing protein), IL17BR (interleukin 17 receptor B), and CHDH (choline dehydrogenase, GenBank accession number A1240933) that were significantly associated with clinical outcome [77]. They then hypothesized that a two gene expression index (HOXBOX13:IL17BR) might be a novel biomarker for predicting treatment outcome in tamoxifen monotherapy. This tumor bank study enrolled 852 patients and demonstrated that HOXBOX13:IL17BR index is a strong independent prognostic factor for ER+ node-negative patients irrespective of tamoxifen therapy [78]. In another study, 206 postmenopausal women with ER+ breast cancer from a randomized adjuvant tamoxifen trial demonstrated that the two gene index was predictive of both early relapse and death in node negative patients, but not in node positive patients [78]. This test in now commercially available and developed by Quest laboratories called Quest H:I ratio test. Results are reported as normalized H:I expression ratio along with categorization of low or high risk for breast cancer at 5 years [79]. The routine use of this assay is not recommended since no published studies have evaluated its ability to predict chemotherapy benefit in comparison with conventional criteria [27].

Rotterdam Signature

The Rotterdam Signature is a gene expression test that consists of 76 gene microarray. In one validation study of 180 lymph node negative patients of all ages and tumor size groups, the authors confirmed that the 76 gene signature is a strong prognostic factor in subgroups of estrogen receptor positive patients, pre- and postmenopausal patients, and patients with tumor size 20 mm or smaller [80]. The routine use of this microarray is not recommend in clinical practice since the tissue collection and preparation requirements are problematic and since the results of this assay have not been validated in core biopsy specimens or whole sections [27].

Bone Marrow Micrometastases

Bone marrow micrometastases in breast cancer patients is defined as epithelial cells found within a bone marrow aspirate that may or may not be breast derived, malignant, or viable [27]. Although many methods can be used, IHC staining of bone marrow epithelial cells from aspirates is the most frequently used method to detect micrometastases. Many studies have showed that bone marrow micrometastases predict higher risk of relapse and worse survival in univariate analysis but not multivariate analysis. In addition, the studies show that metastases are linked to tumor size, grade, or nodal status. Therefore, these patients will already be treated with adjuvant therapy regardless of bone marrow micrometastasis [79, 81–91].

Circulating Tumor Cells

Circulating tumor cells are those cells present in the blood that possess antigenic or genetic characteristics of a specific tumor type. The presence of these cells in breast cancer patients may predict for the presence of a micrometastasis of an aggressive primary tumor. There have been several approaches for detection of these cells. The most frequent used method is immunomagnetic beads that are coated with an antibody specific for a cell surface, epithelial, or cancer-related antigen. After cell selection, the isolated cells are then characterized by immunocytochemistry or by gene expression analysis for the presence of cytokeratins and tumor antigens. Another method of circulating tumor cell detection is to remove leukocytes from the blood sample by positive selection of those cells, and then to interrogate the remaining cells by immunocytochemistry or gene expression analysis using RT-PCR methodology. Yet another method is RT-PCR that can be applied directly to whole blood to assess gene expression [27].

The most compelling evidence to support the use of CTC comes from an initial study of 177 patients with metastatic breast cancer where it was found that the presence of CTC's at baseline and follow-up represented a strong independent prognostic factor for progression free and overall survival [92, 93].

Summary and Recommendations

Table 2.1 summarizes the prognostic and predictive markers for breast cancer that have been well validated and have demonstrated clinical value. The guidelines and recommendations from the American Society of Clinical Oncology (ASCO) for the use of makers in breast cancer are [27]:

- ER, PR, should be evaluated on every primary breast cancer and used to guide endocrine therapy decisions.
- HER2 overexpression should be evaluated on every primary breast cancer and used to guide trastuzumab in metastatic and adjuvant setting. In addition, it can be used to guide anthracycline containing therapy. However, it should not be used for determining prognosis in patients with early breast cancer.
- Multiparameter gene expression analysis (Onco*type* DX assay) can be used to predict the risk of recurrence in women with newly diagnosed, node negative,

Table 2.1 Validated prognostic and predictive markers in breast cancer

Marker	Prognostic value	Predictive value
Histologic		
Tumor size	Yes	No
Grade	Yes	Yes
Type	Yes	Yes
Lymph node involvement	Yes	No
Molecular markers		
ER/PR	Yes	Yes
HER2	Yes	Yes
uPA/PAI-1	Yes	Yes
Gene expression assays		
Oncotype	Yes	Yes
Mammaprint	Yes	No

ER+ breast cancer who will be receiving tamoxifen. Patients with low recurrence risk score can obtain most benefit from tamoxifen alone while patients with high risk recurrence score benefit more from chemotherapy then tamoxifen. The use of other assays is not recommended.

- Measurement of Urokinase plasminogen activator and plasminogen activator inhibitor-1 by ELISA on at least 300 mg of fresh or frozen tissue may be used for determination of prognosis in patients with newly diagnosed, node-negative breast cancer. Low levels of both markers are associated with low risk of recurrence in ER/PR positive disease who will receive adjuvant hormone therapy that additional benefit of chemotherapy is minimal.
- S-phase or other flow cytometry or IHC based markers of proliferation in breast tissue are not recommended for prognostic stratification.
- P53 and cathepsin D is not recommended for management of patients with breast cancer.
- Bone marrow micrometastases or assay for circulating tumor cells in not recommended for management of patients with breast cancer.

References

1. Gasparini G, Pozza F, Harris A. Evaluating the potential usefulness of new prognostic and predictive indicators in node negative breast cancer patients. J Natl Cancer Inst. 1993;85:1206.
2. Hayes DF, Trock B, Harris AL. Assessing the clinical impact of prognostic factors: when is "statistically significant" clinically useful? Breast Cancer Res Treat. 1998;52:305.
3. NIH Consensus Conference. Treatment of early-stage breast cancer. *JAMA*. 1991;265:391.
4. Elledge RM, McGuire WL. Prognostic factors and therapeutic decisions in axillary node negative breast cancer. Annu Rev Med. 1993;44:201–10.
5. Page DL. Prognosis and breast cancer. Recognition of lethal and favorable prognostic types. Am J Surg. 1991;15:334.
6. Rakha EA, El-Sayed ME, Lee AH, et al. Prognostic significance of Nottingham histologic grade in invasive breast cancer. J Clin Oncol. 2008;26:3153.

7. Smith 3rd JA, Gamez-Araujo JJ, Gallager HS, White EC, McBride CM. Carcinoma of the breast: analysis of total lymph node involvement versus level of metastasis. Cancer. 1977;39(2):527–32.
8. Fitzgibbons PL, Page DL, Weaver D, et al. Prognostic factors in breast cancer. College of American pathologists consensus statement 1999. Arch Patho Lab Med. 2000;124:966.
9. Early Breast Cancer Trialists' Collaborative Group (EBCTCG). Effects of chemotherapy and hormonal therapy for early breast cancer on recurrence and 15-year survival: an overview of the randomized trials. Lancet. 2005;365:1687–717.
10. Ravdin PM, Green S, Dorr TM, et al. Prognostic significance of progesterone receptor levels in estrogen receptor-positive patients with metastatic breast cancer treated with tamoxifen: results of a prospective Southwest Oncology Group Study. J Clin Oncol. 1999;10:1284–91.
11. Sommer S, Fuqua SA. Estrogen receptor and breast cancer. Semin Cancer Biol. 2001;11:339–52.
12. Kuiper GG, Enmark E, Pelto-Huikko M, Nilsson S, Gustafsson JA. Cloning of a novel receptor expressed in rat prostate and ovary. Proc Natl Acad Sci USA. 1996;93:5925–30.
13. Esteva JF, Hortobagyi GN. Prognostic molecular markers in early breast cancer. Breast Cancer Res. 2004;6:109–18.
14. Donegan WL. Prognostic factors: stage and receptor status in breast cancer. Cancer. 1992;70:1755–64.
15. Hammond ME, Hayes DF, Dowsett M, et al. American Society of Clinical Oncology/College of American Pathologists guideline recommendations for immunohistochemical testing of estrogen and progesterone receptors in breast cancer. J Clin Oncol. 2010;28:2784–95.
16. Consensus Conference on the Classification of Ductal Carcinoma In Situ. The consensus conference committee. Cancer. 1997;80:1798–802.
17. Colozza M, Azambuja E, Cardoso F, et al. Proliferative markers as prognostic and predictive tools in early breast cancer: Where are we now? Ann Oncol. 2005;16:1723–39.
18. Mandard AM, Denoux Y, Herlin P, et al. Prognostic value of DNA cytometry in 281 premenopausal patients with lymph node negative breast carcinoma randomized in a control trial: Multivariate analysis with Ki-67 index, mitotic count, and microvesseldensity. Cancer. 2000;89:1748–57.
19. Michels JJ, Duigou F, Marnay J. Flow cytometry in primary breast carcinomas: prognostic impact of proliferative activity. Breast Cancer Res Treat. 2000;62:117–26.
20. Chassevent A, Jourdan ML, Romain S, et al. S-phase fraction and DNA ploidy in 633 T1T2 breast cancers: a standardized flow cytometric study. Clin Cancer Res. 2001;7:909–17.
21. Malmström P, Bendahl PO, Boiesen P, et al. S-phase fraction and urokinase plasminogen activator are better markers for distant recurrences than Nottingham Prognostic Index and histologic grade in a prospective study of premenopausal lymph nodenegative breast cancer. J Clin Oncol. 2001;19:2010–9.
22. Lackowska B, Niezabitowski A, Rys J, et al. S-phase fraction and menopausal status as the most important prognostic factors of disease-free survival for node negative patients with breast cancer: a prospective study. Pol J Pathol. 2003;54:101–10.
23. Pinto AE, Andre S, Soares J. Short-term significance of DNA ploidy and cell proliferation in breast carcinoma: a multivariate analysis of prognostic markers in a series of 308 patients. J Clin Pathol. 1999;52:604–11.
24. Prasad AR, Divine G, Zarbo RJ. Two-color, cytokeratin-labeled dna flow cytometric analysis of 332 breast cancers: lack of prognostic value with 12-year follow-up. Arch Pathol Lab Med. 2001;125:364–74.
25. Harbeck N, Dettmar P, Thomssen C, et al. Risk-group discrimination in node-negative breast cancer using invasion and proliferation markers: 6-year median follow-up. Br J Cancer. 1999;80:419–26.
26. Reed Jr DN, Johnson J, Richard P, et al. DNA flow cytometry does not predict 5- or 10-year recurrence rates for T1-2 node-negative breast cancer. Arch Surg. 2000;135:1422–6.
27. Harris L, Fristche H, Mennel R, et al. American Society of Clinical Oncology 2007 update of recommendations for the use of tumor markers in breast cancer. J Clin Oncol. 2007;25:5287.
28. Slamon DJ, Clark GM, Wong SG, et al. Human breast cancer: correlation of relapse and survival with amplification of the HER-2/neu oncogene. Science. 1987;235:177–82.

29. Paik S, Hazan R, Fisher ER, et al. Pathologic findings from the National Surgical Adjuvant Breast and Bowel Project: prognostic significance of erbB-2 protein overexpression in primary breast cancer. J Clin Oncol. 1990;8:103–12.
30. Taucher S, Rudas M, Mader RM, et al. Do we need HER-2/neu testing for all patients with primary breast carcinoma? Cancer. 2003;98:2547.
31. Tandon AK, Clark GM, Chamness GC, et al. HER-2/neu oncogene protein and prognosis in breast cancer. J Clin Oncol. 1989;7:1120.
32. Chia S, Norris B, Speers C, et al. Human epidermal growth factor receptor 2 overexpression as a prognostic factor in a large tissue microarray series of node-negative breast cancers. J Clin Oncol. 2008;26:5697.
33. Baselga J, Norton L, Albanell J, et al. Recombinant humanized anti-HER2 antibody (Herceptin) enhances the antitumor activity of paclitaxel and doxorubicin against HER2/neu overexpressing human breast cancer xenografts. Cancer Res. 1998;58:2825–31.
34. Slamon DJ, Leyland-Jones B, Shak S, et al. Use of chemotherapy plus a monoclonal antibody against HER2 for metastatic breast cancer that overexpresses HER2. N Engl J Med. 2001;344:783–92.
35. Menard S, Valagussa P, Pilotti S, et al. Response to cyclophosphamide, methotrexate, and fluorouracil in lymph node-positive breast cancer according to HER2 overexpression and other tumor biologic variables. J Clin Oncol. 2001;19:329–35.
36. Moliterni A, Menard S, Valagussa P, et al. HER2 overexpression and doxorubicin in adjuvant chemotherapy for resectable breast cancer. J Clin Oncol. 2003;21:458–62.
37. Pritchard KI, Shepgerd LE, O'Malley FP, et al. HER2 and responsiveness of breast cancer to adjuvant chemotherapy. N Engl J Med. 2006;354:2103–11.
38. Press MF, Sauter G, Buyse M, et al. Alteration of topoisomerase ii-alpha gene in human breast cancer: association with responsiveness to anthracycline-based chemotherapy. J Clin Oncol. 2011;29:859–67.
39. Harris LN, Broadwater G, Lin NU, et al. Molecular subtypes of breast cancer in relation to paclitaxel response and outcomes in women with metastatic disease: results from CALGB 9342. Breast Cancer Res. 2006;8:R66.
40. Konecny GE, Thomssen C, Luck HJ, et al. Her-2/neu gene amplification and response to paclitaxel in patients with metastatic breast cancer. J Natl Cancer Inst. 2004;96:1141–51.
41. Berry DA, Muss HB, Thor AD, et al. HER-2/neu and p53 expression versus tamoxifen resistance in estrogen receptor-positive, node-positive breast cancer. J Clin Oncol. 2000;18:3471–9.
42. De Placido S, De Laurentiis M, Carlomagno C, et al. Twenty-year results of the Naples GUN randomized trial: predictive factors of adjuvant tamoxifen efficacy in early breast cancer. Clin Cancer Res. 2003;9(3):1039–46.
43. Ellis MJ, Coop A, Singh B, et al. Letrozole is more effective neoadjuvant endocrine therapy than tamoxifen for ErbB-1- and/or ErbB-2-positive, estrogen receptor-positive primary breast cancer: Evidence from a phase III randomized trial. J Clin Oncol. 2001;19:3808–16.
44. Dowsett M, Allred DC. Relationship between quantitative ER and PgR expression and HER2 status with recurrence in the ATAC trial. San Antonio, TX: Presented at San Antonio Breast Cancer Symposium; 2006.
45. Dowsett M, Ebbs SR, Dixon JM, et al. Biomarker changes during neoadjuvant anastrozole, tamoxifen, or the combination: Influence of hormonal status and HER-2 in breast cancer—a study from the IMPACT trialists. J Clin Oncol. 2005;23:2477–92.
46. Ebeling FG, Stieber P, Untch M, et al. Serum CEA and CA 15-3 as prognostic factors in primary breast cancer. Br J Cancer. 2002;86:1217–22.
47. Gion M, Boracchi P, Dittadi R, et al. Prognostic role of serum CA15.3 in 362 node-negative breast cancers: an old player for a new game. Eur J Cancer. 2002;38:1181–8.
48. Molina R, Filella X, Alicarte J, et al. Prospective evaluation of CEA and CA 15.3 in patients with locoregional breast cancer. Anticancer Res. 2003;23:1035–41.
49. Khatcheressian JL, Wolff AC, Smith TJ, et al. American Society of Clinical Oncology 2006 update of the breast cancer follow-up and management guidelines in the adjuvant setting. J Clin Oncol. 2006;24:5091–7.

50. Kokko R, Holli K, Hakama M. Ca 15-3 in the follow-up of localised breast cancer: a prospective study. Eur J Cancer. 2002;38:1189–93.
51. Stephens RW, Brunner N, Janicke F, et al. The urokinase plasminogen activator system as a target for prognostic studies in breast cancer. Breast Cancer Res Treat. 1998;52:99–111.
52. Look MP, van Putten WL, Duffy MJ, et al. Pooled analysis of prognostic impact of urokinase type plasminogen activator and its inhibitor PAI-1 in 8377 breast cancer patients. J Natl Cancer Inst. 2002;94:116–28.
53. Jänicke F, Prechtl A, Thomssen C, et al. Randomized adjuvant chemotherapy trial in high risk, lymph node-negative breast cancer patients identified by urokinase-type plasminogen activator and plasminogen activator inhibitor type 1. J Natl Cancer Inst. 2000;93:913–20.
54. Olivier M, Langerod A, Carrieri P, et al. The clinical value of somatic TP53 gene mutations in 1,794 patients with breast cancer. Clin Cancer Res. 2006;12:1157–67.
55. Joensuu H, Isola J, Lundin M, et al. Amplification of erbB2 and erbB2 expression are superior to estrogen receptor status as risk factors for distant recurrence in pT1N0M0 breast cancer: a nationwide population-based study. Clin Cancer Res. 2003;9:923–30.
56. Reed W, Hannisdal E, Boehler PJ, et al. The prognostic value of p53 and c-erb B-2 immunostaining is overrated for patients with lymph node negative breast carcinoma: a multivariate analysis of prognostic factors in 613 patients with a follow-up of 14–30 years. Cancer. 2000;88:804–13.
57. Ferrero JM, Ramaioli A, Formento JL, et al. P53 determination alongside classical prognostic factors in node-negative breast cancer: an evaluation at more than 10-year follow-up. Ann Oncol. 2000;11:393–7.
58. Mansour EG, Ravdin PM, Dressler L. Prognostic factors in early breast cancer. Cancer. 1994;74:381.
59. Rosen PP, Lesser ML, Arroyo CD, et al. p53 is node negative breast carcinoma: an immunohistochemical study of epidemiologic risk factors, histologic features, and prognosis. J Clin Oncol. 1995;13:821.
60. Foekens JA, Look MP, Bolt-de Vries J, et al. Cathepsin-D in primary breast cancer: prognostic evaluation involving 2810 patients. Br J Cancer. 1999;79:300–7.
61. Hwang HC, Clurman BE. Cyclin E in normal and neoplastic cell cycles. Oncogene. 2005;24:2776–86.
62. Porter DC, Zhang N, Danes C, et al. Tumor specific proteolytic processing of cyclin E generates hyperactive lower-molecular-weight forms. Mol Cell Biol. 2001;21:6254–69.
63. Wingate H, Zhang N, McGarhen MJ, et al. The tumor-specific hyperactive forms of cyclin E are resistant to inhibition by p21 and p27. J Biol Chem. 2005;280:15148–57.
64. Sieuwerts AM, Look MP, Meijer-van Gelder ME, et al. Which cyclin E prevails as prognostic marker for breast cancer? Results from a retrospective study involving 635 lymph node-negative breast cancer patients. Clin Cancer Res. 2006;12:3319–28.
65. Keyomarsi K, Tucker SL, Buchholz TA, et al. Cyclin E and survival in patients with breast cancer. N Engl J Med. 2002;347:1566–75.
66. Wang L, Shao ZM. Cyclin e expression and prognosis in breast cancer patients: a meta-analysis of published studies. Cancer Invest. 2006;24:581–7.
67. Porter PL, Barlow WE, Yeh IT, et al. P27(Kip1) and cyclin E expression and breast cancer survival after treatment with adjuvant chemotherapy. J Natl Cancer Inst. 2006;98:1723–31.
68. Sørlie T, Perou CM, Tibshirani R, et al. Gene expression patterns of breast carcinomas distinguish tumor subclasses with clinical implications. Proc Natl Acad Sci USA. 2001;98: 10869–74.
69. Paik S, Shak S, Tang G, et al. A multigene assay to predict recurrence of tamoxifen treated, node-negative breast cancer. N Engl J Med. 2004;351:2817.
70. Paik S, Tang G, Shak S, et al. Gene expression and benefit of chemotherapy in women with node-negative, estrogen receptor–positive breast cancer. J Clin Oncol. 2006;24:3726–34.
71. Hornberger J, Cosler LE, Lyman GH. Economic analysis of targeting chemotherapy using a 21-gene RT-PCR assay in lymph-node-negative, estrogen-receptor-positive, early-stage breast cancer. Am J Manag Care. 2005;11:313–24.

72. Albain KS, Barlow WE, Shak S, et al. Prognostic and predictive value of the 21-gene recurrence score assay in postmenopausal women with node-positive, oestrogen-receptor-positive breast cancer on chemotherapy: a retrospective analysis of a randomised trial. Lancet Oncol. 2010;11(1):55–65.
73. van't Veer LJ, Dai H, van de Vijver MJ, et al. Gene expression profiling predicts clinical outcome of breast cancer. Nature. 2002;415:530–6.
74. van de Vijver MJ, He YD, van't Veer LJ, et al. A gene-expression signature as a predictor of survival in breast cancer. N Engl J Med. 2002;347:1999–2009.
75. Buyse M, Loi S, van't Veer L, et al. Validation and clinical utility of a 70-gene prognostic signature for women with node-negative breast cancer. J Natl Cancer Inst. 2006;98:1183–92.
76. Ma X-J, Wang Z, Ryan PD, et al. A two-gene expression ratio predicts clinical outcome in breast cancer patients treated with tamoxifen. Cancer Cell. 2004;5:607–16.
77. Ma X-J, Hilsenbeck SG, Wang W, et al. The *HOXB13:IL17BR* expression ratio is a prognostic factor in early-stage breast cancer. J Clin Oncol. 2006;24:4611–9.
78. Goetz M, Suman V, Ingle JN, et al. A two gene expression ratio of *HOXB13* and IL-17BR for prediction of recurrence and survival in women receiving adjuvant tamoxifen. Clin Cancer Res. 2006;12:2080–7.
79. Foekens JA, Atkins D, Zhang Y, et al. Multicenter validation of a gene expression-based prognostic signature in lymph node-negative primary breast cancer. J Clin Oncol. 2006; 24:1665–71.
80. Braun S, Cevatli BS, Assemi C, et al. Comparative analysis of micrometastasis to the bone marrow and lymph nodes of node-negative breast cancer patients receiving no adjuvant therapy. J Clin Oncol. 2001;19:1468–75.
81. Braun S, Kentenich C, Janni W, et al. Lack of effect of adjuvant chemotherapy on the elimination of single dormant tumor cells in bone marrow of high-risk breast cancer patients. J Clin Oncol. 2000;18:80–6.
82. Braun S, Muller M, Hepp F, et al. Re: micrometastatic breast cancer cells in bone marrow at primary surgery—prognostic value in comparison with nodal status. J Natl Cancer Inst. 1998;90:1099–101.
83. Cote RJ, Rosen PP, Lesser ML, et al. Prediction of early relapse in patients with operable breast cancer by detection of occult bone marrow micrometastases. J Clin Oncol. 1991;9:1749–56.
84. Diel IJ, Cote RJ. Bone marrow and lymph node assessment for minimal residual disease in patients with breast cancer. Cancer Treat Rev. 2000;26:53–65.
85. Diel IJ, Kaufmann M, Costa SD, et al. Micrometastatic breast cancer cells in bone marrow at primary surgery: prognostic value in comparison with nodal status. J Natl Cancer Inst. 1996;88:1652–8.
86. Funke I, Schraut W. Meta-analyses of studies on bone marrow micrometastases: an independent prognostic impact remains to be substantiated. J Clin Oncol. 1998;16:557–66.
87. Gebauer G, Fehm T, Merkle E, et al. Micrometastases in axillary lymph nodes and bone marrow of lymph node-negative breast cancer patients: prognostic relevance after 10 years. Anticancer Res. 2003;23:4319–24.
88. Harbeck N, Untch M, Pache L, et al. Tumour cell detection in the bone marrow of breast cancer patients at primary therapy: results of a 3-year median follow-up. Br J Cancer. 1994;69:566–71.
89. Mansi JL, Gogas H, Bliss JM, et al. Outcome of primary-breast-cancer patients with micrometastases: a long-term follow-up study. Lancet. 1999;354:197–202.
90. Merkle E, Bahr J, Henke A, et al. Immunocytochemical detection of tumor cells in bone marrow as a prognostic factor in breast carcinoma [in German]. Geburtshilfe Frauenheilkd. 1994;54:662–9.
91. Gaforio JJ, Serrano MJ, Sanchez-Rovira P, et al. Detection of breast cancer cells in the peripheral blood is positively correlated with estrogen-receptor status and predicts for poor prognosis. Int J Cancer. 2003;107:984–90.
92. Weigelt B, Bosma AJ, Hart AA, et al. Marker genes for circulating tumour cells predict survival in metastasized breast cancer patients. Br J Cancer. 2003;88:1091–4.
93. Cristofanilli M, Budd GT, Ellis MJ, et al. Circulating tumor cells, disease progression, and survival in metastatic breast cancer. N Engl J Med. 2004;351:781–91.

Chapter 3
Predictive Markers in Lung Cancer

Stephen V. Liu and Barbara J. Gitlitz

Introduction

Non-small-cell lung cancer (NSCLC) is the leading cause of cancer related death in the United States [1]. Chemotherapy has been shown to prolong survival in patients with advanced NSCLC and improve patients' quality of life [2, 3]. Unfortunately, the balance between benefit and toxicity can be difficult to manage and traditional cytotoxic chemotherapy has offered only a modest improvement in outcomes. The development of novel therapeutic agents has provided additional treatment options for these patients, but enthusiasm for their use is tempered by a lack reliable predictive markers. A landmark randomized trial comparing four common platinum doublets (cisplatin and paclitaxel, cisplatin and gemcitabine, cisplatin and docetaxel, or carboplatin and paclitaxel) showed no significant difference between these regimens [4]. As a result, standard first-line chemotherapy often varies by physician and institution. Recently, the development of targeted agents has fueled the search for predictive markers to guide treatment decisions. This strategy has met with early success, particularly with regard to the tyrosine-kinase inhibitors (TKI) erlotinib, gefitinib, and crizotinib. In addition, recent studies have revisited the use of traditional cytotoxic agents and uncovered several promising predictive markers. Several clinicopathologic features have also shown predictive power, though closer study may reveal these as surrogates for molecular markers.

S.V. Liu, M.D. • B.J. Gitlitz, M.D. (✉)
Division of Medical Oncology, Department of Internal Medicine, Norris Comprehensive Cancer Center, Keck School of Medicine, University of Southern California, 1441 Eastlake Avenue, Suite 3447, Los Angeles, CA 90042, USA
e-mail: gitlitz@usc.edu

H.-J. Lenz (ed.), *Biomarkers in Oncology: Prediction and Prognosis*,
DOI 10.1007/978-1-4419-9755-5_3,

The rapid identification of novel therapeutic targets and the efficient development of targeted agents promise to improve the outcomes for patients with NSCLC, but without reliable predictive markers, these benefits will be diluted and potentially hidden. The paradigm of personalized medicine demands that these markers be uncovered and exploited to rationally employ the agents at hand. While there are few validated predictive markers at this time, there is both great promise and rapid advancement in this evolving field.

Bevacizumab and Anti-VEGF Antibody Therapy

Several trials have validated VEGF as a viable target in the treatment of advanced NSCLC. Bevacizumab is a monoclonal antibody targeting VEGF that has demonstrated benefit in patients with nonsquamous NSCLC. Eastern Cooperative Oncology Group (ECOG) study E4599 randomized 878 patients with advanced, nonsquamous NSCLC to receive six cycles of carboplatin and paclitaxel with either bevacizumab or placebo [5]. Bevacizumab was continued until progression or toxicity. This trial met its primary endpoint of OS with a median survival of 12.3 months in the bevacizumab arm and 10.3 months in the placebo arm ($p = 0.003$). PFS was also improved in the bevacizumab arm (6.2 vs. 4.5 months, $p < 0.001$). The phase III AVAiL trial compared six cycles of cisplatin and gemcitabine alone with the same combination plus bevacizumab until progression or toxicity [6]. While the primary endpoint of PFS was met, this did not translate into a significant OS benefit. However, based on the confirmed PFS benefit and the OS benefit seen in E4599, bevacizumab has become a common addition to first-line therapy of NSCLC.

Most clinicians would agree that a specific subpopulation exists in whom bevacizumab and anti-VEGF therapy is more efficacious. Unfortunately, predicting this subpopulation has proven difficult. Baseline plasma VEGF levels were measured in E4599 but did not correlate with outcome. The significance of plasma VEGF levels was further explored in a study of 45 patients with advanced NSCLC treated with platinum-based chemotherapy and bevacizumab [7]. In this analysis, baseline VEGF levels as measured by ELISA did not correlate with outcome. However, low post-treatment VEGF levels, drawn 6 weeks after therapy, were associated with a longer median OS. These findings have not yet been validated. While VEGF is a rational biomarker, its study raises several concerns regarding the proper cutoff for high versus low levels, the specificity for response to anti-VEGF based therapy and its overall clinical utility. Currently, plasma VEGF has no established utility as a predictive marker for bevacizumab in NSCLC.

Certain clinical characteristics have been explored as potential biomarkers of benefit from bevacizumab. An unplanned analysis of E4599 suggested that females did not derive a survival benefit from bevacizumab. Closer analysis of gender in this study revealed several demographic differences between males and females and controlling for these factors eliminated any significant differences by sex, suggesting that gender is not a negative predictive marker in this setting [8]. Other subset analyses showed that age was also not a predictive marker [9]. While there was a higher likelihood of grade 3 and higher toxicity for patients 70 years of age and older, there was no statistically significant difference in response or survival when compared to younger patients. Histology may help predict response. Patients with squamous cell NSCLC are not eligible to receive bevacizumab, largely due to the increased toxicity. Early studies identified squamous cell histology as a predictive marker for hemorrhage. In the phase II study which included squamous histology, the incidence of grade 3 or greater pulmonary hemorrhage was 9.1% whereas the phase III E4599, which excluded patients with squamous histology, noted an incidence of only 2.3% [10]. While other histology subtypes are eligible to receive bevacizumab, one analysis suggested that patients with adenocarcinoma derived greater benefit than patients with large cell undifferentiated, bronchoalveolar, "not otherwise specified" or "other" histologies [11]. The lack of central pathology review and the retrospective nature of this analysis warrant caution in interpreting these findings. While interesting and hypothesis-generating, clinical features are likely surrogates for other molecular markers that have yet to be described.

There is some promise in the study of genetic variation in predicting response to bevacizumab. An analysis of the patients treated on E4599 explored the association between clinical outcome and single nucleotide polymorphisms (SNPs) in genes involved in angiogenesis and DNA repair [12]. Only 133 samples were available from eligible patients, but analysis did demonstrate a treatment effect that differed by genotype for polymorphisms in VEGF, ICAM1, WNK1, EGF, and CXCR2. Prospective analysis will offer further insight into the potential of SNPs as predictive markers for bevacizumab. Another potential predictive marker is the presence of hypertension after initiation of therapy. While this marker cannot be evaluated before starting therapy, it does seem to correlate with outcomes. Retrospective analysis of patients on E4599 demonstrated that high blood pressure (defined as > 150/100 or at least a 20 mmHg increase in diastolic blood pressure) did correlate with outcomes [13]. The improvement in OS with bevacizumab was greater in patients with high blood pressure (HR 0.60, 95% CI 0.43–0.81) compared to those who did not have high blood pressure (HR 0.86, 95% CI 0.74–1.00). This is felt to represent an effect of the reduction in nitric oxide synthesis seen with bevacizumab. While there does seem to be an association with benefit from bevacizumab, prospective validation is lacking and high blood pressure should not be considered a predictive marker at this time.

While bevacizumab does provide benefit to some patients, our ability to prospectively identify those patients is limited. As a result, bevacizumab is often administered empirically to all eligible patients, though only a fraction will derive benefit. Predictive markers for bevacizumab and VEGF-targeted therapy remain an unmet need and the search for a reliable biomarker in this area continues.

EGFR Targeted Agents

Epidermal growth factor receptor (EGFR) plays an essential role in NSCLC. EGFR activation leads to homodimerization with another EGFR or heterodimerization with a different receptor from the HER family [14]. Different ligands can induce different dimerization patterns and this allows for a diverse series of downstream events resulting in the various signals required for survival and proliferation. Agents targeting EGFR have secured a prominent role in the management of advanced NSCLC. There are two major classes of agents targeting EGFR: monoclonal antibodies such as cetuximab and TKIs such as erlotinib and gefitinib. While the target of these agents is the same, the mechanisms are quite different, as are their effects and the predictive biomarkers that accompany them. These classes will be discussed separately.

Anti-EGFR Antibody Therapy

Cetuximab is an IgG1 monoclonal antibody that targets EGFR and has demonstrated efficacy in the treatment of colorectal and head and neck cancers [15, 16]. A phase II study of cetuximab monotherapy in patients with pretreated NSCLC yielded a response rate of only 4.5% [17]. More impressive outcomes were seen when cetuximab was combined with chemotherapy. Two phase III trials compared chemotherapy with and without cetuximab in previously untreated NSCLC. The FLEX trial, randomized patients to receive six cycles of cisplatin and vinorelbine either alone or in combination with cetuximab [18]. Cetuximab was continued until progression or toxicity. Patients who received cetuximab had a longer median OS (11.3 vs. 10.1 months, $p=0.044$). The other phase III study, BMS099, used a chemotherapy backbone of carboplatin with either paclitaxel or docetaxel and randomized patients to receive cetuximab, which was administered until progression or toxicity [19]. This trial did not meet its primary endpoint of an improvement in PFS though cetuximab was associated with a higher response rate (25.7 vs. 17.2%, $p=0.007$) and a trend toward an increase in median OS. These studies demonstrate the potential efficacy of cetuximab in the treatment of NSCLC, though this agent is not yet approved in this setting by the FDA. Efforts to identify patient subsets with a higher likelihood of benefit have not met with great success.

In the treatment of colon cancer, a powerful negative predictive marker for benefit from cetuximab is KRAS mutation status [20]. In NSCLC, however, KRAS mutation status does not have the same predictive power. Analysis of the 225 available tumor specimens from patients treated on BMS099 demonstrated a KRAS mutation rate of 17% but there was no significant association between the presence of a KRAS mutation and outcome [21]. This analysis also explored EGFR expression by IHC (present in 89% of samples), EGFR copy number by FISH (positive in 51.9% of samples), and EGFR mutations (present in 10% of samples). Unfortunately, none of these biomarkers correlated with PFS, OS or RR in this study. The FLEX trial required EGFR expression by IHC in at least one tumor cell and conducted analysis of KRAS mutation and EGFR copy number by FISH. The KRAS mutation rate was 19% in both arms of this study but the presence of a KRAS mutation did not negatively predict a difference in OS, PFS or RR by treatment. This also held true for EGFR copy number by FISH status [18]. These data echo the results of two phase II studies conducted by the Southwest Oncology Group (SWOG). The first of these studies, SWOG S0342, randomized patients to receive either concurrent chemotherapy and cetuximab or sequential chemotherapy and cetuximab, both followed by maintenance cetuximab [22]. The other study was SWOG S0536, which explored the addition of bevacizumab to chemotherapy plus cetuximab [23]. A combined analysis of these studies examined the predictive role of KRAS mutations and benefit from cetuximab [24]. There was no significant negative association between KRAS mutation and outcome. Based on the lack of compelling data to suggest otherwise, there is currently no predictive role for KRAS mutation and cetuximab therapy in patients with NSCLC.

One potential clinical biomarker is the development of an acne-like rash during therapy. The FLEX trial included a prospective analysis of patients who developed a rash during the first cycle of therapy [25]. Among the 518 patients included for analysis, 290 (56%) developed a rash (grade 1–3) during the first 21 days. Patients who developed a rash had a median OS of 15.0 months while those who did not develop a rash had a median OS of 8.8 months ($p<0.001$). Patients who did not receive cetuximab had a median OS of 10.3 months. Intensity of rash did not correlate with outcomes. The optimal management of patients who do not develop a rash is unclear. In the FLEX study, all patients continued therapy and while their outcomes were worse compared to patients who developed a rash, one cannot determine if continuation of cetuximab provided benefit in this subgroup since there is no comparator arm. This could be addressed in a study that randomized patients who did not develop a rash to either continue or stop cetuximab. In the absence of these data, the development of a rash should not be considered a true predictive biomarker, though these associations are interesting and hypothesis-generating. A reliable predictive marker to guide the use of EGFR monoclonal antibodies like cetuximab is still lacking but efforts continue.

EGFR TKI Therapy

Clinical Predictors

Erlotinib and gefitinib are oral EGFR TKIs that competitively bind the ATP binding site. While early studies have shown benefit from these agents in unselected populations, efficacy is far greater in specific subsets of patients. There have been many efforts to identify these enriched subsets and they have met with variable amounts of success [26]. Several clinicopathologic characteristics were identified in early trials. The IDEAL 1 trial was a phase II study of two different doses of gefitinib in patients with pretreated NSCLC [27]. Both doses demonstrated similar efficacy, with a RR of 18.4–19.0% and a median OS of 7.6–8.0 months. Subset analysis of this study demonstrated a greater response rate in Japanese patients (27.5 vs. 10.4%, $p=0.0023$). Gender and histology also correlated with outcomes; females were 2.5 times more likely to respond than men and patients with adenocarcinoma were almost 3.5 times more likely to respond than patients with other histologies. Histology also correlated with outcome in the WJTOG0203 and the BR.21 trials. WJTOG0203 randomized patients with advanced, untreated NSCLC to either six cycles of platinum-doublet therapy or three cycles of platinum-doublet therapy followed by gefitinib until progression [28]. This trial failed to meet its primary outcome of OS, however the subset of patients with adenocarcinoma did derive benefit from gefitinib, with a longer median OS (HR 0.79; 0.65–0.98, $p=0.03$). The BR.21 study demonstrated a survival benefit to erlotinib compared to placebo in the second-line setting for NSCLC [29]. Subset analysis showed a greater benefit to erlotinib in patients who had never smoked [30]. Smoking history has repeatedly been shown to correlate with EGFR TKI response. The TALENT trial randomized 1,172 patients to receive six cycles of gemcitabine plus cisplatin with either placebo or erlotinib [31]. The addition of erlotinib did not improve outcomes, though the small subset of patients that never smoked did have an increased OS and PFS with erlotinib. Many trials have also confirmed the predictive nature of ethnicity. The ISEL trial compared gefitinib with placebo in 1,692 patients with pretreated NSCLC [32]. In this unselected population, median OS did not differ between the two arms (5.6 vs. 5.1 months, $p=0.087$). However, in a preplanned subset analysis, median OS was greater for patients of Asian origin (9.5 vs. 5.5 months, $p=0.01$) [33]. These clinical and pathologic features had the potential to serve as predictive markers for EGFR TKIs in NSCLC and indeed, have guided therapy for many treating physicians. Subsequent studies, however, revealed the importance and reliability of molecular markers in predicting outcome.

KRAS Mutation

As further clinical studies consistently demonstrated small subsets of patients who displayed rapid and dramatic response to EGFR TKIs, the search for molecular correlates intensified. Based largely on its predictive power with cetuximab in other tumors, KRAS mutation status was explored in this setting. Analysis of samples from the BR.21 trial demonstrated a 15% incidence of KRAS mutations. In this trial, patients with KRAS mutations did not demonstrate a survival benefit from erlotinib while patients with wild-type KRAS did derive benefit (HR 0.69, $p=0.03$) [34]. While this relationship did not persist on multivariate analysis, other studies have demonstrated similar findings. A small retrospective analysis of patients treated with gefitinib noted the absence of KRAS mutations in any responders while mutations were noted in 30% of patients with progressive disease on gefitinib [35]. Another retrospective review analyzed 60 specimens from patients with adenocarcinoma who were treated with either gefitinib or erlotinib [36]. Of the 60 specimens, nine KRAS mutations were noted and none of these patients demonstrated a response to gefitinib or erlotinib. Many similar studies support the negative predictive value of KRAS mutations for response to EGFR TKI therapy. These have been summarized in a meta-analysis that included 1,008 patients from 17 studies of patients with advanced NSCLC treated with either single agent gefitinib or erlotinib [37]. Of the 1,008 patients included, 165 had KRAS mutations and the presence of a KRAS mutation was strongly associated with a lack of response to EGFR TKIs (specificity 94%, sensitivity 21%). The presence of a KRAS mutation is a negative predictive marker to benefit from EGFR TKI therapy, though the absence of this mutation does not predict EGFR TKI efficacy.

EGFR Expression

EGFR protein expression, as measured by IHC, was an early candidate predictive marker for EGFR TKIs. In an analysis of patients treated on the BR.21 trial, expression of EGFR did correlate with response [29]. Patients whose tumor was found to overexpress EGFR had a higher response rate than those with EGFR negative tumors ($p=0.03$), but EGFR expression was not a predictor of survival. Analysis of the ISEL trial did reveal a correlation between EGFR overexpression and survival [38]. Patients with EGFR overexpression had a decreased risk of death with gefitinib (HR 0.77; 0.56–1.08) compared to patients with an EGFR-negative tumor (HR 1.57; 0.86–2.87). In the SATURN trial studying maintenance erlotinib following first-line platinum doublet chemotherapy, erlotinib prolonged PFS when compared to placebo [39]. The subset of patients with EGFR overexpression by IHC had superior outcomes with erlotinib [40]. Unfortunately, EGFR IHC has not been a consistent predictive marker. Analysis of 50 patients treated with gefitinib found EGFR expression was more common in squamous cell carcinoma, though none of these patients achieved a response [41]. Among patients with adenocarcinoma, there was a weak correlation between EGFR expression and response but not disease control. Overall, EGFR expression did not correlate with response or survival with gefitinib and in light of other more consistent markers, the predictive role of IHC remains undefined.

EGFR Copy Number

EGFR copy number, as measured by FISH, has also been an inconsistent predictive marker in this setting. In multivariate analysis of the BR.21 trial, EGFR amplification was predictive of survival benefit from erlotinib ($p=0.005$) [34]. EGFR amplification also correlated with OS with gefitinib in the ISEL trial [38]. The INTEREST trial, however, did not demonstrate a benefit from gefitinib in patients with a high EGFR gene copy number. This open-label phase III study randomized patients with pretreated, advanced NSCLC to receive either docetaxel or gefitinib [42]. This study established a noninferior survival of gefitinib to docetaxel, but the subset of patients with a high EGFR copy number did not demonstrate superior outcomes with gefitinib compared to docetaxel. The INVITE trial compared first-line gefitinib with vinorelbine in elderly patients (age ≥ 70 years) and interestingly, patients with a high EGFR copy number had inferior outcomes with gefitinib and derived greater benefit from vinorelbine [43]. The IPASS study, discussed in detail below, compared gefinitib to chemotherapy in untreated patients. While EGFR copy number appeared to correlate with PFS, this association was abrogated when EGFR mutation status was considered [44]. EGFR copy number does not yield consistent predictive power in this setting and has been replaced with EGFR mutation analysis.

EGFR Mutations

Somatic mutations in the tyrosine kinase domain of the EGFR gene have emerged as the most promising predictive marker for EGFR TKIs. These mutations typically reside near the ATP binding pocket of the EGFR which is targeted by these agents. Most of these mutations are in-frame deletions in exon 19 including codons 746 to 750 (E746 to A750) or amino acid substitutions in exon 21 at codon 858 (L858R), though amino acid substitutions in exon 18 are also encountered. In the initial report, EGFR mutations were identified in eight of the nine patients who achieved a response with gefitinib [45]. Four of the eight mutations were exon 19 deletions and the remaining mutations were point mutations, three in exon 21 and one in exon 18. EGFR mutations were absent in all of the seven patients that did not achieve a response with gefitinib. This group then conducted in vitro functional analysis of these mutations. EGFR with an exon 19 deletion and EGFR with the L858R exon 21 missense mutation were expressed in cultured cells and compared to cells bearing wild type EGFR. The mutations did not affect protein stability and neither mutated nor wild-type EGFR demonstrated autophosphorylation in the absence of serum growth factors. The effect of the mutations was only seen when EGF was added, as activation of both mutant EGFRs was two- to threefold greater than wild-type EGFR. Furthermore, wild-type EGFR was downregulated after 15 min but the mutant receptors showed continued activation for up to 3 h. Importantly, this heightened activation translated to a greater in vitro sensitivity to gefitinib when compared to wild-type EGFR. For wild-type EGFR, 50% inhibition was achieved at a concentration of 0.1 μM whereas the same inhibition was achieved in the mutant EGFR at the much lower concentration of 0.015 μM. Studies of KRAS and EGFR mutations consistently show a lack of overlap between these two markers. In a small series of 41 patients, none of the samples with EGFR mutations contained KRAS mutations, and these findings have been observed in several trials [35].

Multiple studies have since confirmed the association between EGFR mutation status and response to EGFR TKI monotherapy. The initial data were in pretreated patients. One retrospective review included 60 adenocarcinoma specimens from patients treated with either gefitinib or erlotinib [36]. In this study, 17 specimens harbored EGFR mutations and all 17 demonstrated a response to gefitinib or erlotinib. In the BR.21 trial, the response rate to second line erlotinib was significantly higher for patients with a mutant EGFR as compared to wild type (27 vs. 7%, $p = 0.03$) [34]. Analysis of patients treated on the INTEREST trial showed that patients with an EGFR mutation had an improved PFS and response rate with gefitinib compared to docetaxel in the second line setting [46]. Analysis of samples from the IDEAL-1 and IDEAL-2 trials also confirmed the relationship between EGFR mutation and response to gefitinib. These studies tested two different doses of gefitinib in patients with pretreated NSCLC. IDEAL-1 was a European and Japanese study that described a 19% PR rate and IDEAL-2 was conducted in the United States and described a 10% PR rate [27, 47]. Pooled analysis of available samples from these studies showed that patients with an EGFR mutation had a better response to gefitinib with an odds ratio of 6 of 13 (46%), compared to 6 of 61 (10%) for those with no mutation [48].

The predictive nature of an activating EGFR mutation was then confirmed in first-line trials (Table 3.1). The OPTIMAL trial included 165 patients with untreated NSCLC that carried an activating EGFR mutation and randomized patients to either erlotinib monotherapy or up to four cycles of carboplatin plus gemcitabine (Fig. 3.1) [49]. The RR was superior in the erlotinib arm (83 vs. 36%) as was the median PFS (13.1 months vs. 4.6 months).

WJTOG 3405 was an open label, phase III study of gefitinib compared to cisplatin plus docetaxel limited to patients with untreated NSCLC that harbored an EGFR mutation [50]. In these patients, PFS favored the gefitinib group (HR 0.49, 95% CI 0.34–0.71). The First-SIGNAL trial also examined the efficacy of first-line gefitinib, comparing it to the doublet of cisplatin and gemcitabine in nonsmokers with adenocarcinoma. Overall, the gefitinib arm had a superior PFS (HR 0.737, 95% CI 0.58–0.94) [51]. However, this was much more pronounced in those patients with an EGFR mutation (HR 0.385, 95% CI 0.208–0.711) and was not evident in patients without an EGFR mutation (HR 1.223, 95% CI 0.65–2.31). The NEJ002 trial randomized patients with advanced, untreated NSCLC that had an EGFR mutation to receive either gefitinib or chemotherapy with carboplatin and paclitaxel [52]. Though the study was designed to accrue 320 patients, an interim analysis performed 4 months after the first 200 patients were entered led to early termination of this study. This was due to a significantly longer PFS in the gefitinib arm (HR 0.30, 95% CI 0.22–0.41). Final analyses showed a 1 year PFS rate favoring gefitinib (42.1 vs. 3.2%) and a response rate favoring gefitinib (73.7 vs. 30.7%, $p < 0.0001$) but there was no difference in median OS (30.5 months vs. 23.6 months, $p = 0.31$), likely due to high cross-over rates. This trial confirmed the benefit to EGFR TKI therapy in patients with EGFR mutations.

The phase III IPASS trial was essential in securing EGFR mutation status as a powerful predictive marker for EGFR TKI therapy [53]. IPASS was limited to patients with advanced, untreated NSCLC and only included light ex-smokers or never-smokers in Asia. This study randomized 1,217 patients to either gefitinib or the combination of carboplatin plus paclitaxel. Demographic analysis shows that 79% of the patients were female and 94% were never-smokers. The gefitinib arm was superior, with a 12-month PFS rate of 24.9%, compared to 6.7% with carboplatin and paclitaxel. In this study, 85.3% of patients were included in biomarker analyses.

Table 3.1 Overview of selected studies demonstrating the predictive nature of EGFR mutations in patients with NSCLC receiving first-line EGFR TKI monotherapy compared to chemotherapy

Study	Treatment arms	PFS with EGFR mutation	PFS without EGFR mutation	OS with EGFR mutation	OS without EGFR mutation
IPASS Mok et al. [53]	Gefitinib vs. Carboplatin + Paclitaxel	*N* = 261 HR 0.48 (0.36–0.64)	*N* = 176 HR 2.85 (2.05–3.98)	*N* = 261 HR 1.00 (0.76–1.33)	*N* = 176 HR 1.18 (0.86–1.63)
First-SIGNAL Lee et al. [51]	Gefitinib vs. Cisplatin + Gemcitabine	*N* = 42 HR 0.62 (0.31–1.22)	*N* = 54 HR 1.52 (0.88–2.61)	*N* = 42 HR 0.82 (0.35–1.92)	*N* = 54 HR 1.20 (0.57–2.52)
WJTOG 3405 Mitsudomi et al. [50]	Gefitinib vs. Cisplatin + Docetaxel	*N* = 172 HR 0.49 (0.34–0.71)	N/A	N/A	N/A
NEJ 002 Maemondo et al. [52]	Gefitinib vs. Carboplatin + Paclitaxel	*N* = 228 HR 0.30 (0.22–0.41)	N/A	*N* = 228 HR NS	N/A
OPTIMAL Zhou et al. [49]	Erlotinib vs. Carboplatin + Gemcitabine	*N* = 154 HR 0.16 (0.10–0.26)	N/A	NR	N/A
EURTAC Rosell et al. [55]	Erlotinib vs. Platinum (Cisplatin or Carboplatin) with either Docetaxel or Gemcitabine	*N* = 154 HR 0.37 (0.25–0.54)	N/A	*N* = 154 HR 0.80 (0.47–1.37)	N/A

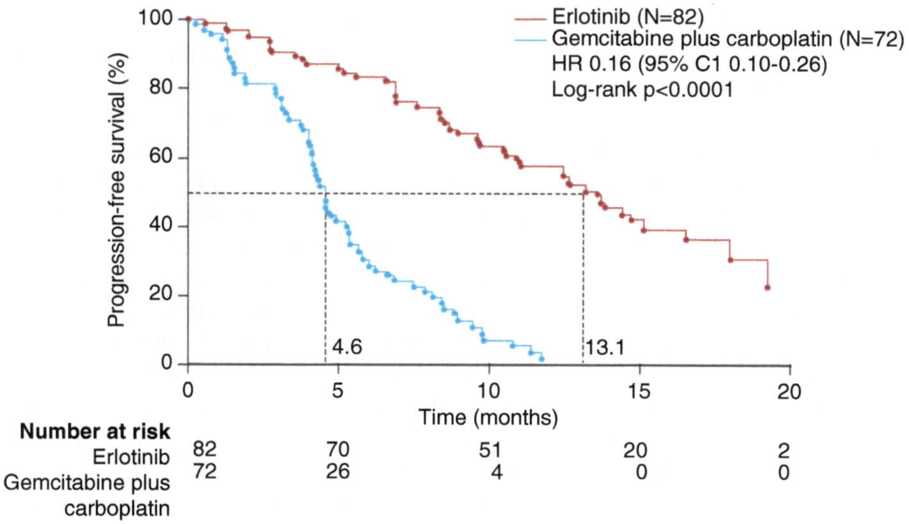

Fig. 3.1 Kaplan-Meier curves for PFS by treatment. Untreated patients with EGFR mutations were randomized to either erlotinib or the doublet of carboplatin with gemcitabine. (Left) PFS was superior with erlotinib as compared to platinum-based chemotherapy (reprinted from [49] with permission from Elsevier)

EGFR mutation status was available for 35.9% of the patients enrolled and of these 437 samples, 59.7% harbored an EGFR mutation. Analysis by type of mutation revealed that 53.6% had exon 19 deletions, 42.5% had the L858R mutation at exon 21, 4.2% had a T790M mutation (discussed below) at exon 20 and 3.8% had other mutations. There was a significant association between EGFR mutation status and outcome. Patients with an EGFR mutation had a significantly longer PFS with gefitinib compared to carboplatin plus paclitaxel (HR 0.48; 95% CI 0.36–0.64, $p<0.001$). In addition, patients without an EGFR mutation who received gefitinib compared to carboplatin plus paclitaxel had a shorter PFS (HR 2.85; 2.05–3.98, $p<0.001$). Similar trends were seen in analysis of response and OS. This study solidified the principle that the presence of an activating EGFR mutation predicts response to EGFR TKI monotherapy.

A meta-analysis of IPASS, WJTOG 3405, NEJ002 and First-SIGNAL confirmed these results [54]. These studies, however, had been largely limited to Asian patients. The phase II trial conducted by the Spanish Lung Cancer Group explored the use of first-line erlotinib in European patients with EGFR mutations and noted a robust 90% response rate [55]. The phase III EURTAC trial compared erlotinib with platinum based chemotherapy in patients with EGFR mutated NSCLC but in a Caucasian population [56]. Interim results demonstrate a superior response rate with erlotinib (54.5 vs. 10.5%, $p<0.0001$) and a superior PFS (HR 0.37, 95% CI 0.25–0.54). These data are assuring and help confirm the predictive nature of EGFR mutation, regardless of ethnicity.

EGFR mutations may also predict outcomes in patients receiving EGFR TKIs in combination with chemotherapy. The phase III TRIBUTE trial treated 1,059 patients with untreated, advanced NSCLC with six cycles of carboplatin and paclitaxel and randomized patients to receive concurrent erlotinib or placebo, with continuation of erlotinib maintenance until toxicity or progression [57]. In an unselected population, erlotinib did not confer a survival advantage. Specimens were available for analysis in 274 of these patients. Activating EGFR mutations were detected in 13% of the specimens and were associated with a better prognosis and predicted a higher response rate with erlotinib [58]. This is in contrast to analysis of the INTACT trials. INTACT-1 and INTACT-2 were phase III studies that compared chemotherapy (cisplatin plus gemcitabine or carboplatin plus paclitaxel, respectively) with and without gefitinib [59, 60]. Neither of these studies described a difference in survival between chemotherapy alone and chemotherapy with gefitinib. In patients with EGFR mutations, the addition of gefitinib did not serve as a predictive marker for gefitinib therapy. A study of erlotinib with and without chemotherapy (CALGB 20406) did not show a significant difference in efficacy between these regimens and while patients with EGFR mutations had better outcomes than those without mutations, the lack of a nonerlotinib arm precludes comment on any predictive power in this study [61]. While many studies show the predictive power of EGFR mutations for EGFR TKI monotherapy, their role in combination therapy remains unclear.

Maintenance therapy with erlotinib has been explored as well. The aforementioned SATURN trial included 889 patients who did not have progressive disease after four cycles of platinum based chemotherapy and randomized patients to receive continuous erlotinib maintenance therapy or placebo [39]. In the entire cohort, the erlotinib arm had a longer median PFS (HR 0.71, 95% CI 0.62–0.82) and a longer median OS (HR 0.81, 95% CI 0.70–0.95). Analysis by EGFR mutation status was performed. Erlotinib prolonged PFS in both mutant and wild-type cases however the impact in patients with EGFR mutations (HR 0.10, 95% CI 0.04–0.25) was more noticeable than in patients with wild-type EGFR (HR 0.78, 95% CI 0.63–0.96).

Some studies suggest that the different EGFR mutations confer different sensitivity to EGFR TKIs. In the phase II Spanish Lung Cancer Group trial, 297 patients were screened and 37 (12.5%) had EGFR mutations: 25 were exon 19 deletions and the remainder were exon 21 point mutations (L858R) [55]. Analysis by mutation showed that all 25 patients with exon 19 mutations demonstrated a response (100%) compared to the 75% response rate seen in patients with the L858R mutation. Another small series of 41 patients detected EGFR mutations in 13 samples (32%) [35]. Nine of the 13 mutations were in-frame deletions in exon 19, most frequently a 15-base pair deletion. The remaining mutations were point mutations in either exon 21 or 18. All of the patients with an exon 19 mutation had either a complete or partial response, though most of the patients with any mutation derived benefit. However, not all studies show a difference in response by type of EGFR mutation. A Japanese study of 16 patients with EGFR mutations receiving first-line gefitinib did not observe differences in survival by type of EGFR mutation [62]. Again, EGFR mutations were more likely in female patients and never or light smokers. In this population, gefitinib had a high efficacy, with a response rate of 75%, though no difference was noted between the nine patients with exon 19 deletions and the seven patients with the L858R mutation in exon 21. In the NEJ002 trial, analysis by type of mutation revealed no significant difference between patients harboring an exon 19 deletion and those with the L858R mutation with median PFS of 11.5 and 10.8 months, respectively, and response rates of 82.8% and 67.3%, respectively [52]. Based on the current evidence, EGFR mutation is a positive predictive marker for EGFR TKI therapy but the type of mutation may not offer additional predictive information.

Not all EGFR mutations are positive predictive markers. One mutation in exon 20 (T790M) has been frequently identified in patients that develop resistance to gefitinib or erlotinib [63]. Position 790 is located in the catalytic cleft of the EGFR tyrosine kinase domain and is critical for proper TKI binding. This mutation has been elegantly explored with in vitro studies in cells with either wild type or mutated EGFR (exon 19 deletion or L858R) [64]. Introduction of the T790M mutation into these cells does not alter EGFR expression or phosphorylation. However, the sensitivity to gefitinib and erlotinib was significantly inhibited with this mutation. While this is often seen in patients who develop resistance during TKI therapy, the mutation can occur de novo, prior to therapy. In the IPASS trial, which included only untreated patients, 4.2% of patients with an EGFR mutation harbored a T790M mutation.

After initiation of therapy, another potential predictive marker may emerge. Though not quite as clinically useful, the development of an acneiform-like rash after initiation of EGFR TKI therapy appears to be an early sign of efficacy. In a study of patients with pretreated EGFR-positive NSCLC, administration of erlotinib resulted in an overall response rate of 12.3% [65]. All of the patients who achieved an objective response experienced a rash, as did 95% of the patients with stable disease. Among patients who had progressive disease, only 54% of patients experienced a rash. Analysis of patients on the BR.21 trial demonstrated an association between the presence of any rash and longer OS and PFS [66]. The association was stronger with a higher grade of rash. Patients who developed a grade 1 rash survived 144% longer than those with no rash and those with at least a grade 2 rash survived 245% longer. In the TRIBUTE study, patients in the erlotinib arm who experienced a grade 2 rash had a median OS of 13.2 months, compared to 10.8 months for patients with a grade 1 rash and 8.4 months for patients with no rash [67]. Similar findings were noted in the TALENT study. While these findings are interesting, further study is needed to define the role of rash development in guiding the use of EGFR TKIs.

Proteomics

Serum proteomics have emerged as a potential predictive marker for EGFR-TKI therapy. Reproducible proteomic signatures can be obtained from pretreatment patient serum and classified based on laser desorption ionization times for flight mass spectrometry [68]. Mass spectrum analysis identifies various peaks which correspond to ions which are predominantly peptides and proteins. A prediction algorithm was generated using a training set of 139 patients with NSCLC treated with gefitinib. This classification algorithm generates a VeriStrat score that is reported as either "good" or "poor." This technique was then validated using samples from ECOG 3503, a trial that studied the benefit of erlotinib in patients with advanced, untreated NSCLC [69]. The trial included 137 patients but only 102 patients had analyzable serum samples and only 43 had analyzable biopsy specimens. Median survival in this unselected population was 7.9 months with a response rate of only 6.9%. Analysis of the biopsy specimens revealed that only three patients (7%) had EGFR mutations, all of which were located in exon 21. These three patients all achieved SD. Thus, in this small study, no difference in RR was noted but presence of the mutation did correlate with a higher disease control rate (100 vs. 34%, $p=0.05$) and trended toward a longer median OS (33 vs. 6 months, $p=0.054$) with erlotinib. In the same study, VeriStrat score was found to correlate with survival. Patients with a good VeriStrat score had a risk of death that was 36% of that for patients with a poor VeriStrat score. Furthermore, VeriStrat score was found to predict outcomes with erlotinib therapy independent of EGFR mutation. While the lack of a proper comparator arm precludes establishing this score as a true predictive marker, these early data are encouraging and prospective, confirmatory trials are underway.

In summary, many clinical features have been shown to predict response to EGFR TKIs including histology, gender, ethnicity and smoking status. Molecular analysis suggests that these may actually be surrogate markers for EGFR mutations. In an analysis that included 617 NSCLC specimens, mutation status was compared with several clinicopathologic variables [70]. In this unselected population, EGFR mutations were detected in 21% of cases, as compared to nearly 60% in the enriched IPASS population. EGFR mutation status was not associated with age or stage. As expected, though, EGFR mutations were far more common in never smokers compared to ever smokers (51 vs. 10%), in adenocarcinoma compared to other histologies (40 vs. 3%), in East Asian ethnicity compared to other ethnicities (30 vs. 8%) and in females compared to males (42 vs. 14%, all $p<0.001$) but not all patients with EGFR mutations will fall into these categories. When available, EGFR mutation status should be used to guide first-line therapy over other features including EGFR expression, EGFR copy number and any clinical characteristics. While female patients, Asian patients, and patients who have never smoked may be more likely to harbor an EGFR mutation, a significant proportion of patients who do not match this clinical profile will still have an activating EGFR mutation and testing of patients who do not fit the classic profile, including men and smokers, is still warranted in the first-line setting.

Crizotinib

The development of crizotinib and its predictive biomarker, the EML4-ALK translocation, is a prime demonstration of the potential of personalized medicine. The creation of a viral complementary DNA library from a resected NSCLC specimen aided in the discovery of an inversion in chromosome 2 that fuses the echinoderm microtubule-associated protein-like 4 (EML4) with the kinase domain of the anaplastic lymphoma kinase (ALK) [71]. The resulting fusion protein (EML4-ALK) was then expressed in vitro and led to the transformation of cells in culture and the development of tumors in mouse models. These data, published in 2007, had successfully identified a therapeutic target with a potential predictive biomarker that was under clinical study only 2 years later.

Subsequent studies showed that EML4-ALK is not a common finding in NSCLC. In a population of Chinese patients with resected NSCLC that was primarily adenocarcinoma, 4.9% were found to have EML4-ALK [72]. This population was similar to the population studied in IPASS and indeed, the rate of EGFR mutation was similar (58%). It is worth noting that there was no overlap between EML4-ALK and EGFR mutation detection. Since 91% of these patients were found to be never or light smokers, another study used these clinical characteristics to further enrich a population. A study examined outcomes of patients with EML4-ALK in a population of patients with NSCLC that had at least two of the following characteristics: female sex, Asian ethnicity, never or light smoking history and adenocarcinoma histology [73]. In this population, the incidence of EGFR mutation was 22% and the incidence of EML4-ALK was 13%. Analysis demonstrated that patients with EML4-ALK tumors were more likely to be younger and more likely to be men. In addition, EML4-ALK was associated with a resistance to EGFR TKIs. This is consistent with the observation that EML4-ALK and EGFR mutations appear to be mutually exclusive [74].

The main relevance of EML4-ALK is its ability to serve as a therapeutic target. Preclinical studies that demonstrated the efficacy of ALK inhibition in cell lines with ALK mutations led to the development of the oral ALK inhibitor crizotinib. The phase I/II study of crizotinib has produced encouraging and exciting results. Out of 1,500 patients with NSCLC, 82 eligible patients were identified that had ALK rearrangements in their tumor [75]. Patients with these rearrangements were more likely to be younger, to be never or light smokers and to have adenocarcinoma histology. Treatment was well tolerated and the overall RR in this largely pretreated population was 57% with an additional 33% achieving stable disease. While there was no placebo comparator arm in this study, a recent comparison between these patients and matched historical controls offers some insight into the impact of crizotinib on survival and the role of ALK rearrangement as a predictive marker [76]. The 82 ALK+patients who received crizotinib had a 2-year OS of 64% while 37 patients with the ALK rearrangement who did not receive crizotinib had a 2-year OS of 33%. This treatment effect would surely have been missed in an unselected population, but the use of the ALK rearrangement as a predictive marker has allowed the potential benefit of crizotinib to be realized.

There are several variants of the EML4-ALK inversion. Analysis of 8 variants demonstrated a constant ALK and tyrosine kinase domain but each EML4 transcript was unique [77]. This is a potential challenge in screening patients for ALK rearrangements and the heterogeneity warrants technical expertise and standardization [78]. With the vast majority of patients with EML4-ALK NSCLC deriving benefit from crizotinib, this agent has quickly moved into randomized studies and is likely to be incorporated into the standard treatment algorithm for these patients. While not yet approved, the journey from identifying a potential target to developing and implementing a targeted agent with a predictive biomarker has been exemplified by crizotinib in EML4-ALK-positive NSCLC and has established a template for future drug development.

Cytotoxic Chemotherapy

Targeted agents often have rational predictive markers that can guide their use. Recent studies have suggested that a similar paradigm can be applied to traditional cytotoxic chemotherapy. While their original efficacy was based on empiric use, identification of patient subsets may further improve outcomes and the likelihood of benefit from first-line therapy. While ongoing studies promise to deliver novel targets and agents, important work is also reshaping our use of existing agents.

Platinum-Based Therapy

Standard first-line chemotherapy consists of a platinum doublet, including either cisplatin or carboplatin. Platinum agents mediate their cytotoxicity through the formation of DNA adducts. Cells can repair this type of DNA damage through the activity of excision repair cross-complementation 1 (ERCC1), a DNA repair endonuclease. There appears to be an inverse relationship between pretreatment ERCC1 expression and platinum sensitivity. A retrospective study of 70 patients with advanced NSCLC showed that low levels of ERCC1 gene expression correlated with a longer survival among patients treated with cisplatin [79]. Analysis of patients on the International Adjuvant Lung Trial (IALT) who received platinum-doublet adjuvant therapy also demonstrated an association between ERCC1 expression and outcomes [80]. The survival benefit to adjuvant therapy was noted in patients with ERCC1-negative tumors (HR 0.65, 95% CI 0.50–0.86) but was not evident in ERCC1-positive patients (HR 1.14, 95% CI 0.84–1.55). Another study of 56 patients with advanced NSCLC treated with gemcitabine and cisplatin demonstrated a significant association between survival and ERCC1 expression [81]. Median OS in patients with low ERCC1 expression was 61.6 weeks compared to 20.4 weeks in patients with high ERCC1 expression. Prospective use of ERCC1 has shown promise. In the Genotypic International Lung Trial (GILT), 346 patients with advanced NSCLC were randomized to standard cisplatin plus docetaxel or to receive treatment based on ERCC1 status: patients with low ERCC1 expression received cisplatin and docetaxel but patients with high ERCC1 expression received docetaxel and gemcitabine [82]. While there was no difference in median OS, response was significantly higher in the group guided by ERCC1 expression. These studies are encouraging and additional study will further define the role of ERCC1 in guiding platinum therapy for NSCLC.

Gemcitabine Therapy

Gemcitabine is an agent often used in the empiric therapy of NSCLC. High expression of one of the targets of gemcitabine, ribonucleotide reductase M1 (RRM1) has been associated with gemcitabine resistance and has the potential to serve as a predictive marker for gemcitabine therapy. Retrospective analysis has demonstrated an association between high RRM1 expression and poor survival with cisplatin and gemcitabine [79]. A study of patients with locally advanced NSCLC correlated pretreatment RRM1 levels with response after two cycles of gemcitabine with carboplatin [83]. RRM1 expression was inversely associated with response ($p = 0.002$).

The use of these biomarkers in combination to guide chemotherapy selection is appealing. One study that demonstrates the feasibility of this approach is the Molecular Analysis-Directed Individualized Therapy (MADeIT) trial [84]. This prospective phase II study of patients with advanced NSCLC required a dedicated biopsy for ERCC1 and RRM1 expression. These data were used to select the first-line chemotherapy regimen. If ERCC1 was overexpressed, platinum was withheld and patients received docetaxel plus gemcitabine (if RRM1 was low) or vinorelbine (if RRM1 was high). If ERCC1 was not overexpressed, patients received cisplatin with either gemcitabine or vinorelbine, based on RRM1 expression. Outcomes were encouraging, with a median OS of 13.3 months. This led to the phase III study that randomized patients to a standard approach or this biomarker driven strategy [85]. Preliminary results demonstrate a longer median OS in patients treated with the personalized approach (12.3 vs. 8.1 months) but longer follow-up in this study and additional validation are needed.

Pemetrexed Therapy

Pemetrexed inhibits several enzymes involved in folate metabolism, including thymidylate synthase (TS) and dihydrofolate reductase (DHFR). Pemetrexed has demonstrated efficacy in the treatment of mesothelioma when combined with cisplatin [86] and as a single agent in the second-line treatment of NSCLC [87]. The phase III trial of cisplatin with either pemetrexed or gemcitabine in the first-line setting demonstrated a comparable efficacy between the two regimens [88]. Prespecified subset analyses, however, demonstrated superior outcomes with pemetrexed for patients with nonsquamous histology. Patients with adenocarcinoma had a longer median OS with pemetrexed compared to gemcitabine (12.6 vs. 10.9 months) as did patients with large cell carcinoma (10.4 vs. 6.7 months). In addition, squamous histology predicted inferior outcomes with pemetrexed. Patients with squamous cell histology had a decreased survival with pemetrexed compared to gemcitabine (10.8 vs. 9.4 months). These data support the role of squamous and nonsquamous histologies as predictive markers for pemetrexed use in NSCLC. Further subset analyses were conducted in an attempt to identify additional clinicopathologic predictors of outcome. While the predictive power of histology was confirmed, other factors including gender, ethnicity, disease stage, smoking history, and performance status were not found to be predictive of benefit in either arm, though they did demonstrate prognostic potential [89]. Histology also predicted benefit from pemetrexed maintenance therapy. This was demonstrated in the phase III trial of maintenance pemetrexed versus placebo in patients with advanced NSCLC treated with four cycles of platinum-based chemotherapy [90]. Maintenance therapy with pemetrexed improved both PFS (4.3 vs. 2.6 months, $p<0.0001$) and OS (13.4 vs. 10.6 months, $p=0.012$) when compared to placebo. Prespecified analyses by histology revealed an OS benefit for patients with nonsquamous histology (15.5 vs. 10.3 months, $p=0.002$) but no benefit over placebo for patients with squamous histology (9.9 vs. 10.8 months, $p=0.678$).

One hypothesis addressing the predictive impact of histology is that squamous cell tumors are more likely to overexpress TS and histology is actually a surrogate for TS expression. In vitro analysis demonstrated that cells sensitive to pemetrexed had decreased expression of TS and DHFR while the least sensitive cell lines overexpressed TS and DHFR [91]. Analysis of 56 specimens from patients with NSCLC revealed that TS expression, as measured by both messenger RNA and protein levels, was much higher in squamous cell carcinoma compared with adenocarcinoma [92]. The potential role of TS was further explored in a retrospective analysis of pretreatment biopsies from patients treated on the phase III study of cisplatin with either pemetrexed or gemcitabine [93]. In this study, 232 patients had tissue samples, with gene expression available in 69 patients and immunohistochemistry (IHC) available in 181 patients. In this limited analysis, there was a significant interaction between low TS expression and pemetrexed treatment effect. TS expression has significant potential as a predictive marker for pemetrexed benefit, though standardized methods of assessment as well as prospective validation are required before the clinical applicability of TS in this setting can be properly defined.

Conclusion

The heterogeneity of lung cancer is clearly demonstrated by the unique molecular signatures of the various subsets already described and the countless more awaiting discovery. The paradigm shift throughout oncology is the personalization of cancer care and chemotherapy delivery to account for these important differences. This approach can improve the likelihood of response and minimize the use of inefficient therapies that would otherwise offer toxicity without benefit and delay initiation of effective therapy. It is only by employing reliable predictive biomarkers that personalized medicine can reach its potential in the treatment of NSCLC. While the development of novel agents is always welcome, their appeal is much greater if they are accompanied by a predictive marker. Novel MET-inhibitors, like the oral agent ARQ 197, have shown efficacy in early studies, but their emergence is more exciting with the discovery that MET amplification can identify a subset of patients more likely to derive benefit from these agents [94].

When considering the role of predictive biomarkers, one must bear in mind the source of these markers. In patients with recurrent or refractory disease, biomarker testing is often performed on archived tissue specimens. It is possible that the active tumor profile bears little resemblance to the original biopsy sample due in part to the selective pressure of prior therapy. While it is unlikely that a tumor that originally harbored an EGFR mutation would mutate to wild type EGFR, the inverse is certainly possible as is the possibility of acquiring additional mutations that may impact therapeutic decisions. Since repeat biopsies are often impractical and occasionally not possible, other means of detection are being actively sought. One area of intense research is in the field of circulating tumor cells (CTC). Studies have shown that these cells can be captured and early studies of KRAS mutation detection and EGFR expression on CTC have been successful [95]. Whether the biomarkers found on these cells retain their predictive power has yet to be determined but these advances have the potential to improve the accuracy, accessibility, and clinical utility of these biomarkers. Predictive biomarkers have radically changed the use of available agents in NSCLC, and more importantly, they have changed the approach to developing the novel agents this field so desperately needs.

References

1. Jemel A, Siegel R, Xu J, Ward E. Cancer statistics, 2010. CA Cancer J Clin. 2010;60: 277–300.
2. Marino P, Pampallona S, Preatoni A, Cantoni A, Invernizzi F. Chemotherapy vs. supportive care in advanced non-small-cell lung cancer: results of a meta-analysis of the literature. Chest. 1994;106:861–5.
3. Cullen M, Billingham J, Woodroffe C, Chetiyawardana AD, Gower NH, Joshi R, Ferry DR, Rudd RM, Spiro SG, Cook JE, Trask C, Bessell E, Connolly CK, Tobias J, Souhami RL. Mitomycin, ifosfamide, and cisplatin in unresectable non-small-cell lung cancer: effects on survival and quality of life. J Clin Oncol. 1999;17:3188–94.
4. Schiller JH, Harrington D, Belani CP, Langer C, Sandler A, Krook J, Zhu J, Johnson DH. Comparison of four chemotherapy regimens for advanced non-small-cell lung cancer. N Engl J Med. 2002;346:92–8.
5. Sandler A, Gray R, Perry MC, Brahmer J, Schiller JH, Dowlati A, Lilenbaum R, Johnson DH. Paclitaxel-carboplatin alone or with bevacizumab for non-small-cell lung cancer. N Engl J Med. 2006;355:2542–50.
6. Reck M, von Pawel J, Zatloukal P, Ramlau R, Gorbounova V, Hirsh V, Leighl N, Mezger J, Archer V, Moore N, Manegold C, BO17704 Study Group. Overall survival with cisplatin-gemcitabine and bevacizumab or placebo as first-line therapy for nonsquamous non-small-cell lung cancer: results from a randomised phase III trial (AVAiL). Ann Oncol. 2010;21:1804–9.
7. An SJ, Huang YS, Chen ZH, Su J, Yang Y, Chen JG, Yan HH, Lin QX, Yang JJ, Yang XN, Zhou Q, Zhang XC, Wu YL. Post treatment plasma VEGF levels may be associated with the

overall survival of patients with advanced non-small-cell lung cancer treated with bevacizumab plus chemotherapy. Med Oncol. 2012;29(2):627–32.
8. Brahmer JR, Dahlberg SE, Gray RJ, Schiller JH, Perry MC, Sandler A, Johnson DH. Sex differences in outcome with bevacizumab therapy: analysis of patients with advanced-stage non-small cell lung cancer treated with or without bevacizumab in combination with paclitaxel and carboplatin in the Eastern Cooperative Oncology Group trial 4599. J Thorac Oncol. 2011;6:103–8.
9. Ramalingam SS, Dahlberg SE, Langer CJ, Gray R, Belani CP, Brahmer JR, Sandler AB, Schiller JH, Johnson DH. Outcomes for elderly, advanced-stage non-small-cell lung cancer patients treated with bevacizumab in combination with carboplatin and paclitaxel: analysis of Eastern Cooperative Oncology Group trial 4599. J Clin Oncol. 2008;26:60–5.
10. Johnson DH, Fehrenbacher L, Novotny WF, Herbst RS, Nemunaitis JJ, Jablons DM, Langer CJ, DeVore RF, Gaudreault J, Damico LA, Holmgren E, Kabbinavar F. Randomized phase II trial comparing bevacizumab plus carboplatin and paclitaxel with carboplatin and paclitaxel alone in previously untreated locally advanced or metastatic non-small-cell lung cancer. J Clin Oncol. 2004;22:2184–91.
11. Sandler A, Yi J, Dahlberg S, Kolb MM, Wang L, Hambleton J, Schiller J, Johnson DH. Treatment outcomes by tumor histology in Eastern Cooperative Oncology Group study 4599 of bevacizumab with paclitaxel/carboplatin for advanced non-small cell lung cancer. J Thorac Oncol. 2010;5:1416–23.
12. Zhang W, Dahlberg SE, Yang D, Sandler AB, Brahmer JR, Schiller JH, Carbone DP, Johnson DH, Lenz H. Genetic variants in angiogenesis pathway associated with clinical outcome in NSCLC patients (pts) treated with bevacizumab in combination with carboplatin and paclitaxel: subset pharmacogenetic analysis of ECOG 4599. J Clin Oncol. 2009;27:15S. suppl; abstr 8032.
13. Dahlberg SE, Sandler AB, Brahmer JR, Schiller JH, Johnson DH. Clinical course of advanced non-small-cell lung cancer patients experiencing hypertension during treatment with bevacizumab in combination with carboplatin and paclitaxel on ECOG 4599. J Clin Oncol. 2010;28:949–54.
14. Olayioye MA, Neve RM, Lane HA, Hynes NE. The ErbB signaling network: receptor heterodimerization in development and cancer. EMBO J. 2000;19:3159–67.
15. Sobrero AF, Maurel J, Fehrenbacher L, Scheithauer W, Abubakr YA, Lutz MP, Vega-Villegas ME, Eng C, Steinhauer EU, Prausova J, Lenz HJ, Borg C, Middleton G, Kroning H, Luppi G, Kisker O, Zubel A, Langer C, Kopit J, Burris 3rd HA. EPIC: phase III trial of cetuximab plus irinotecan after fluoropyrimidine and oxaliplatin failure in patients with metastatic colorectal cancer. J Clin Oncol. 2008;26:2311–9.
16. Vermorken JB, Mesia R, Rivera F, Remenar E, Kawecki A, Rottey S, Erfan J, Zabolotnyy D, Kienzer HR, Cupissol D, Peyrade F, Benasso M, Vynnychenko I, De Raucort D, Bokemeyer C, Schueler A, Amellal N, Hitt R. Platinum-based chemotherapy plus cetuximab in head and neck cancer. N Engl J Med. 2008;359:1116–27.
17. Hanna N, Lilenbaum R, Ansari R, Lynch T, Govindan R, Janne PA, Bonomi P. Phase II trial of cetuximab in patients with previously treated non-small-cell lung cancer. J Clin Oncol. 2006;24:5253–8.
18. Pirker R, Pereira JR, Szczesna A, von Pawel J, Krzakowski M, Ramlau R, Vynnychenko I, Park K, Yu CT, Ganul V, Roh JK, Bajetta E, O'Bryne K, de Marinis F, Eberhardt W, Goddemeier T, Emig M, Gatzemeier U. Cetuximab plus chemotherapy in patients with advanced non-small-cell lung cancer (FLEX): an open label randomised phase III trial. Lancet. 2009;373:1525–31.
19. Lynch TJ, Patel T, Dreisbach L, McCleod M, Heim WJ, Hermann RC, Paschold E, Iannotti NO, Dakhil S, Gorton S, Pautret V, Weber MR, Woytowitz D. Cetuximab and first-line taxane/carboplatin chemotherapy in advanced non-small-cell lung cancer: results of the randomized multicenter phase III trial BMS099. J Clin Oncol. 2010;28:911–7.

20. Karapetis CS, Khambata-Ford S, Jonker DJ, O'Callaghan CJ, Tu D, Tebbutt NC, Simes RJ, Chalchal H, Shapiro JD, Robitaille S, Price TJ, Shepherd L, Au HJ, Langer C, Moore MJ, Zalcberg JR. K-ras mutations and benefit from cetuximab in advanced colorectal cancer. N Engl J Med. 2008;359:1757–65.
21. Khambata-Ford S, Harbison CT, Hart LL, Awad M, Xu LA, Horak CE, Dakhil S, Hermann RC, Lynch TJ, Weber MR. Analysis of potential predictive markers of cetuximab benefit in BMS099, a phase III study of cetuximab and first-line taxane/carboplatin in advanced non-small-cell lung cancer. J Clin Oncol. 2010;28:918–27.
22. Herbst RS, Kelly K, Chansky K, Mack PC, Franklin WA, Hirsch FR, Atkins JN, Dakhil SR, Albain KS, Kim ES, Redman M, Crowley JJ, Gandara DR. Phase II selection design trial of concurrent chemotherapy and cetuximab versus chemotherapy followed by cetuximab in advanced-stage non-small-cell lung cancer: Southwest Oncology Group study S0342. J Clin Oncol. 2010;28:4747–54.
23. Gandara D, Kim ES, Herbst RS, Moon J, Redman MW, Dakhil SR, Hirsch F, Mack PC, Franklin W, Kelly K. S0546: Carboplatin, paclitaxel, cetuximab, and bevacizumab followed by cetuximab and bevacizumab maintenance in advanced non-small cell lung cancer (NSCLC): a SWOG phase II study. J Clin Oncol. 2009;27:15S. suppl; abstr 8015.
24. Mack PC, Holland WS, Redman M, Lara PN, Snyder LJ, Hirsch FR, Franklin WA, Kim ES, Herbst RS, Gandara DR. KRAS mutation analysis in cetuximab-treated advanced stage non-small cell lung cancer (NSCLC): SWOG experience with S0342 and S0536. J Clin Oncol. 2009;27:15S. supple; abstr 8022.
25. O'Byrne KJ, Bondarenko I, Barrios C, Eschbach C, Martens U, Hotko Y, Kortsik C, Celik I, Stroh C, Pirker R. Molecular and clinical predictors of outcome for cetuximab in non-small cell lung cancer (NSCLC): data from the FLEX study. J Clin Oncol. 2009;27:15s. suppl; abstr 8007.
26. Ray M, Salgia R, Vokes EE. The role of EGFR inhibition in the treatment of non-small-cell lung cancer. Oncologist. 2009;14:1116–30.
27. Kris MG, Natale RB, Herbst RS, Lynch TJ, Prager D, Belani C, Schiller JH, Kelly K, Spiridonidis H, Sandler A, Albain KS, Cella D, Wolf MK, Averbuch SD, Ochs JJ, Kay AC. Efficacy of gefitinib, an inhibitor of the epidermal growth factor receptor tyrosine kinase, in symptomatic patients with non-small cell lung cancer: a randomized trial. JAMA. 2003;290:2149–58.
28. Takeda K, Hida T, Sato T, Ando M, Seto T, Satouchi M, Ichinose Y, Katakami N, Yamamoto N, Kudoh S, Sasaki J, Matsui K, Takayama K, Kashii T, Iwamoto Y, Sawa T, Okamoto I, Kurata T, Nakagawa K, Fukuoka M. Randomized phase III trial of platinum-doublet chemotherapy followed by gefitinib compared with continued platinum-doublet chemotherapy in Japanese patients with advanced non-small-cell lung cancer: results of a West Japan Thoracic Oncology Group trial (WJTOG0203). J Clin Oncol. 2009;28:753–60.
29. Shepherd FA, Rodrigues Pereira J, Ciuleanu T, Tan EH, Hirsh V, Thongprasert S, Campos D, Maoleekoonpiroj S, Smylie M, Martins R, van Kooten M, Dediu M, Findlay B, Tu D, Johnston D, Bezjak A, Clark G, Santabarbara P, Seymour L, National Cancer Institute of Canada Clinical Trials Group. Erlotinib in previously treated non-small-cell lung cancer. N Engl J Med. 2005;353:123–32.
30. Tsao MS, Sakurada A, Cutz JC, Zhu CQ, Kamel-Reid S, Squire J, Lorimer I, Zhang T, Liu N, Daneshmand M, Marrano P, Da Cunha Santos G, Lagarde A, Richardson F, Seymour L, Whitehead M, Ding K, Pater J, Shepherd FA. Erlotinib in lung cancer - molecular and clinical predictors of outcome. N Engl J Med. 2005;353:133–44.
31. Gatzemeier U, Pluzanska A, Szczesna A, Kaukel E, Roubec J, De Rosa F, Milanowski J, Karnicka-Mlodkowski H, Pesek M, Serwatowski P, Ramlau R, Janaskova T, Vansteenkiste J, Strausz J, Manikhas GM, Von Pawel J. Phase III study of erlotinib in combination with cisplatin and gemcitabine in advanced non-small-cell lung cancer: the Tarceva lung cancer investigation trial. J Clin Oncol. 2007;25:1545–52.

32. Thatcher N, Chang A, Parikh P, Rodrigues-Pereira J, Ciuleanu T, von Pawel J, Thongprasert S, Tan EH, Pemberton K, Archer V, Carroll K. Gefitinib plus best supportive care in previously treated patients with refractory advanced non-small-cell lung cancer: results from a randomised, placebo-controlled, multicentre study (Iressa Survival Evaluation in Lung Cancer). Lancet. 2005;366:1527–37.
33. Chang A, Parikh P, Thongprasert S, Tan EH, Perng RP, Ganzon D, Yang CH, Tsao CJ, Watkins C, Botwood N, Thatcher N. Gefitinib (IRESSA) in patients of Asian origin with refractory advanced non-small cell lung cancer: subset analysis from the ISEL study. J Thorac Oncol. 2006;1:847–55.
34. Zhu CQ, Da Cunha Santos G, Ding K, Sakurada A, Cutz JC, Liu N, Zhang T, Marrano P, Whitehead M, Squire JA, Kamel-Reid S, Seymour L, Shepherd FA, Tsao MS. Role of KRAS and EGFR as biomarkers of response to erlotinib in National Cancer Institute of Canada clinical trials group study BR.21. J Clin Oncol. 2008;26:4268–75.
35. van Zandwijk N, Mathy A, Boerrigter L, Ruijter H, Tielen I, de Jong D, Baas P, Burgers S, Nederlof P. EGFR and KRAS mutations as criteria for treatment with tyrosine kinase inhibitors: retro- and prospective observations in non-small-cell lung cancer. Ann Oncol. 2007;18:99–103.
36. Pao W, Wang TY, Riely GJ, Miller VA, Pan Q, Ladanyi M, Zakowski MF, Heelan RT, Kris MG, Varmus HE. KRAS mutations and primary resistance of lung adenocarcinomas to gefitinib or erlotinib. PLoS Med. 2005;2:e17.
37. Linardou H, Dahabreh IJ, Kanaloupiti D, Siannis F, Bafaloukos D, Kosmidis P, Papadimitriou CA, Murray S. Assessment of somatic k-RAS mutations as a mechanism associated with resistance to EGFR-targeted agents: a systematic review and meta-analysis of studies in advanced non-small-cell lung cancer and metastatic colon cancer. Lancet Oncol. 2008;9:962–72.
38. Hirsch FR, Varella-Garcia M, Bunn PA, Franklin WA, Dziadziuszko R, Thatcher N, Chang A, Parikh P, Pereira JR, Ciuleanu T, von Pawel J, Watkins C, Flannery A, Ellison G, Donald E, Knight L, Parums D, Botwood N, Holloway B. Molecular predictors of outcome with gefitinib in a phase III placebo-controlled study in advanced non-small-cell lung cancer. J Clin Oncol. 2006;24:5034–42.
39. Cappuzzo F, Ciuleanu T, Stelmakh L, Cicenas S, Szczesna A, Juhasz E, Esteban E, Molinier O, Brugger W, Melezinek I, Klingelschmitt G, Klughammer B, Giaccone G. SATURN Investigators. Erlotinib as maintenance treatment in advanced non-small-cell lung cancer: a multicentre, randomised, placebo-controlled phase 3 study. Lancet Oncol. 2010;11:521–9.
40. Brugger W, Triller N, Blasinska-Morawiec M, Curescu S, Sakalauskas R, Manikhas G, Mazieres J, Whittom R, Rohr K, Cappuzzo F. Biomarker analyses from the phase III placebo-controlled SATURN study of maintenance erlotinib following first-line chemotherapy for advanced NSCLC. J Clin Oncol. 2009;27:15S. suppl; abstr 8020.
41. Parra HS, Cavina R, Latteri F, Zucali PA, Campagnoli E, Morenghi E, Grimaldi GC, Roncalli M, Santoro A. Analysis of epidermal growth factor receptor expression as a predictive factor for response to gefitinib ('Iressa', ZD1839) in non-small-cell lung cancer. Br J Cancer. 2004;91:208–12.
42. Kim ES, Hirsh V, Mok T, Socinski MA, Gervais R, Wu YL, Li LY, Watkins CL, Sellers MV, Lowe ES, Sun Y, Liao ML, Osterlind K, Reck M, Armour AA, Shepherd FA, Lippman SM, Douillard JY. Gefitinib versus docetaxel in previously treated non-small-cell lung cancer (INTEREST): a randomised phase III trial. Lancet. 2008;372:1809–18.
43. Crino L, Cappuzzo F, Zatloukal P, Reck M, Pesek M, Thompson JC, Ford HE, Hirsch FR, Varella-Garcia M, Ghiorghiu S, Duffield EL, Armour AA, Speak G, Cullen M. Gefitinib versus vinorelbine in chemotherapy-naïve elderly patients with advanced non-small-cell lung cancer (INVITE): a randomized, phase II study. J Clin Oncol. 2008;26:4253–60.
44. Fukuoka M, Wu Y, Thongprasert S, Yang C, Chu D, Saijo N, Watkins C, Duffield E, Armour A, Mok T. Biomarker analyses from a phase III, randomized, open-label, first-line study of gefitinib (G) versus carboplatin/paclitaxel (C/P) in clinically selected patients (pts) with

advanced non-small cell lung cancer (NSCLC) in Asia (IPASS). J Clin Oncol. 2009;27:15S. suppl; abstr 8006.

45. Lynch TJ, Bell DW, Sordella R, Gurubhagavatula S, Okimoto RA, Brannigan BW, Harris PL, Haserlat SM, Supko JG, Haluska FG, Louis DN, Christiani DC, Settleman J, Haber DA. Activating mutations in the epidermal growth factor receptor underlying responsiveness of non-small-cell lung cancer to gefitinib. N Engl J Med. 2004;350:2129–39.
46. Douillard JY, Shepherd FA, Hirsh V, Mok T, Socinski MA, Gervais R, Liau ML, Bischoff H, Reck M, Sellers MV, Watkins CL, Speake G, Armour AA, Kim ES. Molecular predictors of outcome with gefitinib and docetaxel in previously treated non-small-cell lung cancer: data from the randomized phase III INTEREST trial. J Clin Oncol. 2010;28:744–52.
47. Fukuoka M, Yano S, Giaccone G, Tamura T, Nakagawa K, Douillard JY, Nishiwaki Y, Vansteenkiste J, Kudoh S, Rischin D, Eek R, Horai T, Noda K, Takata I, Smit E, Averbuch S, Macleod A, Feyereislova A, Dong RP, Baselga J. Multi-institutional randomized phase II trial of gefitinib for previously treated patients with advanced non-small-cell lung cancer. J Clin Oncol. 2003;21:2237–46.
48. Bell DW, Lynch TJ, Haserlat SM, Harris PL, Okimoto RA, Brannigan BW, Sgroi DC, Muir B, Riemenschneider MJ, Iacona RB, Krebs AD, Johnson DH, Giaccone G, Herbst RS, Manegold C, Fukuoka M, Kris MG, Baselga J, Ochs JS, Haber DA. Epidermal growth factor receptor mutations and gene amplification in non-small-cell lung cancer: molecular analysis of the IDEAL/INTACT gefitinib trials. J Clin Oncol. 2005;23:8081–92.
49. Zhou C, Wu YL, Chen G, Feng J, Liu X, Wang C, Zhang S, Wang J, Zhou S, Ren S, Lu S, Zhang L, Hu C, Hu C, Luo Y, Chen L, Ye M, Huang J, Zhi X, Zhang Y, Xiu Q, Ma J, Zhang L, You C. Erlotinib versus chemotherapy as first-line treatment for patients with advanced EGFR mutation-positive non-small-cell-lung cancer (OPTIMAL, CTONG 0802): a multicentre, open-label, randomized, phase 3 study. Lancet Oncol. 2011;12:735–42.
50. Mitsudomi T, Morita S, Yatabe Y, Negoro S, Okamoto I, Tsurutani J, Seto T, Satouchi M, Tada H, Hirashima T, Asami K, Katakami N, Takada M, Yoshioka H, Shibata K, Kudoh S, Shimizu E, Saito H, Toyooka S, Nakagawa K, Fukuoka M. Gefitinib versus cisplatin plus docetaxel in patients with non-small-cell lung cancer harbouring mutations of the epidermal growth factor receptor (WJTOG3405): an open label, randomized phase 3 trial. Lancet Oncol. 2010;11:121–8.
51. Lee JS, Park K, Kim SW, Lee DH, Kim HT, Han JY, Yun T, Ahn JS, Suh C, Lee JS, Han JH, Yu SY, Lee JW, Jo SJ. A randomized phase III study of gefitinib versus standard chemotherapy (gemcitabine plus cisplatin) as a first-line treatment for never-smokers with advanced or metastatic adenocarcinoma of the lung. J Thorac Oncol. 2009;4:1. suppl; abstr PRS4.
52. Maemondo M, Inoue A, Kobayashi K, Sugawara S, Oizumi S, Isobe H, Gemma A, Harada M, Yoshizawa H, Kinoshita I, Fujita Y, Okinaga S, Hirano H, Yoshimori K, Harada T, Ogura T, Ando M, Miyazawa H, Tanaka T, Saijo Y, Hagiwara K, Morita S, Nukiwa T. Gefitinib or chemotherapy for non-small-cell lung cancer with mutated EGFR. NEJM. 2010;362:2380–8.
53. Mok TS, Wu YL, Thongprasert S, Yang CH, Chu DT, Saijo N, Sunpaweravong P, Han B, Margono B, Ichinose Y, Nishiwaki Y, Ohe Y, Yang JJ, Chewaskulyong B, Jiang H, Duffield EL, Watkins CL, Armour AA, Fukuoka M. Gefitinib or carboplatin-paclitaxel in pulmonary adenocarcinoma. N Engl J Med. 2009;361:947–57.
54. Ku GY, Haaland BA, de Lima Lopes Jr G. Gefitinib vs. chemotherapy as first-line therapy in advanced non-small cell lung cancer: Meta-analysis of phase III trials. Lung Cancer. 2011;74(3):469–73.
55. Rosell R, Gervais R, Vergnenegre A, Massuti B, Felip E, Cardenal F, Garcia Gomez R, Pallares C, Sanchez JM, Porta R, Cobo M, Di Seri M, Garrido Lopez P, Insa A, De Marinis F, Corre R, Carreras M, Carcereny E, Taron M, Paz-Ares LG. Erlotinib versus chemotherapy (CT) in advanced non-small cell lung cancer (NSCLC) patients (p) with epidermal growth factor receptor (EGFR) mutations: Interim results of the European Erlotinib Versus Chemotherapy (EURTAC) phase III randomized trial. J Clin Oncol. 2011;29. suppl; abstr 7503.
56. Herbst RS, Prager D, Hermann R, Fehrenbacher L, Johnson BE, Sandler A, Kris MG, Tran HT, Klein P, Li X, Ramies D, Johnson DH, Miller VA. TRIBUTE: a phase III trial of erlotinib

hydrochloride (OSI-774) combined with carboplatin and paclitaxel chemotherapy in advanced non-small-cell lung cancer. J Clin Oncol. 2005;23:5892–9.

57. Eberhard DA, Johnson BE, Amler LC, Goddard AD, Heldens SL, Herbst RS, Ince WL, Janne PA, Januario T, Johnson DH, Klein P, Miller VA, Ostland MA, Ramies DA, Sebisanovic D, Stinson JA, Zhang YR, Seshagiri S, Hillan KJ. Mutations in the epidermal growth factor receptor and in KRAS are predictive and prognostic indicators in patients with non-small-cell lung cancer treated with chemotherapy alone and in combination with erlotinib. J Clin Oncol. 2005;23:5900–9.
58. Giaccone G, Herbst RS, Manegold C, Scagliotti G, Rosell R, Miller V, Natale RB, Schiller JH, von Pawel J, Pluzanska A, Gatzemeier U, Grous J, Ochs JS, Averbuch SD, Wolf MK, Rennie P, Fandi A, Johnson DH. Gefitinib in combination with gemcitabine and cisplatin in advanced non-small-cell lung cancer: a phase III trial—INTACT 1. J Clin Oncol. 2004;22:777–84.
59. Herbst RS, Giaccone G, Schiller JH, Natale RB, Miller V, Manegold C, Scagliotti G, Rosell R, Oliff I, Reeves JA, Wolf MK, Krebs AD, Averbuch SD, Ochs JS, Grous J, Fandi A, Johnson DH. Gefitinib in combination with paclitaxel and carboplatin in advanced non-small-cell lung cancer: a phase III trial—INTACT 2. J Clin Oncol. 2004;22:785–94.
60. Janne PA, Wang XF, Socinski MA, Crawford J, Capelletti M, Edelman MJ, Villalona-Calero MA, Kratzke RA, Vokes EE, Miller VA. Randomized phase II trial of erlotinib (E) alone or in combination with carboplatin/paclitaxel (CP) in never or light former smokers with advanced lung adenocarcinoma: CALGB 20406. J Clin Oncol. 2010;28:15S. suppl; abstr 7503.
61. Paz-Ares L, Sanchez JM, Garcia-Velasco A, Massuti B, Lopez-Vivanco G, Provencio M, Montes A, Isla D, Amador ML, Rosell R. A prospective phase II trial of erlotinib in advanced non-small cell lung cancer (NSCLC) patients (p) with mutations in the tyrosine kinase (TK) domain of the epidermal growth factor receptor (EGFR). J Clin Oncol. 2006;18S:7020.
62. Inoue A, Suzuki T, Fukuhara T, Maemondo M, Kimura Y, Morikawa N, Watanabe H, Saijo Y, Nukiwa T. Prospective phase II study of gefitinib for chemotherapy naïve patients with advanced non-small-cell lung cancer with epidermal growth factor receptor gene mutations. J Clin Oncol. 2006;24:3340–6.
63. Pao W, Miller VA, Politi KA, Riely GJ, Somwar R, Zakowski MF, Kris MG, Varmus H. Acquired resistance of lung adenocarcinomas to gefitinib or erlotinib is associated with a second mutation in the EGFR kinase domain. PloS. 2005;2:e73.
64. Kobayashi S, Boggon TJ, Dayaram T, Janne PA, Kocher O, Meyerson M, Johnson BE, Eck MJ, Tenen DG, Halmos B. EGFR mutation and resistance of non-small-cell lung cancer to gefitinib. N Engl J Med. 2005;352:786–92.
65. Perez-Soler R, Chachoua A, Hammond LA, Rowinsky EK, Huberman M, Karp D, Rigas J, Clark GM, Santabarbara P, Bonomi P. Determinants of tumor response and survival with erlotinib in patients with non-small-cell lung cancer. J Clin Oncol. 2004;22(16):3238–47.
66. Wacker B, Nagrani T, Weinberg J, Witt K, Clark G, Cagnoni PJ. Correlation between development of rash and efficacy in patients treated with epidermal growth factor receptor tyrosine kinase inhibitor erlotinib in two large phase III studies. Clin Cancer Res. 2007;13:3913–21.
67. Perez-Soler R, Saltz L. Cutaneous adverse effects with HER1/EGFR-targeted agents: is there a silver lining? J Clin Oncol. 2005;23:5235–46.
68. Taguchi F, Solomon B, Gregorc V, Roder H, Gray R, Kasahara K, Nishio M, Brahmer J, Spreafico A, Ludovini V, Massion PP, Dziadziuszko R, Schiller J, Grigorieva J, Tsypin M, Hunsucker SW, Caprioli R, Duncan MW, Hirsch FR, Bunn Jr PA, Carbone DP. Mass spectrometry to classify non-small-cell lung cancer patients for clinical outcome after treatment with epidermal growth factor receptor tyrosine kinase inhibitors: a multicohort cross-institutional study. J Natl Cancer Inst. 2007;99:838–46.
69. Amann JM, Lee JW, Roder H, Brahmer J, Gonzalez A, Schiller JH, Carbone DP. Genetic and proteomic features associated with survival after treatment with erlotinib in first-line therapy of non-small cell lung cancer in Eastern Cooperative Oncology Group 3503. J Thorac Oncol. 2010;5:169–78.
70. Shigematsu H, Lin L, Takahashi T, Nomura M, Suzuki M, Wistuba II, Fong KM, Lee H, Toyooka S, Shimizu N, Fujisawa T, Feng Z, Roth JA, Herz J, Minna JD, Gazdar AF. Clinical and biological features associated with epidermal growth factor receptor gene mutations in lung cancer. J Natl Cancer Inst. 2005;97:339–46.

71. Soda M, Choi YL, Enomoto M, Takada S, Yamashita Y, Ishikawa S, Fujiwara S, Watanabe H, Kurashina K, Hatanaka H, Bando M, Ohno S, Ishikawa Y, Aburatani H, Niki T, Sohara Y, Sugiyama Y, Mano H. Identification of the transforming EML4-ALK fusion gene in non-small-cell lung cancer. Nature. 2007;448:561–6.
72. Wong DW, Leung EL, So KK, Tam IY, Sihoe AD, Cheng LC, Ho KK, Au JS, Chung LP, Wong MP. The EML4-ALK fusion gene is involved in various histologic types of lung cancer from nonsmokers with wild-type EGFR and KRAS. Cancer. 2009;115:1723–33.
73. Shaw AT, Yeap BY, Mino-Kenudson M, Digumarthy SR, Costa DB, Heist RS, Solomon B, Stubbs H, Admane S, McDermott U, Settleman J, Kobayashi S, Mark EJ, Rodig SJ, Chirieac LR, Kwak EL, Lynch TJ, Iafrate AJ. Clinical features and outcome of patients with non-small-cell lung cancer who harbor EML4-ALK. J Clin Oncol. 2009;27:4247–53.
74. Inamura K, Takeuchi K, Togashi Y, Nomura K, Ninomiya H, Okui M, Satoh Y, Okumura S, Nakagawa K, Soda M, Choi YL, Niki T, Mano H, Ishikawa Y. EML4-ALK fusion is linked to histological characteristics in a subset of lung cancers. J Thorac Oncol. 2008;3:13–7.
75. Kwak EL, Bang YJ, Camidge R, Shaw AT, Solomon B, Maki RG, Ou SH, Dezube BJ, Janne PA, Costa DB, Varella-Garcia M, Kim WH, Lynch TJ, Fidias P, Stubbs H, Engelman JA, Sequist LV, Tan WW, Gandhi L, Mino-Kenudson M, Wei GC, Shreeve M, Ratain MJ, Settleman J, Christensen JG, Haber DA, Wilner K, Salgia R, Shapiro GI, Clark JW, Iafrate AJ. Anaplastic lymphoma kinase inhibition in non-small-cell lung cancer. N Engl J Med. 2010;363: 1693–703.
76. Shaw AT, Yeap BY, Solomon BJ, Riely GJ, Iafrate AJ, Shapiro G, Costa DB, Butaney M, Ou SI, Maki RG, Bang Y, Varella-Garcia M, Salgia R, Wilner KD, Kulig K, Selaru P, Tang Y, Kwak EL, Clark JW, Camidge DR. Impact of crizotinib on survival in patients with advanced, ALK-positive NSCLC compared with historical controls. J Clin Oncol 2011; 29 (suppl; abstr: 7507).
77. Sasaki T, Rodig SJ, Chirieac LR, Janne PA. The biology and treatment of EML4-ALK non-small cell lung cancer. Eur J Cancer. 2010;46:1773–80.
78. Camidge DR, Kono SA, Flacco A, Tan AC, Doebele RC, Zhou Q, Crino L, Franklin WA, Varella-Garcia M. Optimizing the detection of lung cancer patients harboring anaplastic lymphoma kinase (ALK) gene rearrangements potentially suitable for ALK inhibitor treatment. Clin Cancer Res. 2010;16:5581–90.
79. Ceppi P, Volante M, Novello S, Rapa I, Danenberg KD, Danenberg PV, Cambieri A, Selvaggi G, Saviozzi S, Calogero R, Papotti M, Scagliotti GV. ERCC1 and RRM1 gene expressions but not EGFR are predictive of shorter survival in advanced non-small-cell lung cancer treated with cisplatin and gemcitabine. Ann Oncol. 2006;17:1818–25.
80. Olaussen KA, Dunant A, Fouret P, Brambilla E, Andre F, Haddad V, Taranchon E, Filipits M, Pirker R, Popper HH, Stahel R, Sabatier L, Pignon JP, Tursz T, Le Chevalier T, Soria JC. IALT Bio Investigators. DNA repair by ERCC1 in non-small-cell lung cancer and cisplatin-based adjuvant chemotherapy. N Engl J Med. 2006;355:983–91.
81. Lord RV, Brabender J, Gandara D, Alberola V, Camps C, Domine M, Cardenal F, Sanchez JM, Gumerlock PH, Taron M, Sanchez JJ, Danenberg KD, Danenberg PV, Rosell R. Low ERCC1 expression correlates with prolonged survival after cisplatin plus gemcitabine chemotherapy in non-small cell lung cancer. Clin Cancer Res. 2002;8:2286–91.
82. Cobo M, Isla D, Massuti B, Montes A, Sanchez JM, Provencio M, Vinolas N, Paz-Ares L, Lopez-Vivanco G, Munoz MA, Felip E, Alberola V, Camps C, Domine M, Sanchez JJ, Sanchez-Ronco M, Danenberg K, Taron M, Gandara D, Rosell R. Customizing cisplatin based on quantitative excision repair cross-complementing 1 mRNA expression: a phase III trial in non-small-cell lung cancer. J Clin Oncol. 2007;25:2747–54.
83. Bepler G, Kusmartseva I, Sharma S, Gautam A, Cantor A, Sharma A, Simon G. RRM1 modulated in vitro and in vivo efficacy of gemcitabine and platinum in non-small-cell lung cancer. J Clin Oncol. 2006;24:4731–7.
84. Simon GR, Williams CC, Chiappori AA, Haura EB, Tanvetyanon T, Antonia SJ, Bepler G. Molecular analysis-directed individualized therapy (MADeIT) in advanced non-small cell lung cancer (NSCLC). J Clin Oncol. 2007;25:18S. suppl; abstr 7502.

85. Simon GR, Kim J, Schell M, Bepler G. Personalized chemotherapy may favorably alter intrinsic disease biology to produce a higher proportion of long term survivors in patients with advanced NSCLC. J Thorac Oncol 2009; 4 (suppl; abstract D7.6).
86. Vogelzang NJ, Rusthoven JJ, Symanowski J, Denham C, Kaukel E, Ruffie P, Gatzemeier U, Boyer M, Emri S, Manegold C, Niyikiza C, Paoletti P. Phase III study of pemetrexed in combination with cisplatin versus cisplatin alone in patients with malignant pleural mesothelioma. J Clin Oncol. 2003;21:2636–44.
87. Hanna N, Shepherd FA, Fossella FV, Pereira JR, De Marinis F, von Pawel J, Gatzemeier U, Tsao TC, Pless M, Muller T, Lim HL, Desch C, Szondy K, Gervais R, Shaharyar, Manegold C, Paul S, Paoletti P, Einhorn L, Bunn PA Jr. Randomized phase III trial of pemetrexed versus docetaxel in patients with non-small-cell lung cancer previously treated with chemotherapy. J Clin Oncol 2004;22:1589–97
88. Scagliotti GV, Parikh P, von Pawel J, Biesma B, Vansteenkiste J, Manegold C, Serwatowski P, Gatzemeier U, Digumarti R, Zukin M, Lee JS, Mellemgaard A, Park K, Patil S, Rolski J, Goksel T, de Marinis F, Simms L, Sugarman KP, Gandara D. Phase III study comparing cisplatin plus gemcitabine with cisplatin plus pemetrexed in chemotherapy-naïve patients with advanced-stage non-small-cell lung cancer. J Clin Oncol. 2008;26:3543–51.
89. Syrigos KN, Vansteenkiste J, Parikh P, von Pawel J, Manegold C, Martins RG, Simms L, Sugarman KP, Visseren-Grul C, Scagliotti GV. Prognostic and predictive factors in a randomized phase III trial comparing cisplatin-pemetrexed versus cisplatin-gemcitabine in advanced non-small-cell lung cancer. Ann Oncol. 2010;21:556–61.
90. Ciuleanu T, Brodowicz T, Zielinski C, Kim JH, Krzakowski M, Laack E, Wu YL, Bover I, Begbie S, Tzekova V, Cucevic B, Pereira JR, Yang SH, Madhavan J, Sugarman KP, Peterson P, John WJ, Krejcy K, Belani CP. Maintenance pemetrexed plus best supportive care versus placebo plus best supportive care for non-small-cell lung cancer: a randomised, double-blind, phase 3 study. Lancet. 2009;374:1432–40.
91. Giovannetti E, Mey V, Nannizzi S, Pasqualetti G, Marini L, Del Tacca M, Danesi R. Cellular and pharmacogenetics foundation of synergistic interaction of pemetrexed and gemcitabine in human non-small-cell lung cancer cells. Mol Pharmacol. 2005;68:110–8.
92. Ceppi P, Volante M, Saviozzi S, Rapa I, Novello S, Cambieri A, Iacono ML, Cappia S, Papotti M, Scagliotti GV. Squamous cell carcinoma of the lung compared with other histologies shows higher messenger RNA and protein levels for thymidylate synthase. Cancer. 2006;107: 1589–96.
93. Scagliotti G, Kaiser C, Biesma B, Manegold C, Gatzemeier U, Serwatowski P, Syrigos K, Balint B, Smit H, Vansteenkiste J. Correlations of biomarker expression and clinical outcome in a large phase III trial of pemetrexed plus cisplatin or gemcitabine plus cisplatin in chemonaive patients with locally advanced or metastatic non-small-cell lung cancer (NSCLC): C6-01. J Thorac Oncol. 2007;2:S375.
94. Schiller JH, Akerley WL, Brugger W, Ferrari D, Garmey EG, Gerber DE, Orlov SV, Ramlau R, von Pawel J, Sequist LV. Results from ARQ 197-209: a global randomized placebo-controlled phase II clinical trial of erlotinib plus ARQ 197 versus erlotinib plus placebo in previously treated EGFR inhibitor-naive patients with locally advanced or metastatic non-small cell lung cancer (NSCLC). J Clin Oncol. 2010;28:18S. suppl; abstr LBA7502.
95. Punnoose EA, Atwal SK, Spoerke JM, Savage H, Pandita A, Yeh RF, Pirzkall A, Fine BM, Amler LC, Chen DS, Lackner MR. Molecular biomarker analysis using circulating tumor cells. PLoS One. 2010;5:e12517.

Chapter 4
Prostate Cancer: Predictive Markers in Clinical Development

Courtney K. Phillips and Daniel P. Petrylak

Introduction

Prostate cancer is the most common cancer in men and is the second most common cause of male cancer-related deaths. When prostate specific antigen (PSA) was described and came into general use for screening, it was seen as a huge achievement in cancer detection. But since the early 1980s when this marker came into widespread use, several of its shortcomings have become apparent. Despite the fact that PSA is produced almost entirely in the prostate, elevation of this marker can occur in both benign and malignant conditions. Additionally, even though higher PSA values correlate with more aggressive and advanced disease, lower values fail to differentiate clinically indolent disease from clinically significant disease. In short, PSA screening has been a double edged sword: it has increased the numbers of patients diagnosed with prostate cancer, but has led to the overtreatment of patients. Additionally, whether its use has affected cancer-related mortality is a subject of heated debate. Among governing bodies such as the American Cancer Society, the American Urologic Association, and the United States Preventive Services Task Force, there has never been a consensus whether PSA screening should be performed regularly. Two large, multi-center, randomized studies have recently looked at the impact of PSA screening on survival [1, 2]. The results of both studies showed similar death rates in screening and control groups and underscored the large number of patients who need to be screened before a life is saved. This has led the United States Preventative Task Force recommending against routine PSA screening for men

---

C.K. Phillips, M.D.
Department of Urology, Mount Sinai School of Medicine, 5 East 98th Street, Box 1272, New York, NY 10029, USA

D.P. Petrylak, M.D. (✉)
Signal Transduction Program, 333 Cedar Street, New Haven, CT 20832, USA
e-mail: daniel.petrylak@yale.edu

H.-J. Lenz (ed.), *Biomarkers in Oncology: Prediction and Prognosis*,
DOI 10.1007/978-1-4419-9755-5_4,

With all of the shortcomings of PSA and its adjuncts such as PSA velocity, density, and free PSA, the need for additional markers to diagnose prostate cancer and predict its clinical course is evident. Much work has been done in this area. This chapter focuses on many of the newest serum and urinary markers of prostate cancer. While biomarkers used to predict prognosis are covered in another chapter, in many cases markers are being used for both purposes.

Sarcosine and the TMPRSS2:ERG Translocation

High-throughput technology has allowed scientists to quickly evaluate the entire genetic, gene transcript, and protein milieus of different cells. And while gene array technology has produced a plethora of information, use of this technology often leads to prolific amounts of dead-end data. One of the newer approaches being utilized to identify interesting molecular targets is metabolomics. Metabolomics allows scientists to survey the cells' metabolites, which are, ultimately, the end-products of genes and their transcripts [3]. Additionally, these metabolites give a more complete picture of the active physiology and biochemistry of the cell.

Metabolome profiling of serum and urine in patients with and without prostate cancer has thus far been low yield [4]. In serum, only 20 of 478 metabolites were differentially expressed, with 99% of the 20 being deemed false discoveries. Similarly in urine, 36 of 583 metabolites were either up or down-regulated in cancer patients; but again, the false discovery rate was high: 67%. Tissue metabolomes produced the most interesting results on profiling. Sixteen adjacent benign tissues, 12 localized cancers, and 14 metastatic lesions were profiled. A total of 626 metabolites were identified and 60 of these were present in cancer and metastatic lesions but not in benign tissue. Not unexpectedly metastatic lesions exhibited more metabolic alterations than localized lesions. After analysis, six metabolites were found to be increasingly produced with disease progression: sarcosine, uracil, kynurenine, glycerol-3-phosphate, leucine, and proline. When the metabolic pathways of these substances were analyzed, the overall physiologic picture produced was one of increased nitrogen breakdown and amino acid metabolism. In particular, metastatic lesions demonstrated upregulation of metabolites involved with methyltransferase activity.

Because of these findings, sarcosine became the primary focus for follow-up studies. Sarcosine is produced when glycine *N*-methyl transferase (GNMT) methylates glycine and is converted back to glycine by sarcosine dehydrogenase (SARDH). Sarcosine can also be produced when dimethylglycine dehydrogenase (DMGDH) acts on dimethylglycine. Researchers had already demonstrated that blocking sarcosine production via knockdown of GNMT slowed prostate cancer progression. Similarly, increasing sarcosine, either by addition of exogenous sarcosine or knockdown of SARDH, transformed benign prostate epithelial cells into invasive phenotypes.

Sarcosine was detected in 79% of metastatic lesions and 42% of localized lesions. It was not detected in benign tissue nor was it measurable in the benign tissue next to metastatic lesions. Sarcosine was measurable in urine supernatants and sediments and was significantly higher in both in prostate cancer patients. Despite this, sarcosine's ability to predict prostate cancer was modest, with its area under the ROC (AUC) being 0.71 in urine sediment and 0.67 in urine supernatant. For patients with PSA values of 2–10 ng/ml, sarcosine did perform better than PSA (AUC = 0.69 vs. 0.53, respectively).

In cell culture, sarcosine concentrations were significantly higher in cancer cell lines than in benign cell lines ($p = 0.0218$). Additionally when sarcosine was added to noninvasive benign epithelial cells, it imparted an invasive phenotype and increased cell motility. There were no changes in cell cycle progression or proliferation. When RNA interference was used to knock down the enzymes involved in sarcosine production, GNMT and DMGDH, sarcosine levels and cell invasiveness declined. In contrast, when the enzyme responsible for sarcosine catabolism, SARDH, was knocked down, sarcosine concentration increased three times and cell invasion increased over 3.5-fold.

Genetic translocations, such as the Philadelphia chromosome, have been identified in patients with chronic myelogenous leukemia. The fusion protein that resulted from this translocation has oncogenic potential, and is a therapeutic target. Similarly, gene translocation has also been identified in prostate cancer. [5] This translocation fuses a member of the E26 transformation specific (ETS) family of transcription factors, usually ERG, or less commonly ETV1, to the promoter region of TMPRSS2. ERG and ETV1 have already been implicated in Ewing's sarcoma and myeloid leukemias, and a recent study demonstrated that up to 72% of prostate cancers overexpress ERG [6]. TMPRSS2, which is expressed in both normal and neoplastic prostate tissue, is androgen sensitive. This fusion translocation, which is found in 40% of primary prostate tumors, initiates androgen induced production of the ETS transcription factor involved in the translocation. This change was theorized by the original researchers to be sufficient enough to initiate malignant transformation, but a follow-up study in a murine model with prostate specific overexpression of ERG did not produce neoplasia [7]. A malignant phenotype was, however, produced when ERG was overexpressed in the presence of haploinsufficiency of PTEN [8, 9].

Interestingly, there is an intimate link between the ETS family of transcription factors and sarcosine metabolism. When VCaP cells, which express ERG, and LNCaP cells, which are ETV1 positive, were each incubated with androgen for 48 h, GNMT expression was up-regulated while SARDH expression was down-regulated. Chromatin immunoprecipitation sequencing of the VCaP cells revealed that ERG and androgen receptor were bound to the promoter of GNMT, while ERG alone was bound to the SARDH promoter. In LNCaP cells, AR was bound to the promoter of both GNMT and SARDH.

Studies characterizing sarcosine's role in prostate cancer progression and as a biomarker are in their infancy. Sarcosine appears to play a critical role in prostate cancer progression and is found in the urine, however, the heterogeneity of mechanisms which initiate malignant transformation and cause disease progression may limit its role as a diagnostic marker. But, much like HER2 in breast cancer, sarcosine may eventually play a role in select subsets of patients.

Prostate Specific Membrane Antigen

Prostate specific membrane antigen (PSMA) is a membrane bound glycoprotein which was initially discovered in 1987 during antibody characterization of LNCaP cell membranes [10]. It is found in both benign and hyperplastic prostate tissue as well as HGPIN and malignant prostate epithelial cells, though its expression is higher in malignant cells. It is also found in small quantities in other extraprostatic tissues and other types of tumors [11, 12]. PSMA's early clinical use was plagued by the fact that standard ELISA and Western Blot analysis of this marker was difficult to reliably reproduce. As such, many of the initial reports examining PSMA's function as a prognostic marker yielded conflicting results [13–16].

In the late 1990s, an antibody, 7E11C5.3, which detects the intracellular portion of PSMA was tagged with Indium [17]. This radiolabeled antibody became known as Prostascint©. Because this antibody binds to the intracellular portion of PSMA, it cannot be used as a serum or urine biomarker. When first introduced, Prostascint's utility was limited by both clinician experience and the single photon emission computed tomography being used. But with the advent of dual head gamma cameras, bowel preps, longer delays between injection and imaging, and red blood cell pooling and fusion, Prostascint scanning has found a small but growing niche in detecting soft tissue metastasis in prostate cancer patients. But because of its limitations, PSMA has not found a role as a widely used biomarker.

Human Kallikrein Related Peptidase 2

Like PSA, human kallikrein-related peptidase 2 (KLK2), also known as human glandular kallikrein 2, is a secreted serine protease [18]. KLK2 is from the same family of genes as PSA and is largely expressed in the prostate [19]. But unlike PSA, KLK2 is often expressed at such low levels in healthy men that it is undetectable [20]. In men with cancer, KLK2 is expressed at significantly higher levels than in those with BPH. Several studies demonstrated that, when added to PSA or fPSA, KLK2 can increase the sensitivity and specificity of prostate cancer detection [21–23]. In 740 men undergoing biopsy during the first round of the European Randomized Study for the Screening of Prostate Cancer, multiple combinations of age, PSA, digital rectal exam, and KLK2 levels were used to predict the risk of prostate cancer on biopsy. A total of 192 men were diagnosed with prostate cancer in this round of biopsies. Patients with cancer had significantly higher levels of tPSA and KLK2 than those without cancer; however there was no significant difference in free or intact PSA between those two groups. Two multivariate analyses were performed. One compared age and total PSA (AUC 0.68) to age, tPSA, fPSA, intact PSA, and KLK2 (AUC 0.83, $p<0.0005$). The second analysis added DRE to both arms. The area under the ROC curves for age, tPSA and DRE was 0.72 vs. 0.84 when DRE was added to the full panel of serine proteases ($p<0.0005$).

Despite its promise, the addition of KLK2 did not improve risk assessment. In one study 461 men underwent radical prostatectomy for localized prostate cancer. Preoperative KLK2 did not improve the predictive accuracy of biochemical recurrence (BCR) over standard Kattan nomogram parameters [24]. Three years later the same group published follow-up data [25]. They restructured their study as a case–control study and identified 146 patients who experienced BCR out of 1,356 in the total cohort. Biochemical recurrence was defined as having a tPSA$\geq$0.40. They compared these 146 patients to 436 control patients who were matched by age and year of surgery. The median follow-up for patients who did not experience BCR was 3.2 years. Clinical stage and Gleason sums were significantly worse in the group experiencing BCR. Additionally, median levels of all markers (tPSA, fPSA and KLK2) were significantly higher in those patients who experienced a BCR than in those who did not. In a univariate analysis, all variables were significantly associated with BCR. However in a multivariate analysis, stage, grade and tPSA had an impressive AUC of 0.786. Addition of both fPSA and KLK2 produced an insignificant increase in AUC to 0.798 ($p=0.053$), the majority of this effect contributed by fPSA and not KLK2. A similar trend was seen in patients with tPSA$\leq$10 ng/ml. A second base analysis model was created using pathologic parameters, including surgical Gleason score as well as the presence of extracapsular extension, seminal vesicle invasion, lymph node involvement, and surgical margin status. Again, when fPSA and KLK2 were added to this baseline prediction model, there was no significant addition to predictive accuracy.

KLK2 may be a useful adjunct to PSA in the diagnosis of prostate cancer, but, like other markers, KLK2 does not appear to provide valuable prognostic information or differentiate between clinically significant and insignificant disease. A large, randomized study is needed to compare the utility of KLK2 with other novel markers in this setting.

Prostate Cancer Antigen 3 (PCA3)

Prostate Cancer Antigen 3 (PCA3), also known as Differential Display 3 (DD3), is a noncoding segment of RNA which is expressed almost entirely in the prostate and is upregulated in prostate cancer and its metastatic lesions [18]. In radical prostatectomy specimens, RT-PCR of normal, BPH and cancer specimens revealed that human prostate cancer cells had a median of 66 times, and up to a 1,487 times, the amount of PCA3 mRNA copies of normal prostate cells from the same patient. Normal and BPH prostate samples had similar copy numbers of PCA3 [26]. A subsequent pilot study was then performed on patients' urine sediment. A total of 108 consecutive patients who were referred for prostate biopsy due to a serum PSA of >3 ng/ml were recruited into the study. Each patient underwent a prostatic massage and voided urine samples were tested for both PCA3 and PSA transcripts in the urine sediment. Patients were then biopsied, and a total of 24 were found to have cancer, while the remaining 84 patients had negative biopsy results. The resulting area under the ROC curve calculated for PCA3 transcripts in urine sediment was 0.72, with a specificity of 83% and sensitivity of 67%. In a larger multicenter trial these results were validated. A similar methodology was employed in 583 men with a PSA of 3–15. Of the usable samples (92%), the area under the ROC curve for PCA3 was 0.66 while that of PSA was only 0.57 [27].

Another prospective, multicenter study was done in 570 men undergoing prostate biopsy for serum PSA ≥ 2.5 ng/ml, family history of prostate cancer, abnormal digital rectal exam or another risk factor. This study used a PCA3 score in lieu of absolute mRNA copy numbers [28]. This PCA3 score was the number of PCA3 mRNA copies normalized to PSA mRNA copies in the same sample [(PCA3 mRNA/PSA mRNA) × 1,000]. Of the 570 men, 206 (or 36%) were found to have prostate cancer. There was a direct correlation with PCA3 score and positive biopsy. In this study, 277 subjects were undergoing an initial biopsy while another 280 were undergoing a repeat biopsy after a prior negative biopsy. For first-time biopsy patients, the AUC was 0.703 while the AUC for men undergoing repeat biopsy was 0.684. Patients were then stratified according to pathology. Men with no disease or BPH had a median score of 15, while patients with inflammation had a median score of 13. Patients with PIN and/or atypical small acinar proliferation (ASAP) had median scores of 23–27, while the median score for men with cancer was 38. An analysis of variance revealed that men diagnosed with cancer had significantly higher PCA3 scores than men with either no pathology or PIN/ASAP ($p < 0.0001$ in both cases). These results were consistent among men undergoing first or repeat biopsy. There was, however, no significant difference in PCA3 score between men with Gleason sum 6 or Gleason sum ≥7 cancers (median PCA3 score 38 and 41, respectively).

Of the 570 men in this study, prostate volume data was available for 552 patients. Not surprisingly, PSA was directly related to volume in both men with and without cancer ($p < 0.0001$). PCA3 score did not, however, correlate with prostate volume ($p = 0.54$). When stratified by serum PSA (<4 ng/ml, 4–10 ng/ml and >10 ng/ml), PCA3 scores had a 50–61% sensitivity and a 71–80% specificity (overall sensitivity 54% and specificity 74%). Within each PSA group, the 95% confidence intervals were similar, indicating similar accuracy of PCA3 score at all serum PSA levels. In a logistic regression model, the combination of prostate volume, digital rectal exam, log of serum PSA, and log of PCA3 score led to the highest AUC (0.752). The AUC for PCA3 score was similar to the AUC for prostate volume, DRE and log of serum PSA, which was 0.672. The AUC for PSA alone was only 0.547 in this model.

Even though PCA3 copy numbers or scores did not appear to correlate with prognosis in biopsy studies, a prostatectomy study showed otherwise. Post-DRE urine samples were collected from 72 men prior to undergoing radical prostatectomy for confirmed prostate cancer [29]. PCA3 scores were calculated as previously described and tumors were Gleason graded, staged and stratified by size (<0.5, 0.5–2, >2.0 cm). PCA3 scores were then correlated with pathologic outcomes. Of the 72 men in the study, 70.9% had pT2 disease while 20.8% had pT3a disease. The remainder (8.3%) had pT3b disease. The majority (58.3%) of lesions were Gleason 3+3=6/10 prostate cancer while 27.8% were Gleason 3+4 and only 4.1% were Gleason 4+3. The remaining 9.7% were either Gleason 8 or 9 out of 10. In a univariate analysis, PCA3 score was significantly associated with tumor volume. Additionally, patients with extracapsular extension had significantly higher PCA3 scores than those who did not (48.8 vs. 18.7, $p=0.02$). A multivariate logistic analysis was constructed, and Gleason sum (≤6 or >6), PCA3 score and PSA were all predictive of extracapsular extension (AUC=0.90). The AUC of PCA3 alone was 0.732.

These findings were not duplicated, however, in a similar study published that same year. This study included 62 men about to undergo radical prostatectomy, and it did not find any significant correlation between PCA3 score and Gleason score, tumor volume, pathologic stage or clinical "significance" (defined by stage, grade and volume) [30].

In 2009, a small study of 96 men referred for prostate biopsy was reported [31]. Of these patients, 26 were diagnosed with BPH on biopsy while 70 were found to have cancer. Levels of PCA3 and PSA were measured in post-rectal exam urinary sediment prior to biopsy. In this study, cancer patients had normalized PCA3 scores which were 37 times that of BPH patients ($p<0.0001$). PSA was significantly up-regulated in cancer patients as well, though only by a factor of 7 ($p<0.0001$). Not surprisingly, when the two parameters were combined in a logistic regression model, the two markers together had a diagnostic sensitivity of 80.2% and specificity of 100%.

Though PCA3 studies in patients receiving androgen deprivation therapy (ADT) or in those with hormone refractory disease have not yet been done, in vitro studies suggest that PCA3 is androgen inducible. Real-time PCR of both androgen dependent LnCaP cells and androgen independent PC3 cells' expression of PCA3 and PSA revealed that PC3 cells expressed neither marker, while LnCaP cells expressed both. When androgen was added to culture medium, PSA mRNA transcripts increased 36–58 times in a dose dependent manner. PCA3 transcripts were also upregulated up to 56 times by androgen.

PCA3 is a relatively sensitive and specific marker, which has the added benefit of not being affected by prostate volume or inflammation. Further studies have demonstrated that it may be an androgen inducible gene product. While early studies indicate that it may be useful in risk stratification, these results have not been consistent. A larger, randomized study is needed to determine whether PCA3 can be used to differentiate indolent disease from aggressive disease and predict progression and recurrence in both hormone sensitive and hormone refractory disease.

α Methylacyl CoA Racemase

Originally called P504S, α-methylacyl-coenzyme A (AMACR) is a mitochondrial and peroxisomal enzyme that is involved in the metabolism of branched chain fatty acids and bile acids. Like many other potential biomarkers, AMACR was first identified as a potential biomarker via high-throughput analysis. In an early study, increased expression of AMACR in prostate cancer specimens was found in three out of four DNA microarrays [32]. This finding was confirmed with RT-PCR as well as immunohistochemistry. Immunohistochemistry studies revealed that while 108 benign prostate cancer specimens had a mean staining intensity (SI) of only 1.31, PIN's SI was 2.67, and localized cancer and metastatic cancer had mean SI's of 3.2 and 2.5, respectively ($p<0.001$). In an immunohistochemistry survey of 263 cancer specimens, including 38 prostate cancers, Nassar and colleagues found that 34 out of 38 (89.5%) stained positively for AMACR [33].

One of the unfortunate aspects of AMACR is that assays have not detected it appreciable amounts of this enzyme in serum [34]. To circumvent this obstacle, Sreekumar and colleagues analyzed sera for a humoral response to AMACR and PSA. Sera from 46 men with biopsy proven prostate cancer and 28 healthy controls were analyzed with protein microarrays and immunoblots. After incubation with patient sera, it was found that all control patients' sera and 42 of the cancer patients' sera tested positive for PSA autoantibodies and there were no statistically significant differences in immunoreactivity between control and cancer patients. For AMACR, however, patients with cancer had significantly higher immunoreactivity than control patients (mean 2602.1 relative units versus 1116.3 relative units, respectively, $p<0.009$). These results were validated in a larger study set using both high-throughput immunoblot analysis and ELISA. When results were correlated with PSA, Gleason score, pathologic stage and risk of recurrence, no significant relationships between AMACR immunoreactivity and these parameters were found. When ROC curves were constructed for AMACR and PSA, AMACR was found to have 71.8% specificity at a 61.6% sensitivity (AUC 0.663, $p<0.001$). AMACR could also discriminate cancer from benign pathology in patients with intermediate PSA's of 4–10 ng/ml ($p<0.001$), while PSA could not ($p=0.888$). For this subset, the AUC for a humoral response to AMACR was 0.789, while PSA's was 0.492.

In 2006, Zehentner and coworkers used a different method to approach measuring AMACR in human blood [35]. Instead of measuring whole blood or an immune response, they used cell surface antibodies to isolate circulating tumor cells and then measured AMACR transcripts in this fraction with RT-PCR. They collected blood from 76 healthy male controls as well as 69 patients with lung cancer, 23 with breast cancer, and 24 with ovarian cancer. Another group of 28 men had benign prostatic or genitourinary diseases including two with prostatitis, five with urethritis and nine with BPH. Among the 163 prostate cancer patients, 88 had localized disease and 58 had metastatic disease and were receiving chemotherapy. A third group of 17 patients was categorized as "in remission" and had undergone either prostatectomy or had a response to chemotherapy.

In this study, a distribution of AMACR copies in the blood of healthy controls was analyzed and a cutoff value of 73.6 copies, which was 3 standard deviations above the mean, was used for the remainder of the study. Based on in vitro cell culture studies, this copy number was theorized to be equivalent to 1 tumor cell per 10 cc of blood. None of the patients with breast, ovarian or lung cancer had were positive for AMACR and only 2 of the 76 normal healthy controls (2.6%) tested positive. In men with benign prostatic diseases, 37% had positive values. 44.5 and 48.2% of patients with organ confined and metastatic prostate cancer, respectively, tested positive. And, though this study was not correlated with long-term outcomes, only one of 17 patients (5.9%) who were clinically considered to be in remission had a positive AMACR level. Unfortunately, this small study assumed a normal distribution and used the chi-squared test which makes the significance of their statistical results unclear, but their novel technique to detect AMACR in peripheral blood was interesting.

Other groups developed different methods to circumvent the lack of AMACR in human serum. One study examined the post prostate biopsy voided urines of 26 men [36]. AMACR was detected with Western blot analysis. In this small pilot study, 18 out of the 26 men had AMACR in their urine. All 12 of the patients diagnosed with prostate cancer tested positive for AMACR, while 5 of 12 patients without cancer did as well. One of the two patients with atypia also tested positive, yielding an overall sensitivity of 100% and specificity of 58%.

Zielie and colleagues assessed the presence of AMACR in post-prostatic massage urinary prostatic secretions [37]. This small study included a total of 21 patients: 10 had biopsy proven cancer, 2 had high-grade PIN, and 9 were benign. Total RNA was extracted from urine sediment and quantitative RT-PCR was used to detect both PSA and AMACR. A relative value score (RVS) for AMACR was created by normalizing AMACR transcripts to PSA transcripts. In this study, the absolute value of PSA and AMACR transcripts did not correlate with the presence of cancer. However when the RVS for AMACR was calculated, the mean RVS for cancer patients was much higher than the RVS for control patients (189.6 ± 253.2 vs. 15.2 ± 8.5). When a cutoff point of 32, which is 2 standard deviations above the mean control RVS was used, all nine healthy controls fell below the cutoff point. Of the ten cancer patients, seven had prostatic secretion AMACR RVS above the cutoff. Two of the patients with cancer who had AMACR RVS below 32 had, at time of prostatectomy, what the authors considered clinically insignificant disease: one focus of Gleason 6 disease involving less than 5% of the entire prostate. Both HGPIN patients were above the cutoff.

With several novel markers in development, utilization of combinations of these markers, preferably from the same body fluid, may potentially provide improved diagnostic or prognostic utility over one marker alone. In 2009, Ouyang and coworkers measured AMACR and PCA3 (see prior section) in urine sediment and compared these tests' efficacy to that of serum PSA [38]. The study cohort included 92 patients: 43 patients with prostate cancer and 49 patients without prostate cancer. Quantitative real time PCR was used to calculate transcript levels of AMACR and

PCA3 in the sediment of urine collected after digital rectal exam. Transcript levels were normalized to PSA transcript levels, resulting in AMACR and PCA3 scores.

In a univariate analysis, both AMACR and PCA3 were able to discern patients with prostate cancer, from those without prostate cancer ($p=0.006$ and 0.014, respectively), while serum PSA could not ($p=0.306$). Based upon an ROC curve for AMACR and PCA3, cutoff points of 10.7 for AMACR and 19.9 for PCA3 were established. These cutoff points resulted in a sensitivity and specificity of 70 and 71% for AMACR and 72 and 59% for PCA3. The AUC for AMACR was 0.67 ($p<0.01$) and 0.65 for PCA3 ($p<0.01$), while the AUC for PSA was only 0.59 ($p>0.05$). When elevation of at least one of the two (AMACR or PCA3) markers was the criteria for a positive test, the sensitivity and specificity of the combination was 81 and 84%.

Serum testing of AMACR is technically difficult and urine analysis can be performed in a number of different ways. Despite this, these early tests indicate that AMACR may have a role in diagnosis and prognosis. Assay standardization, inter-operator variability studies and further randomized studies are going to be needed before this marker can be used in widespread practice.

Urokinase Plasminogen Activator and Receptor

Urokinase Plasminogen Activator Receptor (uPAR) is a membrane receptor that is critical in degrading the extracellular matrix allowing cancer to spread [39]. Increasing levels of serum uPAR have been related to poor prognosis in breast colon and non-small-cell lung cancer [40, 41], and overexpression of uPAR has been demonstrated in prostate cancer as well [42, 43]. Early studies failed to show any significant difference between levels of soluble uPAR in benign and cancerous prostate conditions [44], but as improved assays for detecting the various isotypes of uPAR were developed [45], significant differences were detected. In one study, uPAR fragments were measured in 355 patients referred for prostate biopsy [46]. In univariate and multivariate analyses, uPAR levels were a significant predictor of prostate cancer diagnosis.

In another study by Milanese and coworkers, serum was taken from 79 consecutive patients prior to prostate biopsy and tested for full length and cleaved forms of uPAR with ELISA [47]. Out of 79 patients, 30 (38%) were diagnosed with prostate cancer. Patients with prostate cancer were found to have significantly higher levels of uPAR than those without cancer (median 2.6 ng/ml vs. 1.5 ng/ml, respectively, $p<0.0001$). Almost half (46.9%) of patients with negative biopsies had some evidence of prostatitis on biopsy. Patients with prostatitis and no evidence of cancer had significantly higher PSA's than patients without cancer and prostatitis; prostatitis did not, however, increase uPAR levels. On a multivariate analysis, uPAR was not an independent predictor of prostate cancer ($p=0.163$), but did have a 90%

sensitivity and 63% specificity when a 1.54 ng/ml cutoff was used. All 30 patients with prostate cancer underwent radical prostatectomy. In a multivariate analysis, uPAR levels were closely correlated to the presence of extra-prostatic extension, seminal vesicle invasion and perineural invasion ($p=0.027$, 0.048 and 0.040, respectively).

uPAR appears to be an interesting marker for prostate cancer diagnosis and prognosis. While Milanese's study did not demonstrate that uPAR was a significant predictor of prostate cancer, it did demonstrate that uPAR was helpful in predicting the presence of poor pathologic characteristics at prostatectomy. Additionally uPAR was not elevated in prostatitis, a condition that frequently produces falsely elevated PSA levels. Additional studies are warranted to further characterize this marker.

EGF Receptor

Endothelial growth factor receptor (EGF-r) is a 170 kDa transmembrane glycoprotein which is part of the erbB protooncogene family [47]. It plays a critical role in several cellular pathways, including those which regulate angiogenesis, motility, and apoptosis [48]. EGF-r is overexpressed in many malignancies, including prostate cancer, and appears to be closely linked to uPAR (see prior section). Multiple in vitro and in vivo models have shown that EGF-r can regulate prostate cancer progression if uPAR is expressed [49–51]. In prostate cancer cells, EGF-r inhibitors can inhibit cell growth and decrease metastatic potential [49, 50, 52].

Because of this close relationship, Milanese and coworkers also characterized serum EGF-r levels in their uPAR study [47]. In the 79 consecutive patients who had undergone prostate biopsy, patients with biopsy proven prostate cancer had significantly higher serum levels of EGF-r ($p \leq 0.0001$) and there was a significant correlation between uPAR and EGF-r levels (ρ 0.628, $p \leq 0.0001$). Neither of these markers correlated with PSA. Additionally, patients without cancer but with biopsy proven prostatitis did not have elevated EGF-r levels. On a multivariate analysis, EGF-r was the only significant independent predictor of prostate cancer, conferring a 1.9-fold increase in relative risk when elevated (95% CI 1.235–2.991). When a cutoff of 67.84 ng/ml was used, EGF-r's sensitivity and specificity for diagnosing prostate cancer were 93.3% and 98%, respectively.

Thirty of the original 79 patients biopsied had prostate cancer and all underwent radical prostatectomy. Like uPAR, EGF-r correlated with pathologic stage ($p \leq 0.0001$) while PSA did not. EGF-r levels were also significantly higher in patients with extraprostatic extension ($p=0.001$), seminal vesicle invasion ($p \leq 0.0001$), Gleason>6 ($p=0.013$), more positive cores at time of biopsy ($p \leq 0.0001$), and lymphovascular invasion ($p=0.005$).

EGF-r may be a promising marker for both prostate cancer diagnosis and prognosis however the literature on this biomarker is very limited. Larger, randomized studies are necessary to determine if this marker has true clinical utility, if it is useful in all ethnic groups, and if it can be used in the post-treatment setting to monitor for recurrence.

Huntingtin Interacting Protein-1

Identified in 1997, Huntingtin Interacting Protein-1 (HIP-1) was initially characterized during studies with the Huntingtin protein, which, when mutated, produces Huntington's disease [53]. HIP-1 is a 116 kDa protein which plays a role in clathrin mediated endocytosis and trafficking [54]. Subsequent evidence demonstrated that a chromosomal translocation producing a fusion of HIP-1 and platelet-derived growth factor β receptor was a common mutation in chronic myelomonocytic leukemia [55]. In a subsequent Western Blot survey of 60 different cancer cell lines, HIP-1 was found to be overexpressed in the majority of solid tumors. Immunohistochemistry in malignant and nonmalignant human tissue demonstrated that HIP-1 was expressed in normal small vessel endothelium, many secretory epithelia, and distal renal tubular epithelium. In tumor microarrays, there was significant staining in central nervous system, breast, lung, colon, ovarian, melanoma and prostate cancers. When comparing normal and benign tissues from these organs, the majority of benign tissues stained HIP-1 positive while their malignant counterparts did not; the notable exceptions to this being prostate and colon cancer. Both normal colonic and prostatic epithelium did not stain for HIP-1. In fact, when benign tissue, HGPIN, and prostate cancer tissue were surveyed, 95% of all benign epithelium did not stain for HIP-1, and the remaining 5% only exhibited weak staining. Only 25% of HGPIN samples demonstrated moderate or strong staining, while 51% of clinically localized prostate cancer samples stained positive. Among samples from patients with hormone refractory prostate cancer, there was a 70% staining rate.

The prior arrays were constructed from multiple samples from the same patients. A second survey in multiple patients demonstrated that primary tumors from patients with metastatic prostate cancer stained positive for HIP-1 100% of the time, while 88% of localized prostate cancer tumor samples stained positively. Only 50% of HGPIN samples stained HIP-1 positive. These results were then correlated with progression, which was defined as PSA > 0.2 ng/ml after radical prostatectomy. None of the patients with negative HIP-1 staining developed a PSA recurrence, whereas 28% of the HIP-1 positive patients did ($p = 0.05$). In a multivariate Cox regression analysis which also included PSA, Gleason score and pathologic stage, HIP-1 expression was an independent predictor of PSA recurrence. Additionally, even though pretreatment PSA (<4.0 ng/ml) was a significant predictor of PSA recurrence, pretreatment PSA did not correlate with HIP-1 expression.

Three years later, the same group described a serum antibody test to HIP-1 [56]. They first demonstrated the importance of HIP-1 to tumorigenesis in the TRAMP (transgenic adenocarcinomas of the mouse prostate) model. HIP-1 knockout TRAMP mice developed fewer prostate tumors than their wild-type TRAMP counterparts. They then examined the sera of TRAMP mice. Because HIP-1 is a cytoplasmic protein, the antigen itself was not detected in serum. They then created recombinant HIP-1 to test for serum antibodies to HIP-1 and found that HIP-$1^{+/+}$ TRAMP mice had anti-HIP-1 antibodies while TRAMP/HIP-$1^{-/-}$ mice did not. In chronologic studies, it was found that HIP-1 antibodies developed at 4 months of age, prior to tumor development which usually occurred at 6.5 months of age. None of the control (normal) mice developed HIP-1 antibodies.

When the sera of 97 prostate cancer patients and 211 age matched controls were assayed by Western blot, 46% of prostate cancer patients and 27% of controls tested positive for HIP-1 autoantibodies. Similar results were attained when ELISA was used to assay for antibodies. When the two tests were combined, only 24% of prostate cancer patients' sera and 12% of controls were positive for HIP-1 antibodies on both assays, resulting in a low sensitivity, but a specificity of 88%. There was no correlation between a positive test result and poorer clinical parameters. When compared to the anti-α-methylacyl CoA racemase (AMACR) serum assay, the HIP-1 assay had similar sensitivity and specificity for prostate cancer. When AMACR and HIP-1 were used in combination with PSA, specificity increased to 97%.

As a molecular and pathologic marker, HIP-1 is interesting because its expression correlates with both the presence and severity of prostate cancer. Its prognostic ability did not appear to persist in serum assays, and, despite its high specificity, its sensitivity was very low. Perhaps with improved assays or larger studies, HIP-1 will live up to its original promise, but currently it suffers from many of the limitations of other serum biomarkers.

Chromogranin A and Neuron-Specific Enolase

Because prostatic adenocarcinoma is a result of the malignant transformation of prostatic epithelial cells, the vast majority of research has focused on these cells. Recently, however, the role of the cell's milieu, or microenvironment, has been cited as an increasingly important factor in tumorigenesis and progression. Prostate tissue is comprised of stroma and three types of cells: basal cells, secretory epithelial cells and neuroendocrine cells [57]. Neuroendocrine cells have sparked particular interest because they are not androgen dependent and recent studies have revealed that this subset of cells is resistant to apoptosis, potentially via overexpression of survivin [58, 59]. Though the proportion of prostate cells which are neuroendocrine changes over a male's lifetime, neuroendocrine cells within the prostate always produce Chromogranin A (CgA) and Neuron-specific Enolase (NSE). CgA is a 49 kDa protein coded on chromosome 14 that is measurable in plasma with either ELISA or radioimmunoassay and is stable at room temperature [60]. After undergoing tissue-specific proteolysis, CgA becomes peptides that act as autocrine or paracrine hormones. Though stable in serum, CgA levels can be artificially increased by renal and hepatic failure, type A gastritis, essential hypertension and proton pump inhibitors.

NSE is an isomer of enolase found in the neurons. Like CgA, NSE is a marker of neuroendocrine tissues and tumors and is used as a marker for Merkel-cell tumors and non-small-cell lung cancers. It is measurable in the serum and is also used as an immunohistochemistry marker.

In 2006, Tropea and colleagues published a small pilot study measuring serum levels of CgA in patients with a variety of nonneuroendocrine tumors [60]. Several groups had already noted that serum CgA levels are elevated in prostate cancer patients [61–63]. Serum was collected from 151 patients with metastatic nonneuroendocrine tumors. Of these, nine patients were classified as having "genitourinary" tumors: five prostate, three bladder and one kidney. Two thirds of this group of patients had elevated serum CgA levels, though the investigators did not specify what type of tumors these six patients had. There were eight patients with extreme CgA elevations (>150 μ/l), two of whom had prostate cancer. Both of these patients had positive Indium [17] labeled Octreotide scans (somatostatin receptor scintigraphy, OctreoScan©). All five of the patients who tested positive for somatostatin receptor tumors, including the two with prostate cancer, were given long acting Octreotide. Though the authors hint at somewhat positive results, they do not give enough details or have sufficient objective measures to adequately describe outcomes after treatment.

A second study published in the same year examined three groups of males: 57 had biopsy confirmed prostatic adenocarcinoma, 61 had BPH and 44 were otherwise healthy control patients [57]. CgA and NSE were measured in the serum of all study participants and clinical parameters were recorded. Among the three groups, there were no significant differences between age, blood pressure, heart rate, and body weight. Patients with prostate cancer did have significantly higher levels of CgA than BPH and control patients (mean CgA 140.1 ± 53.2 ng/ml vs. 77 ± 32 ng/ml vs. 45.8 ± 23.2 ng/ml, respectively, $p<0.0001$). PSA's were also significantly higher in the prostate cancer group ($p<0.0001$). For NSE, while the differences between the groups were statistically significant, the results were harder to interpret in the clinical setting because patients with BPH had the highest levels of NSE, and patients with cancer had NSE levels which fell between BPH and control patients (4.8 ± 1.7 μg/l vs. 3.8 ± 2.1 μg/l and 2.4 ± 0.9 μg/l, respectively).

Among the cancer patients, the 19 patients with high grade (Gleason grade 7–10) disease had significantly higher levels of CgA than the 15 patients with intermediate (Gleason 5–6) disease or the 23 patients with low grade (Gleason Grade 2–4) disease (mean CgA 174.63 ± 42.9 vs. 140.7 ± 34.5 vs. 111.0 ± 54 ng/ml, respectively, $p<0.001$ and $p<0.0001$). There was also a statistically significant difference in PSA levels between these three groups ($p<0.01$ and $p<0.0001$), however NSE did not vary with Gleason grade ($p=0.408$ and $p=0.313$ and $p=0.880$).

Results were also correlated with clinical stage (T1, T2, T3 or Tx). There were significantly higher levels of serum CgA, PSA and NSE in patients with T2 vs. T1 disease ($p<0.01$, $p=0.032$ and $p<0.0001$, respectively). When patients with T2 vs. T3 disease were compared, there were significantly higher levels of CgA and NSE in T3 patients ($p=0.003$ and $p=0.028$), but PSA levels were not significantly different ($p=0.769$).

One aspect that makes CgA particularly compelling as a marker is its link to neuroendocrine cells instead of epithelial cells. Patients treated with androgen deprivation therapy (ADT) often have a marked initial decrease in androgen sensitive tissue, however neuroendocrine cells are not androgen sensitive and are not ablated during ADT. This increase in the relative amount of neuroendocrine cells is believed by many to play a role in progression to hormone refractory disease.

Supporting this theory is a 2005 study by Berruti and colleagues in which serum CgA levels were measured in 108 consecutive patients with newly diagnosed HRPC [61]. Hormone refractory disease was defined as having two consecutive rises in serum PSA levels or the development of a new bone or soft tissue lesion in the presence of castrate levels of testosterone. Of these patients, 97% had bone metastases and 10% had soft tissue metastases. Median survival was 16.7 months and, at the time of last follow-up, 74.1% of the patients had died. Upon development of hormone refractory disease, 41.7% of patients had elevated serum CgA levels while 84.2% had elevated PSA's. A univariate analysis of these patients revealed that elevated serum CgA levels were correlated with poorer survival (10.2 months in patients with elevated serum CgA versus 22.6 months in patients with normal serum CgA, $p=0.0002$). The negative impact that serum CgA levels had on survival was only significant for those patients with serum PSA's below the median PSA level of 97 ng/ml. On multivariate analysis, serum CgA levels were again a significant negative prognostic factor when performance status, Gleason score, hemoglobin, and serum alkaline phosphate, albumin and LDH were adjusted for ($p=0.05$).

Serial serum CgA and PSA levels were also measured at 3, 6, and 9 months in a subset of 50 patients who underwent chemotherapy. The article does not specify how these patients were chosen or if these patients had baseline clinical and pathologic characteristics similar to the initial group of 108 patients. Because these patients were recruited in 1998–2003, prior to the publication of SWOG 99-16 [64] and TAX327 [65] in 2004, they received a variety of chemotherapy regimens: 20 patients received docetaxel and estramustine, 15 patients received epirubicin, and 15 received estramustine only. All patients were continued on LHRH agonists and none were on antiandrogens, as this was part of the initial inclusion criteria for the study. Only 36% of these 50 patients had a PSA response. Median serum CgA levels were 13.3 U/l at baseline, 19.1 U/l at 3 months, 20.8 U/l at 6 months and 39.4 U/l at 9 months ($p<0.01$). Additionally, the proportion of patients with elevated CgA levels increased as well. At baseline, 3, 6, and 9 months, the proportion of patients with elevated CgA levels were 34, 46, 52, and 68% ($p<0.005$). Stratification by PSA response did not affect these results.

These results were further supported by data from the Cancer and Leukemia Group B 9480 Study (CALGB 9480) [66]. This study, performed in patients with HRPC, was a Phase III study of suramin, a polysulphonated naphthylurea which is a multicytokine receptor blocker. As an ancillary metric, the investigators also measured the pretreatment levels of CgA in 321 of the 390 subjects. This study had a median follow-up of 35.23 months, and 96% of study participants died. Among patients who died, the median level of CgA was 12 U/l. When this was used as a cut-off in a univariate analysis, elevated levels of CgA had an inverse correlation with survival (17 months for patients with CgA < 12 U/l and 11 months for patients with CgA ≥ 12 U/l, $p = 0.014$). A CgA cutoff of 9.5 U/l also yielded a statistically significant difference in survival as well ($p = 0.021$) in a univariate analysis. In a multivariate analysis adjusting for serum CgA, PSA, LDH and performance status, CgA was again significantly correlated with poor survival when a cutoff of 9.5 U/l was used ($p = 0.0203$); however, performance status, PSA and serum LDH were all stronger predictors of survival than CgA, though.

Subsequently, the Berruti group reported a study of 211 intermediate to high risk prostate cancer patients who underwent androgen deprivation therapy (ADT) alone or in combination as first line treatment [67]. Prostate biopsy specimens were tested for CgA expression and serum CgA levels were measured at the time of diagnosis and at 12 and 24 months after diagnosis. All of these patients had ≥T2b cancer, Gleason sum ≥7 or PSA ≥10. Patients were excluded if they were taking medication or had any condition which could alter serum CgA levels. Patients enrolled in the study received LHRH agonists as first line treatment and an antiandrogen was added if PSA increased. If, after second line hormonal manipulation, patients had >25% increase in PSA on two consecutive tests at least 2 weeks apart or if they developed a bone or measurable lesion in the presence of castrate levels of testosterone, the patient was defined as hormone refractory.

Of the 211 patients, 46% demonstrated evidence of neuroendocrine differentiation on immunohistochemistry, with 41% demonstrating CgA expression in <30% of tumor cells. Only 175 patients underwent serum CgA analysis because the remaining 36 took medications or had medical conditions which could affect serum CgA levels. Sixty percent of patients with elevated serum CgA had evidence of CgA expression on immunohistochemistry, while only 30% of patients with normal serum CgA showed evidence of tissue CgA expression. The remaining 10% showed no evidence of tissue CgA expression but did have increased levels of serum CgA.

The patients received one of three types of treatment: 35% underwent ADT alone, 23% underwent prostatectomy and adjuvant ADT, while the remaining 42% underwent external beam radiation with adjuvant ADT. At a median follow-up of 55 months, 112 (53%) patients had developed hormone refractory disease and 81 (38%) had died of their disease. In a univariate analysis, tissue expression of CgA was significantly related to shorter survival and decreased time to the development of hormone refractory disease ($p = 0.007$ and $p = 0.0003$, respectively). When patients were stratified by treatment type, tissue CgA expression still correlated with the development of hormone refractory disease. In a multivariate model which included serum PSA, stage and Gleason score, any tissue CgA expression was still significantly associated with time to develop hormone refractory disease ($p = 0.03$ for CgA in <30%, $p = 0.001$ for CgA in >30%). Having >30% of cells stain positively for CgA was significantly related to poor survival ($p = 0.01$).

After primary treatment, serum CgA levels were measured in 129 patients after 1 year and 93 patients after 2 years. Between 0 and 1 years, 14 patients developed HRPC and another 10 patients developed hormone refractory disease between years 1 and 2. At each time point there were increasing numbers of patients with elevated serum CgA levels: 23% of patients at baseline had elevations, while 32 and 33% were elevated at 1 and 2 years, respectively. Elevation of baseline serum CgA was significantly related to time to the development of hormone refractory disease (HR 3.0, 95% CI 1.8–5.2, $p=0.000$) and overall survival (HR 2.4, 95% CI 14-3.9, $p=0.000$). These significant relationships were seen at all time points, with elevated serum CgA producing the highest hazard ratios for survival and hormone refractory disease at year one (HR 5.8, 95% CI 3.1–10.8, $p=0.000$ and HR 4.8, 95% CI 2.9–7.9, $p=0.000$).

CgA is a promising biomarker for prostate cancer, however its utility appears to be time sensitive. Its relatively low sensitivity in early stage disease may limit its value in prostate cancer diagnosis. As was demonstrated by Sciarra and colleagues, [68] 35% of patients with localized disease had serum CgA levels >60 ng/ml while 100% of patients with metastatic cancer had elevated serum CgA levels. Its utility is also limited by a number of extraprostatic conditions and medications which can alter serum CgA levels. Its benefit may be greater at later stages of disease progression or after androgen deprivation therapy. Its utility in all treatment settings is unclear, however. A small study of 40 HRPC patients who received carboplatin and etoposide after failing first-line docetaxel treatment failed to demonstrate any significant prognostic value for serum CgA or NSE [69]. Further studies are necessary to determine in what clinical setting, if any, CgA is a useful marker.

Prostate Secretory Protein 94 (PSP94) and Prostat Secretory Protein 94 Binding Protein

Prostate secretory protein of 94 amino acids (PSP94) is a secreted 10.7 kDa protein found in high levels in semen [70]. Although the exact role of PSP94 is unclear, it has been implicated in a number of diverse roles. Studies have linked it to the regulation of sperm motility, apoptosis and growth of prostate cancer cells, and circulating FSH levels [71–73]. It also binds to immunoglobulins in the female reproductive tract [74]. Thus far, binding sites for PSP94 have been identified in the testes, pituitary gland and prostate, however a receptor has yet to be characterized [70].

In normal control male patients, circulating levels of PSP94 are usually 0–20 ng/ml and only slightly higher in urine [75]. A 1988 study by Teni and coworkers found that serum levels of PSP94 were significantly higher in patients with BPH and prostate cancer, while urine levels were lower in cancer patients and higher in BPH and control patients. In a separate study published 5 years later by Huang and colleagues, circulating PSP94 was elevated in several men with prostate cancer, but its sensitivity for the disease was lower than PSA's [76]. With low sensitivity and conflicting results, PSP94 lost some momentum as a biomarker. Subsequent studies, however, discovered that prostate cancer patients largely express a different isoform of PSP94 that has a higher molecular weight of 60–150 kDa, due to either aggregation or serum protein binding. Once this isoform was characterized, scientists realized that the antibodies used in earlier studies did not have high avidity for the higher molecular weight version of PSP94 [75–79].

Molecular studies reported the same year, demonstrated that PSP94 expression is downregulated in prostate cancer, [80] and in 2005 when a new sandwich ELISA designed to detect both the free and complexed PSP94 isoforms was developed [70], Nam and colleagues performed a study looking for the high molecular weight form of the protein. The study looked at 1,212 men who were referred for either an abnormal digital rectal exam or a PSA of 4.0 ng/ml or greater. In this cohort of men, with a mean age of 65.4 years and mean PSA of 12.0 ng/ml (median 8.1 ng/ml), 49.2% (596 patients) were diagnosed with prostate cancer. Of these men, 3.7% had Gleason grade 2–5 disease while 31.4, 49.7 and 8.7% had Gleason grade 6, 7, and 8 disease, respectively. The remaining 6.5% had Gleason 9 or 10 disease, and 7.4% of patients presented with locally advanced or metastatic prostate cancer.

Sandwich ELISA revealed that patients with prostate cancer had significantly lower levels of serum PSP94 than control patients (2.6 ng/ml, rage 0.5–26 ng/ml vs. 3.4 ng/ml, range 0.5–35.6, respectively, $p<0.0001$). In a multivariate logistic regression, the AUC of PSA, rectal exam, ethnicity and age was 0.66. Adding the ratio of free to total PSA or PSP94 increased the AUC to 0.72 in both instances, while the combination of all three serum parameters increased the AUC to 0.74. When PSP94 was correlated with Gleason sum and stage, it was found that patients with Gleason sums of 7 or more or those with metastatic disease had significantly lower levels of PSP94 ($p=0.007$ and 0.04, respectively). PSA and free to total PSA values were not significantly different between these groups. Additionally, after stratifying patients into aggressive (Gleason sum ≥7 and/or locally advanced/metastatic disease) and nonaggressive groups, it was found that a PSP cutoff of 4.5 ng/ml (which provided an 85% sensitivity) had an odds ratio of 2.74 while a cutoff <5.2 ng/ml (90% sensitivity) had an odds ratio of 3.33, both of which were statistically significant. Neither PSA nor free to total PSA ratio were able to significantly predict increased risk of aggressive or advanced disease.

A smaller study done in 185 prostate cancer patients treated with radical prostatectomy was reported the same year [81]. Though smaller, this study correlated clinical variables such as total PSA, Gleason score, surgical margin status, clinical stage, total PSP94, free PSP94, the ratio of bound to free PSP94 and PSP94 binding protein (PSPBP) with time to recurrence over a median follow-up time of 48 months. There was no correlation between age or family history and any serum marker. PSP94 (free, total and ratio) levels were significantly lower in the black patients in the study, while PSA showed no difference. Unlike the prior study, none of the PSP94 measurements was correlated with advanced clinical stage or high Gleason sum, though total PSA was. Of the 185 patients enrolled in the study, 31 patients showed evidence of biochemical recurrence in the follow-up period. Clinical stage, pretreatment PSA, Gleason sum, margin status, and a high PSP94 bound to free ratio were significantly associated with risk of recurrence. PSPBP was negatively associated with recurrence, and had a stronger correlation with recurrence than the ratio (PSPBP $p=0.005$ and bound to free PSP94 ratio $p=0.008$). In a multivariate Cox proportional hazards analysis, PSPBP was a significant independent predictor of recurrence in models which also included PSA, Gleason score and a combination of the two. The ratio of bound to free PSP94 was also an independent marker of recurrence in this model, but PSPBP had stronger significance.

PSP94, its isoforms, and PSPBP may potentially play a role in risk stratification as well as prostate cancer diagnosis. Early studies' failure to detect high molecular weight isoforms and bound versions resulted in initial underestimation of this biomarker, highlighting the role a faulty assay plays in characterization of any biomarker. While the two largest studies to date show some conflicting results, a large randomized clinical trial is warranted to determine this marker's utility in diagnosis and risk stratification.

Cysteine Rich Secretory Protein 3

Initially identified in neutrophils, Cysteine Rich Secretory Protein 3 (CRISP-3), was first reported by the name Specific-granule protein of 28 kDa (SGP28) in 1996 [82]. Like many other markers, CRISP-3 was initially identified as a potential biomarker in prostate cancer using high-throughput technology. One early report examined a library of expressed sequence tags (EST) in normal and prostate cancer specimens and found that the gene with the most up-regulated expression in prostate cancer is CRISP-3 [83]. CRISP-3 belongs to a large family of highly conserved proteins that is found in fungi, plants, insects and vertebrates [83]. Its name comes from the fact that its COOH terminus region contains a cysteine-rich domain. In humans, the three genes in the CRISP family are found on chromosome 6, with the majority of the CRISP-3 being expressed in prostate, pancreas and salivary glands. Smaller amounts are also found in the thymus, ovary, testes, colon, epididymis, and lacrimal glands [83, 84].

In an initial study to establish CRISP-3's possible role as a biomarker, an analysis of prostate cancer libraries identified 37 EST's from prostate [83]. Of these 37, 32 were found in libraries from microdissected prostate cancer specimens. The remaining five were from normal bulk prostate tissue libraries. In studies normalizing the amount of CRISP-3 mRNA to total mRNA expression, CRISP-3 was found to represent approximately 0.2% of all mRNA transcripts in prostate cancer libraries. Because noninvasive biomarkers must be secreted, the group then sought to confirm whether CRISP-3 was secreted. Sequence analysis subsequently revealed that the first 20 residues were a secretory signal. A tagged CRISP-3 vector was then created and transfected into HEK293 cells. The cell culture supernatant was analyzed with Western Blot 60 h after transfection, and CRISP-3 was detected in the fluid.

Using in situ hybridization, prostate cancer specimens of Gleason patterns 3 and 5 were then analyzed and both were found to have strong staining for CRISP-3. Normal and BPH tissues had variable but weak signal patterns. Several benign and Gleason 3 pattern epithelial cells were subsequently laser capture microdissected. RT-PCR on these samples demonstrated that CRISP-3 expression was much higher in malignant epithelium than normal epithelium. These findings were confirmed using real-time RT-PCR.

Using a similar microdissection technique, Ernst and colleagues analyzed the mRNA of 17 untreated prostate cancer specimens and 9 normal specimens adjacent to cancer [85]. Quantitative real-time RT-PCR was used to analyze 12,600 mRNA sequences and a validation set was also analyzed. A total of 63 genes were upregulated at least 2.5 times in cancer as compared to benign tissue while 153 genes were down-regulated at least 2.5 times. The most upregulated gene, specific granule protein 28, or CRISP-3, exhibited a 21.1-fold increase in expression.

Bjartell and coworkers confirmed these results [86]. They performed immunohistochemistry on 20 prostatectomy specimens, 150 TURP specimens (many of which were from patients with hormone refractory disease), 15 malignant pelvic lymph nodes and 15 metastatic bone lesions obtained from laminectomy. Serum collected prior to biopsy from 152 patients with prostate cancer and another 81 with BPH was also analyzed. Twenty of the patients diagnosed with cancer underwent orchiectomy as first line therapy and serum CRISP-3 levels were measured 2–5 months post-operatively. In whole mount prostatectomy specimens, CRISP-3 was detected in the majority of HGPIN and malignant lesions, but not in benign tissues. In microarrays constructed from TURP, lymph node and bone metastasis specimens, CRISP-3 staining was strongest in areas of high grade (Gleason grade 4 and 5) disease. PSA staining was not more intense in these areas. Out of the metastatic lesions, 11/15 lymph nodes and 12/15 bone lesions stained positively for CRISP-3. Unlike tissue samples, serum CRISP-3 levels were not significantly different between cancer and BPH patients.

Interestingly, immunoprecipitation studies of seminal fluid identified a bound form of CRISP-3. These complexes are formed by a strong noncovalent bond between CRISP-3 and PSP94, also known as β-microseminoprotein (MSP). Because of this, the Bjartell group expanded their initial study and stained prostatectomy tissue from 945 patients for both of these markers. They correlated these results with biochemical recurrence. Biochemical recurrence was defined as a PSA >0.2 ng/ml, confirmed at least once. In this study, with a median follow-up time of 6 years for survivors, 224 of the 945 patients developed a biochemical recurrence. Initial analysis indicated that staining intensity alone was not correlated to recurrence, and ultimately positive staining definitions for both markers included both staining intensity and percentage of positively staining tumor cells. For CRISP-3 positive staining was defined by staining intensity ≥1.5 and ≥80% of tumor cells staining positive. For PSP94, the cutoff was staining intensity ≥1 and ≥20% of tumor cells staining positive.

Utilizing these definitions in a univariate analysis, patients staining positive for CRISP-3 were more likely to experience biochemical recurrence, with a hazard ratio of 1.53 ($p=0.010$), while patients staining positive for PSP94 were less likely to experience a recurrence (HR 0.63, $p=0.004$). In a multivariate model including pretreatment PSA, Gleason grade, pathologic stage, extracapsular extension, seminal vesicle invasion, positive margins, lymph node involvement and marker staining, both CRISP-3 and PSP94 staining were significantly associated with biochemical recurrence. CRISP-3 staining, however, did not increase predictive accuracy of biochemical recurrence while PSP94 staining did. Based on the apparent inverse expression patterns of PSP94 and CRISP-3 in prostate cancer, the two markers were examined in all specimens, but there was no association between staining patterns of the two markers. Additionally, neither CRISP-3 nor PSP94 staining were correlated with Gleason score ($p=0.3$ and 0.6, respectively).

Thus far, CRISP-3's limited utility lies as a molecular, rather than as a serum or urine, biomarker. Studies examining its ability to improve diagnostic accuracy are lacking. And, while CRISP-3 immunohistochemistry is associated with risk of recurrence, the scoring technique is cumbersome, subject to significant interoperator variability, and ultimately did not improve accuracy above and beyond the parameters already currently used. As it stands now, the data does not support CRISP-3's utility in diagnosis or risk stratification though, these studies do add further support to the use of PSP94 in post-treatment risk stratification.

Annexin A3

Annexin A3 is a calcium and phospholipid binding protein which functions in cellular differentiation, migration, bone metabolism and immune response [87]. Though the exact role of Annexin A3 in the biology and progression of prostate cancer has not been fully characterized, it is clear that unlike most markers, Annexin A3 has an inverse relationship to prostate cancer. In an initial differential expression study, Wozny and coworkers found that benign tissue had significantly higher levels of Annexin A3 expression than cancer specimens [88]. A follow-up study by the same group looking at a tissue microarray of 1,589 prostate cancer specimens as well as benign and HGPIN specimens confirmed these results [89]. In a subsequent multi-center blinded clinical trial of 591 patients who were scheduled to undergo prostate biopsy [90], the group examined serum complexed, free and total PSA prior to digital rectal exam (DRE) as well as density normalized post-DRE urinary Annexin A3 levels. Of the 591 patients recruited into the study, 368 (62.3%) were subsequently diagnosed with prostate cancer, while 223 were not. Of the 223 patients without demonstrable cancer, 13 had PIN. The addition of density normalized Annexin A-3 to total PSA, free PSA, complexed PSA, percent free PSA and percent total PSA had significantly higher AUC's than each of the PSA parameters alone ($p<0.001$–0.0013). In the sub-group of patients with intermediate total PSA levels of 2–6 ng/ml, the combination of density normalized Annexin A3, and PSA had an AUC of 0.812 while Annexin A3 itself had an AUC of 0.725 and PSA alone was 0.679. In those patients with difficult to interpret PSA levels of 4–10 ng/ml, Annexin A3 also had significant diagnostic value. In these patients, a combination of density normalized Annexin A3 and free PSA resulted in an AUC of 0.832. This value was again higher than any of the PSA parameters alone in this subgroup (total PSA 0.587, complexed PSA 0.582, percent complexed PSA 0.641, and percent free PSA 0.716, $p<0.0001$).

The highest AUC in this study was seen in patients with a normal DRE and PSA levels of 4–10 ng/ml. In these patients, the combination of density normalized Annexin A3 and complexed PSA was 0.844.

The authors of this study only performed 10-core prostate biopsies and acknowledged that the lower detection rate of this method, as opposed to 12-core biopsies, could have potentially deteriorated their results. Additionally, again lacking is evidence that this marker can reliably distinguish clinically relevant from indolent disease. At this time, Annexin A3 appears to warrant further testing and may be particularly useful in those patients with low PSA levels or negative DRE results.

Leptin, Adiponectin, Insulin-Like Growth Factor 1, Interleukin-6, Tumor Necrosis Factor-α and Adiposity Related Genes

The profound and devastating impact of obesity on health has been known for decades. A major breakthrough in the study of this condition occurred in 1995, when two groups described an obesity gene, whose protein product appeared to increase metabolic rate and body temperature while decreasing body weight, body fat percentage, food intake and serum glucose and insulin levels [91, 92]. The product of the *obese* gene, which was named leptin, was later identified to be a hormone which plays a key role in food intake. The discovery of this gene, in conjunction with anecdotal and epidemiologic evidence linking obesity and prostate cancer led to a the hypothesis that leptin and other obesity related hormones could potentially be markers of prostate cancer.

For years, evidence had indicated that obesity increased prostate cancer prevalence and that populations with burgeoning rates of obesity often times had increasing rates of prostate cancer. Adding to this anecdotal and epidemiologic evidence was basic science evidence linking leptin to the reproductive tract: leptin and its receptors were found in reproductive tissue and were characterized as important to the development of these tissues as well as angiogenesis [93–98]. Additional studies continued to link obesity to prostate cancer. In China, a country which historically has always had one of the lowest incidences of prostate cancer, increased rates of prostate cancer have coincided with increasing rates of obesity, Western diet habits and waist to hip ratios [99–101]. In 2001, the group which reported many of these trends in men from Shanghai, China reported their findings on obesity associated markers and prostate cancer [102]. In this study, which included 128 Shanghaiese men with prostate cancer and 306 healthy Shanghaiese controls, anthropomorphic measurements as well as serum leptin, insulin, sex hormones and insulin-like growth factor-1 (IGF-1) were measured and correlated with prostate cancer risk. In a multivariate analysis, when body mass index (BMI), waist to hip ratio (WHR), IGF-1 and sex hormone levels were adjusted for, elevated serum insulin levels were significantly associated with increased risk of prostate cancer ($p < 0.001$). There was no statistically significant correlation between serum leptin and prostate cancer.

In that same year, a second group compared the serum leptin concentrations in men who had low volume (≤ 0.5 cc) tumors with men who had nonmetastatic, high volume disease (>0.5 cc tumors or extraprostatic extension) [103]. There were 48 men with low volume disease and 151 men with high volume disease. The two groups were matched by age (±5 years) and year of diagnosis (±1 year). As would be expected, leptin levels correlated closely with weight and BMI in all groups. In a univariate analysis, the median leptin level for low volume cases was 4.65 while the median for high volume cases was 7.04 ($p = 0.008$). In a multivariate analysis, which adjusted for BMI and testosterone, men with high plasma leptin levels had a greater risk of having high volume disease. When the model stratified men by height, obesity, and testosterone, it was found that having either elevated serum leptin or serum testosterone levels increased the risk of high volume disease (high leptin only OR=2.59, 95% CI 1.01–6.61 versus high testosterone only OR=2.49, 95% CI 1.00–6.21). In men with both high leptin and high testosterone, the risk of being diagnosed with high volume prostate cancer was even greater (OR=9.73, 95% CI 2.05–46.24).

Though the trends in these studies were interesting, not all studies supported these findings. Freedland and colleagues did not find a correlation between serum leptin and pathologic stage in 225 men who were undergoing radical prostatectomy [104]. And many other factors appear to play a role in weight and fat homeostasis. Both interleukin-6 (IL-6) and tumor necrosis factor-α (TNF-α) are proinflammatory adipokines [105]. Adiponectin is another cytokine which was characterized after leptin. Unlike leptin, which appears to promote obesity, adiponectin is secreted by adipocytes and increases sensitivity to insulin and increases fat catabolism; but similar to leptin, adiponectin has not demonstrated a consistent relationship with the development or progression of prostate cancer [106–110].

As an alternative approach, one group hypothesized that the lack of a high penetrance genetic alteration in familial cases of prostate cancer suggests that prostate cancer is caused by the accumulation of multiple low penetrance mutations. They felt that it was not the absolute serum concentrations of these adipokines that affected prostate cancer risk and progression, but it was alleles of each of the markers which may be more critical. In an effort to address these controversies, a large genetic study was conducted using the serum of 1,053 Finnish men with prostate cancer and 1,053 age-matched Finnish controls to examine the distribution of relatively prevalent (>5% prevalence in Caucasian males) and functional (e.g., located in coding exons) single nucleotide polymorphisms (SNP) found in the genes coding for leptin (*LEP*), the leptin receptor (*LEPR*), TNF-α (*TNF*), and adiponectin (*ADIPOQ*). Additionally, in a smaller subset of 196 control patients, these allelic variations were correlated to serum levels of adiposity markers such as serum insulin, serum glucose, IGF binding protein-3 (IGFBP-3) and IGF-1 [105]. After analysis, three of six SNP's in *LEP* were significantly correlated with an approximate 20% reduction in prostate cancer risk. Homyozogosity of a fourth allele in the *LEP* gene was associated with an increase in prostate cancer risk which was on the borderline of statistical significance. There were no allelic variations in any of the other genes studied that appeared to impact prostate cancer risk positively or negatively. In the smaller subset of 196 controls whose serum markers were quantified, there were no significant relationships between serum markers or BMI and genotype.

A second more comprehensive study examined 17 common SNP's in multiple classes of genes [111]. These included adiposity related genes: *LEP* and *ADIPOQ* as well as genes involved in the immune response: RNase-L (*RNASEL*) and toll-like receptor-4 (*TLR4*). The inflammation modulators interleukin-1B, interleukin-6, interleukin-8, TNF, and interleukin-10 (*IL10*) were also included. The patient cohort was extracted from a prospective study (CLUE II) based in Washington County, Maryland. Similar to the Finnish study, the cohort was predominantly Caucasian (98%). Out of all of the alleles examined, only the -1,082G>A allele of *IL10* was significantly associated with an increased risk of prostate cancer ($p=0.02$), though the hazard ratios for men carrying one A allele (OR 1.69, 95% CI 1.10–2.60) or two A alleles (OR 1.81, 95% CI 1.11–2.96) were low.

Despite tremendous amounts of resources being placed into obesity research, the mechanisms behind obesity are complex and still not well understood. The epidemiologic research linking prostate cancer and obesity is compelling, but may be due to other factors including increased screening and socioeconomic class.

Golgi Protein GOLM1

Golgi Membrane Protein 1 (GOLM1) is a Golgi membrane protein originally shown to be up-regulated in patients with acute or chronic hepatitis or hepatocellular carcinoma [17]. To date, GOLM1's function is not entirely understood. Subsequent studies have demonstrated that GOLM1 expression was increased in prostate cancer [112] and GOLM1 was also detectable in the urine of patients with prostate cancer [113]. Quantitative PCR on the cDNA of 11 benign, 27 localized and eight metastatic prostate cancer specimens demonstrated marked upregulation of GOLM1 in localized prostate cancer and only moderate up-regulation in metastatic prostate cancer specimens [114]. These findings were confirmed via Western blot on laser capture microdissected samples of BPH, HGPIN, localized prostate cancer and metastatic hormone refractory prostate cancer. Immunofluorescence staining on tissue microarrays further characterized high grade PIN as having intermediate up-regulation of GOLM1. When the urine of patients both with and without prostate cancer was immunoblotted for GOLM1 protein, it was found that patients with prostate cancer had significantly higher GOLM1 reactivity than those without cancer (2.77 vs. 0.96, $p<0.0001$). The AUC for urinary GOLM1 was 0.785 ($p<0.0001$) and had a sensitivity of 75% and a specificity of 72%. Additionally, the urine of 333 patients was analyzed via quantitative RT-PCR for GOLM1 transcripts. GOLM1 transcript detection had an AUC of 0.622, which was higher than that of PSA (AUC=0.495).

There is very little research on GOLM1 as a biomarker for prostate cancer. Until the results of this study are validated and additional randomized studies are done, GOLM1 should be used on an experimental basis only.

Endoglin CD105

In 2008 Pavlovich and coworkers used a cytokine array to examine cytokine content in the prostatic fluid of men with prostate cancer [115]. One of the cytokines most upregulated in high volume prostate cancer was a type I transmembrane glycoprotein named endoglin, or CD105 [116]. CD105 acts as an accessory TGF-β receptor that is usually expressed in vascular endothelial cells during inflammation and tumor neovascularization. Immunohistochemical studies confirmed that endoglin can also be found in the endothelial cells associated with prostate cancer, as well as the epithelial cells and stroma associated with PIN and prostate cancer [117]. That same year, a different group found that serum endoglin levels correlated with risk of lymph node metastases at time of prostatectomy and biochemical recurrence after prostatectomy [118, 119].

The Pavlovich group subsequently examined the urine of 99 patients who were either at high risk for prostate cancer or who had been previously diagnosed with the disease. They also examined the serum of 89 patients: 20 low risk patients with negative biopsy results and 69 preprostatectomy patients with biopsy proven cancer. As assessed by ELISA, there was no difference in serum endoglin levels between men with and without biopsy proven prostate cancer (16.9 ± 2.6 ng/ml vs. 18.1 ± 2.6 ng/ml, respectively). Among biopsy proven prostate cancer patients, however, patients with non-organ-confined disease (≥ pT3) did have significantly higher serum endoglin levels than their organ confined (< pT2) counterparts (18.0 ± 3.6 nl/ml vs. 15.4 ± 2.3 ng/ml, respectively, $p < 0.01$).

Among the patients from whom urine was collected, 67.7% had prostate cancer. Urinary endoglin levels were normalized to both urinary protein and creatinine concentrations. With both normalization methods, urinary endoglin was significantly higher in patients with cancer than those without. Mean urinary endoglin was 73.2 ± 77 pg/ml for patients without cancer and 132.4 ± 121.4 pg/ml for patients with cancer. When normalized to total urinary protein, urinary endoglin was 13.4 ± 14.4 pg/ml and 5.18 ± 6.8 pg/ml for cancer and noncancer patients, respectively. Among the 67 men who had prostate cancer, 34 underwent radical prostatectomy. Levels of urinary endoglin were significantly higher in patients with high volume tumors than in those with low volume tumors (9.73 ± 7.35 pg/ug vs. 3.25 ± 5.05 pg/ug, respectively, $p = 0.008$). Urinary endoglin did not correlate with Gleason score, cancer stage, PSA or age. For all patients, the AUC was 0.72 (95% CI 0.61–0.82) for urinary endoglin and only 0.5 (95% CI 0.37–0.63) for PSA ($p < 0.01$).

The authors acknowledge that there is no standardized method for detecting endoglin and that serum endoglin is of limited utility in localized disease. Urinary endoglin, while valuable, must be performed immediately after DRE, which results in a certain degree of intervention bias. For now, urinary endoglin appears to be potential marker in prostate cancer diagnosis, while serum endoglin, is more likely useful for prognosis.

Prostate Stem Cell Antigen

Prostate stem cell antigen (PSCA) was initially reported in 1998 after being identified as a cell surface marker which was overexpressed in a murine prostate cancer xenograft model, LAPC-4 [120]. PSCA is a 123 amino acid protein coded for on chromosome 8. Its 30% homology to stem cell antigen-2 led to its misleading name: PSCA is not expressed solely in the prostate and it is not a marker of stem cells. Though it is known that PSCA is a member of the Thy-1/Ly-6 family of glycosylphosphatidylinositol anchored cell surface proteins, its exact function is unclear. PSCA does not appear to be critical for reproductive or genitourinary development or function. Homozygous PSCA knockout mice are fertile and have normal reproductive capabilities. Additionally they do not have an increased risk of prostate cancer, even after exposure to gamma-irradiation [121]. PSCA is predominantly expressed in the prostate, however its mRNA has also been detected in placenta, bladder, stomach, colon, kidney and small intestine. [120, 122, 123] Within the prostate, PSCA is expressed in basal and secretory epithelial cells as well as neuroendocrine cells [122].

One of the first studies of PSCA and prostate cancer found that 81% of prostate tumors expressed PSCA [120]. Immunohistochemical analysis showed that only 6% of tumors did not stain positively for PSCA, while 21% exhibited strong staining and 63% stained moderately [122]. PSCA is also detectable by immunohistochemistry in metastatic lesions [122, 124]. Additional studies have demonstrated a significant relationship between PSCA expression and Gleason score, tumor stage, disease progression as well as seminal vesicle and capsular invasion [125]. Another study in patients with advanced prostate cancer, noted that patients who expressed PSCA transcripts had a worse disease-free survival than their PSCA negative counterparts [126]. Supporting this was a second study which examined the prostate chips obtained after transurethral resection of prostate for BPH [127]. Of the 288 patients in the study, 32.3% expressed PSCA. Of PSCA positive patients, 23.7% were diagnosed with prostate cancer in the follow-up period, versus only 1% of PSCA negative patients. Among the patients expressing PSCA who developed prostate cancer, a significant relationship between PSCA expression and Gleason score and clinical stage was noted. Interest in PSCA naturally proceeded to detection in body fluids. Unfortunately only 13.8% of prostate cancer patients in one study had PSCA transcripts detectable in blood [128].

The extremely low sensitivity of serum PSCA may ultimately undermine its role as a noninvasive, diagnostic biomarker. Certainly indirect and alternative methods could be tested for serum detection. Like other markers, its sensitivity, specificity

Table 4.1 Table of biomarkers

Biomarker	Biologic source	Advantage	Disadvantage
Sarcosine	Tissue Urine supernatants & sediments	Slightly better than PSA for prostate cancer detection Present in 79% of metastatic lesions	Low predictive value
Prostate specific membrane antigen (PSMA)	Normal and benign prostate, extraprostatic tissue, other tumors	Development of labeled antibodies (Prostascint) are used in radiologic testing	No value as a predictive or prognostic biomarker at the current time
Human Kallikrein related peptidase 2 (KLK2)	Blood	Can be detected in blood When used in combination with PSA, can add to detection specificity	Has no prognostic value
Prostate cancer antigen 3 (PCA3)	Tissue, Urine Sediment	Does not correlate with prostate volume or inflammation	Low sensitivity, with higher specificity Controversial prognostic value
α Methylacyl CoA racemase (AMACR)	Tissue Anti-AMACR antibodies can be detected in blood Circulating tumor cells Urine sediment	Sensitivity and specificity vary by detection modality	Elevated AMACR in CTC's can be found in benign conditions Optimal assay and metric for AMACR not established
Urokinase plasminogen activator (uPAR)	Serum	Not influenced by prostatitis May be more valuable for prognosis	Lower value for detection
Endothelial growth factor receptor (EGF-r)	Serum	Has high sensitivity and specificity Correlates with pathologic stage	Very limited data available
Huntington interacting protein-1 (HIP-1)	Tissue Serum	As a tissue marker, may have role in detection and prognosis As a serum marker may be useful in combination with other markers	Low sensitivity as a serum marker

(continued)

Table 4.1 (continued)

Biomarker	Biologic source	Advantage	Disadvantage
Chromogranin A (CgA)& Neuron specific enolase (NSE)	Serum	A neuroendocrine marker, CgA may be more useful in advanced disease stages	Less useful for localized disease
Prostate secretory protein 94 (PSP94) and binding protein (PSPBP)	Serum Urine	May have a role in risk stratification Early studies skewed by failure to detect all isoforms	Studies conflict as to the value of this family of markers
Cysteine rich secretory protein 3 (CRISP-3)	Tissue	Immunohistochemistry staining may be correlated with recurrence	Cumbersome scoring techniques for cell staining Only found in tissue
Annexin A3	Urine Tissue	May be useful when used in combination with PSA, especially in patients with PSA's of 4–10	Limited studies available
Adiposity related genes	Varies by marker	Several genetic polymorphisms may help assess risk of developing prostate cancer once more studies are done	There are several mechanisms for obesity; thus far there are no biomarkers identified
Golgi membraine protein 1 (GOLM1)	Tissue Urine	Very early testing indicates that this may have good sensitivity and specificity	Very limited studies available
Endoglin (CD105)	Urine Serum	May have a role in prognosis; studies are limited	Urine must be collected after DRE Serum levels are of limited use in localized disease
Prostate stem cell antigen (PSCA)	Tissue Serum		Very low sensitivity as a serum biomarker Overall unclear significance

and prognostic accuracy may be more useful when it is used as a tissue based marker. Further studies are needed to examine PSCA's potential role in prostate cancer diagnosis and risk stratification. (Table 4.1)

Conclusion

The search for a novel, noninvasive biomarker for prostate cancer which does not have the same pitfalls as PSA has been heavily studied. While many markers have been characterized, lack of standardized methods of detection, interoperator variability, lack of secretion into the serum or urine, and small study cohorts continue to plague this area of study. Certainly many of the marker described may add to the sensitivity and specificity of PSA when used as part of a diagnostic panel, preferably from the same body fluid. However the silver bullet markers that would diagnose prostate cancer and/or differentiate clinically indolent disease from clinically significant disease, has not yet been characterized.

References

1. Andriole GL, Crawford ED, Grubb 3rd RL, et al. Mortality results from a randomized prostate-cancer screening trial. N Engl J Med. 2009;360:1310–9.
2. Schroder FH, Hugosson J, Roobol MJ, et al. Screening and prostate-cancer mortality in a randomized European study. N Engl J Med. 2009;360:1320–8.
3. Abate-Shen C, Shen MM. Diagnostics: the prostate-cancer metabolome. Nature. 2009;457:799–800.
4. Sreekumar A, Poisson LM, Rajendiran TM, et al. Metabolomic profiles delineate potential role for sarcosine in prostate cancer progression. Nature. 2009;457:910–4.
5. Tomlins SA, Rhodes DR, Perner S, et al. Recurrent fusion of TMPRSS2 and ETS transcription factor genes in prostate cancer. Science. 2005;310:644–8.
6. Petrovics G, Liu A, Shaheduzzaman S, et al. Frequent overexpression of ETS-related gene-1 (ERG1) in prostate cancer transcriptome. Oncogene. 2005;24:3847–52.
7. Carver BS, Tran J, Chen Z, et al. ETS rearrangements and prostate cancer initiation. Nature. 2009;457:E1. discussion E2-3.
8. King JC, Xu J, Wongvipat J, et al. Cooperativity of TMPRSS2-ERG with PI3-kinase pathway activation in prostate oncogenesis. Nat Genet. 2009;41:524–6.
9. Carver BS, Tran J, Gopalan A, et al. Aberrant ERG expression cooperates with loss of PTEN to promote cancer progression in the prostate. Nat Genet. 2009;41:619–24.
10. Horoszewicz JS, Kawinski E, Murphy GP. Monoclonal antibodies to a new antigenic marker in epithelial prostatic cells and serum of prostatic cancer patients. Anticancer Res. 1987;7:927–35.
11. Chang SS, O'Keefe DS, Bacich DJ, Reuter VE, Heston WD, Gaudin PB. Prostate-specific membrane antigen is produced in tumor-associated neovasculature. Clin Cancer Res. 1999;5:2674–81.
12. Taneja SS. ProstaScint(R) scan: contemporary Use in clinical practice. Rev Urol. 2004;6 Suppl 10:S19–28.

13. Xu T, Chen X, Wang XF, et al. Study of PSA, PSMA and hK2 mRNA in peripheral blood of prostate cancer patients and its clinical implications. Beijing da xue xue bao Yi xue ban. J Peking Univ. 2004;36:164–8.
14. Murphy GP, Kenny GM, Ragde H, et al. Measurement of serum prostate-specific membrane antigen, a new prognostic marker for prostate cancer. Urology. 1998;51:89–97.
15. Marchal C, Redondo M, Padilla M, et al. Expression of prostate specific membrane antigen (PSMA) in prostatic adenocarcinoma and prostatic intraepithelial neoplasia. Histol Histopathol. 2004;19:715–8.
16. Kurek R, Nunez G, Tselis N, et al. Prognostic value of combined "triple"-reverse transcription-PCR analysis for prostate-specific antigen, human kallikrein 2, and prostate-specific membrane antigen mRNA in peripheral blood and lymph nodes of prostate cancer patients. Clin Cancer Res. 2004;10:5808–14.
17. Kladney RD, Bulla GA, Guo L, et al. GP73, a novel Golgi-localized protein upregulated by viral infection. Gene. 2000;249:53–65.
18. Sardana G, Dowell B, Diamandis EP. Emerging biomarkers for the diagnosis and prognosis of prostate cancer. Clin Chem. 2008;54:1951–60.
19. Ramirez ML, Nelson EC, Evans CP. Beyond prostate-specific antigen: alternate serum markers. Prostate Cancer Prostatic Dis. 2008;11:216–29.
20. Becker C, Piironen T, Pettersson K, et al. Discrimination of men with prostate cancer from those with benign disease by measurements of human glandular kallikrein 2 (HK2) in serum. J Urol. 2000;163:311–6.
21. Partin AW, Catalona WJ, Finlay JA, et al. Use of human glandular kallikrein 2 for the detection of prostate cancer: preliminary analysis. Urology. 1999;54:839–45.
22. Nam RK, Diamandis EP, Toi A, et al. Serum human glandular kallikrein-2 protease levels predict the presence of prostate cancer among men with elevated prostate-specific antigen. J Clin Oncol. 2000;18:1036–42.
23. Becker C, Piironen T, Pettersson K, Hugosson J, Lilja H. Testing in serum for human glandular kallikrein 2, and free and total prostate specific antigen in biannual screening for prostate cancer. J Urol. 2003;170:1169–74.
24. Steuber T, Vickers AJ, Haese A, et al. Risk assessment for biochemical recurrence prior to radical prostatectomy: significant enhancement contributed by human glandular kallikrein 2 (hK2) and free prostate specific antigen (PSA) in men with moderate PSA-elevation in serum. Int J Cancer. 2006;118:1234–40.
25. Wenske S, Korets R, Cronin AM, et al. Evaluation of molecular forms of prostate-specific antigen and human kallikrein 2 in predicting biochemical failure after radical prostatectomy. Int J Cancer. 2009;124:659–63.
26. Hessels D, Klein Gunnewiek JM, van Oort I, et al. DD3(PCA3)-based molecular urine analysis for the diagnosis of prostate cancer. Eur Urol. 2003;44:8–15. discussion -6.
27. van Gils MP, Hessels D, van Hooij O, et al. The time-resolved fluorescence-based PCA3 test on urinary sediments after digital rectal examination; a Dutch multicenter validation of the diagnostic performance. Clin Cancer Res. 2007;13:939–43.
28. Deras IL, Aubin SM, Blase A, et al. PCA3: a molecular urine assay for predicting prostate biopsy outcome. J Urol. 2008;179:1587–92.
29. Whitman EJ, Groskopf J, Ali A, et al. PCA3 score before radical prostatectomy predicts extracapsular extension and tumor volume. J Urol. 2008;180:1975–8. discussion 8-9.
30. van Gils MP, Hessels D. Hulsbergen-van de Kaa CA, et al. Detailed analysis of histopathological parameters in radical prostatectomy specimens and PCA3 urine test results. Prostate. 2008;68:1215–22.
31. Mearini E, Antognelli C, Del Buono C, et al. The combination of urine DD3PCA3 mRNA and PSA mRNA as molecular markers of prostate cancer. Biomarkers. 2009;14:235–43.
32. Rubin MA, Zhou M, Dhanasekaran SM, et al. alpha-Methylacyl coenzyme A racemase as a tissue biomarker for prostate cancer. JAMA. 2002;287:1662–70.

33. Nassar A, Amin MB, Sexton DG, Cohen C. Utility of alpha-methylacyl coenzyme A racemase (p504s antibody) as a diagnostic immunohistochemical marker for cancer. Appl Immunohistochem Mol Morphol. 2005;13:252–5.
34. Sreekumar A, Laxman B, Rhodes DR, et al. Humoral immune response to alpha-methylacyl-CoA racemase and prostate cancer. J Natl Cancer Inst. 2004;96:834–43.
35. Zehentner BK, Secrist H, Zhang X, et al. Detection of alpha-methylacyl-coenzyme-A racemase transcripts in blood and urine samples of prostate cancer patients. Mol Diagn Ther. 2006;10:397–403.
36. Rogers CG, Yan G, Zha S, et al. Prostate cancer detection on urinalysis for alpha methylacyl coenzyme a racemase protein. J Urol. 2004;172:1501–3.
37. Zielie PJ, Mobley JA, Ebb RG, Jiang Z, Blute RD, Ho SM. A novel diagnostic test for prostate cancer emerges from the determination of alpha-methylacyl-coenzyme a racemase in prostatic secretions. J Urol. 2004;172:1130–3.
38. Ouyang B, Bracken B, Burke B, Chung E, Liang J, Ho SM. A duplex quantitative polymerase chain reaction assay based on quantification of alpha-methylacyl-CoA racemase transcripts and prostate cancer antigen 3 in urine sediments improved diagnostic accuracy for prostate cancer. J Urol. 2009;181:2508–13. discussion 13-4.
39. Steuber T, Helo P, Lilja H. Circulating biomarkers for prostate cancer. World J Urol. 2007;25:111–9.
40. Pappot H, Hoyer-Hansen G, Ronne E, et al. Elevated plasma levels of urokinase plasminogen activator receptor in non-small cell lung cancer patients. Eur J Cancer. 1997;33:867–72.
41. Stephens RW, Nielsen HJ, Christensen IJ, et al. Plasma urokinase receptor levels in patients with colorectal cancer: relationship to prognosis. J Natl Cancer Inst. 1999;91:869–74.
42. Usher PA, Thomsen OF, Iversen P, et al. Expression of urokinase plasminogen activator, its receptor and type-1 inhibitor in malignant and benign prostate tissue. Int J Cancer. 2005;113:870–80.
43. Cozzi PJ, Wang J, Delprado W, et al. Evaluation of urokinase plasminogen activator and its receptor in different grades of human prostate cancer. Hum Pathol. 2006;37:1442–51.
44. McCabe NP, Angwafo 3rd FF, Zaher A, Selman SH, Kouinche A, Jankun J. Expression of soluble urokinase plasminogen activator receptor may be related to outcome in prostate cancer patients. Oncol Rep. 2000;7:879–82.
45. Piironen T, Laursen B, Pass J, et al. Specific immunoassays for detection of intact and cleaved forms of the urokinase receptor. Clin Chem. 2004;50:2059–68.
46. Steuber T, Vickers A, Haese A, et al. Free PSA isoforms and intact and cleaved forms of urokinase plasminogen activator receptor in serum improve selection of patients for prostate cancer biopsy. Int J Cancer. 2007;120:1499–504.
47. Milanese G, Dellabella M, Fazioli F, et al. Increased urokinase-type plasminogen activator receptor and epidermal growth factor receptor in serum of patients with prostate cancer. J Urol. 2009;181:1393–400.
48. Shariat SF, Roehrborn CG, McConnell JD, et al. Association of the circulating levels of the urokinase system of plasminogen activation with the presence of prostate cancer and invasion, progression, and metastasis. J Clin Oncol. 2007;25:349–55.
49. Festuccia C, Angelucci A, Gravina GL, et al. Epidermal growth factor modulates prostate cancer cell invasiveness regulating urokinase-type plasminogen activator activity. EGF-receptor inhibition may prevent tumor cell dissemination. Thromb Haemostasis. 2005;93:964–75.
50. Angelucci A, Gravina GL, Rucci N, et al. Suppression of EGF-R signaling reduces the incidence of prostate cancer metastasis in nude mice. Endocr Relat Cancer. 2006;13:197–210.
51. Jo M, Thomas KS, Takimoto S, et al. Urokinase receptor primes cells to proliferate in response to epidermal growth factor. Oncogene. 2007;26:2585–94.
52. Unlu A, Leake RE. The effect of EGFR-related tyrosine kinase activity inhibition on the growth and invasion mechanisms of prostate carcinoma cell lines. Int J Biol Markers. 2003;18:139–46.

53. Wanker EE, Rovira C, Scherzinger E, et al. HIP-I: a huntingtin interacting protein isolated by the yeast two-hybrid system. Hum Mol Genet. 1997;6:487–95.
54. Rao DS, Hyun TS, Kumar PD, et al. Huntingtin-interacting protein 1 is overexpressed in prostate and colon cancer and is critical for cellular survival. J Clin Invest. 2002;110:351–60.
55. Ross TS, Bernard OA, Berger R, Gilliland DG. Fusion of Huntingtin interacting protein 1 to platelet-derived growth factor beta receptor (PDGFbetaR) in chronic myelomonocytic leukemia with t(5;7)(q33;q11.2). Blood. 1998;91:4419–26.
56. Bradley SV, Oravecz-Wilson KI, Bougeard G, et al. Serum antibodies to huntingtin interacting protein-1: a new blood test for prostate cancer. Cancer Res. 2005;65:4126–33.
57. Ranno S, Motta M, Rampello E, Risino C, Bennati E, Malaguarnera M. The chromogranin-A (CgA) in prostate cancer. Arch Gerontol Geriatr. 2006;43:117–26.
58. Fixemer T, Remberger K, Bonkhoff H. Apoptosis resistance of neuroendocrine phenotypes in prostatic adenocarcinoma. Prostate. 2002;53:118–23.
59. Xing N, Qian J, Bostwick D, Bergstralh E, Young CY. Neuroendocrine cells in human prostate over-express the anti-apoptosis protein survivin. Prostate. 2001;48:7–15.
60. Tropea F, Baldari S, Restifo G, Fiorillo MT, Surace P, Herberg A. Evaluation of chromogranin A expression in patients with non-neuroendocrine tumours. Clin Drug Investig. 2006;26:715–22.
61. Berruti A, Mosca A, Tucci M, et al. Independent prognostic role of circulating chromogranin A in prostate cancer patients with hormone-refractory disease. Endocr Relat Cancer. 2005;12:109–17.
62. Cussenot O, Villette JM, Valeri A, et al. Plasma neuroendocrine markers in patients with benign prostatic hyperplasia and prostatic carcinoma. J Urol. 1996;155:1340–3.
63. Deftos LJ, Nakada S, Burton DW, di Sant'Agnese PA, Cockett AT, Abrahamsson PA. Immunoassay and immunohistology studies of chromogranin A as a neuroendocrine marker in patients with carcinoma of the prostate. Urology. 1996;48:58–62.
64. Petrylak DP, Tangen CM, Hussain MH, et al. Docetaxel and estramustine compared with mitoxantrone and prednisone for advanced refractory prostate cancer. N Engl J Med. 2004;351:1513–20.
65. Tannock IF, de Wit R, Berry WR, et al. Docetaxel plus prednisone or mitoxantrone plus prednisone for advanced prostate cancer. N Engl J Med. 2004;351:1502–12.
66. Taplin ME, George DJ, Halabi S, et al. Prognostic significance of plasma chromogranin a levels in patients with hormone-refractory prostate cancer treated in Cancer and Leukemia Group B 9480 study. Urology. 2005;66:386–91.
67. Berruti A, Mosca A, Porpiglia F, et al. Chromogranin A expression in patients with hormone naive prostate cancer predicts the development of hormone refractory disease. J Urol. 2007;178:838–43. quiz 1129.
68. Sciarra A, Di Silverio F, Autran AM, et al. Distribution of high chromogranin A serum levels in patients with nonmetastatic and metastatic prostate adenocarcinoma. Urol Int. 2009;82:147–51.
69. Loriot Y, Massard C, Gross-Goupil M, et al. Combining carboplatin and etoposide in docetaxel-pretreated patients with castration-resistant prostate cancer: a prospective study evaluating also neuroendocrine features. Ann Oncol. 2009;20:703–8.
70. Reeves JR, Xuan JW, Arfanis K, et al. Identification, purification and characterization of a novel human blood protein with binding affinity for prostate secretory protein of 94 amino acids. Biochem J. 2005;385:105–14.
71. Sheth AR, Arabatti N, Carlquist M, Jornvall H. Characterization of a polypeptide from human seminal plasma with inhibin (inhibition of FSH secretion)-like activity. FEBS Lett. 1984;165:11–5.
72. Chao CF, Chiou ST, Jeng H, Chang WC. The porcine sperm motility inhibitor is identical to beta-microseminoprotein and is a competitive inhibitor of Na+, K(+)-ATPase. Biochem Biophys Res Commun. 1996;218:623–8.

73. Garde SV, Basrur VS, Li L, et al. Prostate secretory protein (PSP94) suppresses the growth of androgen-independent prostate cancer cell line (PC3) and xenografts by inducing apoptosis. Prostate. 1999;38:118–25.
74. Hirano M, Kamada M, Maeda N, Yamamoto S, Aono T, Koide SS. Presence of immunoglobulin binding factor on human sperm surface as sperm coating antigen. Arch Androl. 1996;37:163–70.
75. Teni TR, Sheth AR, Kamath MR, Sheth NA. Serum and urinary prostatic inhibin-like peptide in benign prostatic hyperplasia and carcinoma of prostate. Cancer Lett. 1988;43:9–14.
76. Huang CL, Brassil D, Rozzell M, Schellhammer PF, Wright Jr GL. Comparison of prostate secretory protein with prostate specific antigen and prostatic acid phosphatase as a serum biomarker for diagnosis and monitoring patients with prostate carcinoma. Prostate. 1993;23:201–12.
77. Abrahamsson PA, Andersson C, Bjork T, et al. Radioimmunoassay of beta-microseminoprotein, a prostatic-secreted protein present in sera of both men and women. Clin Chem. 1989;35: 1497–503.
78. von der Kammer H, Krauhs E, Aumuller G, Scheit KH. Characterization of a monoclonal antibody specific for prostatic secretory protein of 94 amino acids (PSP94) and development of a two-site binding enzyme immunoassay for PSP94. Clin Chim Acta. 1990;187:207–19.
79. Wu D, Guo Y, Chambers AF, Izawa JI, Chin JL, Xuan JW. Serum bound forms of PSP94 (prostate secretory protein of 94 amino acids) in prostate cancer patients. J Cell Biochem. 1999;76:71–83.
80. Liu AY, Bradner RC, Vessella RL. Decreased expression of prostatic secretory protein PSP94 in prostate cancer. Cancer Lett. 1993;74:91–9.
81. Reeves JR, Dulude H, Panchal C, Daigneault L, Ramnani DM. Prognostic value of prostate secretory protein of 94 amino acids and its binding protein after radical prostatectomy. Clin Cancer Res. 2006;12:6018–22.
82. Kjeldsen L, Cowland JB, Johnsen AH, Borregaard N. SGP28, a novel matrix glycoprotein in specific granules of human neutrophils with similarity to a human testis-specific gene product and a rodent sperm-coating glycoprotein. FEBS Lett. 1996;380:246–50.
83. Asmann YW, Kosari F, Wang K, Cheville JC, Vasmatzis G. Identification of differentially expressed genes in normal and malignant prostate by electronic profiling of expressed sequence tags. Cancer Res. 2002;62:3308–14.
84. Kratzschmar J, Haendler B, Eberspaecher U, Roosterman D, Donner P, Schleuning WD. The human cysteine-rich secretory protein (CRISP) family. Primary structure and tissue distribution of CRISP-1, CRISP-2 and CRISP-3. Eur J Biochem. 1996;236:827–36.
85. Ernst T, Hergenhahn M, Kenzelmann M, et al. Decrease and gain of gene expression are equally discriminatory markers for prostate carcinoma: a gene expression analysis on total and microdissected prostate tissue. Am J Pathol. 2002;160:2169–80.
86. Bjartell A, Johansson R, Bjork T, et al. Immunohistochemical detection of cysteine-rich secretory protein 3 in tissue and in serum from men with cancer or benign enlargement of the prostate gland. Prostate. 2006;66:591–603.
87. Gerke V, Creutz CE, Moss SE. Annexins: linking Ca2+ signalling to membrane dynamics. Nat Rev. 2005;6:449–61.
88. Wozny W, Schroer K, Schwall GP, et al. Differential radioactive quantification of protein abundance ratios between benign and malignant prostate tissues: cancer association of annexin A3. Proteomics. 2007;7:313–22.
89. Kollermann J, Schlomm T, Bang H, et al. Expression and prognostic relevance of annexin A3 in prostate cancer. Eur Urol. 2008;54:1314–23.
90. Schostak M, Schwall GP, Poznanovic S, et al. Annexin A3 in urine: a highly specific noninvasive marker for prostate cancer early detection. J Urol. 2009;181:343–53.
91. Pelleymounter MA, Cullen MJ, Baker MB, et al. Effects of the obese gene product on body weight regulation in ob/ob mice. Science. 1995;269:540–3.

92. Halaas JL, Gajiwala KS, Maffei M, et al. Weight-reducing effects of the plasma protein encoded by the obese gene. Science. 1995;269:543–6.
93. Mantzoros CS, Flier JS, Rogol AD. A longitudinal assessment of hormonal and physical alterations during normal puberty in boys. V. Rising leptin levels may signal the onset of puberty. J Clin Endocrinol Metab. 1997;82:1066–70.
94. Mounzih K, Lu R, Chehab FF. Leptin treatment rescues the sterility of genetically obese ob/ob males. Endocrinology. 1997;138:1190–3.
95. Hassink SG, Sheslow DV, de Lancey E, Opentanova I, Considine RV, Caro JF. Serum leptin in children with obesity: relationship to gender and development. Pediatrics. 1996;98: 201–3.
96. Zamorano PL, Mahesh VB, De Sevilla LM, Chorich LP, Bhat GK, Brann DW. Expression and localization of the leptin receptor in endocrine and neuroendocrine tissues of the rat. Neuroendocrinology. 1997;65:223–8.
97. Hoggard N, Mercer JG, Rayner DV, Moar K, Trayhurn P, Williams LM. Localization of leptin receptor mRNA splice variants in murine peripheral tissues by RT-PCR and in situ hybridization. Biochem Biophys Res Commun. 1997;232:383–7.
98. Sierra-Honigmann MR, Nath AK, Murakami C, et al. Biological action of leptin as an angiogenic factor. Science. 1998;281:1683–6.
99. Hsing AW, Devesa SS, Jin F, Gao YT. Rising incidence of prostate cancer in Shanghai, China. Cancer Epidemiol Biomarkers Prev. 1998;7:83–4.
100. Hsing AW, Tsao L, Devesa SS. International trends and patterns of prostate cancer incidence and mortality. Int J Cancer. 2000;85:60–7.
101. Hsing AW, Deng J, Sesterhenn IA, et al. Body size and prostate cancer: a population-based case-control study in China. Cancer Epidemiol Biomarkers Prev. 2000;9:1335–41.
102. Hsing AW, Chua Jr S, Gao YT, et al. Prostate cancer risk and serum levels of insulin and leptin: a population-based study. J Natl Cancer Inst. 2001;93:783–9.
103. Chang S, Hursting SD, Contois JH, et al. Leptin and prostate cancer. Prostate. 2001;46:62–7.
104. Freedland SJ, Sokoll LJ, Mangold LA, et al. Serum leptin and pathological findings at the time of radical prostatectomy. J Urol. 2005;173:773–6.
105. Moore SC, Leitzmann MF, Albanes D, et al. Adipokine genes and prostate cancer risk. Int J Cancer. 2009;124:869–76.
106. Baillargeon J, Platz EA, Rose DP, et al. Obesity, adipokines, and prostate cancer in a prospective population-based study. Cancer Epidemiol Biomarkers Prev. 2006;15:1331–5.
107. Goktas S, Yilmaz MI, Caglar K, Sonmez A, Kilic S, Bedir S. Prostate cancer and adiponectin. Urology. 2005;65:1168–72.
108. Michalakis K, Williams CJ, Mitsiades N, et al. Serum adiponectin concentrations and tissue expression of adiponectin receptors are reduced in patients with prostate cancer: a case control study. Cancer Epidemiol Biomarkers Prev. 2007;16:308–13.
109. Freedland SJ, Sokoll LJ, Platz EA, et al. Association between serum adiponectin, and pathological stage and grade in men undergoing radical prostatectomy. J Urol. 2005;174: 1266–70.
110. Arisan ED, Arisan S, Atis G, Palavan-Unsal N, Ergenekon E. Serum adipocytokine levels in prostate cancer patients. Urol Int. 2009;82:203–8.
111. Wang MH, Helzlsouer KJ, Smith MW, et al. Association of IL10 and other immune response- and obesity-related genes with prostate cancer in CLUE II. Prostate. 2009;69:874–85.
112. Lapointe J, Li C, Higgins JP, et al. Gene expression profiling identifies clinically relevant subtypes of prostate cancer. Proc Natl Acad Sci USA. 2004;101:811–6.
113. Laxman B, Morris DS, Yu J, et al. A first-generation multiplex biomarker analysis of urine for the early detection of prostate cancer. Cancer Res. 2008;68:645–9.
114. Varambally S, Laxman B, Mehra R, et al. Golgi protein GOLM1 is a tissue and urine biomarker of prostate cancer. Neoplasia. 2008;10:1285–94.

115. Fujita K, Ewing CM, Chan DY, et al. Endoglin (CD105) as a urinary and serum marker of prostate cancer. Int J Cancer. 2009;124:664–9.
116. Fujita K, Ewing CM, Sokoll LJ, et al. Cytokine profiling of prostatic fluid from cancerous prostate glands identifies cytokines associated with extent of tumor and inflammation. Prostate. 2008;68:872–82.
117. Kassouf W, Ismail HR, Aprikian AG, Chevalier S. Whole-mount prostate sections reveal differential endoglin expression in stromal, epithelial, and endothelial cells with the development of prostate cancer. Prostate Cancer Prostatic Dis. 2004;7:105–10.
118. Karam JA, Svatek RS, Karakiewicz PI, et al. Use of preoperative plasma endoglin for prediction of lymph node metastasis in patients with clinically localized prostate cancer. Clin Cancer Res. 2008;14:1418–22.
119. Svatek RS, Karam JA, Roehrborn CG, Karakiewicz PI, Slawin KM, Shariat SF. Preoperative plasma endoglin levels predict biochemical progression after radical prostatectomy. Clin Cancer Res. 2008;14:3362–6.
120. Reiter RE, Gu Z, Watabe T, et al. Prostate stem cell antigen: a cell surface marker overexpressed in prostate cancer. Proc Natl Acad Sci USA. 1998;95:1735–40.
121. Moore ML, Teitell MA, Kim Y, et al. Deletion of PSCA increases metastasis of TRAMP-induced prostate tumors without altering primary tumor formation. Prostate. 2008;68:139–51.
122. Gu Z, Thomas G, Yamashiro J, et al. Prostate stem cell antigen (PSCA) expression increases with high gleason score, advanced stage and bone metastasis in prostate cancer. Oncogene. 2000;19:1288–96.
123. Cunha AC, Weigle B, Kiessling A, Bachmann M, Rieber EP. Tissue-specificity of prostate specific antigens: comparative analysis of transcript levels in prostate and non-prostatic tissues. Cancer Lett. 2006;236:229–38.
124. Lam JS, Yamashiro J, Shintaku IP, et al. Prostate stem cell antigen is overexpressed in prostate cancer metastases. Clin Cancer Res. 2005;11:2591–6.
125. Han KR, Seligson DB, Liu X, et al. Prostate stem cell antigen expression is associated with gleason score, seminal vesicle invasion and capsular invasion in prostate cancer. J Urol. 2004;171:1117–21.
126. Raff AB, Gray A, Kast WM. Prostate stem cell antigen: a prospective therapeutic and diagnostic target. Cancer Lett. 2009;277:126–32.
127. Zhigang Z, Wenlu S. The association of prostate stem cell antigen (PSCA) mRNA expression and subsequent prostate cancer risk in men with benign prostatic hyperplasia following transurethral resection of the prostate. Prostate. 2008;68:190–9.
128. Hara N, Kasahara T, Kawasaki T, et al. Reverse transcription-polymerase chain reaction detection of prostate-specific antigen, prostate-specific membrane antigen, and prostate stem cell antigen in one milliliter of peripheral blood: value for the staging of prostate cancer. Clin Cancer Res. 2002;8:1794–9.

[illegible]

Chapter 5
Biomarkers in GIST

Howard J. Lim and Charles D. Blanke

Introduction

Gastrointestinal Stromal Tumors' (GISTs) represent a specific mesenchymal neoplasm arising from the GI tract. Advances in molecular techniques and research have dramatically changed the treatment paradigm for this disease in two specific ways. First, the strategy of investigating the specific molecular pathogenesis underlying the disease, and the subsequent development of therapy targeted against the malignant process has become a model for future solid tumor research. Next, molecular analysis has provided predictive biomarkers that have helped refine the use of the first effective therapy, imatinib mesylate, in this disease. Both of these steps have furthered the ultimate goal of individualizing treatment for those with solid tumors.

With the advent of newer targeted medications and biotechnology, biomarkers are increasingly being utilized not only to determine the potential odds of response to therapy, but to select that therapy itself. For example, with breast cancer, markers such as estrogen receptor and HER2 neu allow for the selection of antiestrogen therapy and trastuzumab. This goal has not yet been achieved in GIST; however, molecular studies looking at the mutational status of the *KIT* gene have identified biomarkers allowing treating physicians to select the optimal dose of imatinib. Further studies should enable clinicians to determine which patients would derive benefit from different drugs. The following section reviews the identification and development of clinical use of biomarkers and targeted therapies in GIST.

H.J. Lim, M.D., Ph.D., F.R.C.P.C. (✉)
Department of Medical Oncology, British Columbia Cancer Agency,
600 West 10th Avenue, Vancouver, BC V5Z 4E6, Canada
e-mail: hlim@bccancer.bc.ca

C.D. Blanke, M.D.
Division of Medical Oncology, British Columbia Cancer Agency,
Vancouver, BC, Canada

H.-J. Lenz (ed.), *Biomarkers in Oncology: Prediction and Prognosis*,
DOI 10.1007/978-1-4419-9755-5_5, © Springer Science+Business Media New York 2013

Molecular Markers in Gastrointestinal Stromal Tumors

KIT (CD 117) is a transmembrane glycoprotein tyrosine kinase receptor coded by the *KIT* gene, a homolog of the viral oncogene v-*KIT*. It is a type III receptor kinase and is part of the normal functioning in mast cells, hematopoietic cells, germ cells, interstitial cell of Cajal, ductal breast epithelium, and melanocytes [1–5]. KIT is expressed in numerous human malignancies such as GIST, small-cell lung cancer, breast cancer, melanoma, ovarian cancer, and leukemia. Several mechanisms of KIT activation have been investigated [6–17]: (1) autocrine and/or paracrine activation of the receptor by its ligand, cytokine stem cell factor, or steel factor, (2) cross-activation via other receptor kinases, and (3) the presence of activating mutations.

Genotyping analysis for *KIT* and *PDGFRA* has evolved substantially. Currently pathologic review of the tumor material is required to ensure that sufficient material has been obtained. Extraction of the DNA from frozen or paraffin-embedded tissue using standard methodology is then performed and genes of interest are amplified via polymerase chain reaction. Screening for mutations can occur via a variety of methods. These include the use of direct sequencing, denaturing HPLC, mutation specific PCR and melting analysis. Previous technology limited analysis to a select number of genes or exons; however, with recent advances, sequencing is now done at a faster rate allowing for greater innovation. Gene expression profiling, use of single nucleotide polymorphisms (SNPs), micro-RNA (miRNA) profiling, and the use of mass spectrometry to detect changes in protein or even DNA have refined and expanded the biomarker field. Newer methodologies have made the screening of tumor for predictive biomarkers affordable and accessible.

There are several mutations of the *KIT* gene that lead to tyrosine kinase activity and GIST oncogenesis (see Fig. 5.1). The most common are exon 11 mutations (70–75% of mutations), which affect the juxtamembrane region. Several mutations exist. The most common is an in-frame deletion which can be associated with point mutations or small insertions affecting the amino acids before or after the deletion or both. This portion of the receptor serves as an antidimerization domain, so mutations within this region lead to increased kinase activity due to ligand-independent receptor coupling [18–21]. Exon 9 mutations (15–20% of mutations) occur within the extracellular portion of KIT, leading to ligand independent activation [22–24]. The exon 13 K462E mutation (5% of mutations) occurs within the KIT tyrosine kinase domain, also allowing ligand-independent activation of the receptor has been described in tumor formation in nude mice [25]. Point mutations in exon 17 (2% of mutations) occur in the cytoplasmic tyrosine kinase 2 domain are also responsible for gain of function [20].

Platelet derived growth factor receptor A (*PDGFRA*) activation is an alternative mechanism for malignant potential in GIST [26, 27]. *KIT* and *PDGFRA* mutation are mutually exclusive in GIST. *PDGFRA* activate the signaling pathway involving protein kinase B, mitogen-activated protein kinase and signal transducers and activators of transcription proteins. *PDGFRA* mutants tend to occur in non-KIT expressing tumors and represent approximately 8% of the GIST population. Missense mutations (D842V) are the most common (62.6%). In frame deletions resulting in

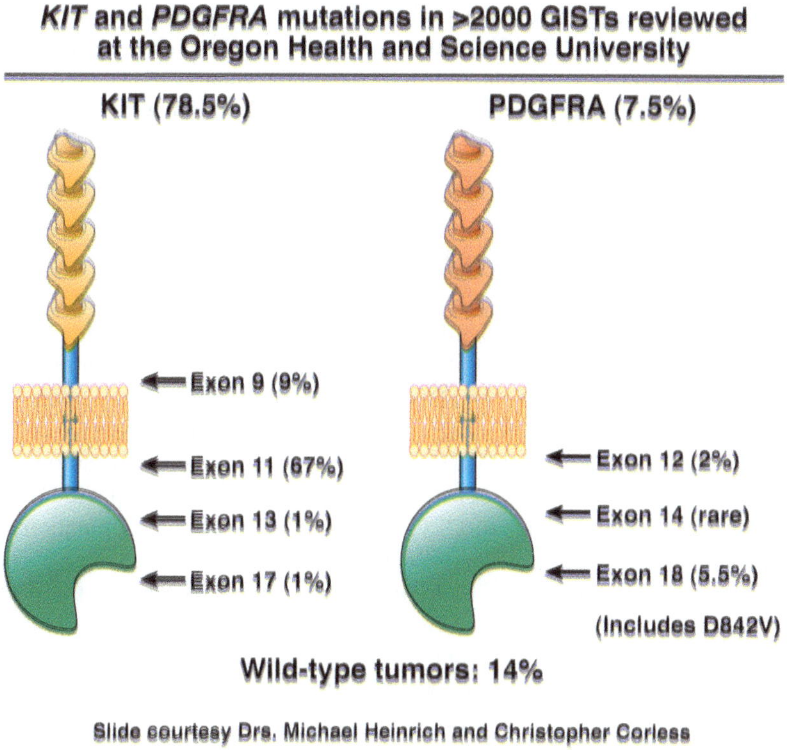

Fig. 5.1 KIT and PDGFRA mutations in GIST

the loss of amino acid residues 842–845 (DIMH) that occur within the activation loop (exon 18) or IMHD 843–846 are the next most common (14.9%). Mutations also occur within the juxtamembrane region (exon 12) with insertion (ER 561–562) and deletion type mutations (RVIES560-564) or (SPDGHE566-571R). In vitro studies using *PDGFRA* isoforms in Chinese hamster ovary cells as well as transfected BA/F3 cells demonstrated that the D842 mutants (with exception to D842Y) are significantly resistance to imatinib at levels that achieved in patients [26].

Newer markers have been recently been described [28]. DOG-1, a protein with unknown function, was discovered using GIST cDNA microarrays. The genes FLJ10261 encodes this protein and specifically is expressed in GIST with immunoreactivity recently described in 136 of 139 cases of scorable GIST. This novel marker may play a role in diagnosis, especially in *KIT* negative tumors but its predictive role is undefined. Insulin-like growth factor 1 and 2 may also be useful biomarkers. These ligands bind to the IGF family, composed of 2 insulin growth factor receptors and 6 binding proteins. This triggers activation of PI3K and MAPK pathways responsible for cellular proliferation and antiapoptosis. In 94 patients with GIST, strong IGF1 expression was seen in 40 cases, correlating with a higher mitotic index, larger, higher risk, metastatic and relapsed GISTs [29]. Strong IGF2 expression was present in 30 cases and correlated with higher mitotic index and higher risk GIST. Disease free survival (DFS) was measured in the high risk groups and IGF1 negative patients trended towards improved outcomes versus IGF1 positive patients (median DFS not reached versus 5.4 years). This was similar with IGF2 (median DFS 10.6 vs. 3.8 years).

Additional Clinical Evidence

Mutations in *KIT* resulting in gain of function and implication in GIST were described by Hirota et al. in 1998 [11]. Using in vitro assays, the c-kit mutations that were found in GIST wild type *c-kit* cDNA were transfected into interleukin 3 (IL-3) dependent Ba/F3 murine lymphoid cell lines. While wild type transfected cells grew only when exposed to IL-3, the Ba/F3 cells with mutated c-kit grew autonomously without IL-3. This indicated the constitutive activation of the tyrosine kinase receptor leading to the pathogenesis of GIST. The involvement of *KIT* mutations in the pathogenesis of GIST, make *KIT* a rationale target.

However, the development of many of drugs useful in GIST was not primarily designed to exploit *KIT* inhibition. For example, imatinib mesylate (see below) was initially developed as a BCR-ABL inhibitor for use in chronic myelogenous leukemia. This myeloproliferative disease is associated with a translocation (t(9;22)(q34;q11)), also known as the Philadelphia chromosome. Due to this abnormality, the gene fusion product BCR-ABL, a constitutively active tyrosine kinase, is formed and is responsible for the pathogenesis of this disease. However, in addition to blocking BCR-ABL, imatinib also inhibited c-kit and PDGFRA. The initial patient with rapidly progressive GIST who was treated with imatinib was reported in 2001 [30]. The diagnosis was confirmed with CD117 immunostaining and was found to have an exon 11 mutation. There was a dramatic response with the liver lesions decreasing in size from 112.5 to 28 cm^2 at 8 months with 400 mg of imatinib. This changed the landscape for the treatment of GIST.

The realization that specific *KIT* and *PDGFRA* mutations might affect GIST responses to small-molecule TK inhibitors has subsequently been extensively explored. Tumors from 127 patients who were enrolled in a multicenter, open-label randomized phase II study of imatinib treatment for metastatic GIST (400 vs. 600 mg daily) were analyzed for *KIT* and *PDGFRA* mutations and correlated to response [31]. Of the enrolled patients, 88.2% had an activating mutation in KIT, most commonly in exon 11(66.9%), followed by exon 9 (18.1%). *PDGFRA* mutations were found in 4.7% of patients. Wild type patients were 11.8%. Patients with wild type disease or with a *PDGFRA* mutation exhibited a PR 47.8% ($p=0.006$) vs. 0.0%, ($p<0.0001$), stable disease 33.3 vs. 0% and progressive disease in 55.6% vs. 66.7% respectively. Patients with exon 11 mutations experienced partial response rates of 83.5 vs. 47.8% for patients with exon 9 mutations ($p=0.0006$), stable disease of 8.2 vs. 26.1%, event free survival of 687 vs. 200 days. Wild type patients had event free survival of 82 days. Overall survival was improved in exon 11 mutations versus exon 9 ($p=0.0034$) or wild type ($p<0.0001$). Based on the proportional hazards model, exon 11 mutation was a strong prognostic factor reducing the risk of death by more than 95%.

The EORTC also conducted a phase I/II study with patients receiving imatinib 400 mg twice daily. Of the 51 patients in the phase II portion, 27 had GIST while the remaining had soft tissue sarcomas [32]. Of the patients with GIST, 4% had a CR, 67% a PR, 18% SD and 11% PD. The median TTP was 58 days. A smaller correlative sub-study from the EORTC phase I/II study of imatinib in advanced GIST was also performed [33]. Tumors from 37 patients were analyzed. *KIT* and *PDGFRA* mutations were found in 78 and 6% of the samples, respectively. Exon 11 and 9 mutations were most common (83% and 14% respectively). The majority of exon 11 mutations were in-frame deletions; the exon 9 mutations were AY502-503 duplication and exon 13 Lys-Glu missense mutation. PDGFRA demonstrated Asp-Glu substitution. Patients with exon 11 mutations: 83% achieved a partial response, 13% stable disease, and 4% progressive disease. Patients with Exon 9 mutations: 25% had a partial response, 75% stable disease. Wild type patients: 33% had partial response, 33% had stable disease, and 33% progressive disease. Event free survival was longer in patients with exon 11 mutations versus other mutations (849 vs. 327 days).

More data supporting the predictive role for *KIT* and *PDGFRA* mutations came from two phase III trials, plus their combined meta-analysis. Seven hundred forty six patients with metastatic GIST were enrolled in the North American CALGB 150105 study of imatinib in advanced GIST, were treated with either 400 mg or 800 mg of imatinib daily [34]. After a median follow-up of 4.5 years, progression free survival was 18 and 20 months for patients on the 400 vs. 800 mg doses respectively. Tumors from 397 patients were analyzed for *KIT* and *PDGFRA* mutations [35]. Exon 11 mutations were the most common (71.3%), while exon 9 and *PDGFRA* mutations were seen in 8.2% and 1.2% respectively. Patients were more likely to achieve a CR/PR with an exon 11 mutation versus an exon 9 mutation (71.7 vs. 44.4%; $p=0.007$) versus those whose tumors were wild type (71.7 vs. 44.6%; $p=0.0002$). There was no difference comparing wild-type to exon 9 (44.6 vs. 44.4%). The improvement in response rates also translated to a significant increase in time to progression. Patients whose tumors contained an exon 11 mutation had an increased time to progression of 24.7 months versus exon 9 (16.7 months) and 12.8 months for wild type ($p=0.0013$ and $p=0.005$ respectively). Overall survival was also improved: 60 vs. 38.4 months and 49 months for the *KIT* exon 11 mutation, exon 9 and wild type ($p=0.011$ and $p=0.49$ respectively).

The dose of imatinib had differential importance in subsets of GIST patients on this trial. Response rates were higher for those with exon 9 mutations when given 800 vs. 400 mg (CR/PR 17 vs. 67%, $p=0.02$). Wild type and exon 11 mutants did not demonstrate any objective differences (42 vs. 50% and 71 vs. 72% respectively) between higher and lower dose. The increased response rate in exon 9 patients did not translate to a statistically significant difference in time to progression (9.4 vs. 18 months, $p=0.97$), though that may have been an artifact related to the low number of samples. Overall survival was nearly identical (38.6 vs. 38.4 months) likely due to salvage with the increase in imatinib dosing. Additionally, there was no significant difference in time to progression or overall survival between the 400 and 800 mg doses for the exon 11 mutant and wild type tumors.

In the EORTC-ISG-AGITG phase III imatinib dosing trial for those with incurable GIST, 946 patients were treated with 400 mg or 800 mg of imatinib [36]. With a median follow-up of 760 days, Progression occurred in 56% of the low dose versus 50% of the high dose group (p=0.026) and a 2 year overall survival of 69 and 74% in the low versus high dose groups (p=NS). Samples from 377 patients, treated with either 400 mg or 800 mg on imatinib were analyzed [37]. *KIT* mutations were seen in 83.6% of the patient population, of which 65.8% of the total population were exon 11, 15.4% exon 9, 1.6% exon 13 and 0.8% exon 17), 15.4% were wild type and 2.6% were *PDGFRA* mutants. In patients who expressed an exon 9 mutation, had a significantly worse progression free survival and overall survival than exon 11 mutant with a relative risk increase of 171 and 190% (p 0.0001 for both end points). However, exon 9 mutants demonstrated an improved progression-free survival with a 61% relative risk reduction (p=0.0013) when treated with 800 vs. 400 mg. Time to progression was not different between the two dose groups in the exon 11 mutation or wild type.

Within the EORTC-ISG-AGITG study, of the 248 patients that expressed the exon 11 mutation an exploratory prognostic factor analysis was also conducted to determine the mechanism of response and resistance to imatinib. Mutations and/or deletion of codons 562, 565, 566, 567, and 579 demonstrated significant prognostic value (p 0.01) in the univariate analysis. Specifically mutation or deletion of codon 579 was an independent prognostic factor.

A meta-analysis of these two trials was conducted [38]. Overall, although there was a small progression free survival advantage for the high dose group (HR=0.89, p=0.04), this did not translate into an overall survival (HR 1.00, p=0.97). In the combined mutational analysis, those with exon 11 mutants demonstrated a more favorable prognosis than exon 9 mutations, other mutations or wild type (p<0.0001). An analysis of predictive factors showed that PFS was significantly longer (p=0.017) with exon 9 mutations however this did not translate in to an overall survival advantage (p=0.15).

The suggestion that mutations in *KIT* may be prognostic has also been demonstrated in patients who underwent surgical resection for localized GIST [39]. Of the 48 patients 8.3% were wild type, 12.5% had exon 9 mutation, 52.1% had a deletion or insertion in exon 11, 18% had a missense in exon 11, 4.2% exon 13, and 4.2% had an exon 176 mutation. Patients with missense exon 11 mutations had a 5-year recurrence free survival of 89±10% compared to 40±8% for GISTs with other mutations types, while wild type patients had a 5 year recurrence-free survival of 100%.

This was further explored in the intergroup phase III trial ACOSOG Z9001 randomizing patients with resected primary GIST to 1 year of 400 mg imatinib versus placebo. Seven hundred and thirteen patients with KIT-expressing, >3 cm GIST tumors were enrolled. After a median follow-up of 20 months 2 year recurrence free survival (RFS) was 74% (placebo) versus 91% (imatinib). KIT and PDGFRA

Table 5.1 Summary of trials of unresectable GIST treated with imatinib and mutation status

Study		Exon 11	Exon 9	PDGFRA	Wild type
Heinrich et al. [31] Phase II 127 pt samples	Percentage of patients	66.9	18.1	4.7	11.8
	PR	83.5%	47.8%	33.3%	0
	Event free survival	687 days	200 days	Not reported	82 days
Debiec-Rychter et al. [33] Phase I/II 37 pt samples	Percentage of patients	83	14	5	3
	PR	83%	23%	Not reported	33%
	Progression free at week 104	75%	6%	0%	12%
	Event free survival	849 days	327 days (included as other)		
Heinrich et al. [35] Phase III/ CALGB 150105—overall 397 pt samples (400 mg subgroup) (800 mg subgroup)	Percentage of patients	71.3	8.2	1.2	
	CR/PR	71.7%	44.4%	40%	44.6%
	TTP months	24.7	16.7	Not reported	12.8
	OS months	60	38.4	Not reported	49
	CR/PR	71%	17%	Not reported	42%
	TTP months	27.2	9.4	Not reported	15.6
	OS months	60.0	38.6	Not reported	49.0
	CR/PR	72%	67%	Not reported	50%
	TTP months	23.9	18.0	Not reported	9.8
	OS months	Not reached	38.4	Not reported	39.5
Debiec-Rychter [37] Phase III/ EORTC-ISG-AGITG 377 pt samples	Percentage of patients	65.8	15.4	2.6	15.4
	CR/PR	67.74%	34.48%	30%	23.08%
	Hazard Ratio 400 vs. 800 mg	0.821	0.392	Not reported	1.823

mutations analysis was performed centrally. KIT exon 11 mutation was the most common at 68%. On multivariate analysis of the placebo arm, exon 11 mutation was associated with a worse RFS (HR 3.0 $p<0.05$). Two year RFS was 65 vs. 91% ($p<0.0001$) for placebo and imatinib respectively in the exon 11 mutation analysis. In the PDGFRA mutation analysis, RFS was 76 vs. 100% ($p<0.01$) for placebo and imatinib respectively. Patient with exon 9 mutations had a 1 year RFS of 80 vs. 100% for placebo and imatinib respectively.

In summary, exon 9 and11 mutations offer both prognostic and predictive value. In the metastatic setting, untreated exon 11 mutations are associated with worse survival; however, treated exon 11 patients enjoy the best responses and survival. Exon 9 mutations are useful in guiding dosing of imatinib (longer PFS with 800 vs. 400 mg dosing). Table 5.1 summarizes and outlines the various mutations in comparison to wild type. This information helps guide treatment decision making with respect to proper dosing, as well as estimation of prognostic timelines for the patient.

Table 5.2 Small molecules currently investigated in GIST

Drug	Target	Phase
Nilotinib	BCR-ABL, PDGFR, *KIT*	Phase II/III
Masitinib	*KIT*, stem cell factor receptor, PDGFR, fibroblast growth factor, focal adhesion kinase	Phase III
Sorafenib	RAF kinase, VEGFR-2/PDGFR-beta	Phase II
Dasatinib	BCR-ABL, SRC kinase	Phase II
STA-9090	Heat Shock protein 90 inhibitor	Phase II
BIIB021	Heat Shock protein 90 inihibitor	Phase II

Sunitinib malate is less specific than imatinib, targeting KIT, PDGFRA, vascular endothelial growth factor (VEGF), FMS-like tyrosine kinase 3 (FLT3), and colony-stimulating factor 1 receptor (CSF-1R). This is now approved for imatinib-refractory or intolerant GIST. Samples from 78 of 97 incurable patients from an early phase I/II trial were analyzed [40, 41]. Patients who were resistant or intolerant to imatinib, received sunitinib 50 mg/day for 4 weeks with a 2 week break. Overall, 32 patients had a continued clinical benefit as defined as partial response or stable disease for greater than 6 months. After a median treatment of 1 year, six patients had progressive disease. Clinical benefit was demonstrated in exon 9 mutant (58%), exon 11 mutant (34%) and wild type tumors (56%). Progression free survival was longer in the exon 9 mutants and wild type versus exon 11 mutants (19.4 months and 19.0 vs. 5.1 months p=0.0005 and 0.0356 respectively). Overall survival benefits were also seen with exon 9 mutants (26.9 months) or wild-type (30.5 months) versus exon 11 (12.3 months, p=0.12 and 0.0132 respectively). Several other agents are being investigated in clinical trials (see Table 5.2) exploiting the pathogenesis of GIST.

The lack of sensitivity of imatinib in tumors with exon 9 mutations may be explained by the structural differences due to the mutation. Exon 9 mutations upregulate activity via ligand-mediated receptor dimerization [42], while exon 11 mutations affect the intracellular juxtamembrane domain [43]. Analysis of in vitro models using an isogenic BaF3 model, the IC50 in exon 9 mutations was almost eight times higher than that of exon 11 V559D mutations [44]. This is confirmed in in vitro studies with Chinese hamster ovary cells, exon 11 V560D mutations demonstrated an IC50 that was ten times less than that of those with an exon 9 mutation 22. However, these exon 9 mutants were more sensitive to sunitinib both in vitro and in vivo whereas patients with acquired secondary kinase mutations resulting in imatinib resistance were less sensitive to sunitinib. This demonstrates a clear difference in the mechanism of the mutations and the binding pockets of these drugs.

The use of circulating levels of soluble *KIT* (s*KIT*) has also been evaluated in a phase III trial of sunitinib after imatinib failure in advanced gastrointestinal stromal tumors [45]. Three hundred and twelve patients were randomized in a 2:1 fashion to receive sunitinib (n=207) or placebo [46]. The median TTP was 27.3 vs. 6.4 weeks in favor of sunitinib ($p<0.0001$). Progression free survival at 26 weeks was 16 vs. 1% in favor sunitinib and overall survival had not been reached at the time of the analysis. Of the patients in the sunitinib group 7% had a partial response, 58% had stable disease and 19% had progressive disease versus within the placebo the rate were 0%, 48%, and 37% respectively. Plasma s*KIT* levels were sampled every 2 weeks in cycle 1 and on days 1 and 28 and analyzed by ELISA. Decreases in s*KIT* levels at the end of cycle 2 had a median time to progression of 34.3 vs. 16.0 weeks in patients with elevated levels. The median overall survival was also increased in patients with reduced s*KIT* on Cycle 1 day 28, cycle 2 day 28 and cycle 3 day 1 were 80.6, 99.3 and 92.4 weeks versus 44.3, 40.3, 41.4 weeks with patients with increased s*KIT* levels ($p=0.0001$, $p<0.0001$, and $p=0.0016$ respectively). This suggests that s*KIT* may also be a predictive marker for sunitinib and future study would be warranted.

Functional Imaging

During monitoring of treatment response, conventional CT scans sometimes can be misleading, as GISTs can increase in size due to intratumoral bleeding or necrosis. The changes in the densities of fluid seen on CT scan are more important but are difficult to interpret. In general, the use of Response Evaluation Criteria in Solid Tumors (RECIST) in the use of GIST has been debated. Another method (the MD Anderson criteria) combines the use of a 10% decrease in tumor size or more than 15% decrease in tumor density at 2 months of treatment). This method was studied comparing CT findings with PET, a total 172 lesions were evaluated in 40 patients with metastatic GIST treated with imatinib [47]. This method resulted in a sensitivity of 97% and specificity of 100% in identifying PET responders versus 52 and 100% by RECIST. Use of the MDACC criteria also correlated with TTP ($p=0.0002$) and disease specific survival ($p=0.04$) better than RECIST [48].

Positive Electron Transmission imaging (PET) with the use of F18-fludoxyglucose (FDG) has become a useful tool in predicting response. PET scanning has increased the accuracy of determining the response of GISTs to treatment. A decrease in FDG activity is clearly seen with successful therapy, even within 24 h of starting therapy [49]. PET was used to follow the response of 64 patients with advanced GIST to imatinib over a 16 month period. At 21–40 days 79% of the patients demonstrated a decrease in SUV to <2.0 and were still in remission at 16 months. Patients with an SUV >2.0 were deemed as progression (15%) or progressed after a temporary response (6%) (see Fig. 5.2). This is in contrast to conventional CT scanning, which take weeks or months to determine a demonstrable response. A comparison of PET/CT to PET and CT for monitoring of imatinib therapy in advanced GIST [50]. Tumor response was correctly assessed in 95% of patients at 1 month, 100% at 3 and 6 months, versus 85, 100, and 100% for PET and 44, 60 and 57% for CT scanning respectively. It should noted that the study

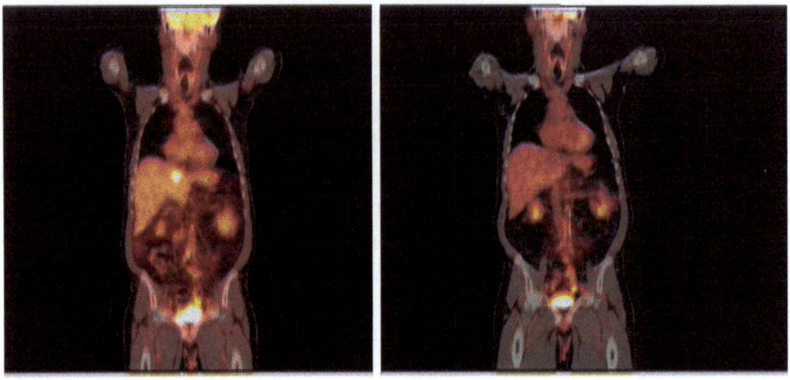

Fig. 5.2 18F-FDG-PET/CT images demonstrating a hypermetabolic left lobe metastasis (*left*). The *right* scan was performed after 1 month of treatment of imatinib therapy showing complete resolution

progression via RECIST versus the MDACC criteria. PET also predicts response to sunitinib. PET was performed in 23 patients who received at least 1 cycle of sunitinib, before and after the first 4 weeks of sunitinib therapy. PFS correlated with early PET metabolic response with 29 weeks for metabolic partial response, 16 weeks for metabolically stable disease and 4 weeks with metabolically progressive disease. Patients who had metabolically progressive disease subsequently progressed according to RECIST criteria [51].

Conclusions

Tyrosine kinase therapy for GISTs represents rational drug design developed through an understanding of the molecular pathogenesis of the disease. Within this framework, both prognostic and predictive biomarkers have been identified. *KIT* exon 9 and 11 mutations are of particular importance, and their best utilization in clinical care of patients with GIST is still evolving. Timing and patterns of drug resistance, in addition to this molecular classification, will also help guide therapy, particularly with respect to changing to a new second or third line therapy versus dose escalating imatinib. This is significantly different than the current treatments with traditional cytotoxics, where therapy is changed based on progression.

Advances in biotechnology have also changed GIST clinical trial design to essentially mandate tissue collection, to prospectively validate potential future biomarkers. Built-in functional imaging requirements should also help clarify timing and choice of best treatment. Hopefully future GIST therapies will be designed based on sophisticated tumor analysis, enabling oncologists to spare patients potential side effects and select the best treatment for the individual with cancer.

References

1. Arber DA, Tamayo R, Weiss LM. Paraffin section detection of the c-*KIT* gene product (CD117) in human tissues: value in the diagnosis of mast cell disorders. Hum Pathol. 1998;29:498–504.
2. Lammie A, Drobnjak M, Gerald W, et al. Expression of c-*KIT* and *KIT* ligand proteins in normal human tissues. J Histochem Cytochem. 1994;42:1417–25.
3. Tsuura Y, Hiraki H, Watanabe K, et al. Preferential localization of c-*KIT* product in tissue mast cells, basal cells of skin, epithelial cells of breast, small cell lung carcinoma and seminoma/dysgerminoma in human: immunohistochemical study on formalin-fixed, paraffin-embedded tissues. Virchows Arch. 1994;424:135–41.
4. Natali PG, Nicotra MR, Sures I, et al. Expression of c-*KIT* receptor in normal and transformed human nonlymphoid tissues. Cancer Res. 1992;52:6139–43.
5. Matsuda R, Takahashi T, Nakamura S, et al. Expression of the c-*KIT* protein in human solid tumors and in corresponding fetal and adult normal tissues. Am J Pathol. 1993;142:339–46.
6. Turner AM, Zsebo KM, Martin F, et al. Nonhematopoietic tumor cell lines express stem cell factor and display c-*KIT* receptors. Blood. 1992;80:374–81.
7. Tian Q, Frierson HFJ, Krystal GW, et al. Activating c-*KIT* gene mutations in human germ cell tumors. Am J Pathol. 1999;154:1643–7.
8. Beghini A, Cairoli R, Morra E, et al. In vivo differentiation of mast cells from acute myeloid leukemia blasts carrying a novel activating ligand-independent C-*KIT* mutation. Blood Cells Mol Dis. 1998;24:262–70.
9. Ning Z-Q, Li J, Arceci RJ. Activating mutations of c-*KIT* at Asp816 are associated with constitutive activation of Stat signal transduction pathways in acute myeloid leukemia. Blood. 1999;94:264a. abstr.
10. Timeus F, Crescenzio N, Valle P, et al. Stem cell factor suppresses apoptosis in neuroblastoma cell lines. Exp Hematol. 1997;25:1253–60.
11. Hirota S, Isozaki K, Moriyama Y, et al. Gain-of-function mutations of c-*KIT* in human gastrointestinal stromal tumors. Science. 1998;279:577–80.
12. DiPaola RS, Kuczynski WI, Onodera K, et al. Evidence for a functional *KIT* receptor in melanoma, breast, and lung carcinoma cells. Cancer Gene Ther. 1997;4:176–82.
13. Cohen PS, Chang JP, Lipkunskaya M, et al. Expression of stem cell factor and c-*KIT* in human neuroblastoma. Blood. 1994;84:3465–72.
14. Sekido Y, Takahashi T, Ueda R, et al. Recombinant human stem cell factor mediates chemotaxis of small-cell lung cancer cell lines aberrantly expressing the c-*KIT* protooncogene. Cancer Res. 1993;53:1709–14.
15. Sekido Y, Obata Y, Ueda R, et al. Preferential expression of c-*KIT* protooncogene transcripts in small cell lung cancer. Cancer Res. 1991;51:2416–9.
16. Kondoh G, Hayasaka N, Li Q, et al. An in vivo model for receptor tyrosine kinase autocrine/paracrine activation: Auto-stimulated *KIT* receptor acts as a tumor promoting factor in papilloma virus induced tumorigenesis. Oncogene. 1995;10:341–7.
17. Caceres-Cortes JR, Alvarado-Moreno JA, Waga K, et al. Implication of tyrosine kinase receptor and steel factor in cell density dependent growth in cervical cancers and leukemias. Cancer Res. 2001;61:6281–9.
18. Ma Y, Cunningham ME, Wang X, et al. Inhibition of spontaneous receptor phosphorylation by residues in a putative alpha-helix in the *KIT* intracellular juxtamembrane region. J Biol Chem. 1999;274:13399–402.
19. Irusta PM, DiMaio D. A single amino acid substitution in a WW-like domain of diverse members of the PDGF receptor subfamily of tyrosine kinases causes constitutive receptor activation. EMBO J. 1998;17:6912–23.
20. Kitayama H, Kanakura Y, Furitsu T, et al. Constitutively activating mutations of c-*KIT* receptor tyrosine kinase confer factor independent growth and tumorigenicity of factor-dependent hematopoietic cell lines. Blood. 1995;85:790–8.

21. Fenski R, Mizuki M, Gruning W, et al. Internal tandem duplications of the Flt3 juxtamembrane domain results in factor independent growth of 32D cells. Blood. 1999;94:591a. abstr.
22. Lux ML, Rubin BP, Biase TL, et al. *KIT* extracellular and kinase domain mutations in gastrointestinal stromal tumors. Am J Pathol. 2000;156:791–5.
23. Lasota J, Wozniak A, Sarlomo-Rikala M, et al. Mutations in exons 9 and 13 of *KIT* gene are rare events in gastrointestinal stromal tumors: a study of 200 cases. Am J Pathol. 2000;157:1091–5.
24. Hirota S, Nishida T, Isozaki K, et al. Gain-of-function mutation at the extracellular domain of *KIT* in gastrointestinal stromal tumors. J Pathol. 2001;193:505–10.
25. Isozaki K, Terris B, Belghiti J, et al. Germline-activating mutation in the kinase domain of *KIT* gene in familial gastrointestinal stromal tumors. Am J Pathol. 2000;157:1581–5.
26. Corless CL, Schroeder A, Griffith D, et al. PDGFRA mutations in gastrointestinal stromal tumors: frequency, spectrum and in vitro sensitivity to imatinib. J Clin Oncol. 2005;23(23):5357–64.
27. Heinrich MC, Corless CL, Duensing A, et al. PDGFRA activating mutations in gastrointestinal stromal tumors. Science. 2003;299(5607):708–10.
28. West RB, Corless CL, Chen X, et al. The novel marker, DOG1, is expressed ubiquitously in gastrointestinal stromal tumors irrespective of *KIT* or PDGFRA mutation status. Am J Pathol. 2004;165(1):107–13.
29. Braconi C, Bracci R, Bearzi I, et al. Insulin-like growth factor (IGF) 1 and 2 help to predict disease outcome in GIST patients. Ann Oncol. 2008;19(7):1293–8.
30. Joensuu H, Roberts PJ, Sarlomo-Rikala M, et al. Effect of the tyrosine kinase inhibitor STI571 in a patient with a metastatic gastrointestinal stromal tumor. N Engl J Med. 2001;344:1052–6.
31. Heinrich MC, Corless CL, Demetri GD, et al. Kinase mutations and imatinib response in patients with metastatic gastrointestinal stromal tumor. J Clin Oncol. 2003;21(23):4342–9.
32. Verweij J, van Oosterom A, Blay JY, et al. Imatinib mesylate (STI-571 Glivec, Gleevec) is an active agent for gastrointestinal stromal tumors, but does not yield responses in other soft-tissue sarcomas that are unselected for a molecular target. Results from an EORTC Soft Tissue and Bone Sarcoma Group phase II study. Eur J Cancer. 2003;39(14):2006–11.
33. Debiec-Rychter M, Dumez H, Judson I, et al. Use of c-*KIT*/PDGFRA mutational analysis to predict the clinical response to imatinib in patients with advanced gastrointestinal stromal tumours entered on phase I and II studies of the EORTC Soft Tissue and Bone Sarcoma Group. Eur J Cancer. 2004;40(5):689–95.
34. Blanke CD, Rankin C, Demetri GD, et al. Phase III randomized, intergroup trial assessing imatinib mesylate at two dose levels in patients with unresectable or metastatic gastrointestinal stromal tumors expressing the *KIT* receptor tyrosine kinase: S0033. J Clin Oncol. 2008;26(4):626–32.
35. Heinrich MC, Owzar K, Corless CL, et al. Correlation of kinase genotype and clinical outcome in the North American Intergroup Phase III Trial of imatinib mesylate for treatment of advanced gastrointestinal stromal tumor: CALGB 150105 Study by Cancer and Leukemia Group B and Southwest Oncology Group. J Clin Oncol. 2008;26(33):5360–7.
36. Verweij J, Casali PG, Zalcberg J, et al. Progression-free survival in gastrointestinal stromal tumours with high-dose imatinib: randomized trial. Lancet. 2004;364:1127–34.
37. Debiec-Rychter M, Sciot R, Le Cesne A, et al. *KIT* mutations and dose selection for imatinib in patients with advanced gastrointestinal stromal tumours. Eur J Cancer. 2006;42(8):1093–103.
38. Gastrointestinal Stromal Tumor Meta-Analysis Group (MetaGIST). Comparison of two doses of imatinib for the treatment of unresectable or metastatic gastrointestinal stromal tumors: a meta-analysis of 1,640 patients. J Clin Oncol. 2010;28:1247–53.
39. Singer S, Rubin BP, Lux ML, et al. Prognostic value of *KIT* mutation type, mitotic activity, and histologic subtype in gastrointestinal stromal tumors. J Clin Oncol. 2002;20(18):3898–905.

40. Maki RG, Fletcher JA, Heinrich MC, et al. Results from a continuation trial of SU11248 in patients with imatinib-resistant gastrointestinal stromal tumor (GIST). J Clin Oncol. 2005;23:818s. suppl; abstr 9011.
41. Heinrich MC, Maki RG, Corless CL, et al. Primary and secondary kinase genotypes correlate with the biological and clinical activity of sunitinib in imatinib-resistant gastrointestinal stromal tumor. J Clin Oncol. 2008;26(33):5352–9.
42. Yuzawa S, Opatowsky Y, Zhang Z, et al. Structural basis for activation of the receptor tyrosine kinase *KIT* by stem cell factor. Cell. 2007;130:323–34.
43. Dibb NJ, Dilworth SM, Mol CD. Switching on kinases: oncogenic activation of BRAF and the PDGFR family. Nat Rev Cancer. 2004;4:718–27.
44. Guo T, Agaram NP, Wong GC, et al. Sorafenib inhibits the imatinib-resistant *KIT*T670I gatekeeper mutation in gastrointestinal stromal tumor. Clin Cancer Res. 2007;13(16):4874–81.
45. Deprimo SE, Huang X, Blackstein ME, et al. Circulating levels of soluble *KIT* serve as a biomarker for clinical outcome in gastrointestinal stromal tumor patients receiving sunitinib following imatinib failure. Clin Cancer Res. 2009;15(18):5869–77.
46. Demetri GD, van Oosterom AT, Garrett CR, et al. Efficacy and safety of sunitinib in patients with advanced gastrointestinal stromal tumor after failure of imatinib: a randomized controlled trial. Lancet. 2006;368(9544):1329–38.
47. Choi H, Charnsangavej C, Faria SC, et al. Correlation of computed tomography and positron emission tomography in patients with metastatic gastrointestinal stromal tumor treated at a single institution with imatinib mesylate: proposal of new computed tomography response criteria. J Clin Oncol. 2007;25(13):1753–9.
48. Benjamin RS, Choi H, Macapinlac HA, et al. We should desist using RECIST, at least in GIST. J Clin Oncol. 2007;25(13):1760–4.
49. Van den Abbeele AD. GIST Collaborative PET Study Group Dana-Farber Cancer Institute, Boston, Massachusetts; OHSU, Portland, Oregon, Helsinki University Central Hospital, Turku University Central Hospital,Finland, Novartis Oncology. F18-FDG-PET provides early evidence of biological response to STI571 in patients with malignant gastrointestinal stromal tumors (GIST). Proc Am Soc Clin Oncol. 2001;20:362a.
50. Antoch G, Kanja J, Bauer S, et al. Comparison of PET, CT, and dual-modality PET/CT imaging for monitoring of imatinib (STI571) therapy in patients with gastrointestinal stromal tumors. J Nucl Med. 2004;45(3):357–65.
51. Prior JO, Montemurro M, Orcurto MV, et al. Early prediction of response to sunitinib after imatinib failure by 18 F-fluorodeoxyglucose positron emission tomography in patients with gastrointestinal stromal tumor. J Clin Oncol. 2009;27(3):439–45.

Chapter 6
Cytogenetic and Molecular Aberrations as Predictive Biomarkers in Acute Myeloid Leukemia

Steffen Heeg and Cornelius F. Waller

Introduction

Persistent scientific efforts over the last decades have led to a better understanding of the biology of human cancer and the development of new therapeutic options, which significantly improved survival of cancer patients. With the dissection of the cellular pathways and molecular changes involved in malignant transformation of cells, human cancer has been characterized as a highly individual disease that significantly differs among patients.

Acute myeloid leukemia (AML) is a genetically heterogeneous clonal disorder of hematopoietic progenitor cells in which the physiologic mechanisms of self-renewal, proliferation, and differentiation are altered by the accumulation of genetic aberrations [1]. In recent years, several genetic alterations have been identified as potential therapeutic targets and as prognostic parameters for survival of AML patients. A prognostic biomarker provides information about the patients overall outcome, regardless of the therapy [2]. In contrast, the presence or absence of a predictive biomarker can be used to project a patient's response to a certain therapeutic intervention. Predictive biomarkers are therefore helpful tools to indentify the most beneficial treatment regimen for an individual patient and are an important step towards tailored anti-cancer strategies.

Prognostic markers in AML have been identified in numerous studies over the last decade. Marcucci et al. provided a very detailed review on the prognostic and therapeutic implications of genetic alterations in AML in which they accurately integrate the extensive and in part conflicting data published on prognostic markers in AML (Table 6.1) [3].

S. Heeg, M.D. • C.F. Waller, M.D. (✉)
Department of Hematology and Oncology, University of Freiburg Medical Center, Hugstetter Str. 55, Freiburg 79106, Germany
e-mail: cornelius.waller@uniklinik-freiburg.de

H.-J. Lenz (ed.), *Biomarkers in Oncology: Prediction and Prognosis*,
DOI 10.1007/978-1-4419-9755-5_6, © Springer Science+Business Media New York 2013

Table 6.1 Selected genetic aberrations with prognostic and/or predictive significance in AML

Marker	Prognostic significance (according to [52])	Predictive significance
NPM1	Mutated NPM1 without FLT3-ITD predicts a higher CR rate, favorable RFS and OS in younger patients Favorable impact of NPM1 mutations in older patients	Mutated NPM1 without FLT3-ITD predicts sensitivity to ATRA in older AML patients [20]
FLT3		
ITD	Associated with inferior outcome, allogeneic HSCT should be considered	Absence of FLT3-ITD together with NPM1 mutation predicts ATRA sensitivity in older AML patients [20] Controversial data on the significance of FLT3-ITD in the prediction of response to FLT3-tyrosine kinase inhibitors [48–50]
TKD	Prognostic significance controversial	No data available
CEBPA	Double mutations associated with higher CR rate and favorable RFS and OS	No data available
RAS	No prognostic significance shown	Mutant NRAS may predict sensitivity to cytarabine [40]
IDH1, IDH2	IDH1 and possibly IDH2 mutations confer higher risk of relapse and inferior OS in molecular low-risk cytogenetically normal AML	No data available
KIT	Mutations associated with inferior outcome in CBF-AML	No data available

By contrast, the role of predictive biomarkers in AML is less clear. This chapter provides an overview of the current level of knowledge about the value of cytogenetic changes and molecular aberrations in the prediction of response to AML treatment.

Cytogenetics

Clonal chromosomal aberrations can be detected in the majority of patients (55–60%) with acute myeloid leukemia. In recent years the role of different cytogenetic changes in AML has been extensively studied and recognized as the most important prognostic factor for the achievement of complete remission, risk of relapse and overall survival [4, 5]. This led to the classification of AML into three cytogenetic risk groups (Fig. 6.1).

Nevertheless, little is known about the role of cytogenetic abnormalities for the prediction of response to certain AML therapy regimens. The first evidence for a potential role of cytogenetics in response prediction came from a prospective, randomized clinical trial conducted by the Cancer and Leukemia Group B (CALGB) [6],

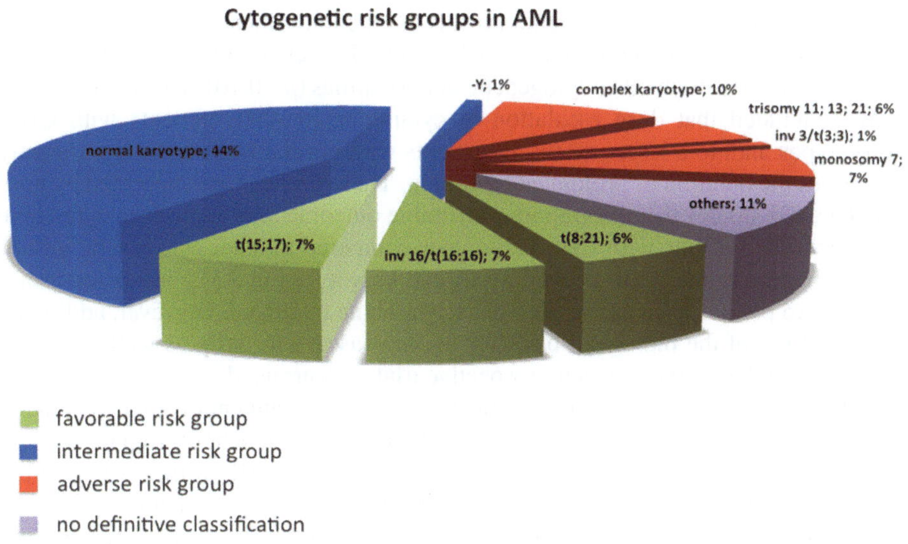

Fig. 6.1 Cytogenetic risk groups in AML (based on data from [5, 51])

evaluating the role of cytarabine dose escalation in postremission therapy of AML. In this trial patients aged 16 years or older with newly diagnosed AML were treated with 3 days of daunorubicin and 7 days of cytarabine. Patients who reached a complete remission were randomly assigned to receive four courses of cytarabine at one of three doses: 100 mg/m^2 of body-surface area per day for 5 days by continuous infusion (group A), 400 mg/m^2 per day for 5 days by continuous infusion (group B), or 3 g/m^2 in a 3-h infusion every 12 h (twice daily) on days 1, 3, and 5 (group C). Indeed, the duration of complete remission for all patients was related to the cytarabine dose. The probability of remaining in continuous complete remission after 4 years for patients 60 years of age or younger was 24% in group A, 29% in group B, and 44% group C, respectively. Bloomfield et al. consecutively assessed the response duration to the various cytarabine regimens by cytogenetic subtype [7]. Patients were categorized to one of three cytogenetic groups:

1. CBF-karyotypes: t(8;21)(q22;q22), t(16;16)(p13;q22), del(16)(q22), or inv(16)(p13q22)) karyotypes.
2. Normal karyotype.
3. Other abnormal karyotype.

It could be demonstrated that not all cytogenetic subgroups benefit from an increased dose of cytarabine. In patients with CBF-karyotypes remission duration was extended with increasing doses of cytarabine with 78% of the patients still in complete remission after 5 years in group C. In group B 57% of the patients were still in complete remission after 5 years compared to only 16% in the low dose AraC group

($p<0.001$). Interestingly, this benefit of cytarabine intensification was less obvious in patients with normal karyotypes (40% versus 37% versus 20%; $p=0.01$) and was absent in patients with other cytogenetic abnormalities ($p=0.10$). The authors therefore concluded that dose escalation of cytarabine in AML patients with CBF-karyotypes and, to a lesser extent, in patients with normal karyotypes significantly increases the duration of prolonged remission. These findings are supported by non-randomized studies that also report a favorable outcome after high-dose cytarabine treatment for patients with CBF-karyotypes compared to other cytogenetic groups [8, 9]. In conclusion, CBF as well as normal karyotypes in AML blasts are useful markers to predict response to high-dose cytarabine treatment. However, additional investigation of the biological basis for the increased sensitivity as well as further validation in larger randomized prospective trials is warranted.

The development of new therapeutic agents for the treatment of AML will inevitably lead to the question which subgroup of patients might benefit from these modern drugs. One of the questions addressed by the MRC AML15 trial was whether patients benefit from the addition of the immuno-conjugate gemtuzumab ozogamicin (GO) to induction or consolidation therapy regimens. Preliminary results support the application of 3 mg/m^2 gemtuzumab ozogamicin with standard- and high-dose cytarabine and anthracyclines for the treatment of de novo AML. While the rate of complete remission showed no significant difference, the risk for relapse could be significantly reduced, resulting in an improved disease-free survival. In particular, favorable and intermediate risk groups benefit from the addition of gemtuzumab ozogamicin with regard to relapse risk and disease free survival, respectively [10, 11]. These promising but rather preliminary results need to be further validated with further follow up of the study as well as in other randomized clinical trials before definitive conclusions can be drawn.

Molecular Markers

Nucleophosmin1 (NPM1)

Nucleophosmin1 (NPM1) is a nucleolar phosphoprotein encoded in the chromosomal region 5q35 with pleiotropic cellular functions. Besides its interaction with the tumor suppressors p53 and p19(Arf) it is thought to be indispensable for ribogenesis, intracellular trafficking of proteins, cell proliferation, and survival after DNA damage. Several alterations of the NPM1 gene such as mutations and deletions have been described in hematologic neoplasms. NPM1 is also involved in chromosomal translocations, e.g., t(5;17) (q35;q21) present in a rare variant of acute promyelocytic leukemia (APL) and resulting in the expression of the NPM1-RARA fusion protein. The fusion protein exhibits abnormal transcriptional activity and has been shown to be sensitive to treatment with all-trans retinoic acid (ATRA) [12, 13]. NPM1 mutations are the most frequent genetic alteration in adult AML but occur less frequently in pediatric AML [1]. They can be found in 45–64% of cytogenetically normal AML.

In 2005, Falini et al. were able to show that NPM1 exon 12 mutations lead to the creation of a new nuclear export signal motif and consecutive cytoplasmic translocation of NPM1 [14]. The loss of nuclear NPM1 is assumed to influence the function of the tumor suppressor p53 leading to genetic instability [15].

It has been demonstrated that NPM1 mutations are associated with a better prognosis in patients with AML [16–18]. However, the advantage of NPM1 mutations is restricted to the subgroup of patients without an additional FLT3-ITD mutation. In a large, retrospective study published by Thiede et al. the rate of cumulative relapse in patients with a normal karyotype harboring a NPM1 mutation was significantly lower compared to NPM1 wild type (25% versus 33%, $p=0,004$). In contrast, no significant difference could be observed in the presence of an additional internal tandem duplication within the FLT3-Gene (FLT3-ITD) constitutively activating the FLT3-receptor tyrosine kinase [16].

While the prognostic value of NPM1 mutations has been shown unanimously in large clinical studies, the role of NPM1 mutations as a marker to predict response to a certain therapy is less clear. The first evidence that NPM1 mutations might also be of predictive value came from the AML 98B trial (German-Austrian AML Study Group). This study demonstrated that administration of ATRA in addition to intensive chemotherapy improved the outcome of patients 61 years of age and older [19]. Furthermore, it could be shown that patients treated with ATRA had a significantly higher rate of complete remission and a better event-free and overall survival, respectively, with a 4-year relapse free survival of 20.9% ($p=0.006$) and an overall survival rate of 10.8% ($p=0.003$) compared to 4.8% and 5% in the standard treatment arm. The authors hypothesized that the beneficial effect of ATRA may be restricted to a specific biological subgroup of AML. To prove that hypothesis data from mutation analyses of the NPM1, CEBPA, FLT3, and MLL genes were correlated with outcome in patients 61 years of age and older treated within the AML HD98B trial. Response was assessed after the second course of induction chemotherapy. 114 (47%) of the 242 patients randomized for ATRA achieved a complete remission. Logistic regression analysis revealed that mutant NPM1 was significantly associated with achievement of complete remission (odds ratio 3.17; 95% CI 1.37–7.35; $p=0.02$). No significant impact was found for the molecular aberrations FLT3-ITD, FLT3-TDK and MLL-PTD. The median follow up for survival was 68.5 months. Survival analyses and evaluation of potential predictive factors for treatment outcome were performed on an intention-to-treat basis and revealed a significant difference in both relapse-free (HR 0.27; CI 0.07–0.95; $p=0.04$) and overall survival (HR 0.28; CI 0.11–0.75; $p=0.01$), respectively in favor of the experimental ATRA arm in patients harboring mutant NPM1 in the absence of a FLT3-ITD [20].

The molecular mechanisms of the ATRA-induced and NPM1-dependent effects in AML remain elusive. Potential explanations imply the role of NPM1 as a transcriptional corepressor during ATRA-induced cell differentiation and a selective downregulation of the mutant NPM1 protein by ATRA [21, 22].

Interestingly, other trials evaluating a potential beneficial effect of ATRA in addition to intensive chemotherapy in AML treatment did not show a positive effect [23–25]. One reason for the discrepant trial results might be the differing schedules of ATRA administration. As suggested by in vitro experimental data, a synergistic effect of ATRA might be only observed when ATRA is administered after exposure to cytotoxic drugs [26, 27]. In these studies the administration of ATRA started prior or simultaneously with chemotherapy. In contrast, in the AML HD98B trial, ATRA was started on the third day of chemotherapy, a time point when a significant proportion of cytotoxic drugs had already been administered. The findings of this study are currently being validated prospectively in patients treated in the AMLSG 07-04 trial protocol to further evaluate the role of mutant NPM1 and other biomarkers as predictive factors for therapy response.

Chevallier et al. investigated the influence of the NPM1/FLT3-ITD status on outcome in relapsed and refractory AML patients with normal karyotype, who received a salvage regimen using gemtuzumab ozogamicin as monotherapy or in combination with other agents. In this smaller series of 57 patients overall survival was increased (78% versus 36% at 2 years, $p=0.026$) in patients with mutant NPM1 in the absence of a FLT3-ITD, indicating a potential role of NPM1 in the prediction of response to treatment with gemtuzumab ozogamicin. However, the differences in rates of complete remission and relapse were not significant and further evaluation in larger studies will be mandatory [28].

Ras Mutations

Alterations in the Ras oncogene family are frequent and well-characterized genetic changes in myeloid disorders [29, 30]. Three human Ras genes encode four different proteins, namely, H-Ras, N-Ras, and the 2 K-Ras splicing variants K-Ras4A and K-Ras4B. Ras functions as a regulatory GTP-hydrolase switching back and forth between its activated and inactivated state. Ras takes the center stage within the Ras-dependent cellular signaling pathways involved in the complex regulation of proliferation, differentiation, and survival. Ras mutations can result in the inactivation of the GTPase reaction leaving Ras in its active GTP-bound state [31, 32]. In this constitutively active state Ras contributes to proliferative and antiapoptotic signals critical for myeloid leukemogenesis.

In AML activating point mutations could be shown to affect almost exclusively N-Ras and K-Ras at codons 12, 13 and 6 [33]. Ras mutations can be found in varying frequencies of about 20% (some authors report more than 48%) of AML being one of the most common genetic alterations in AML [34].

Despite the frequent occurrence of Ras mutations in AML the prognostic significance of Ras mutations has not been firmly established, as existing data remain conflicting. While several studies indicate poor clinical outcomes [35] for patients with Ras mutations other authors reported a similar [36] or even better prognosis [33] compared to patients with wild type Ras. While data on the prognostic significance of Ras mutations remain conflicting, even less is known about its role in the prediction of response to a specific AML therapy. The first line of evidence that activated or mutated Ras may sensitize leukemia and other tumor cells to the treatment with chemotherapeutic agents came from Koo et al. almost 20 years ago. These in vitro-analyses revealed a striking correlation with cytarabine sensitivity in the cell lines harboring Ras mutations compared to tumor lines with wild-type Ras alleles [37]. Later studies showed that Ras mutations indicate poor prognosis in untreated non-small-cell lung cancer (NSCLC), whereas in NSCLC or AML treated with chemotherapy, Ras mutations were associated with a better outcome [33, 38], indicating a role of Ras mutations in sensitization to chemotherapy. The constitutive activation of Ras signaling is not restricted to activating mutations of Ras alone and can also be induced by alterations in receptor tyrosine kinases or other members of the signaling pathway upstream of Ras. In a study correlating Ras mutations and Ras activation with outcome in 191 AML patients treated with chemotherapy including cytarabine, only 22.2% of the patients with Ras mutations showed activated Ras signaling. In this context, Ras mutations also were not associated with treatment response. In contrast, patients with strong Ras activity were more likely to achieve a complete remission than their Ras-inactive counterparts, with the strongest association found in younger patients treated with high-dose cytarabine (89.5% versus 55.6%; $p<0.05$). While an increased overall survival could be observed in this group disease-free survival and relapse rate were not affected [39]. The strong positive correlation of Ras activity and induction of remission in younger AML patients might be explained by the fact that in this study, patients younger than 61 years of age received far higher doses of cytarabine than older patients.

These results demonstrate that higher levels of Ras activity might confer increased sensitivity to the treatment with cytarabine and these patients might benefit from higher doses.

More compelling evidence is coming from a retrospective study by Neubauer et al. that correlates Ras mutation status and outcome in 185 AML patients treated with cytarabine as postremission therapy [40]. Patients were enrolled into the CALGB trial 8525 comparing the duration of complete remission and overall survival after postremission treatment with high (3 g/m^2 or 400 mg/m^2) or standard doses of cytarabine (100 mg/m^2), respectively. While there was no significant difference in outcome between patients who had Ras mutations compared to those with wild-type Ras, results were considerably different when Ras mutation status and cytarabine dosage where taken into account. Although therapy with high-dose cytarabine resulted in a lower rate of relapse both in patients with and without Ras mutations, the dose of cytarabine for consolidation therapy had greater impact on patients with Ras mutations (hazard ratio for high dose versus low dose cytarabine=0.28; $p=0.002$) than on those with wild-type Ras (HR=0.67; $p=0.044$). Notably, more than 50% of patients with mutated Ras treated with high-dose cytarabine remained in remission. The authors claim that this result might be explained by the findings of Koo et al., who demonstrated that cells harboring an activated Ras oncogene fail to arrest in the S-phase of the cell cycle in response to cytarabine treatment which results in their apoptotic death. In contrast, tumor cells with wild-type *RAS* genes undergo marked S-phase growth arrest on exposure to cytarabine that is reversible once the drug is removed. Thus, the presence of Ras mutations may change cellular response to cytarabine from cytostatic to cytotoxic, most likely because of altered cellular checkpoint functions in response to cytarabine [41].

In summary, alterations of the Ras signaling pathway by Ras mutations itself or activation of receptor tyrosine kinases upstream of Ras might constitute a novel molecular marker useful to identify AML patients that would benefit from treatment with high-dose cytarabine. As present data came from retrospective analyses, a large prospective randomized trial will be needed to confirm these promising results and further evaluate the clinical use of Ras as a prognostic as well as a predictive molecular biomarker.

FLT3 Mutations

Mutations in the fms-related tyrosine kinase 3 gene (FLT3) can be found in approximately 40% of patients with cytogenetically normal acute myeloid leukemia (AML), being one of the most frequently affected genes in AML [20].

The FLT3 gene is located in the chromosomal region 13q12, coding for a class III receptor tyrosine kinase, which is mainly involved in differentiation and proliferation of hematopoietic stem cells.

To date, three clusters of activating mutations have been identified: *FLT3* internal tandem duplications (*FLT3*-ITDs) in approximately 30%, point mutations within the activation loop of the second tyrosine kinase domain (*FLT3*-TKD) in 7–10% and, in a very low frequency (~2%), point mutations in the juxtamembrane domain (JMD) as well as in the extracellular domain [42]. In recent years, the prognostic value of FLT3-mutations has been extensively studied. In these studies FLT3-ITDs were associated with a higher risk of relapse and shorter overall and progression-free survival, respectively [43–45]. In contrast, the role of FLT3 mutations as predictive markers for response to certain therapeutic regimens or agents is less clear.

As described earlier in this chapter the absence of a FLT3-ITD in combination with a mutated NPM1 gene is associated with a significantly improved relapse free and overall survival in older patients treated with all-trans retinoic acid (ATRA) [20]. This is the first study on the predictive value of FLT3-ITD indicating that FLT3-ITD might be a useful tool in the prediction of therapy response to ATRA. Data from the AMLSG 07-04 trial in which patients younger than 61 years of age were recruited will help to further characterize the role of FLT3-ITD and NPM1 mutations as predictive biomarkers in that subgroup of patients.

More evidence that FLT3-ITDs alter chemotherapy response and therefore may be a useful predictive biomarker comes from a genetically defined mouse model of AML in which Pardee and coworkers examined the effects of the FLT3-ITDs on response to cytarabine and doxorubicin in vitro and in vivo. In this model FLT3-ITDs conferred resistance to treatment with doxorubicin alone and doxorubicine plus cytarabine, but sensitivity to cytarabine alone. The resistance could be reverted by the treatment with the FLT3-inhibitor sorafenib underlining the role of the FLT3 aberration in that setting [46]. The authors speculate that patients with FLT3-ITD positive AML may not benefit from the treatment with an anthracycline in the absence of a FLT3-inhibitor. Further studies in human in vitro and xenograft models will be needed to prove these findings in human AML and finally warrant clinical trials that analyze the role of FLT3-ITD and FLT3-inhibition in resistance to anthracyclines.

The important role of FLT3 in the development of AML and its association with inferior therapy outcome have made it an attractive molecular target for the development of new therapeutics. In recent years FLT3-inhibitors have been tested in various clinical trials both alone and in combination with chemotherapy. Several studies aimed to analyze the role of FLT3 mutations in the response to treatment with FLT3-inhibitors. Midostaurin is an orally available potent inhibitor of the FLT3-tyrosine kinase that inhibits both wild-type FLT3 and FLT3 with a mutated tyrosine kinase domain or an internal tandem duplication [47]. As FLT3 is overexpressed in many patients with AML, it is possible that inhibition of FLT3 could have therapeutic benefit in patients with either mutant or wild-type FLT3. In a phase-IIb trial Fischer et al. investigated the role of midostaurin in patients with AML and high-risk myelodysplastic (MDS) syndrome with either wild-type or mutated FLT3. Ninety-five patients with AML or MDS with either wild-type ($n=60$) or mutated ($n=35$) FLT3 were randomly assigned to receive oral midostaurin at 50 mg or 100 mg twice daily. Both patients with FLT3-mutant and wild-type responded to midostaurin, but only one patient (1%) showed a partial response and no complete remission has been achieved. In contrast, reduction of blasts (BR) was frequently observed, occurring in 71% of patients with FLT3-mutant and 42% of patients with FLT3 wild-type [48]. Biological responses also occurred in patients with no documented mutation of FLT3, although in a lower frequency compared to the FLT3-mutant population, indicating a role for midostaurin especially in the treatment of FLT3-mutated AML. Interestingly, the investigators observed no differences in the blast responses according to type of FLT3 mutation. In contrast, a previous study demonstrated that the response of blast cells from 11 patients with a mutation in the FLT3-tyrosine kinase domain to the FLT3-inhibitor lestaurtinib was significantly less than that of FLT3/ITD positive cells but similar to FLT3 wild-type cells [49]. Furthermore, Pratz and coworkers demonstrated that ex vivo samples of patients with a high mutant allelic burden were more likely to be responsive to FLT3 inhibition compared to the samples with a low mutant allelic burden [50].

These results have important implications for the potential therapeutic use of FLT3 inhibitors in patients with FLT3-mutant AML and suggest a potential role for FLT3-aberrations in the prediction of response to FLT3-inhibition. The controversial data from preclinical and clinical studies indicate the importance of further investigation to ultimately clarify in which setting FLT3-aberrations can be used as predictive biomarker.

In conclusion, the prognostic significance of several cytogenetic as well as molecular aberrations in AML has been well established. However, their predictive value is less well characterized as summarized in Table 6.1.

The current knowledge has led to the development of the first targeted therapies and predictive information to guide therapeutic decisions is needed to further individualize the treatment of AML patients. The development of new molecular biological techniques such as gene- and micro-RNA-expression profiling or next generation sequencing will provide further insight into the mechanisms of disease and identify new genetic profiles that might be potential candidates in the prediction of treatment response. The translation of this new information into the clinical situation will be a major future challenge that needs to be addressed in collaborative prospective multicenter studies.

References

1. Dohner K, Dohner H. Molecular characterization of acute myeloid leukemia. Haematologica. 2008;93:976–82.
2. Oldenhuis CN, Oosting SF, Gietema JA, de Vries EG. Prognostic versus predictive value of biomarkers in oncology. Eur J Cancer. 2008;44:946–53.
3. Marcucci G, Haferlach T, Dohner H. Molecular genetics of adult acute myeloid leukemia: prognostic and therapeutic implications. J Clin Oncol. 2011;29:475–86.
4. Mrozek K, Marcucci G, Paschka P, Whitman SP, Bloomfield CD. Clinical relevance of mutations and gene-expression changes in adult acute myeloid leukemia with normal cytogenetics: are we ready for a prognostically prioritized molecular classification? Blood. 2007;109: 431–48.
5. Estey E, Dohner H. Acute myeloid leukaemia. Lancet. 2006;368:1894–907.
6. Summers K, Stevens J, Kakkas I, et al. Wilms' tumour 1 mutations are associated with FLT3-ITD and failure of standard induction chemotherapy in patients with normal karyotype AML. Leukemia. 2007;21:550–1 [author reply 2].
7. Bloomfield CD, Lawrence D, Byrd JC, et al. Frequency of prolonged remission duration after high-dose cytarabine intensification in acute myeloid leukemia varies by cytogenetic subtype. Cancer Res. 1998;58:4173–9.
8. Ghaddar HM, Plunkett W, Kantarjian HM, et al. Long-term results following treatment of newly-diagnosed acute myelogenous leukemia with continuous-infusion high-dose cytosine arabinoside. Leukemia. 1994;8:1269–74.
9. Anderlini P, Ghaddar HM, Smith TL, et al. Factors predicting complete remission and subsequent disease-free survival after a second course of induction therapy in patients with acute myelogenous leukemia resistant to the first. Leukemia. 1996;10:964–9.
10. Burnett AK. The addition of gemtuzumab ozogamicin to induction chemotherapy for AML improves disease free survival without extra toxicity. Preliminary analysis of 1115 patients in the MTC AML15 trial. Blood. 2006;106:8a.
11. Gleissner B, Schlenk R, Bornhauser M, Berdel WE. Gemtuzumab ozogamicin (mylotarg) for the treatment of acute myeloid leukemia—ongoing trials. Onkologie. 2007;30:657–62.
12. Redner RL, Corey SJ, Rush EA. Differentiation of t(5;17) variant acute promyelocytic leukemic blasts by all-trans retinoic acid. Leukemia. 1997;11:1014–6.
13. Redner RL, Chen JD, Rush EA, Li H, Pollock SL. The t(5;17) acute promyelocytic leukemia fusion protein NPM-RAR interacts with co-repressor and co-activator proteins and exhibits both positive and negative transcriptional properties. Blood. 2000;95:2683–90.
14. Falini B, Mecucci C, Tiacci E, et al. Cytoplasmic nucleophosmin in acute myelogenous leukemia with a normal karyotype. N Engl J Med. 2005;352:254–66.
15. Chen W, Rassidakis GZ, Medeiros LJ. Nucleophosmin gene mutations in acute myeloid leukemia. Arch Pathol Lab Med. 2006;130:1687–92.

16. Thiede C, Koch S, Creutzig E, et al. Prevalence and prognostic impact of NPM1 mutations in 1485 adult patients with acute myeloid leukemia (AML). Blood. 2006;107:4011–20.
17. Schnittger S, Schoch C, Kern W, et al. Nucleophosmin gene mutations are predictors of favorable prognosis in acute myelogenous leukemia with a normal karyotype. Blood. 2005;106: 3733–9.
18. Dohner K, Schlenk RF, Habdank M, et al. Mutant nucleophosmin (NPM1) predicts favorable prognosis in younger adults with acute myeloid leukemia and normal cytogenetics: interaction with other gene mutations. Blood. 2005;106:3740–6.
19. Schlenk RF, Frohling S, Hartmann F, et al. Phase III study of all-trans retinoic acid in previously untreated patients 61 years or older with acute myeloid leukemia. Leukemia. 2004;18:1798–803.
20. Schlenk RF, Dohner K, Kneba M, et al. Gene mutations and response to treatment with all-trans retinoic acid in elderly patients with acute myeloid leukemia. Results from the AMLSG Trial AML HD98B. Haematologica. 2009;94:54–60.
21. Liu H, Tan BC, Tseng KH, et al. Nucleophosmin acts as a novel AP2alpha-binding transcriptional corepressor during cell differentiation. EMBO Rep. 2007;8:394–400.
22. Martelli MP, Pettirossi V, Manes N, et al. Selective silencing of the NPM1 mutant protein and apoptosis induction upon ATRA in vitro treatment of AML cells carrying NPM1 mutations. Blood. 2007;110:868.
23. Estey EH, Thall PF, Pierce S, et al. Randomized phase II study of fludarabine + cytosine arabinoside + idarubicin +/– all-trans retinoic acid +/– granulocyte colony-stimulating factor in poor prognosis newly diagnosed acute myeloid leukemia and myelodysplastic syndrome. Blood. 1999;93:2478–84.
24. Burnett AK, Milligan D, Prentice AG, et al. A comparison of low-dose cytarabine and hydroxyurea with or without all-trans retinoic acid for acute myeloid leukemia and high-risk myelodysplastic syndrome in patients not considered fit for intensive treatment. Cancer. 2007;109:1114–24.
25. Milligan DW, Wheatley K, Littlewood T, Craig JI, Burnett AK. Fludarabine and cytosine are less effective than standard ADE chemotherapy in high-risk acute myeloid leukemia, and addition of G-CSF and ATRA are not beneficial: results of the MRC AML-HR randomized trial. Blood. 2006;107:4614–22.
26. Ketley NJ, Allen PD, Kelsey SM, Newland AC. Modulation of idarubicin-induced apoptosis in human acute myeloid leukemia blasts by all-trans retinoic acid, 1,25(OH)2 vitamin D3, and granulocyte-macrophage colony-stimulating factor. Blood. 1997;90:4578–87.
27. Andreeff M, Jiang S, Zhang X, et al. Expression of Bcl-2-related genes in normal and AML progenitors: changes induced by chemotherapy and retinoic acid. Leukemia. 1999;13:1881–92.
28. Chevallier P, Prebet T, Pigneux A, et al. Influence of NPM1 and FLT3-ITD status on outcome in relapsed/refractory AML patients receiving salvage therapy including gemtuzumab ozogamicin. Leukemia. 2009;24(2):467–9.
29. Li Q, Haigis KM, McDaniel A, et al. Hematopoiesis and leukemogenesis in mice expressing oncogenic NrasG12D from the endogenous locus. Blood. 2011;117(6):2022–32.
30. Bacher U, Haferlach T, Schoch C, Kern W, Schnittger S. Implications of NRAS mutations in AML: a study of 2502 patients. Blood. 2006;107:3847–53.
31. Vigil D, Cherfils J, Rossman KL, Der CJ. Ras superfamily GEFs and GAPs: validated and tractable targets for cancer therapy? Nat Rev Cancer. 2010;10:842–57.
32. Ahmadian MR, Zor T, Vogt D, et al. Guanosine triphosphatase stimulation of oncogenic Ras mutants. Proc Natl Acad Sci U S A. 1999;96:7065–70.
33. Neubauer A, Dodge RK, George SL, et al. Prognostic importance of mutations in the ras proto-oncogenes in de novo acute myeloid leukemia. Blood. 1994;83:1603–11.
34. Reuter CW, Morgan MA, Bergmann L. Targeting the Ras signaling pathway: a rational, mechanism-based treatment for hematologic malignancies? Blood. 2000;96:1655–69.
35. Kiyoi H, Naoe T, Nakano Y, et al. Prognostic implication of FLT3 and N-RAS gene mutations in acute myeloid leukemia. Blood. 1999;93:3074–80.

36. Ritter M, Kim TD, Lisske P, Thiede C, Schaich M, Neubauer A. Prognostic significance of N-RAS and K-RAS mutations in 232 patients with acute myeloid leukemia. Haematologica. 2004;89:1397–9.
37. Koo HM, Monks A, Mikheev A, et al. Enhanced sensitivity to 1-beta-D-arabinofuranosylcytosine and topoisomerase II inhibitors in tumor cell lines harboring activated ras oncogenes. Cancer Res. 1996;56:5211–6.
38. Rodenhuis S, Boerrigter L, Top B, et al. Mutational activation of the K-ras oncogene and the effect of chemotherapy in advanced adenocarcinoma of the lung: a prospective study. J Clin Oncol. 1997;15:285–91.
39. Illmer T, Thiede C, Fredersdorf A, et al. Activation of the RAS pathway is predictive for a chemosensitive phenotype of acute myelogenous leukemia blasts. Clin Cancer Res. 2005;11:3217–24.
40. Neubauer A, Maharry K, Mrozek K, et al. Patients with acute myeloid leukemia and RAS mutations benefit most from postremission high-dose cytarabine: a Cancer and Leukemia Group B study. J Clin Oncol. 2008;26:4603–9.
41. Koo HM, McWilliams MJ, Alvord WG. Vande Woude GF. Ras oncogene-induced sensitization to 1-beta-D-arabinofuranosylcytosine. Cancer Res. 1999;59:6057–62.
42. Kayser S, Schlenk RF, Correa Londono M, et al. Insertion of FLT3 internal tandem duplication in the tyrosine kinase domain-1 is associated with resistance to chemotherapy and inferior outcome. Blood. 2009;114:2386–92.
43. Frohling S, Schlenk RF, Breitruck J, et al. Prognostic significance of activating FLT3 mutations in younger adults (16 to 60 years) with acute myeloid leukemia and normal cytogenetics: a study of the AML Study Group Ulm. Blood. 2002;100:4372–80.
44. Kottaridis PD, Gale RE, Frew ME, et al. The presence of a FLT3 internal tandem duplication in patients with acute myeloid leukemia (AML) adds important prognostic information to cytogenetic risk group and response to the first cycle of chemotherapy: analysis of 854 patients from the United Kingdom Medical Research Council AML 10 and 12 trials. Blood. 2001;98:1752–9.
45. Stirewalt DL, Kopecky KJ, Meshinchi S, et al. Size of FLT3 internal tandem duplication has prognostic significance in patients with acute myeloid leukemia. Blood. 2006;107:3724–6.
46. Pardee TS, Zuber J, Lowe SW. The Flt3 internal tandem duplication alters chemotherapy response in vitro and in vivo in a p53-dependent manner. Exp Hematol. 2011;39(4):473.e4–85.e4.
47. Sanz M, Burnett A, Lo-Coco F, Lowenberg B. FLT3 inhibition as a targeted therapy for acute myeloid leukemia. Curr Opin Oncol. 2009;21:594–600.
48. Fischer T, Stone RM, Deangelo DJ, et al. Phase IIB trial of oral Midostaurin (PKC412), the FMS-like tyrosine kinase 3 receptor (FLT3) and multi-targeted kinase inhibitor, in patients with acute myeloid leukemia and high-risk myelodysplastic syndrome with either wild-type or mutated FLT3. J Clin Oncol. 2010;28:4339–45.
49. Mead AJ, Gale RE, Kottaridis PD, Matsuda S, Khwaja A, Linch DC. Acute myeloid leukaemia blast cells with a tyrosine kinase domain mutation of FLT3 are less sensitive to lestaurtinib than those with a FLT3 internal tandem duplication. Br J Haematol. 2008;141:454–60.
50. Pratz KW, Sato T, Murphy KM, Stine A, Rajkhowa T, Levis M. FLT3-mutant allelic burden and clinical status are predictive of response to FLT3 inhibitors in AML. Blood. 2010;115: 1425–32.
51. Burnett A, Wetzler M, Lowenberg B. Therapeutic advances in acute myeloid leukemia. J Clin Oncol. 2011;29:487–94.
52. Marcucci G, Mrozek K, Radmacher MD, Garzon R, Bloomfield CD. The prognostic and functional role of microRNAs in acute myeloid leukemia. Blood. 2011;117:1121–9.

Chapter 7
Prognostic Markers in Colon Cancer

Janine M. Davies and Howard L. McLeod

Introduction

Colorectal cancers (CRC) are the fourth most common cancers in the USA and the second most common cause of death from cancer [1]. In 2009, an expected 146,970 new patients will be diagnosed with CRC, of which more than two-thirds will be colon cancers. In this same year, 49,920 will die of this disease [2]. While dramatic improvements have been made in the management of colon cancers including chemotherapy and targeted therapies, surgical resection of primary and metastatic lesions, and the palliation of incurable disease, means to more accurately assess prognosis beyond the standard staging systems have been elusive.

Overall, 5 year survival (OS) with CRC is 68%. However, prognosis is highly dependent on the stage at diagnosis. Among local cancers, i.e., the cancer does not extend beyond the bowel wall, the 5 year survival is 90%, but when lymph nodes are involved, it decreases to 70%, and survival further worsens with metastases, in which only 11% of patients are alive 5 years from diagnosis [2].

J.M. Davies, M.D., B.N., M.Sc. (✉)
Division of Hematology/Oncology, Lineberger Comprehensive Cancer Center,
University of North Carolina at Chapel Hill,
170 Manning Dr, CB 7305, Chapel Hill, NC 27516, USA
e-mail: janine_davies@med.unc.edu

H.L. McLeod, Pharm.D.
Department of Pharmacy, Eshelman School of Pharmacy,
University of North Carolina at Chapel Hill,
Chapel Hill, NC, USA

H.-J. Lenz (ed.), *Biomarkers in Oncology: Prediction and Prognosis*,
DOI 10.1007/978-1-4419-9755-5_7,

Data regarding survival following recurrence in colon cancer can be difficult to elicit due to limitations on collected registry data. The Adjuvant Colon Cancer End Points (ACCENT) data set is a compilation of data from stage II and III patients randomized to clinical trials using 5-fluorouracil (5FU)-based therapy [3]. Among patients initially diagnosed with stage II CRC whose disease eventually recurred, median OS was 18.2 months compared with 12.5 months for patients initially diagnosed with stage III disease (HR 0.70, $p<0.0001$) [3]. This is informative, but does not reflect newer therapies including oxaliplatin, irinotecan, or targeted therapies.

This chapter focuses on prognostic markers, including histologic, molecular, and genetic markers and reviews the data on the most clinically relevant markers and selected markers that may have potential to provide clinical guidance with further evaluation.

Prognostic Markers in Colon Cancer

An independent prognostic marker is one that, in the absence of treatment effects, is able to predict a patient's clinical outcome. An independent prognostic marker must provide additional information to that provided by stage and histologic information and cannot be an intermediary between clinical prognostic factors and outcome [4]. Its effects are best assessed in untreated patients as treatment is prognostic in and of itself and can bias the assessment. The best known prognostic marker in CRC at this time is the AJCC TNM staging system. Independent of treatment, each stage is predictive of prognosis.

In contrast to prognostic biomarkers, a predictive biomarker is one that can predict the clinical benefit of a given treatment in a given context. For example, k-ras mutational status is predictive of benefit from anti-EGFR therapies, but does not otherwise define clinical outcome. Predictive markers are discussed separately.

In the context of CRC, ideal prognostic markers will help guide the clinical management of patients. Based on TNM staging, physicians currently have crude opportunities to individualize treatment options depending on the stage at diagnosis. A prognostic marker developed for use in the preoperative setting may be less important when surgical resectability is technically possible. But postoperatively in stage II and III CRC, prognostic markers would be particularly important to identify those patients at higher risk of recurrence, and potentially determine those for whom adjuvant treatment options may be most relevant. Ideally, prognostic markers in this context would provide a clear distinction between people that do or do not require adjuvant therapy. In unresectable metastatic disease, identification of indolent versus more aggressive behaving phenotypes would be particularly important from both treatment and quality of life perspectives. With potentially resectable metastatic disease, identification of aggressive disease, in which the burden of resection may outweigh the potential benefit of treatment, would be important. Each prognostic biomarker should be tailored to a specific clinical setting during development to ensure rational implementation.

Established Prognostic Markers in Colon Cancers

Currently, established prognostic markers include TNM stage, certain pathologic features, and the number of evaluated lymph nodes (LNs). Other markers have been well evaluated, such as p53, but due to inconsistent findings, the prognostic role of such markers has yet to be elucidated. Lastly, certain markers are promising but have had insufficient evaluation, such as 18qLOH, CIN, and k-ras.

AJCC TNM Staging

Cancer staging is currently the best marker of prognosis in CRC. The TNM staging system by the AJCC provides a four stage classification in which outcome clearly worsens with increasing tumor dissemination, as reflected by increasing stage of disease [5]. The AJCC TNM staging system assesses three factors: (1) the depth of tumor invasion into the bowel wall; (2) the presence or absence of LN invasion and the number of involved nodes; and (3) the presence or absence of distant metastases. A T1 tumor reflects the least amount of tumor invasion (invading the submucosal layer only), and are progressively more invasive up to a T4 tumor in which the tumor penetrates the entire thickness of the bowel wall and invades nearby tissues and/or perforates the visceral peritoneum. LN status evaluation includes metastases in 0 (N0) versus 1–3 (N1) versus 4 or more lymph nodes (N2). Distant metastases are classified dichotomously, present (M1) or absent (M0). The TNM evaluations are then used to determine the stage of disease [5]. Survival is clearly better with lower stage of disease; however, even within stages there remain significant differences in outcomes.

In an evaluation of the AJCC 6th edition staging criteria based on SEER national cancer registry data of 119,363 colon cancer patients from 1991 to 2000, survival worsened with increasing stage of disease [6]. Additionally, within a given stage, outcomes varied significantly based on tumor or nodal status (Fig. 7.1). In fact, 5 year OS for stage IIb and IIIa was not significantly different, although there was a trend to better survival among the stage IIIa patients (i.e., among those with T1/T2 N1 disease vs. T3/4 N0 disease), suggesting that tumor depth of invasion was more important than LN involvement. Within stage III, 5 year OS worsened with increasing nodal status by approximately 20% [6]. This data highlights the importance of staging and nodal status as prognostic markers in colon cancer. This evaluation has not been repeated in the era of the use of adjuvant therapy, but would be particularly informative to evaluate stage II and III patients.

Colon cancer survival is better than that for rectal cancer in a stage for stage comparison. Survival for rectal cancer was evaluated using the National Cancer Data Base which compiled data from US cancer registries of 5,850,000 cancer diagnoses between 1985 and 1995 [7]. Five year survival by stage was 72% for stage I, 52% for stage II, 37% for stage III, and 4% for stage IV [7], all of which are

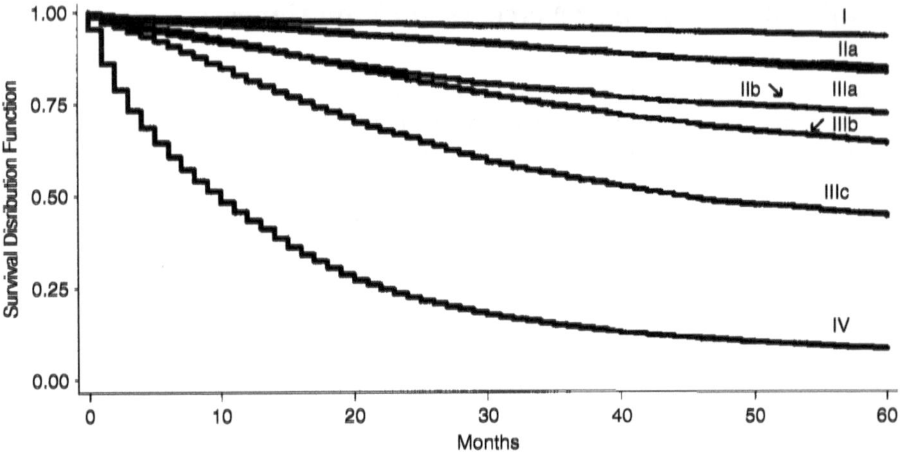

Stage	0 mo		30 mo			60 mo		
	Survival, %	NO.	Survival, %	NO.	*P*	Survival, %	NO.	*P*
I	100	14500	96.1	8,581	–	93.2	4514	–
IIa	100	28535	91.0	2,105	<.001	84.7	8494	<.001
IIb	100	5826	80.2	3,060	<.001*	72.2	1611	<.001*
IIIa	100	1989	91.4	1,120	NS†	83.4	551	NS†
IIIb	100	15946	77.3	7,786	<001‡	64.1	3579	<001‡
IIIc	100	8600	59.1	3,039	<.001	44.3	1250	<.001
IV	100	20802	17.3	1,832	<.001	8.1	432	<.001

Fig. 7.1 Five year overall survival for colon cancer by AJCC stage. (Based on data from ref. [6])

dramatically worse than for colon cancer. Again, this has not been reassessed with the use of adjuvant chemotherapy nor with newer treatments for metastatic disease.

More recently, the MOSAIC study compared adjuvant 5FU/leucovorin (LV) versus FOLFOX chemotherapy in stage II and III colon cancer patients [8]. Number of involved LNs was a prespecified prognostic factor. The improvement in the rate of relapse with the use of adjuvant FOLFOX was similar in patients with 0–3 versus 4 or more involved LNs [8].

While the TNM staging system is highly prognostic, it fails to identify a significant proportion of patients within each stage that recur. The identification of prognostic markers in early stage CRC would help to identify patients that have an increased risk of recurrence that could be further assessed in clinical trials of adjuvant therapy, and those for whom the risk of recurrence does not warrant further therapy.

Number of Evaluated Lymph Nodes

The negative prognostic implication of LNs with metastases has been noted at least since its initial description by Dr. Cuthbert Dukes in 1932 with regards to rectal cancer [9]. Most recently, this was demonstrated in the previously described SEER

Table 7.1 Colon cancer survival statistics based on stage and number of recovered lymph nodes, from the INT 0089 clinical trial

Stage	No. of lymph nodes	Overall survival (%)	P	Cause-specific survival (%)	P	Disease-free survival (%)	P
II	<11	73	<0.001	80	0.015	72	0.11
	11–20	80		85		79	
	>20	87		92		83	
IIIA–IIIB	<11	67	<0.001	74	0.002	65	<0.001
	11–40	74		78		70	
	>40	90		93		93	
IIIC	1–35	51	0.002	55	0.018	48	0.014
	>35	71		71		69	

(Based on data from refs. [10, 11])

data evaluation of the AJCC 6th edition staging classification for colon cancer [6]. An analysis was performed in which the number of involved LNs was subdivided beyond that outlined in the 6th edition: no LN involvement (stages I and II) were compared with 1–3, versus 4 or 5, versus 6–8, and 9 or more metastatic LNs, and with metastatic disease. There was a clear worsening of survival with greater numbers of involved LNs [6]. Interestingly, survival among patients with 1–3 involved LNs was better than that of stage IIb patients, again reflecting the impact of tumor depth of invasion.

The INT 0089 clinical trial assessed adjuvant therapy for stage II and III colon cancer and retrospectively assessed prognostic factors including both the actual number of LNs involved and the overall number of surgically recovered LNs [10]. This was based on retrospective data suggesting a survival benefit from a more thorough lymphadenectomy. Overall, the authors demonstrated that both the number of involved LNs and the number of recovered LNs were independent predictors of survival, and this benefit was present even among LN negative patients (Table 7.1) [10, 11]. However, some retrospective studies have not supported an extended lymphadenectomy to improve survival [12, 13].

Proposed reasons for improved survival with lymphadenectomy include better surgical technique among surgeons that perform a more complete lymphadenectomy, more thorough pathologic LN analysis, and a potential therapeutic benefit of the procedure itself. Additionally, because therapeutic decisions are made based on this information, understaged patients may not have the opportunity to consider adjuvant therapy. On the other hand, the inflammatory reaction may facilitate identification of LNs and inflammation itself may portend a better prognosis. While the Working Party Report to the World Congresses of Gastroenterology determined that a minimum sampling of 12 LNs is required to adequately stage a cancer [14], it is clear from the INT 0089 study that a lymphadenectomy of at least 20 LN is of benefit [10]. Other studies have validated that recovery of 14 or fewer LNs is prognostically negative in T3 and T4 LN negative tumors [15].

As such, the National Cancer Institute panel of experts in oncologic resections recommends that a minimum of 12 LNs should be pathologically examined to ensure that the nodes are not involved, with accuracy in excess of 90% [14].

Histologic and Pathologic Features

Certain histologic features have demonstrated important prognostic benefits in colon cancer.

An evaluation of SEER data demonstrated a statistically better 5 year survival with adenocarcinoma (66%, $p<0.001$) and mucinous adenocarcinoma histologies (62%, $p<0.001$) than with signet ring cell carcinoma (36%) among stage II, III, and IV colon cancer patients, but no difference for stage I patients [6].

By location, survival with colon cancer was better for lesions in the sigmoid colon (5 year OS 70%) than for other tumor locations (right colon 64%, $p<0.001$; transverse colon 65%, $p<0.001$; and left colon 65%, $p<0.001$), which was similarly found by stage in all but stage II colon cancers [6]. This may reflect the better prognosis afforded patients with MSI-H tumors that are more likely to be right-sided lesions and earlier stage.

While the majority of stage II colon cancers will not recur, attempts have been made to identify features that would identify tumors at high risk for recurrence. Pathologic features that are prognostically negative include: tumor penetration of the serosal layer surrounding the colon (T4) [15–17], perforation of the colonic wall [15, 16], bowel obstruction [15, 16], and lymphovascular invasion or perineural invasion [17]. As noted previously, lymphadenectomy of less than 12 LNs is also associated with a higher risk of recurrence.

Carcinoembryonic Antigen

Carcinoembryonic Antigen (CEA) is an oncofetal antigen in a family of related glycoproteins detectable in the serum that is overexpressed by many adenocarcinomas of the colon and rectum [18]. It is an imperfect marker of recurrence as approximately 30% of tumors do not express CEA, particularly among poorly differentiated tumors [18]. Additionally, CEA elevations can also occur with other factors such as smoking, inflammation, hepatitis, and colitis. CEA has an established role in surveillance monitoring following curative therapies for stage II and III CRC, and is reflected in various guidelines including ASCO and EGTM. However, its role as a prognostic factor is more limited.

In the preoperative setting with no detectable metastases, serum CEA levels are prognostic. Independent of stage, CEA levels above 2.5 ng/mL, and more so above 10 ng/mL, portend a poorer prognosis [19]. CEA levels in excess of 2.5 ng/mL were found in 28% of patients with Dukes' A disease, 45% with Dukes' B, 75% with Dukes' C, and 84% with Dukes' D disease [20]. Another early prospective study demonstrated that CEA levels less than 2.5 ng/mL and greater than 10 ng/mL are prognostic [21].

The use of perioperative CEA measurement in the prediction of cure among patients undergoing hepatic resection is a topic of significant interest as surgical techniques and chemotherapeutic agents have evolved. The best prognostic factors in the setting of liver resection, based on an analysis of 1,001 cases, were negative resection margins and the absence of extrahepatic disease [22], although a subsequent study of over 500 patients found that tumor size of less than 5 cm and three or fewer liver metastases were prognostically better, and that tumor margin was not an independent predictor [23]. In the setting of potentially curable metastatic disease, CEA measurement prior to resection is also advisable [24, 25].

In a prospective evaluation of CEA levels pre- and postcurative liver resections (including complete resection of all other known extrahepatic disease), 5 year OS was 36%, with a 5 year DFS rate of 18% [26]. Independent prognostic factors for OS in multivariate analyses were perioperative changes in CEA (RR 3.0, 95% CI 1.4–6.3, $p=0.003$), hepatic pedicle LN metastases (RR 3.9, 95% CI 1.9–8.2, $p<0.001$), and the number and size of liver metastases (RR 2.0, 95% CI 1.2–3.3, $p=0.008$, and RR 1.9, 95% CI 1.1–3.1, $p=0.02$, respectively). These factors were also significant for DFS, in addition to gender. Among initially resectable liver metastases, 5 year OS among patients with normal pre and post operative CEA levels (group A), elevated preoperative and normal postoperative CEA (group B), and elevated pre and post operative CEA levels (group C) were 55, 37, and 0% in groups A, B, and C respectively. Significant differences were noted between groups A and C ($p<0.001$) and groups B and C ($p<0.001$), but not between groups A and B ($p=0.24$). Among patients undergoing a staged hepatectomy, 5 year survival was not reached in group A, was 46% in group B, and 0% in group C, with a significant difference noted between groups B and C ($p=0.007$) [26]. This analysis was hampered by small patient numbers. This study clarifies the role of CEA as a prognostic factor for initially resectable liver metastases, particularly the benefit realized with normalization of postoperative CEA.

The prognostic benefit of preoperative CEA levels prior to colonic and hepatic resection is clear. Overall, the ASCO and EGTM guidelines recommend using a preoperative CEA level as a prognostic marker, including prior to liver resection [24, 25]. The EGTM guidelines specify using this in conjunction with standard prognostic factors.

Inconsistent or Contradictory Evidence

Microsatellite Instability

The mismatch repair (MMR) pathway is one proposed pathway of carcinogenesis. Microsatellites are repeating units of short DNA nucleotide segments that occur throughout the germline. Losses or gains of microsatellites can occur when the MMR enzyme is not functioning or is inactivated, resulting in DNA replication errors, with a consequent loss of function of the associated proteins which then allows malignant growth [27, 28]. An accumulation of mutations of single nucleotides and changes in microsatellite lengths are found in the tumor tissue as compared to adjacent normal tissue. High levels of microsatellite instability are labeled MSI-H; low levels are MSI-L or microsatellite stable (MSS). MSI-H is defined as instability of at least 30% of screened loci, MSI-L as less than 30% instability, and MSS as no evidence of instability at any of the loci, as per the NCI concensus definitions [29]. Since biologically MSI-L and MSS are similar, these categories are generally grouped together for assessment.

Germline mutations of MMR enzymes, predominantly MLH-1, MSH-2, and MSH-6, are found in a familial CRC condition associated with MSI called hereditary nonpolyposis colorectal cancer (HNPCC) or Lynch Syndrome [28], which accounts for 2–5% of CRC diagnoses [27]. Additionally, approximately 15–20% of sporadic colon cancers have a nonhereditary mutation of one of the MMR genes [27]. MSI-H status has been associated with increased OS in several retrospective studies [30–32], although not always as an independent prognostic indicator [33], and not consistently [34, 35].

Characteristic features of MSI-H tumors include right-sided colon cancers [27, 36]; mucinous, signet ring, or medullary histologic type; a pushing tumor border (as opposed to infiltrating); and with lymphocytic or inflammatory infiltration [27, 37–40]. HNPCC is often identified by younger age at diagnosis and a family history of CRC or other associated malignancies [36].

Population-based registry data from Ontario, Canada, was used to assess MSI status with regard to outcomes in patients aged 50 years or less [30]. MSI-L patients (3% of the study sample) were excluded due to insufficient patient numbers. Of 607 specimens, 17% were MSI-H and characterized by the expected features: increased depth of invasion, lower stage, poorly differentiated histology, proximal location, multiple synchronous or metachronous tumors, and younger age. By multivariate analyses, MSI-H and lower tumor depth were independently associated with decreased chance of metastases to LNs or distant organs. Five year OS among MSI-H patients was 76% (±4% SE) compared to 54% (±2% SE, $p<0.001$) for MSS, independent of stage. Prognosis was poorer among mucinous, signet ring, or undifferentiated histology, greater degree of dedifferentiation with increased stage, and MSS. Of note, the high incidence of MSI-H was likely reflective of the young population examined [30].

In a systematic review and meta-analysis of 32 studies reporting MSI status from 7,642 patients with CRC, of which 1,277 had MSI, a survival benefit for patients with MSI-H in comparison to MSS tumors was found (HR 0.65, 95% CI 0.59–0.71, p for heterogeneity = 0.16, p for publication bias >0.1) [41]. This effect was maintained when the data was analyzed by stage (HR 0.67, 95% CI 0.58–0.78, p for heterogeneity = 0.31) [41]. However, to confirm these findings, a prospective validation with a randomized control trial is required.

In the first prospective assessment of MSI status, based on randomized clinical trials for stage II and III CRC that compared adjuvant 5FU-based chemotherapy to no chemotherapy, data was used from five clinical trials: National Cancer Institute of Canada C.03, North Central Cancer Treatment Group protocols 784852 and 874651, Gastrointestinal Intergroup trial 0035 of the National Cancer Institute, and

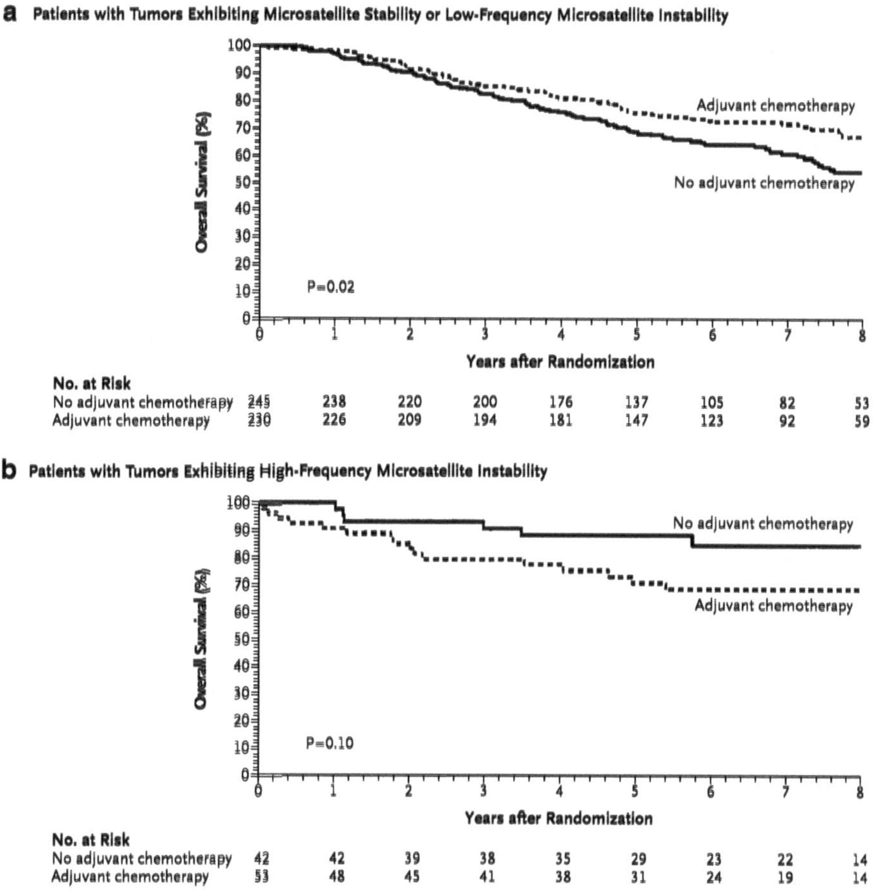

Fig. 7.2 Overall survival of patients with stage II and III CRC by MSI status. (**a**) No adjuvant chemotherapy. (**b**) Adjuvant chemotherapy. [Reprinted from Ribic CM, Sargent DJ, Moore MJ, et al. Tumor microsatellite-instability status as a predictor of benefit from fluorouracil-based adjuvant chemotherapy for colon cancer. N Engl J Med. 2003;349(3):247–257. With permission from Massachusetts Medical Society]

la Fondation Française de Cancérologie Digestive [42]. Overall, 570 specimens were tested, representing almost 30% of the patients on the various trials. Five year OS was 88% for MSI-H (95% CI 78.7–98.4) and 68% for MSS (95% CI 62.7–74.6, $p=0.004$); these patients were not treated with adjuvant chemotherapy (Fig. 7.2a). Multivariate analysis adjusted for stage and grade among patients not treated with adjuvant chemotherapy revealed that MSI-H was associated with improved survival (HR 0.32, 95% CI 0.14–0.75, $p=0.008$) [42]. Interestingly, when treatment effects were assessed, MSI-H patients did not derive benefit from the chemotherapy, whereas patients with MSS tumors seemed to benefit (Fig. 7.2b). This example highlights MSI as a prognostic factor, such that MSI-H tumors have a better prognosis, but as a predictive factor, only MSS tumors fared better with adjuvant chemotherapy.

MSI seems to have a stage associated prognostic benefit. MSI-H tumors have generally, but not entirely consistently, been associated with a better prognosis than MSS tumors, and with conflicting evidence with regards to its predictive ability for benefit from 5FU-based chemotherapy. Among Dukes stage B2 and C patients in one study, MSI-H was found in 26 and 14% of tumors respectively, but only found a survival benefit in the stage C tumors [32]. In mCRC, MSI-H has been identified in a minority of patients including less than 3% of patients with potentially resectable liver metastases [43]. In an evaluation of stage and MSI status, MSI-H tumors made up 14% of advanced cases compared to 53% of stages I through III disease ($p<0.001$), possibly reflecting a lower metastatic potential of these tumors [27]. The authors also hypothesized that the better prognostic outcomes with MSI was related to lymphocytic infiltration which may result in improved surveillance for cancer [27].

Among resectable liver metastases, there is some evidence to suggest that there is a low frequency of MSI-H tumors [43]. In patients with CRC, up to 40% will develop hepatic metastases, either at initial diagnosis or at the time of recurrence [43]. If resectable, a significant proportion of patients experience long term survival or cure, with 3, 5, and 10 year survival of 57, 37, and 22% respectively, based on a consecutive series of 1,001 patients [22]. Among 190 consecutive patients with resected liver metastases, only 5 patients (2.7%) had MSI-H tumors by RT-PCR, all of which were hMLH1 deficient [43]. A trend to improved survival was seen among MSI-H patients compared to MSS, although the study was hampered by small numbers [43]. However, this study suggests that with such a small rate of MSI-H tumors, that MSI status is not a good marker with which to prognosticate in the setting of resectable liver metastases. It is not clear if the low frequency of MSI-H resectable tumors truly reflects a lower rate of metastasis to the liver, versus a reflection of resectability, versus other factors to explain this difference [43].

Overall, as an independent prognostic factor, the evidence suggesting a prognostic benefit of MSI-H tumors is somewhat inconsistent and therefore has not been accepted as a prognostic marker by ASCO [25], the EGTM [24], nor the National Cancer Institute [29]. However, it may be that as a prognostic marker, it is particularly beneficial among lower stage patients.

Lymphocytic Infiltration

Features reflecting a host immune response, including Crohns disease-like peritumoral reaction and intratumoral lymphocytic infiltrate, have been seen in many MSI-H tumors [44]. It has been hypothesized that this immunogenic response may protect against the malignancy [27, 44].

MSI status and lymphocytic infiltration have been evaluated in several studies. One study evaluated the number of tumor-infiltrating lymphocytes (TILs) and

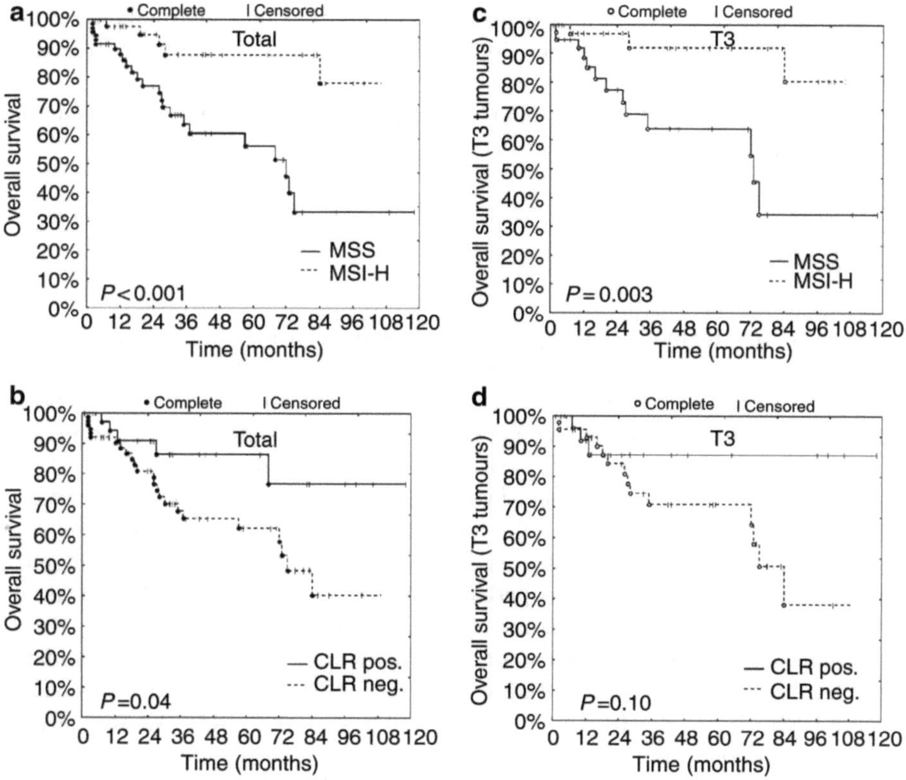

Fig. 7.3 Overall survival for all stages by MSI status (**a**) and Crohn's like reaction (**b**). Overall survival for patients with T3 tumors by MSI status (**c**) and Crohn's like reaction (**d**). [Reprinted from Buckowitz A, Knaebel HP, Benner A, et al. Microsatellite instability in colorectal cancer is associated with local lymphocyte infiltration and low frequency of distant metastases. Br J Cancer. 2005;92(9):1746–1753. With permission from Nature Publishing Group]

compared this to MSI status [39]. MSI-H tumors had increased numbers of TILS compared with MSI-L and MSS tumors ($p<0.0001$) [39]. Another study was a retrospective assessment of MSI and lymphocytic infiltrate (LI) status that suggested MSI-H with presence of LI (LI+) were associated with better 5 year OS (89%) than absence of both features (55%, $p=0.06$) [44]. Multivariate analyses only identified MSI status as an independent predictor of survival, but the analysis was limited by a small number of cases. By stage, improved DFS was notable in the stage II patients with LI+tumors [44].

In a prospective assessment of patients with at least two Amsterdam or Bethesda criteria (reflecting a suspicion of, but not diagnostic for, HNPCC), MSI-H patients were characterized by proximal lesions, earlier stage of disease, and fewer distant metastases [27]. Crohn's-like (lymphocytic) reaction (CLR) was more frequently present and survival was better in MSI-H patients than MSS (Fig. 7.3). In a proportional hazards model to assess the prognostic value of MSI status with regards to stage, presence of CLR, age at diagnosis, and use of 5FU, only age at diagnosis and stage were statistically significant for OS [27]. This may represent a protective effect of lymphocytic invasion.

These findings are intriguing, but require further evaluation prior to considering LI as a prognostic factor.

Clinical Scoring Methods

Clinical scoring methods can help predict which patients may be at higher or lower risk with a given procedure. One such example is a clinical risk score (CRS) for tumor recurrence used to predict 5 year OS of patients with liver metastases based on the number of clinical risk factors [22]. One point is assigned for each of the following negative risk factors: LN positive primary tumor, disease free interval less than 12 months, multiple liver metastases, largest liver metastasis greater than 5 cm, and CEA above 200 ng/mL, with the final CRS ranging from 0 to 5. Survival with no risk factors (CRS 0) was 60% at 5 years, with a median OS of 74 months. However, for the worst prognosis patients with a CRS of 5, the 5 year survival rate of 14% and median OS of 22 months [22] are similar to the prognosis of patients with metastatic disease at initial diagnosis. This scoring system has been validated with retrospective data, demonstrating that a CRS of 0, 1 and 2 had better survival than a CRS of 3 or 4 (HR 2.1, 95% CI 1.2–3.6, $p=0.006$) [45]. Additionally, in comparison to other scoring systems, the CRS differentiated patients by risk score at various survival time points, with 5 year OS for a CRS of 0 through 5 constantly decreasing (5 year OS for CRS 0=42%, CRS 1=39%, CRS 2=36%, CRS 3=25%, CRS 4=13%, and CRS 5=0%, $p=0.006$) [46]. Similarly, a scoring system by Iwatsuki et al. also demonstrated prognostic benefit [46]. These scoring systems now require prospective validation.

Lymph Node Micrometastases

LN micrometastases have been explored as a potential prognostic marker in stage II CRC. LN micrometastases are defined as a solitary or group of tumor cells measuring less than 2 mm within an otherwise negative LN [47]. These cells are thought to herald risk of future tumor spread.

In one study, 192 LNs were assessed from 26 consecutive patients with resected stage II CRC [48]. None of these patients received adjuvant therapy. Overall, half the patients with evidence of LN micrometastases, as assessed by RT-PCR amplification of CEA mRNA, had cancer related deaths compared to 8% in the group without micrometastases. This represented a 5 year OS of 36% versus 75% respectively ($p=0.03$). These differences were attributable to micrometastases when adjusted for pathologic tumor staging, age, and presence or absence of lymphatic invasion [48].

A subsequent study of Dukes' B patients that were not treated with adjuvant chemotherapy found no correlation between the presence of LN micrometastases and survival nor death with disease [47]. Evaluation of LN micrometastases requires further evaluation.

18q Loss of Heterozygosity and Deleted in Colon Cancer

Chromosome 18 contains several important genes involved in carcinogenesis, including Deleted in Colon Cancer (DCC) and SMAD-4 [49]. Loss of chromosome 18q (18qLOH) is associated with chromosomal instability and infrequently associated with MSI [50]. Measurement of loss of chromosome 18q can be done by methods including LOH/allelic imbalance (AI) and DCC gene expression [51].

DCC is a gene at 18q21 that encodes for a protein [52] linked to cell proliferation and differentiation [53]. Decreased expression has been associated with carcinoma [52, 54], and LOH of DCC in malignancies suggests this gene has a tumor suppressor function [52]. In fact, approximately 70% of CRCs have 18q LOH [50, 55, 56]. However, not all in vitro and animal data support the tumor suppressor gene function of DCC [53].

The role of 18qLOH has been assessed in various studies. The prognostic significance of 18qLOH was demonstrated among stage II and III patients [57]. This retrospective study found that 18q allelic loss was more common in stage III than stage II tumors ($p=0.007$). However, only among stage II patients did allelic loss portend a worse prognosis (5 year OS 54% vs. 93%) and was an independent prognostic factor (HR death 2.46, 95% CI 1.06–5.71, $p=0.036$) [57]. With IHC evaluation of DCC in stage II and III CRC, a prognostic benefit to DCC expression was found [58]. Five year OS for DCC stage II positive tumors was 94% versus 62% for DCC negative tumors ($p<0.001$), and among stage III patients, 59% versus 33% respectively ($p=0.03$) [58]. Among sporadic CRCs, 18qLOH was correlated with metastatic potential and specifically hepatic metastasis [59].

A systematic review and meta-analysis of 17 published studies of 2,189 patients assessed the prognostic value of 18qLOH/AI and loss of DCC expression [51]. While this analysis is very limited in the conclusions as they did not include individual patient data, used only published studies, and found significant heterogeneity between the studies, it did provide pooled data to support the hypothesis that 18q LOH has a poor prognostic role (HR 2.0, 95% CI 1.49–2.69, p for heterogeneity <0.0001). There was evidence of publication bias ($p=0.05$, Egger's test), but the benefit remained after adjustment (HR 1.63, CI 1.21–2.20). Loss of chromosome 18q occurred in just over half the patients by any method of analysis. In stages II and III CRC, 18q loss still conferred a poorer prognosis (pooled HR 1.69, 95% CI 1.13–2.54, p for heterogeneity $=0.001$) but could not be assessed in stage IV disease for lack of patient numbers [51].

An evaluation of multiple molecular predictors of survival in colon cancer used data from adjuvant 5FU-based therapy trials of stage II and III patients in two NCI

GI Intergroup clinical trials [60]. Forty-nine percent had 18qLOH evaluated by PCR. P53 mutations (assessed by high labeling index) were found in 71% of tumors. Intact 18q had increased survival compared to 18qLOH (5 year OS 69% vs. 50%, $p=0.005$). Patients with MSS and intact 18q tumors had similarly improved survival over 18qLOH. Patients were treated with adjuvant 5FU based chemotherapy which may therefore confound the prognostic effect of the factor. 18qLOH was associated with a poorer survival and DFS among stage III patients treated with adjuvant chemotherapy, but this was not found in stage II patients [60]. However, other retrospective studies have not replicated this finding [32].

Most recently, the first prospective evaluation of 18qLOH in untreated stage II colon cancer patients reported that intact 18q was associated with a better survival than for 18q LOH (5 year OS HR 0.98 vs. 0.86, $p=0.01$; 5 year DFS HR 0.92 vs. 0.78, $p=0.03$) [61].

Based on the available data, there is insufficient evidence to support the use of 18qLOH or DCC for determining prognosis. Neither the ASCO nor EGTM guidelines recommend using these as prognostic indicators in operable CRC [24, 25]. However, it seems likely that these factors will be prognostically relevant, although the role of 18qLOH vis-à-vis DCC and other genomic regions in carcinogenesis remains unclear.

Chromosomal Instability or Aneuploidy/Polyploidy

Chromosomal instability (CIN), found in at least 50% of CRCs [62], was described initially by Fearon and Vogelstein [52]. It describes genetic processes that occur at various times in the development of an adenoma to carcinoma to metastases [52] that results in a number of structural or numerical chromosomal changes [63]. CINs include MSS, aneuploidy and/or polyploidy, and genetic mutations of genes such as k-ras, APC, and TP53 [52, 64]. Tumors can, although infrequently, have genomic instability of both the chromosomal and microsatellite pathways (3.4% in one series) while 38% have neither [50, 63]. At this point, inconsistent prognostic implications have been found [65–67]. Complicating matters, measurement of CIN is inconsistent, as flow cytometry can identify multiple chromosomal abnormalities, but not differentiate stable from unstable or simple from complex changes, and more specific assessments of CIN are not feasible in such studies [63].

A meta-analysis evaluating CIN as a prognostic factor found that presence of CIN (CIN+) conferred a worse prognosis than when CIN was not present (CIN–) [63]. CIN was measured by flow or image cytometry, and identified by two peaks on the DNA histogram, the first of which represents the diploid cells. CIN+ was found in 60% of tumors from 10,126 patients, 91% of which were stages II and III. Overall, CIN+ was associated with a worse survival (HR 1.45, 95% CI 1.35–1.55, $p<0.001$) and PFS, with no evidence of heterogeneity, and similarly worse in both the colon and rectal subgroups and stage II and III subgroups. Stages I and IV could not be evaluated due to insufficient data. In patients that did not receive adjuvant treatment, CIN+ was again associated with a worse prognosis [63]. The effect of MSI was not assessed.

Overall, a meta-analysis suggests that CIN has a negative prognostic effect in stage II and III disease. The assessment of MSI and CIN should be further evaluated to determine if these are independent prognostic factors, to determine the role of CIN in stage I and IV disease, and to prospectively evaluate the role of CIN. Due to the current uncertainties, neither ASCO nor EGTM guidelines recommend the use of CIN as a prognostic factor.

K-ras

Ras is a family of genes with homologous members (k-, h-, and n-ras) that transduce, and likely integrate, messages from growth factor receptors [68]. K-ras is an intracellular signaling protein from the RAS family. Mutation of k-ras is an early event in the adenoma–carcinoma sequence. K-ras mutations are found in 30–40% of patients with mCRC, in which the protein is constitutively "on," such that the cells can evade apoptosis and continue to proliferate and invade. Ninety percent of k-ras activating mutations in CRC have been found on exon 1 codons 12, 13, and 61 [68, 69].

The potential prognostic significance was assessed with a compilation of data from researchers that had published data on k-ras gene mutations (The Kirsten ras in-colorectal-cancer collaborative group, RASCAL), representing 2,721 patients from 22 centers in 13 countries [70]. Multivariate analyses demonstrated that failure-free survival (FFS) and OS were worse with higher Dukes' stage and any mutation. Figure 7.4 demonstrates the deleterious mutation effects on OS by stage. Any mutation was associated with a 22% increased risk of death (HR 1.22, 95% CI 1.07–1.40, $p=0.004$). This identified that G to T mutations, and particularly glycine to valine codon 12 mutations, were worse prognostically (HR for OS = 1.44, 95% CI 1.18–1.75, $p<0.001$; HR for OS = 1.43, 95% CI = 1.13–1.82, $p=0.004$, respectively). None of the other mutations had a prognostic significance for FFS or OS. Interpretation of the data by histologic grade was limited by missing data [70].

In a follow-up analysis (RASCAL II) to assess specific k-ras mutations at different stages of disease, data from 3,439 patients were analyzed [71]. This confirmed that valine mutations on codon 12 were deleterious in terms of FFS (HR 1.30, 95% CI 1.09–1.54, $p=0.004$) and OS (HR 1.29, 95% CI 1.08–1.55, $p=0.008$), and that guanine to thymidine (G to T) mutations were associated with worse FFS (HR 1.27, 95% CI 1.10–1.47, $p=0.002$) and OS (HR 1.28, 95% CI 1.10–1.50, $p=0.002$), when controlling for stage, age, and center. By stage, valine mutations were neither associated with FFS or OS in Dukes' B carcinoma, but in Dukes' C were associated with worse FFS (HR 1.5, 95% CI 1.13–1.98, $p=0.008$), yet only a trend to significance for OS (HR 1.45, 95% CI 1.07–1.96, $p=0.02$, [significant p value for multiple testing <0.01]). Overall, 8.9% of the patients harbored the codon 12 valine mutation [71].

K-ras status has been evaluated in a number of large clinical trials, although those in which an untreated group was used for comparison are more limited.

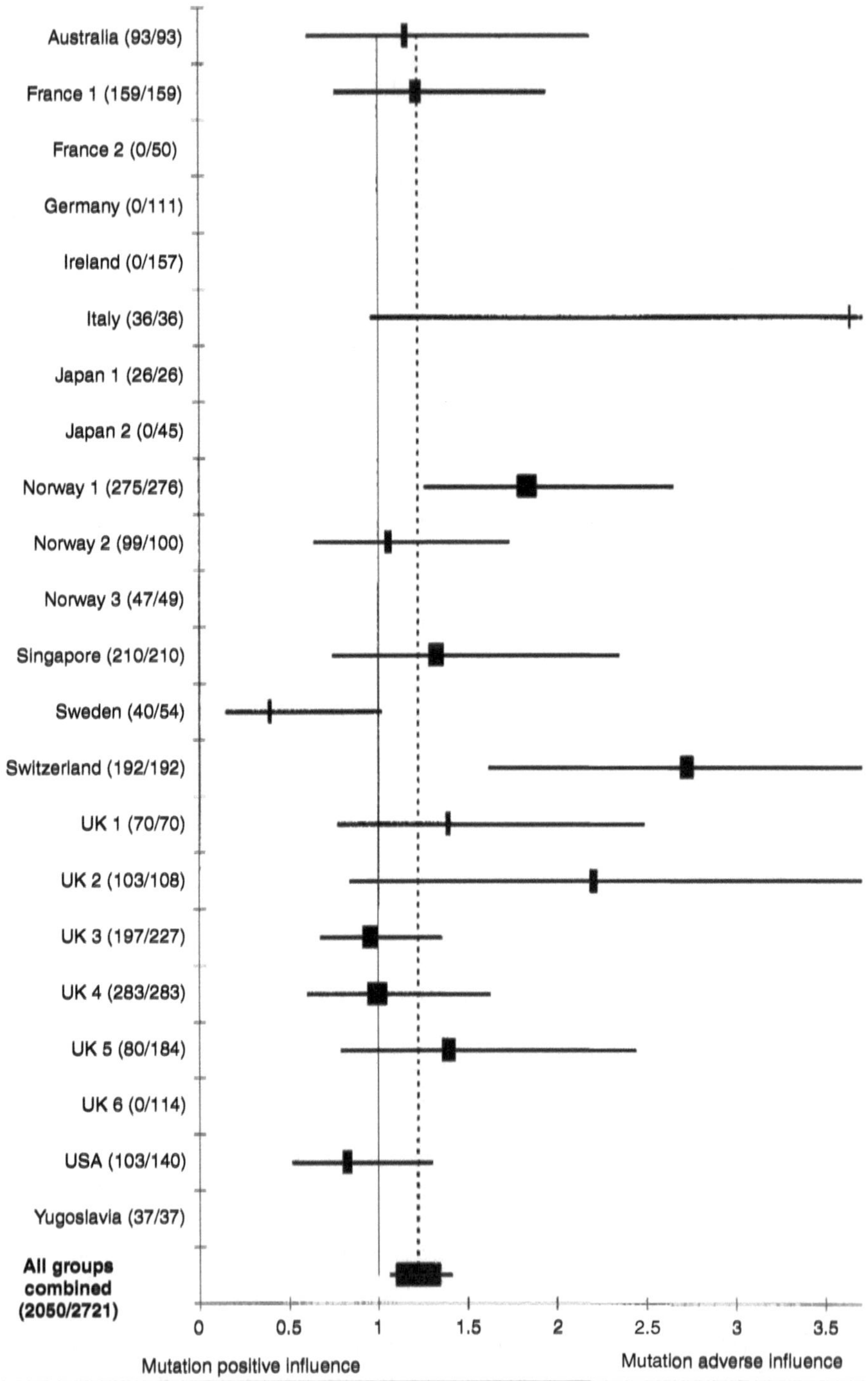

Fig. 7.4 Overall survival by k-ras status, stratified by stage from the RASCAL study. *Bold* = k-ras mutation, *light* = k-ras wild type. [Reprinted from Andreyev HJ, Norman AR, Cunningham D, Oates JR, Clarke PA. Kirsten ras mutations in patients with colorectal cancer: the multicenter "RASCAL" study. J Natl Cancer Inst. 1998;90(9):675–684. With permission from Oxford University Press]

In a large randomized phase III clinical trial evaluating panitumumab versus best supportive care (BSC) in refractory mCRC, a secondary analysis was performed to determine responses by k-ras status [72]. While k-ras WT status was predictive of efficacy, k-ras WT was prognostic for survival in the untreated patients among all BSC patients (mOS 7.6 months vs. 4.4 months, HR 0.68, $p=0.007$) with no difference in PFS, but when restricted to patients that did not cross over to panitumumab therapy, there was no difference in survival [72]. A similar study that evaluated cetuximab in the refractory setting found no difference in survival by k-ras status among those in the best supportive care arms (k-ras WT 4.8 vs. k-ras mutant 4.6 months, HR for death 1.01, $p=0.97$) [73]. Prospective specimen collection in the PETACC-3 clinical trial, in which stage II and III patients were randomized to adjuvant 5FU/LV with or without irinotecan, allowed assessment of the prognostic value of k-ras in these two treated groups [74]. There was no difference in recurrence free survival (RFS) or OS by k-ras mutation status [74]. Overall, these reveal inconsistencies in the prognostic effect of k-ras.

The role of k-ras status in the primary tumor and in the histologically negative LNs has also been evaluated. However, these studies have reached mixed conclusions. Two studies found no association between k-ras mutation and LN micrometastases, and no survival difference based on LN k-ras status [47, 75], while another found that codon 12 k-ras mutations in histologically negative LNs were associated with a worse prognosis than k-ras negative tumors (5 year risk of death 57% vs. 17%, $p=0.036$) [76].

In mCRC, it is more difficult to ascertain the role of k-ras due to conflicting results and many recent studies have evaluated k-ras in conjunction with other genes. Additionally, the presence of treatment effects, such as treatment with EGFR inhibitors cetuximab and panitumumab, makes the determination of k-ras mutational status as an independent prognostic factor in mCRC more difficult [77].

The 2006 ASCO recommendations for the use of tumor markers in GI tumors concluded that there was insufficient evidence to recommend ras oncogene testing in the management of CRC patients [26]. Similarly, the 2007 EGTM cited insufficient evidence for the use of k-ras in predicting prognosis [24]. Certainly, based on the RASCAL data, the negative prognostic effect of specific k-ras mutations is quite possible but requires further evaluation. However, clear clinical significance has not been demonstrated to date.

B-raf

With the understanding of k-ras as a potential prognostic and predictive tool in mCRC, further understanding has developed regarding the role of b-raf in conferring an effect on prognosis, and potentially in predicting effect of EGFR antibody therapies.

K-ras and b-raf mutations are mutually exclusive, that is, tumors do not harbor both mutations, and b-raf mutations are only found in k-ras WT tumors [78–81].

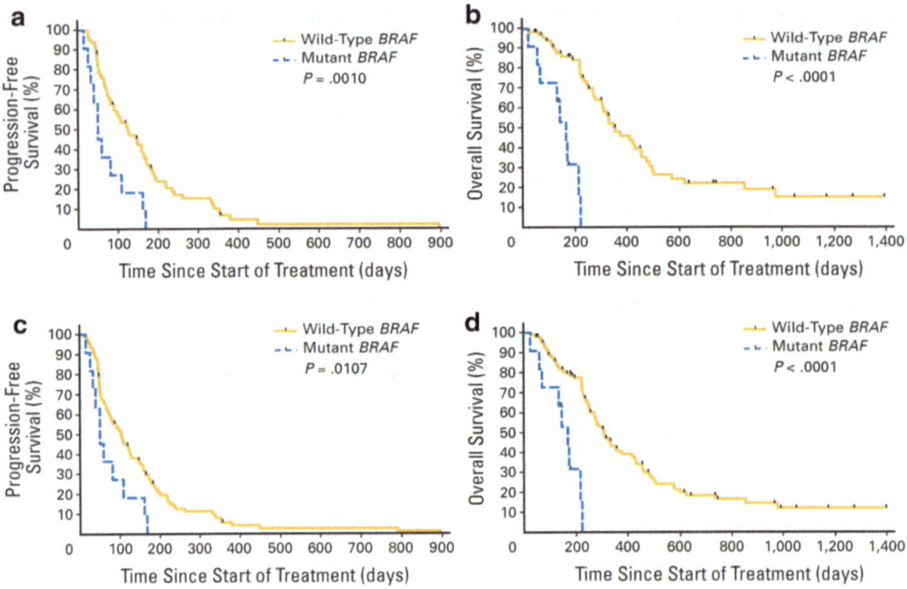

Fig. 7.5 Progression free survival and overall survival of patients with k-ras WT tumors (**a, b**) and all patients (**c, d**), based on b-raf mutation status. [Reprinted from Di Nicolantonio F, Martini M, Molinari F, et al. Wild-type BRAF is required for response to panitumumab or cetuximab in metastatic colorectal cancer. J Clin Oncol. 2008;26(35):5705–5712. With permission from American Society of Clinical Oncology]

Di Nicolantonio et al. [79] assessed b-raf mutational status among k-ras WT patients treated with an anti-EGFR antibody, representing 70% of all patients with mCRC in their retrospective study. B-raf mutations were found in 14% of k-ras WT patients (11 of 79 patients), all of which were the V600E substitution. OS and PFS were better in the b-raf WT patients as compared to the b-raf mutated patients in all patients (k-ras WT and mutant) and specifically in the subset of k-ras WT patients (Fig. 7.5). Further, MSI was not detected in any of the b-raf mutant tumors. In fact, only one of the 75 samples tested was MSI-H (k-ras and b-raf WT) [79]; this certainly corroborates the evidence that MSI is prognostically better and found in earlier disease stage.

A shorter median PFS and OS were also found retrospectively among patients with b-raf mutated tumors compared to WT, whether treated with an anti-EGFR therapy or not [81].

In the previously mentioned PETACC-3 clinical trial, b-raf mutations were associated with worse OS, but there was no difference in RFS [74]. In multivariate analyses, b-raf mutations were statistically significantly associated with right sided tumors, females, age over 60, histological grade 3 or 4, and MSI-H tumors. Treatment effects may be in part responsible for the difference in survival but this argues for continued evaluation of the mutational status of b-raf [74].

These results are intriguing; prospective studies need to continue to evaluate the predictive and prognostic nature of b-raf.

TP53

Under normal circumstances, the tumor suppressor gene p53 is "off" [82]. With cell damage or stress, the p53 protein can initiate cell cycle arrest, allow repair, or initiate apoptosis [53]. It is the most frequent genetic mutation found in cancers [82], present in 30–76% of tumors [53]. However, the prognostic role of p53 has been inconsistently reported.

Loss of function of TP53 is a late event in the adenoma–carcinoma sequence of events [52]. It has been inconsistently reported as a prognostic factor in CRC; however, mutations of exon 7, codon 245, conserved areas, and L3 structural domains have been reported to affect prognosis [83]. Overall, 40–50% of CRC tumors harbor TP53 mutations, the majority of which are GC to AT missense mutations [83].

In a study of patients with resected primary colon cancers, none of whom received adjuvant chemotherapy, p53 positivity was correlated with left sided and higher grade tumors (versus poorly differentiated), but its expression was not associated with OS or DFS in univariate or multivariate analyses [53].

In an analysis of P53 abnormalities detected by IHC or DNA sequence analysis, p53 abnormalities increased the risk of death for patients otherwise predicted to have a good outcome [84].

The TP53-CRC Collaborative Study Group evaluated data on 3,583 CRC patients to assess TP53 as a prognostic tool in CRC, based on tumor site, stage, type of TP53 mutation, and use of adjuvant treatment [83]. Overall, TP53 mutations were found in 42% of patients, more commonly in distal and rectal cancers (45% each) than proximal colon cancers (34%, $p<0.001$). There were no significant differences between types of mutation and tumor sites. There was no evidence of a prognostic significance of TP53 on its own or by tumor site. While there were worse outcomes with certain types of mutations, in multivariate analyses only TP53 mutations with amino acid loss in distal colon tumors was independently associated with worse survival (RR 2.52, 95% CI 1.03–1.79, $p=0.03$) when adjusted for Dukes' stage, LN status, histologic grade, and lymphatic invasion. There was a trend to worse survival with exon 5 mutations in proximal colon tumors [83]. This evidence suggests that TP53 mutations may not all have the same prognostic impact, or tumor site may be an important differentiating factor. However, given the numerous studies assessing TP53, it seems unlikely that a strong effect will be found.

Problems with the data collected to date on P53 include retrospective studies with insufficient power to detect a meaningful prognostic impact, inconsistent methodology, clinical heterogeneity, and interpretation challenges [24, 84]. At this point, given that the evidence is not very strong, p53 status is not recommended as a prognostic marker in CRC.

PIK3CA Gene Mutation

Downstream of Ras, phosphatidylinositol 3-kinase (PI3K) phosphorylates and activates AKT [85], creating a cell survival, proliferation, and metastasis pathway [86–88], and additionally regulates the mTOR pathway [86, 87]. Ten to thirty percent of colon cancers have mutations of PIK3CA [88–90]. Mutations are thought to arise late in the adenoma to carcinoma sequence given the low frequency of PIK3CA mutations found in adenomas [90].

PIK3CA mutations have been associated with inferior survival. In a study of resected CRC cases, PIK3CA mutations of exons 9 and 20 were found in 11.4% ($n = 18$) of untreated stage I, II and III patients [89]. In this small sample, there was no correlation between k-ras mutations and PIK3CA mutations. PIK3CA mutations were associated with shorter disease-specific survival than WT. However, when considering only the stage II and III patients in multivariate analyses, only PIK3CA mutation was an independent prognostic factor for relapse free survival (HR = 2.478, 95% CI 1.028–5.973, $p = 0.0433$) [89].

In an analysis of 450 resected stage I to III colon cancers from two prospective cohort studies, the Nurses' Health Study and the Health Professionals Follow-Up Study, 18% had PIK3CA mutations [85]. There was a trend towards worse colon cancer-specific survival among PIK3CA mutated tumors (HR 1.64, 95% CI 0.95–2.86) but was significant in multivariate analyses (HR 2.23, 95% CI 1.21–4.11), mostly from adjusting for tumor stage, p53 status, and BMI. Overall survival was not different for PIK3CA mutational status. Lack of p53 expression was associated with PIK3CA mutations ($p = 0.01$). Stratified analyses of clinical factors, including age, sex, stage, and other genetic abnormalities, including MSI, b-raf, and p53 status, did not modify the PIK3CA mutation effect. However, PIK3CA mutations were highly associated with k-ras mutations ($p < 0.0001$) compared to PIK3CA WT tumors. Cancer-specific mortality was worse among k-ras WT tumors with PIK3CA mutation (multivariate HR 3.80, 95% CI 1.56–9.27) but was not significant among the k-ras mutated patients or for OS. The test for interaction was not significant ($p = 0.13$), suggesting that the effect was not modulated by k-ras [85].

Mutational activation of the RAS-MAPK and PI3K pathways was assessed to determine the relationship with prognosis [91]. As such, they did not assess the specific gene mutations with prognosis, but rather the impact of any mutation on prognosis. Over half the cases had a mutation in at least one of k-ras, PIK3CA, or b-raf. Activation of the network (i.e., at least one mutation present) was associated with worse 3 year survival than WT tumors (59% vs. 69%, $p = 0.009$), which persisted for multivariate analyses adjusting for age and tumor stage (HR = 1.48, 95% CI 1.07–2.04, $p = 0.017$) [91].

To date, the data for PI3K and mutations of PIK3CA remain insufficiently assessed and will require prospective evaluation to determine the prognostic value of this biomarker.

GUCY2C Expression

A newer strategy of molecular nodal examination is to assess the expression of guanylyl cyclase 2C (GUCY2C), an intestinal tumor suppressor that may be lost early in carcinogenic transformation [92]. Expression of GUCY2C may represent occult metastases. A recent study demonstrated the prognostic ability of the presence or absence of GUCY2C expression in histologically negative LNs, with 21% of patients with GUCY2C expression developing recurrent disease compared to 6% of those without (adjusted HR 4.66, 95% CI 1.11–19.57, $p=0.04$) [92]. This requires further prospective evaluation.

TS, TP, and DPD

In the metabolism of fluoropyrimidines, the enzymes TS, TP, and DPD have fundamental roles.

The thymidylate synthase gene (TYMS) encodes for a protein whose product, thymidylate synthase (TS), catalyzes 5FU metabolism, but is also required for DNA synthesis [53, 93]. TS is an enzyme required for conversion of dUMP to dTMP which results in DNA synthesis. TS is inhibited by the chemotherapeutic agent 5-fluorouracil (5FU), a backbone in the treatment of CRC.

Expression of TS may be discordant between the primary tumor and metastatic lesions [94] and may be higher in pulmonary than hepatic metastases [95]. In contrast, among patients undergoing curative resections, high TS levels in the primary tumor were correlated with improved OS [96].

Evaluation of TYMS gene copies has also been conducted. A high versus low number of TYMS genes per nucleus was associated with both recurrence and worse survival, particularly with stage III disease [97]. This was also found in multivariate analyses when adjusted for stage, vascular tumor invasion, and bowel obstruction at resection, with an increased risk of recurrence (HR 1.6, 95% CI 1.1–2.2, $p=0.02$) and death (HR=1.6, 95% CI 1.1–2.3, $p=0.01$) with high TYMS gene per nucleus [97]. In a systematic review and pooled analysis of published trials assessing TS expression and OS, increased TS levels were associated with decreased survival in both advanced and adjuvant settings (HR 1.74, 95% CI 1.34–2.26, and HR 1.35, 95% CI 1.07–1.80, respectively), with evidence of heterogeneity in both analyses [93]. Of note, in the metastatic setting, all patients received TS inhibitor therapy while in the adjuvant setting, some patients were untreated. Among the advanced disease patients, TS levels assessed from metastatic lesions were more predictive than from the primary tumor [93]. Three studies in the adjuvant setting assessed the role of surgery alone, representing 562 patients. The survival benefit was maintained with low TS levels (HR 1.92, 95% CI 1.12–3.32) and similarly for PFS, but the small number of studies in these analyses requires cautious interpretation [93]. Given the heterogeneity between studies, the use of TS as a prognostic marker is not recommended. Additionally, the lack of standardized methodology for TS assessment limits our current evaluation of the data.

Other enzymes such as thymidine phosphorylase (TP) and dihydropyrimidine dehydrogenase (DPD) have been assessed as potential prognostic markers, but there is insufficient evidence to use these as prognostic markers in CRC.

Gene Signatures in Colon Cancer

With the limited success of intracellular factors to predict outcomes, attention has turned to the molecular fingerprints of the cell, the DNA. DNA is akin to the control center of the cell, which transcribes mRNA, the machinery, in order to produce proteins that are required to perform specific actions. Analyses of RNA are underway to identify means to identify specific tumors and to differentiate tumors with varying characteristics, such as prognostic and predictive signatures. Additionally, microanalysis of RNA can reflect the amount of protein that is made, although RNA and protein levels do not necessarily correlate. Microarray analyses are used to develop gene expression profiles. Current microarray chips can examine over 20,000 genes at once. Identification of these genes and patterns of gene expression (e.g., up and down-regulated genes) can be used to identify features specific to particular cancers, like a picture of a cell at a given point in time. This process requires complex statistical programs to analyze the large volume of data created by such arrays. DNA microarray technology affords the opportunity to identify previously unknown or unassessed genes and their expression to better understand their influence on both prognosis and the prediction of benefit from therapy.

In evaluating gene expression profiles, one of two types of analysis is generally used. Cluster analyses identify genes with similar patterns of expression. With grouping of these genes, a supervised analysis can be performed in which known characteristics are used to predefine groups to develop a signature to differentiate based on those factors. In an unsupervised analysis, similar samples cluster together and are identified in the gene array. Both methods of analysis can be done in order to verify the selected genes and to select the best signature. Both analyses require an initial group of patients (training set) to develop the signature, and a separate group of patients for validation (validation set).

23-Gene Prognostic Signature

A 23-gene prognostic signature was developed for stage II colon cancer patients that were not treated with adjuvant chemotherapy [98]. An unsupervised clustering analysis developed a microarray-based prognosis predictor using the 74 patients, resulting in a group of 54 patients of which 33% relapsed within 3 years compared to the remaining 20 patients, of which 65% relapsed (χ^2 $p=0.028$). Thereafter, two methods were analyzed to determine the gene signature. In one, using the two groups identified from the unsupervised clustering, 23 genes were selected from the lower and higher risk of recurrence groups. In the other, a training set of 38 patients were used to identify genes to predict recurrence; this resulted in a 60 gene set. Finally, the 23 and 60 gene signatures were compared using the 36 patients from the validation set. The 23-gene signature was found to predict poor versus good outcome (Fig. 7.6), with a predictive accuracy of 78%, sensitivity of 72%, and specificity of 83%. The risk of recurrence based on this 23-gene signature was most predictive in

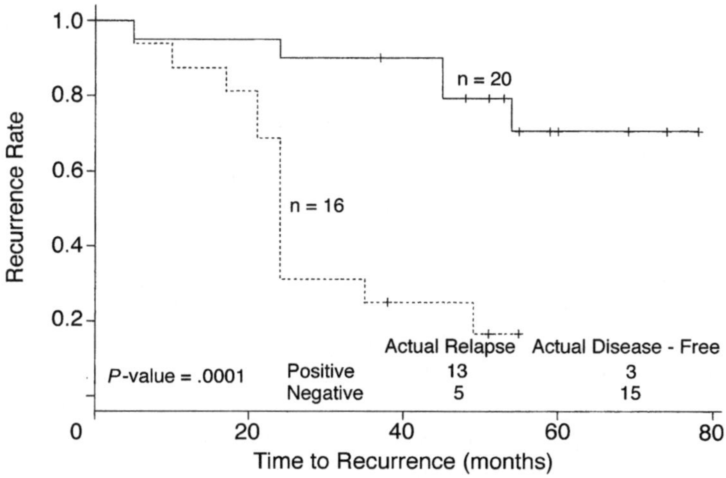

Fig. 7.6 Risk of recurrence based on high versus low risk groups as determined by the 23 gene prognostic signature for stage II colon cancer patients. [Reprinted from Wang Y, Jatkoe T, Zhang Y, et al. Gene expression profiles and molecular markers to predict recurrence of Dukes' B colon cancer. J Clin Oncol. 2004;22(9):1564–1571. With permission from American Society of Clinical Oncology]

multivariate analyses (RR 0.17, 95% CI 0.06–0.51, $p=0.001$) [98]. This is a very promising development in the prognostication of stage II colon cancer patients.

30-Gene Prognostic Predictor

Also using gene expression profiling, a 30-gene prognosis predictor (PP) was developed for stage II MSS colon cancer [99]. Fifty tumors were used, of which 25 patients developed distant metastases. A PP was developed based on whether the disease recurred or not using half the patients, resulting in a 30-gene PP that was validated with the remaining patients, demonstrating 80% accuracy, 75% sensitivity, and 85% specificity. Cross-validation was then performed. Finally, this study validated the 23-gene signature by Wang et al. [98], but found that the 30-gene signature was superior in prognostic prediction accuracy than the 23-gene signature (76% vs. 67% respectively) [99].

26 Gene Signature to Identify Good Versus Poor Prognosis for Dukes' Stage B and C Patients

One method to determine a gene expression signature for CRC was to differentiate poor versus good prognosis patients, based on apriori definitions of survival of less than and greater than 36 months respectively [100]. Seventy-eight tumor samples were evaluated using a 32,000 cDNA microarray, including Dukes' Stage B, C, and D cases, as well as three adenomas. Overall, a cluster analysis using 53 genes delineated two groups (Fig. 7.7a) with different outcomes (Fig. 7.7c), which similarly differentiates the good versus poor prognosis patients (Fig. 7.7e, $p<0.001$). Evaluation by Dukes stage demonstrated that the gene clustering was not simply identifying stage-specific prognosis (Fig. 7.7b, d) [100].

Based on a gene ranking approach called leave-one-out cross-validation, 43 genes were consistently identified statistically. At 36 months, the overall accuracy of this 43 gene set was 90%, with 93% sensitivity, and 84% specificity [100].

In order to validate this signature, an independent set of 95 tumors was evaluated. However, due to methodological differences, only 26 of the 43 gene signature could be used. This signature was able to differentiate good versus poor prognostic patients (Fig. 7.8a), independent of Dukes' stage (Fig. 7.8b), and among Dukes' stage B and C patients, good and poor prognosis groups were identified (Fig. 7.8c) [100].

This 26 gene expression signature requires further validation in other independent data sets. Additionally, only two biologically significant genes were included in the signature, osteopontin and neuregulin. However, while the influence of other genes in CRC may not yet be known, it behooves us to perform adequate validation when a set of genes does not clearly reflect what we currently know about CRC biology. It is interesting that this gene signature did not identify any genes in common with the 23-gene signature determined by Wang et al. [98] for stage II colon cancer. This may represent biologic differences based on the populations studied, specifically Wang et al. [98] assessed stage II disease and colon cancer only, whereas Eschrich et al. [100] assessed Dukes stage B and C and both colon and rectal cancer, but further evaluations will help to clarify these differences.

Recurrence Score Based on Seven Genes for Stage II Colon Cancer

A multigene RT-PCR colon cancer assay demonstrated the predictive validity of these genes for stage II patients [101]. Patients treated with surgery alone from the NSABP CO1 and CO2 trials and from a Cleveland Clinic follow-up study were used to identify the 44 genes (from 761 candidate genes in 1,851 patients) that predicted recurrence. In the end, seven genes predicted recurrence based on a score of 0–100. These 7 genes were biologically plausible as they included stromal

Fig. 7.7 (continued) discrimination between Dukes' B and C, demonstrating that these genes are not just surrogates for stage. (**c**) When gene clusters were evaluated, survival differed between cluster 1 versus cluster 2. (**d**) Survival curves based on stage. (**e**) Survival curves of the validation set demonstrate a clear distinction between those with a good prognosis gene signature versus those with a poor gene signature. [Reprinted from Eschrich S, Yang I, Bloom G, et al. Molecular staging for survival prediction of colorectal cancer patients. J Clin Oncol. 2005;23(15):3526–3535. With permission from American Society of Clinical Oncology]

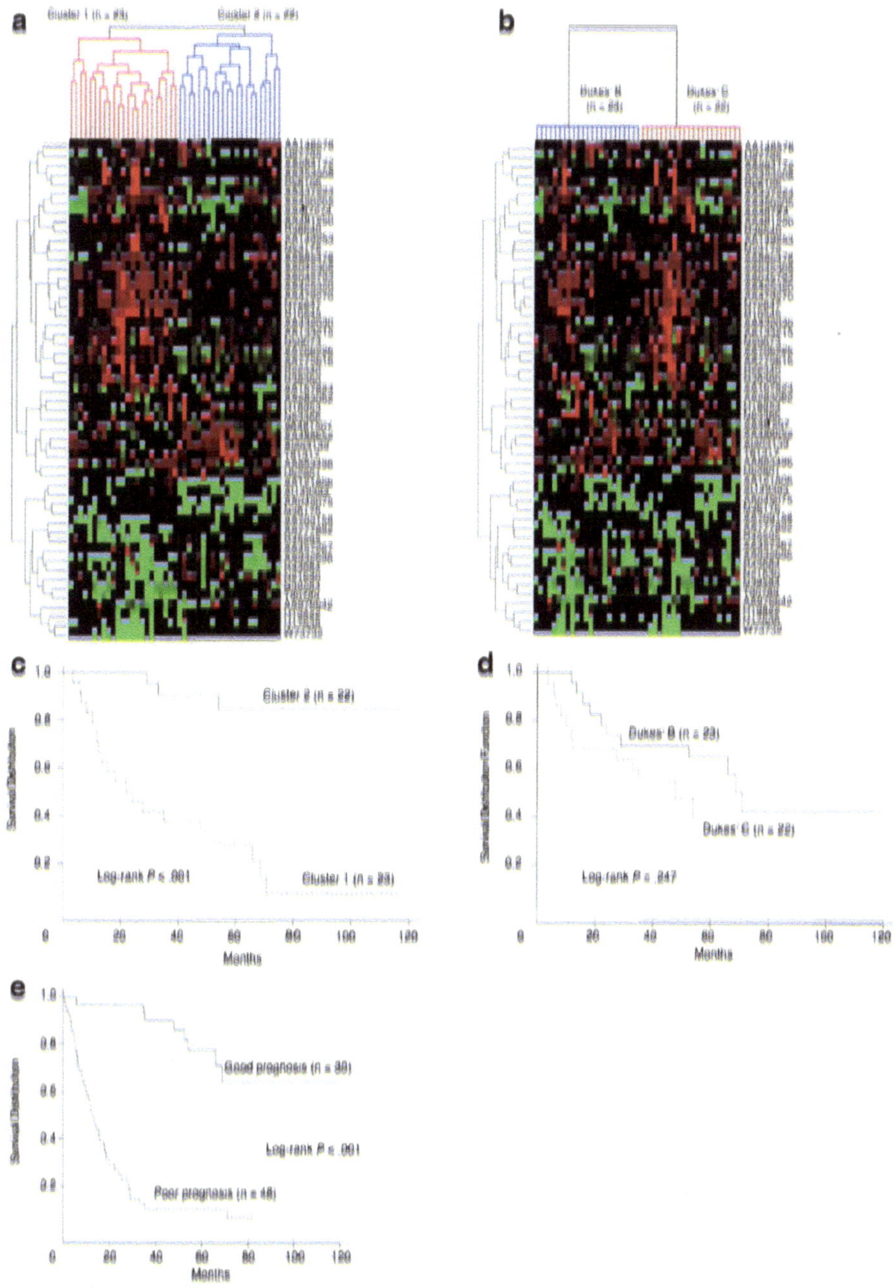

Fig. 7.7 Demonstration of a gene signature distinguishing good from poor prognosis Dukes' stage B and C patients. (**a**) In a cluster analysis, overexpressed genes (*red*) and underexpressed genes (*green*) are depicted from 53 significance analysis of microarrays-selected (SAM) genes. This demonstrates that there is an ability to distinguish patients with a good prognosis from those with a poor prognosis. (**b**) Importantly, when SAM selected genes were clustered by stage, there was no

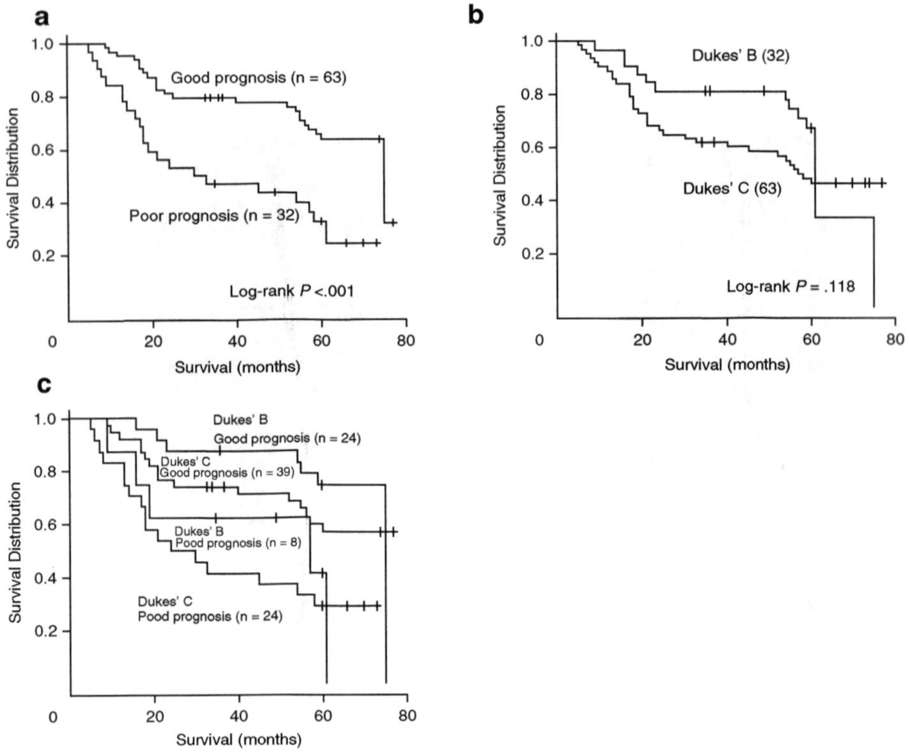

Fig. 7.8 Validation test set for the 26 gene signature. (**a**) Survival curves based on good versus poor prognosis derived from the gene signature ($p<0.001$). (**b**) Survival curves based on Dukes' staging ($p=0.118$). (**c**) Survival curves combining the gene signature with Dukes' staging information provides further differentiation of prognosis. [Reprinted from Eschrich S, Yang I, Bloom G, et al. Molecular staging for survival prediction of colorectal cancer patients. J Clin Oncol. 2005;23(15):3526–3535. With permission from American Society of Clinical Oncology]

genes (FAP, INHBA, and BGN), cell cycle genes (Ki-67, c-MYC, MYBL2), and a DNA repair gene (GAPD45B), and were compared to 5 reference genes. This was then validated using evaluable stage II patients from the QUASAR study population [101].

When risk groups were created, the high risk patients [recurrence score (RS) > 40] had a 22% risk of recurrence at 3 years (95% CI 16–29) compared to 18% for the intermediate group (95% CI 13–24%), and 12% for the low risk group (95% CI 9–16%) [101]. The colon cancer RS predicted the risk of recurrence among low versus high risk groups (HR = 1.47, $p=0.046$). In multivariate analyses, MSS, T4 (vs. T3), and RS (a continuous score per 25 units) were all independent predictors of recurrence [101]. This RS demonstrated that the prediction of recurrence is possible based on a defined set of genes.

At this time, prospective validation of gene signatures must be undertaken to determine their clinical relevance. This will be most appropriate through large clinical

Table 7.2 Summary of prognostic biomarkers

Established prognostic factors	Potential prognostic factors	Limited or inconsistent information as a prognostic factor
TNM Stage	MSI	Chromosomal instability
Number of evaluated lymph nodes	Lymphocytic infiltration	k-ras
	Clinical scoring methods	TP53
Certain histologic factors	Lymph node micrometastases	PIK3CA gene mutation
Preoperative CEA	18q LOH, DCC	GUCY2C expression
	b-raf	TYMS
	Gene expression signatures	

trials group(s) in order to have sufficient numbers of patients and adequate resources to conduct the relevant tests.

Conclusions and Future Challenges

New prognostic markers in CRC are being developed and validated. Recurrent limitations with prognostic studies include small numbers of patients, heterogeneous populations, methodologic inconsistencies, including initial sample processing, and differences in the assessment of primary versus metastatic lesions. Attention to these details will be important when evaluating the relevance of studies aimed to validate initial findings. Molecular heterogeneity is likely responsible for the prognostic differences seen in otherwise clinically and pathologically similar tumors.

By far, the most important marker of prognosis is stage of disease, but other important prognostic information is derived from lymph node status, histologic features, and CEA levels (Table 7.2). Other prognostic markers are encouraging in certain subsets of patients with colon cancer, such as MSI status and lymphocytic infiltration. However, it is anticipated that the most clinically relevant prognostic information will be derived from gene signatures, of which several are in development and are very promising.

References

1. American Cancer Society. Cancer Facts & Figures. Atlanta 2009.
2. Horner M, Ries L, Krapcho M, et al. SEER cancer statistics review, 1975–2006, National Cancer Institute. http://seer.cancer.gov/csr/1975_2006/, based on November 2008 SEER data submission. Accessed 15 Dec 2009.
3. O'Connell MJ, Campbell ME, Goldberg RM, et al. Survival following recurrence in stage II and III colon cancer: findings from the ACCENT data set. J Clin Oncol. 2008;26(14):2336–41.
4. McLeod HL, Murray GI. Tumour markers of prognosis in colorectal cancer. Br J Cancer. 1999;79(2):191–203.
5. Greene FL, Page ID, Fleming DL, et al., editors. AJCC Cancer Staging Manual. 6th ed. Chicago, IL: Springer; 2002.

6. O'Connell JB, Maggard MA, Ko CY. Colon cancer survival rates with the new American Joint Committee on Cancer Sixth Edition staging. J Natl Cancer Inst. 2004;96(19):1420–5.
7. Jessup JM, Stewart AK, Menck HR. The National Cancer Data Base Report on patterns of care for adenocarcinoma of the rectum, 1985–95. Cancer. 1998;83(11):2408–18.
8. Andre T, Boni C, Mounedji-Boudiaf L, et al. Oxaliplatin, fluorouracil, and leucovorin as adjuvant treatment for colon cancer. N Engl J Med. 2004;350(23):2343–51.
9. Dukes C. The classification of cancer of the rectum. J Pathol Bacteriol. 1932;35:323–32.
10. Le Voyer TE, Sigurdson ER, Hanlon AL, et al. Colon cancer survival is associated with increasing number of lymph nodes analyzed: a secondary survey of intergroup trial INT-0089. J Clin Oncol. 2003;21(15):2912–9.
11. Chang GJ, Rodriguez-Bigas MA, Skibber JM, Moyer VA. Lymph node evaluation and survival after curative resection of colon cancer: systematic review. J Natl Cancer Inst. 2007;99(6):433–41.
12. Toyota S, Ohta H, Anazawa S. Rationale for extent of lymph node dissection for right colon cancer. Dis Colon Rectum. 1995;38(7):705–11.
13. Tagliacozzo S, Tocchi A. Extended mesenteric excision in right hemicolectomy for carcinoma of the colon. Int J Colorectal Dis. 1997;12(5):272–5.
14. Nelson H, Petrelli N, Carlin A, et al. Guidelines 2000 for colon and rectal cancer surgery. J Natl Cancer Inst. 2001;93(8):583–96.
15. Burdy G, Panis Y, Alves A, Nemeth J, Lavergne-Slove A, Valleur P. Identifying patients with T3-T4 node-negative colon cancer at high risk of recurrence. Dis Colon Rectum. 2001;44(11):1682–8.
16. Figueredo A, Coombes ME, Mukherjee S. Adjuvant therapy for completely resected stage II colon cancer. Cochrane Database Syst Rev. 2008; (3):CD005390.
17. Quah HM, Chou JF, Gonen M, et al. Identification of patients with high-risk stage II colon cancer for adjuvant therapy. Dis Colon Rectum. 2008;51(5):503–7.
18. Fletcher RH. Carcinoembryonic antigen. Ann Intern Med. 1986;104(1):66–73.
19. Scott NA, Wieand HS, Moertel CG, Cha SS, Beart RW, Lieber MM. Colorectal cancer. Dukes' stage, tumor site, preoperative plasma CEA level, and patient prognosis related to tumor DNA ploidy pattern. Arch Surg. 1987;122(12):1375–9.
20. Wanebo HJ, Rao B, Pinsky CM, et al. Preoperative carcinoembryonic antigen level as a prognostic indicator in colorectal cancer. N Engl J Med. 1978;299(9):448–51.
21. Wolmark N, Fisher B, Wieand HS, et al. The prognostic significance of preoperative carcinoembryonic antigen levels in colorectal cancer. Results from NSABP (National Surgical Adjuvant Breast and Bowel Project) clinical trials. Ann Surg. 1984;199(4):375–82.
22. Fong Y, Fortner J, Sun RL, Brennan MF, Blumgart LH. Clinical score for predicting recurrence after hepatic resection for metastatic colorectal cancer: analysis of 1001 consecutive cases. Ann Surg. 1999;230(3):309–18. discussion 318–321.
23. Pawlik TM, Scoggins CR, Zorzi D, et al. Effect of surgical margin status on survival and site of recurrence after hepatic resection for colorectal metastases. Ann Surg. 2005;241(5):715–22. discussion 722–714.
24. Duffy MJ, van Dalen A, Haglund C, et al. Tumour markers in colorectal cancer: European Group on Tumour Markers (EGTM) guidelines for clinical use. Eur J Cancer. 2007;43(9):1348–60.
25. Locker GY, Hamilton S, Harris J, et al. ASCO 2006 update of recommendations for the use of tumor markers in gastrointestinal cancer. J Clin Oncol. 2006;24(33):5313–27.
26. Oussoultzoglou E, Rosso E, Fuchshuber P, et al. Perioperative carcinoembryonic antigen measurements to predict curability after liver resection for colorectal metastases: a prospective study. Arch Surg. 2008;143(12):1150–8. discussion 1158–1159.
27. Buckowitz A, Knaebel HP, Benner A, et al. Microsatellite instability in colorectal cancer is associated with local lymphocyte infiltration and low frequency of distant metastases. Br J Cancer. 2005;92(9):1746–53.
28. Furlan D, Casati B, Cerutti R, et al. Genetic progression in sporadic endometrial and gastrointestinal cancers with high microsatellite instability. J Pathol. 2002;197(5):603–9.

29. Boland CR, Thibodeau SN, Hamilton SR, et al. A National Cancer Institute workshop on microsatellite instability for cancer detection and familial predisposition: development of international criteria for the determination of microsatellite instability in colorectal cancer. Cancer Res. 1998;58(22):5248–57.
30. Gryfe R, Kim H, Hsieh ET, et al. Tumor microsatellite instability and clinical outcome in young patients with colorectal cancer. N Engl J Med. 2000;342(2):69–77.
31. Thibodeau SN, Bren G, Schaid D. Microsatellite instability in cancer of the proximal colon. Science. 1993;260(5109):816–9.
32. Halling KC, French AJ, McDonnell SK, et al. Microsatellite instability and 8p allelic imbalance in stage B2 and C colorectal cancers. J Natl Cancer Inst. 1999;91(15):1295–303.
33. Lothe RA, Peltomaki P, Meling GI, et al. Genomic instability in colorectal cancer: relationship to clinicopathological variables and family history. Cancer Res. 1993;53(24):5849–52.
34. Curran B, Lenehan K, Mulcahy H, et al. Replication error phenotype, clinicopathological variables, and patient outcome in Dukes' B stage II (T3, N0, M0) colorectal cancer. Gut. 2000;46(2):200–4.
35. Salahshor S, Kressner U, Fischer H, et al. Microsatellite instability in sporadic colorectal cancer is not an independent prognostic factor. Br J Cancer. 1999;81(2):190–3.
36. Lynch HT, de la Chapelle A. Hereditary colorectal cancer. N Engl J Med. 2003;348(10):919–32.
37. Alexander J, Watanabe T, Wu TT, Rashid A, Li S, Hamilton SR. Histopathological identification of colon cancer with microsatellite instability. Am J Pathol. 2001;158(2):527–35.
38. Risio M, Reato G, di Celle PF, Fizzotti M, Rossini FP, Foa R. Microsatellite instability is associated with the histological features of the tumor in nonfamilial colorectal cancer. Cancer Res. 1996;56(23):5470–4.
39. Smyrk TC, Watson P, Kaul K, Lynch HT. Tumor-infiltrating lymphocytes are a marker for microsatellite instability in colorectal carcinoma. Cancer. 2001;91(12):2417–22.
40. Kim H, Jen J, Vogelstein B, Hamilton SR. Clinical and pathological characteristics of sporadic colorectal carcinomas with DNA replication errors in microsatellite sequences. Am J Pathol. 1994;145(1):148–56.
41. Popat S, Hubner R, Houlston RS. Systematic review of microsatellite instability and colorectal cancer prognosis. J Clin Oncol. 2005;23(3):609–18.
42. Ribic CM, Sargent DJ, Moore MJ, et al. Tumor microsatellite-instability status as a predictor of benefit from fluorouracil-based adjuvant chemotherapy for colon cancer. N Engl J Med. 2003;349(3):247–57.
43. Haddad R, Ogilvie RT, Croitoru M, et al. Microsatellite instability as a prognostic factor in resected colorectal cancer liver metastases. Ann Surg Oncol. 2004;11(11):977–82.
44. Chang EY, Dorsey PB, Frankhouse J, et al. Combination of microsatellite instability and lymphocytic infiltrate as a prognostic indicator in colon cancer. Arch Surg. 2009;144(6):511–5.
45. Mala T, Bohler G, Mathisen O, Bergan A, Soreide O. Hepatic resection for colorectal metastases: can preoperative scoring predict patient outcome? World J Surg. 2002;26(11):1348–53.
46. Reissfelder C, Rahbari NN, Koch M, et al. Validation of prognostic scoring systems for patients undergoing resection of colorectal cancer liver metastases. Ann Surg Oncol. 2009;16(12):3279–88.
47. Zauber NP, Wang C, Lee PS, Redondo TC, Bishop DT, Goel A. Ki-ras gene mutations, LOH of the APC and DCC genes, and microsatellite instability in primary colorectal carcinoma are not associated with micrometastases in pericolonic lymph nodes or with patients' survival. J Clin Pathol. 2004;57(9):938–42.
48. Liefers GJ, Cleton-Jansen AM, van de Velde CJ, et al. Micrometastases and survival in stage II colorectal cancer. N Engl J Med. 1998;339(4):223–8.
49. Anwar S, Frayling IM, Scott NA, Carlson GL. Systematic review of genetic influences on the prognosis of colorectal cancer. Br J Surg. 2004;91(10):1275–91.
50. Goel A, Arnold CN, Niedzwiecki D, et al. Characterization of sporadic colon cancer by patterns of genomic instability. Cancer Res. 2003;63(7):1608–14.

51. Popat S, Houlston RS. A systematic review and meta-analysis of the relationship between chromosome 18q genotype, DCC status and colorectal cancer prognosis. Eur J Cancer. 2005;41(14):2060–70.
52. Fearon ER, Vogelstein B. A genetic model for colorectal tumorigenesis. Cell. 1990;61(5): 759–67.
53. Klump B, Nehls O, Okech T, et al. Molecular lesions in colorectal cancer: impact on prognosis? Original data and review of the literature. Int J Colorectal Dis. 2004;19(1):23–42.
54. Itoh F, Hinoda Y, Ohe M, et al. Decreased expression of DCC mRNA in human colorectal cancers. Int J Cancer. 1993;53(2):260–3.
55. Vogelstein B, Fearon ER, Hamilton SR, et al. Genetic alterations during colorectal-tumor development. N Engl J Med. 1988;319(9):525–32.
56. Diep CB, Thorstensen L, Meling GI, Skovlund E, Rognum TO, Lothe RA. Genetic tumor markers with prognostic impact in Dukes' stages B and C colorectal cancer patients. J Clin Oncol. 2003;21(5):820–9.
57. Jen J, Kim H, Piantadosi S, et al. Allelic loss of chromosome 18q and prognosis in colorectal cancer. N Engl J Med. 1994;331(4):213–21.
58. Shibata D, Reale MA, Lavin P, et al. The DCC protein and prognosis in colorectal cancer. N Engl J Med. 1996;335(23):1727–32.
59. Iino H, Fukayama M, Maeda Y, et al. Molecular genetics for clinical management of colorectal carcinoma. 17p, 18q, and 22q loss of heterozygosity and decreased DCC expression are correlated with the metastatic potential. Cancer. 1994;73(5):1324–31.
60. Watanabe T, Wu TT, Catalano PJ, et al. Molecular predictors of survival after adjuvant chemotherapy for colon cancer. N Engl J Med. 2001;344(16):1196–206.
61. Bertagnolli MM, Niedzwiecki D, Hall M, et al. Presence of 18q loss of heterozygosity (LOH) and disease-free and overall survival in stage II colon cancer: CALGB Protocol 9581. ASCO Meet Abstr. 2009;27(15S):4012.
62. Goel A, Nagasaka T, Arnold CN, et al. The CpG island methylator phenotype and chromosomal instability are inversely correlated in sporadic colorectal cancer. Gastroenterology. 2007;132(1):127–38.
63. Walther A, Houlston R, Tomlinson I. Association between chromosomal instability and prognosis in colorectal cancer: a meta-analysis. Gut. 2008;57(7):941–50.
64. Smits KM, Cleven AH, Weijenberg MP, et al. Pharmacoepigenomics in colorectal cancer: a step forward in predicting prognosis and treatment response. Pharmacogenomics. 2008;9(12):1903–16.
65. Yamazoe Y, Maetani S, Nishikawa T, Onodera H, Tobe T, Imamura M. The prognostic role of the DNA ploidy pattern in colorectal cancer analysis using paraffin-embedded tissue by an improved method. Surg Today. 1994;24(1):30–6.
66. Tang R, Ho YS, You YT, et al. Prognostic evaluation of DNA flow cytometric and histopathologic parameters of colorectal cancer. Cancer. 1995;76(10):1724–30.
67. Risques RA, Moreno V, Marcuello E, et al. Redefining the significance of aneuploidy in the prognostic assessment of colorectal cancer. Lab Invest. 2001;81(3):307–15.
68. Jimeno A, Messersmith WA, Hirsch FR, Franklin WA, Eckhardt SG. KRAS mutations and sensitivity to epidermal growth factor receptor inhibitors in colorectal cancer: practical application of patient selection. J Clin Oncol. 2009;27(7):1130–6.
69. Castagnola P, Giaretti W. Mutant KRAS, chromosomal instability and prognosis in colorectal cancer. Biochim Biophys Acta. 2005;1756(2):115–25.
70. Andreyev HJ, Norman AR, Cunningham D, Oates JR, Clarke PA. Kirsten ras mutations in patients with colorectal cancer: the multicenter "RASCAL" study. J Natl Cancer Inst. 1998;90(9):675–84.
71. Andreyev HJ, Norman AR, Cunningham D, et al. Kirsten ras mutations in patients with colorectal cancer: the 'RASCAL II' study. Br J Cancer. 2001;85(5):692–6.
72. Amado RG, Wolf M, Peeters M, et al. Wild-type KRAS is required for panitumumab efficacy in patients with metastatic colorectal cancer. J Clin Oncol. 2008;26(10):1626–34.
73. Karapetis CS, Khambata-Ford S, Jonker DJ, et al. K-ras mutations and benefit from cetuximab in advanced colorectal cancer. N Engl J Med. 2008;359(17):1757–65.

74. Roth AD, Tejpar S, Delorenzi M, et al. Prognostic role of KRAS and BRAF in stage II and III resected colon cancer: results of the translational study on the PETACC-3, EORTC 40993, SAKK 60–00 trial. J Clin Oncol. 2010;28(3):466–74.
75. Clarke GA, Ryan E, Crowe JP, O'Keane JC, MacMathuna P. Tumour-derived mutated K-ras codon 12 expression in regional lymph nodes of stage II colorectal cancer patients is not associated with increased risk of cancer-related death. Int J Colorectal Dis. 2001;16(2):108–11.
76. Belly RT, Rosenblatt JD, Steinmann M, et al. Detection of mutated K12-ras in histologically negative lymph nodes as an indicator of poor prognosis in stage II colorectal cancer. Clin Colorectal Cancer. 2001;1(2):110–6.
77. Lievre A, Bachet JB, Boige V, et al. KRAS mutations as an independent prognostic factor in patients with advanced colorectal cancer treated with cetuximab. J Clin Oncol. 2008;26(3): 374–9.
78. Deng G, Bell I, Crawley S, et al. BRAF mutation is frequently present in sporadic colorectal cancer with methylated hMLH1, but not in hereditary nonpolyposis colorectal cancer. Clin Cancer Res. 2004;10(1Pt1):191–5.
79. Di Nicolantonio F, Martini M, Molinari F, et al. Wild-type BRAF is required for response to panitumumab or cetuximab in metastatic colorectal cancer. J Clin Oncol. 2008;26(35): 5705–12.
80. Frattini M, Balestra D, Suardi S, et al. Different genetic features associated with colon and rectal carcinogenesis. Clin Cancer Res. 2004;10(12Pt1):4015–21.
81. Tol J, Nagtegaal ID, Punt CJ. BRAF mutation in metastatic colorectal cancer. N Engl J Med. 2009;361(1):98–9.
82. Vogelstein B, Lane D, Levine AJ. Surfing the p53 network. Nature. 2000;408(6810):307–10.
83. Russo A, Bazan V, Iacopetta B, Kerr D, Soussi T, Gebbia N. The TP53 colorectal cancer international collaborative study on the prognostic and predictive significance of p53 mutation: influence of tumor site, type of mutation, and adjuvant treatment. J Clin Oncol. 2005;23(30):7518–28.
84. Munro AJ, Lain S, Lane DP. P53 abnormalities and outcomes in colorectal cancer: a systematic review. Br J Cancer. 2005;92(3):434–44.
85. Ogino S, Nosho K, Kirkner GJ, et al. PIK3CA mutation is associated with poor prognosis among patients with curatively resected colon cancer. J Clin Oncol. 2009;27(9):1477–84.
86. Engelman JA, Luo J, Cantley LC. The evolution of phosphatidylinositol 3-kinases as regulators of growth and metabolism. Nat Rev Genet. 2006;7(8):606–19.
87. Manning BD, Cantley LC. AKT/PKB signaling: navigating downstream. Cell. 2007;129(7): 1261–74.
88. Samuels Y, Wang Z, Bardelli A, et al. High frequency of mutations of the PIK3CA gene in human cancers. Science. 2004;304(5670):554.
89. Kato S, Iida S, Higuchi T, et al. PIK3CA mutation is predictive of poor survival in patients with colorectal cancer. Int J Cancer. 2007;121(8):1771–8.
90. Samuels Y, Velculescu VE. Oncogenic mutations of PIK3CA in human cancers. Cell Cycle. 2004;3(10):1221–4.
91. Barault L, Veyrie N, Jooste V, et al. Mutations in the RAS-MAPK, PI(3)K (phosphatidylinositol-3-OH kinase) signaling network correlate with poor survival in a population-based series of colon cancers. Int J Cancer. 2008;122(10):2255–9.
92. Waldman SA, Hyslop T, Schulz S, et al. Association of GUCY2C expression in lymph nodes with time to recurrence and disease-free survival in pN0 colorectal cancer. JAMA. 2009;301(7):745–52.
93. Popat S, Matakidou A, Houlston RS. Thymidylate synthase expression and prognosis in colorectal cancer: a systematic review and meta-analysis. J Clin Oncol. 2004;22(3):529–36.
94. Aschele C, Debernardis D, Tunesi G, Maley F, Sobrero A. Thymidylate synthase protein expression in primary colorectal cancer compared with the corresponding distant metastases and relationship with the clinical response to 5-fluorouracil. Clin Cancer Res. 2000;6(12):4797–802.
95. Gorlick R, Metzger R, Danenberg KD, et al. Higher levels of thymidylate synthase gene expression are observed in pulmonary as compared with hepatic metastases of colorectal adenocarcinoma. J Clin Oncol. 1998;16(4):1465–9.

96. Sanguedolce R, Vultaggio G, Sanguedolce F, et al. The role of thymidylate synthase levels in the prognosis and the treatment of patients with colorectal cancer. Anticancer Res. 1998;18(3A):1515–20.
97. Jensen SA, Vainer B, Witton CJ, Jorgensen JT, Sorensen JB. Prognostic significance of numeric aberrations of genes for thymidylate synthase, thymidine phosphorylase and dihydrofolate reductase in colorectal cancer. Acta Oncol. 2008;47(6):1054–61.
98. Wang Y, Jatkoe T, Zhang Y, et al. Gene expression profiles and molecular markers to predict recurrence of Dukes' B colon cancer. J Clin Oncol. 2004;22(9):1564–71.
99. Barrier A, Boelle PY, Roser F, et al. Stage II colon cancer prognosis prediction by tumor gene expression profiling. J Clin Oncol. 2006;24(29):4685–91.
100. Eschrich S, Yang I, Bloom G, et al. Molecular staging for survival prediction of colorectal cancer patients. J Clin Oncol. 2005;23(15):3526–35.
101. Kerr D, Gray R, Quirke P, et al. A quantitative multigene RT-PCR assay for prediction of recurrence in stage II colon cancer: selection of the genes in four large studies and results of the independent, prospectively designed QUASAR validation study. American Society for Clinical Oncology, Annual Meeting 2009. Abstract #4000.

Chapter 8
Markers in Lung Cancer

Edwin Y. Lin, Ravin Rupani, and Barbara J. Gitlitz

Introduction

Lung cancer remains the most common cause of cancer death in both men and women in the United States with an estimated incidence of 219,440 for 2009 with 159,390 deaths [1]. Despite newer drugs and improved supportive care, the improvement in survival over the past decade has been small. In one review of prior studies, 5 year overall survival for patients with pathologic stage I disease was 64.6% (range 55–72%) and 41.2% for patients with stage II disease (range, 29–51%) [2]. Pathological stage IIIA patients do significantly worse with 77% dying within 5 years [3]. Patient with advanced NSCLC stage IIIB and IV do even worse, with a median overall survival of 10–12 months in recent trials [4, 5]. Thus, overall, prognosis remains poor for the majority of patients with only about 15% alive 5 years after diagnosis. Of note, there appears to be a great amount of variability in survival differences within a particular stage, indicating the presence of modifying factors.

For early stage disease, surgery represents the only current possibility for cure with adjuvant chemotherapy recently showing some benefit in selected populations. There have been multiple trials evaluating the effect of adjuvant chemotherapy following complete surgical resection of NSCLC [6–9]. Although overall there

E.Y. Lin, M.D.
Department of Medical Oncology, Norris Comprehensive Cancer Center,
Keck School of Medicine, University of Southern California, Los Angeles, CA, USA

R. Rupani, M.D.
Department of Hematology and Oncology, Norris Comprehensive Cancer Center,
University of Southern California, Los Angeles, CA, USA

B.J. Gitlitz, M.D. (✉)
Division of Medical Oncology, Department of Medicine, Norris Comprehensive
Cancer Center, Keck School of Medicine, University of Southern California,
1441 Eastlake Avenue, Suite 3452, Los Angeles, CA 90042, USA
e-mail: gitlitz@usc.edu

H.-J. Lenz (ed.), *Biomarkers in Oncology: Prediction and Prognosis*,
DOI 10.1007/978-1-4419-9755-5_8,

appears to be benefit with adjuvant chemotherapy, the benefit is largely seen in those patients with stage II and III disease with small to no benefit in stage I disease. Given this data, it can be inferred that if all patients with stage IB to stage III tumors are treated with adjuvant chemotherapy, there will be many patients that receive adjuvant chemotherapy who may not gain any benefit. Conversely if patients with stage I disease do not receive adjuvant chemotherapy, there may be some who may have actually benefited from the additional therapy. Thus the need for improved prognostic factors is apparent. With the side effects of treatment and rising costs of newer medications, it would be of considerable interest to identify those patients who are unlikely to gain benefit from adjuvant treatment as well as capture those with early stage cancers that may benefit.

The outcome in metastatic disease is even more dismal. Various doublets chemotherapy regimens were shown to be roughly equivocal with median survivals around 10 months. Newer agents such as pemetrexed, bevacizumab, and tyrosine kinase inhibitors have shown improved benefit, but long-term survival remains rare. In this setting, prognostic information can help guide patients and physicians in the decision to pursue therapy.

In this section, we review the promising prognostic molecular markers that have been studied in lung cancer followed by data on combining markers and gene profiling. Finally, we evaluate some of the clinical trials currently in process. Although the majority of data is focused on non-small-cell lung cancer, we also touch briefly on some of the data in small-cell lung cancer.

ERCC1

The ERCC1 gene, located on chromosome 19q, produces a rate-limiting protein essential for nucleotide excision repair (NER) [10]. The importance of NER is in the repair of bulky covalent lesions within the DNA and thus provides a mechanism by which tumors can generate genomic instability as well as a potential mechanism for resistance to platinum-based chemotherapy. ERCC1 helps in the recognition/excision repair of DNA damage. Its importance is underscored by the observations that defective cells have a severe DNA repair deficient phenotype [11] and that ERCC1 knockout mice die before weaning (Fig. 8.1) [12].

Significant focus on the predictive value of ERCC1 in guiding chemotherapy options has resulted from the multiple studies showing resistance to platinum agents with high levels of ERCC1 [13–15], but there have also been many studies showing that ERCC1 carries significant prognostic implications independent of its predictive nature. The evaluation of ERCC1 as a prognostic marker was first described by Simon et al., who utilized quantitative-RT PCT in the specimens of 51 patients who had undergone curative surgical resection for stage IA–IIIB NSCLC [16]. The expression of ERCC1 was found to be greater in nonsmokers and adenocarcinomas in comparison to prior smokers and other NSCLC subtypes. In this study, patients were subdivided by amount of ERCC1 expression with higher expression associated with a statistically significant longer survival (94.6 months vs. 35.5 months,

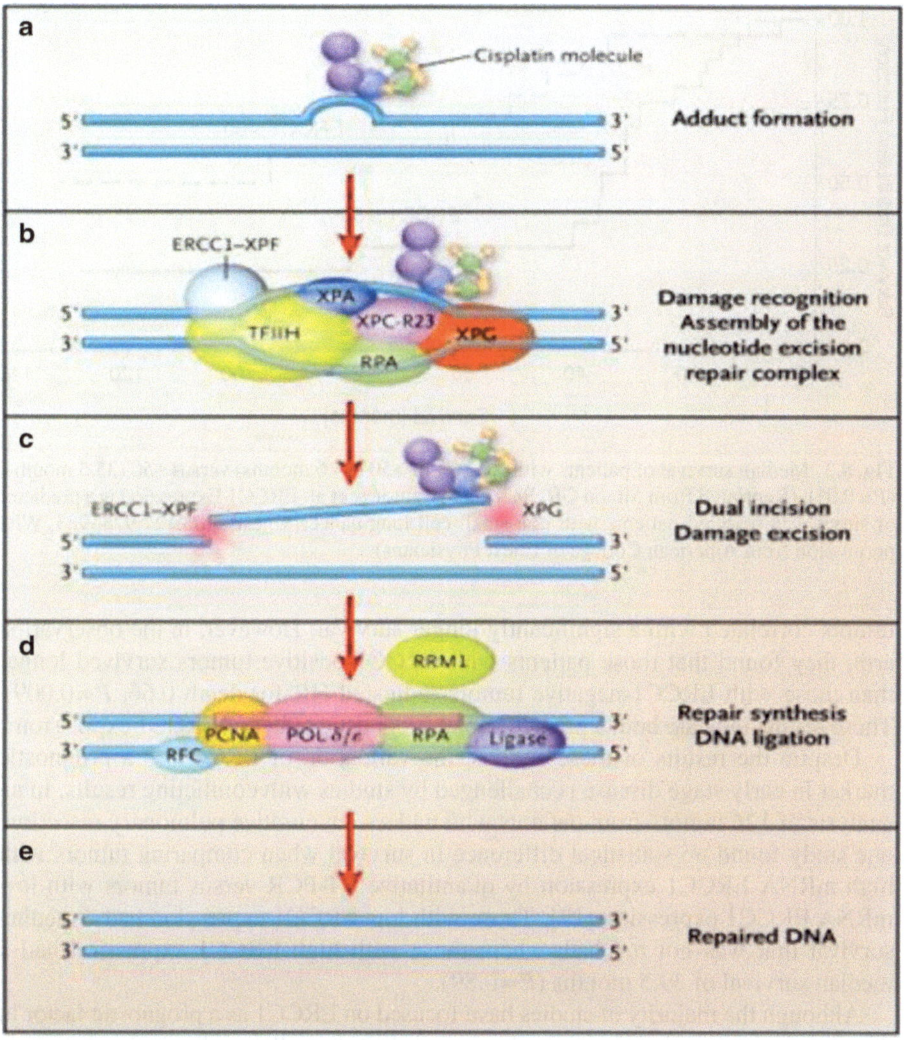

Fig. 8.1 Excision repair modulated by ERCC1 and RRM1. (**a**) Cisplatin binds covalently to form a DNA adduct. In chemoresistant cells with high nucleotide excision repair activity, the adduct may be excised and the DNA repaired. (**b**)Recognition of DNA adducts by the nucleotide excision repair complex. (**c**) Endonucleases create incisions flanking the damaged bases. (**d**) Repair of the excised segment by polymerases, accessory replication proteins, and DNA ligase. The protein RRM1 catalyzes the biosynthesis of the building blocks necessary for repair. (**e**) Repaired DNA. (Reprinted from Gazdar AF. DNA repair and survival in lung cancer—The two faces of Janus. N Eng J Med 2007;356:771–773. With permission from the Massachusetts Medical Society)

$P=0.01$) (Fig. 8.2). More recently, expression of ERCC1 by immunohistochemistry (IHC) has been correlated to survival in patients with resected NSCLC who had been enrolled in the International Adjuvant Lung Cancer Trial (IALT) [15]. Positive ERCC1 expression was demonstrated in 335 out of 761 patients (44%). Among those patients who received adjuvant cisplatin-based chemotherapy, ERCC1-negative

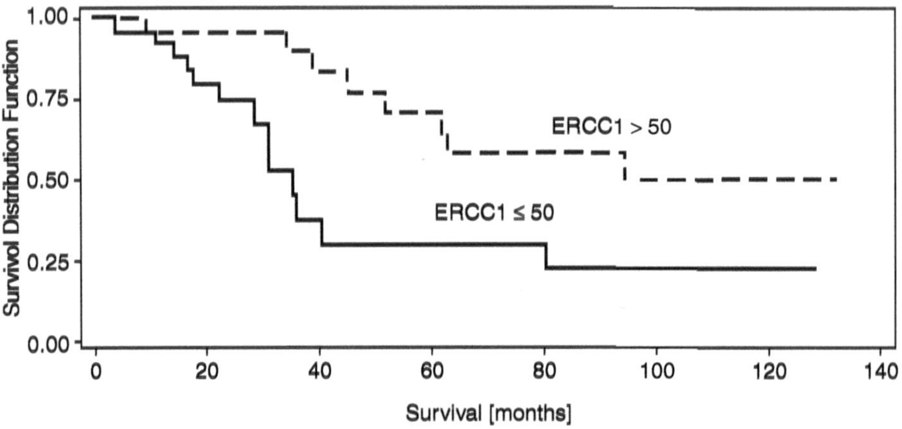

Fig. 8.2 Median survival of patients with ERCC1 of >50 (94.6 months) versus ≤50 (35.5 months) ($P=0.01$). (Reprinted from Simon GR, Sharma S, Cantor A et al. ERCC1 Expression is a predictor of survival in resected patients with non-small-cell lung cancer. Chest 2005;127:978–983. With permission from American College of Chest Physicians)

tumors correlated with a significantly longer survival. However, in the observation arm, they found that those patients with ERCC1-positive tumors survived longer than those with ERCC1-negative tumors (adjusted HR for death 0.66, $P=0.009$). These results indicate both a predictive and prognostic effect of ERCC1 expression.

Despite the results of these studies, the validation of ERCC1 as a prognostic marker in early stage disease is challenged by studies with conflicting results. In an analysis of 126 tumors from patients who underwent curative pulmonary resection, one study found no statistical difference in survival when comparing tumors with high mRNA ERCC1 expression by quantitative RT-PCR versus tumors with low mRNA ERCC1 expression [17]. Those with low ERCC1 expression had a median survival that was not reached, where those with high ERCC1 expression had a median survival of 39.5 months ($P=0.89$).

Although the majority of studies have focused on ERCC1 as a prognostic factor in the adjuvant setting, there have also been a number of smaller studies in the metastatic setting. Lord et al. evaluated ERCC1 mRNA expression by RT-PCR in samples from 56 patients with stage IIIB and IV disease who had received gemcitabine and cisplatin as part of a 3-arm randomized trial [18]. In this analysis, mRNA expression relative to an internal control housekeeping gene β(beta)-actin was determined for each sample with the median expression found to be 6.7×10^{-3}. The median overall survival for patients with tumors expressing ERCC1 below the median level of 6.7×10^{-3} was significantly prolonged in comparison to those with high ERCC1 expressing tumors (median survival 62 weeks vs. 20 weeks $P=0.009$). Given that there was no evaluation of patients who had not received treatment, this difference may in large part reflect the predictive nature or ERCC1 in patients receiving a cisplatin-containing regimen. In another study, ERCC1 expression was evaluated by IHC in samples from 32 patients with NSCLC that had participated in a trial comparing cisplatin/gemcitabine and epirubicin/gemcitabine [19]. Patients were preselected according to survival so that only patients who survived <26 weeks or >78 weeks were included in the analysis. Overall, 14/32 patients showed positive nuclear staining for ERCC1. There was no significant association between ERCC1 expression and survival or response rates.

Overall, the majority of data suggest a positive correlation between high ERCC1 levels and improved prognosis in early stage NSCLC.

RRM1

RRM1, located on chromosome 11p15.5, is a highly conserved gene that encodes the regulatory subunit of ribonucleotide reductase. The discovery of the importance of RRM1 in lung cancer was initiated with the observation of a loss of genetic material in the short arm of chromosome 11 in a variety of tumor types including lung cancer [20]. It was later noted that a large proportion of lung cancers show loss of heterozygosity (LOH) in this region with 88% of small-cell, 57% of squamous-cell, and 40% of adenocarcinomas showing LOH at this site. Clinical correlation with stage was also found in subsequent studies with a trend towards metastatic disease [21]. The structural gene for RRM1 had previously been located in the short arm of chromosome 11 and thus was identified as a key potential regulatory gene in the pathogenesis of a variety of cancers [22]. The activity of ribonucleotide reductase is cell cycle-dependent, reaching its maximum activity during S phase, though levels of the M1 subunit appears constant throughout the cell cycle in contrast to the M2 subunit [23]. In addition to its role in DNA synthesis, data suggests that its interaction with RRM2 and PTEN effects signaling in the regulation of various cell functions such as cellular differentiation and migration (Fig. 8.3) [24–26].

As a prognostic factor in NSCLC, RRM1 gene expression has been evaluated using RT-PCR on tumor specimens from patients with resected NSCLC with validation of results using an additional set of patients [27]. The majority of the 77 patients in the validation set of the study had stage I disease (84.4%) with only one patient in the cohort receiving either neoadjuvant or adjuvant therapy. There were no significant differences in RRM1 expression in the various subsets examined including smoking status, sex, ECOG, pathologic stage, or histopathology. Median survival was not reached in the patients with high expression of RRM1 ($n=39$) and was significantly longer in comparison to those patients with lower expression of RRM1 ($P=0.011$). Using Cox regression analysis RRM1 was found to be a significant independent predictor of survival independent of tumor stage, performance status, and weight loss ($P=0.05$). To further validate this data, a follow-up study by the same group evaluated 187 patients with completely resected, stage I non-small-cell lung cancer for RRM1 protein expression using AQUA scoring (immunofluorescence combined with automated quantitative analysis) [28]. Median disease-free survival for patients with low levels of RRM1 was 54.5 months versus 120 months for those with high levels of RRM1 ($P=0.004$, HR 2.2). Similarly the median overall survival was 60.2 months versus >120 months for those patients with high levels of

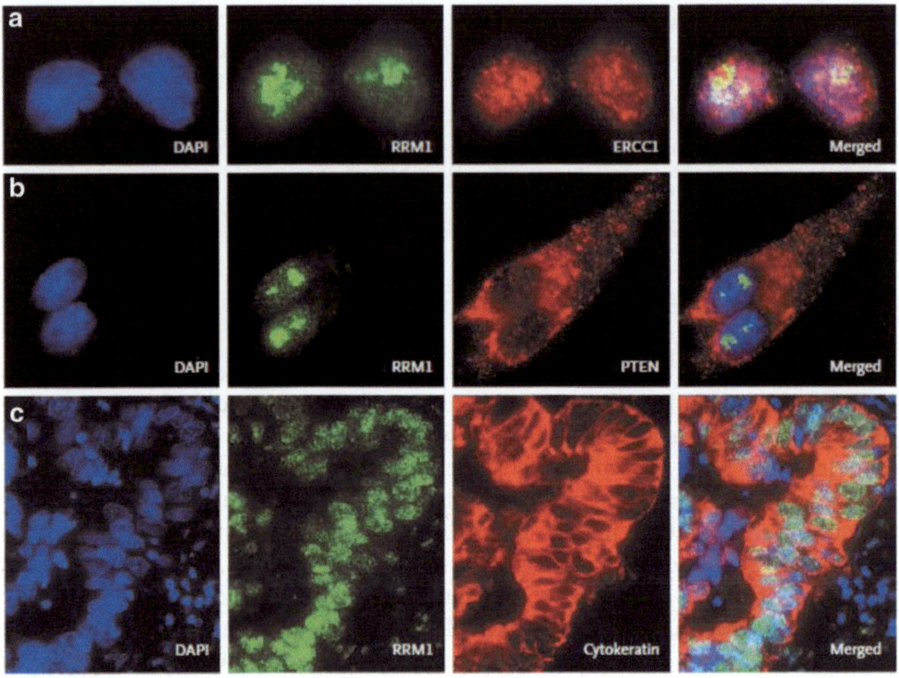

Fig. 8.3 Confocal microscopy of RRM1, ERCC1, and PTEN expression in cell lin NCI-H23. (**a**, **b**) show nuclei labeled with 4 ,6-diamidine-2-phenylindole (DAPI, *blue*). RRM1 was visualized with the use of R1AS-6 labeled with Alexa 488 (*green*). ERCC1 and PTEN were visualized with the use of commercial antibodies labeled with Alexa 555 (*red*). During the interphase, RRM1 is only nuclear, ERCC1 is predominantly nuclear, and PTEN is predominantly cytoplasmic. (**c**) shows multitarget immunofluorescence labeling of formaldehyde-fixed and paraffin-embedded histologic sections of lung cancer. The nuclei are *blue*, RRM1 is *green*, and the tumor cytoplasm is *red*. RRM1 is located in the nucleus and displays a granular pattern. (Reprinted from Zheng Z, Chen T, Li X et al. DNA synthesis and repair genes *RRM1* and *ERCC1* in lung cancer. N Eng J Med 2007;356:800–808. With permission from the Massachusetts Medical Society)

RRM1 ($P=0.02$, HR 1.6). In multivariate analysis including RRM1 expression, stage, ECOG status, sex, and smoking status, RRM1 was the only variable that carried statistical significance for disease-free survival ($P=0.03$). However, association with overall survival did not reach statistical significance ($P=0.11$) (Fig. 8.4).

Overall, high RRM1 expression appears to correlate with improved prognosis in NSCLC both in early stage disease.

BRCA1

BRCA1 mutations have long been known by their relationship to inherited breast and ovarian cancer syndromes. Located on the long arm of chromosome 17, the BRCA1 protein works with other proteins to repair strand breaks in DNA and is considered a key protein participating in cell cycle [29].

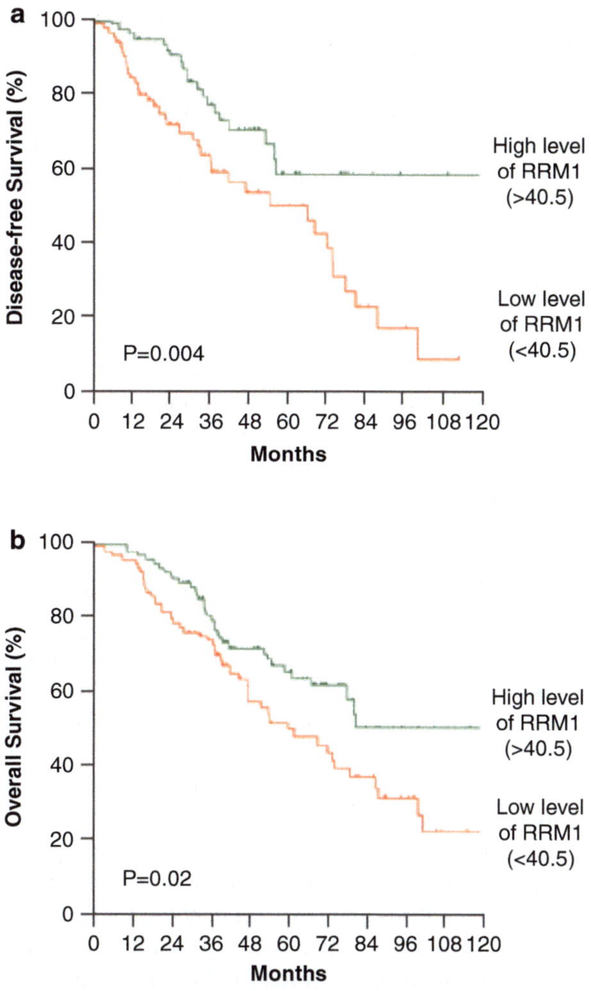

Fig. 8.4 Kaplan–Meier estimates of disease-free survival and overall survival among 187 patients with completely resected, stage I non-small-cell lung cancer, according to rrm1 expression level. The median value for RRM1 protein expression (determined with R1AS-6 and AQUA scoring) was used to divide the patients into high-expression and low-expression groups. (Reprinted from Zheng Z, Chen T, Li X et al. DNA synthesis and repair genes *RRM1* and *ERCC1* in lung cancer. N Eng J Med 2007;356:800–808. With permission from the Massachusetts Medical Society)

BRCA1 gene expression as evaluated by RT-PCR has been strongly associated with poor survival in NSCLC patients who have undergone surgical resection [17]. The identification of BRCA1 expression as a prognostic marker was first examined using samples from an initial cohort of 126 patients. BRCA1 expression was found to be significantly higher in squamous cell cancers in comparison to adenocarcinomas (median value 4.26 vs. 1.50, $P=0.0001$). With a median follow-up of 30 months, the analysis of both event free survival and overall survival demonstrated that high levels of BRCA1 expression correlated with shortened survival (median survival not reached with low expression of BRCA1 vs. 29 months with high expression, $P=0.04$). This finding held in a subset analysis of only stage I patients. Additionally, the prognostic value of BRCA1 was further validated in a second cohort of 58 patients with stage IB–IIB NSCLC patients who had also undergone surgical resection. With a median follow-up of 40 months survival was significantly shorter in patients with high expression of BRCA1 (HR 2.4, 95% CI: 1.01–5.92, $P=0.04$).

Thus, current data demonstrates that high expression of BRCA1 by RT-PCR is associated with a poor prognosis in NSCLC. Data is limited in volume, and therefore this correlation requires further validation in future studies.

p53

The p53 tumor suppressor gene, located on chromosome 17p, has been implicated in the development of numerous tumor types, most commonly breast cancer and sarcoma. It is thought to play a number of roles in various cellular pathways including apoptosis, cell cycle checkpoints, and DNA repair. The frequency of p53 mutations in lung cancer has been estimated at 45%. In one study of NSCLC patients, p53 mutations were found in higher frequency in patients with a history of smoking [30].

The effect of p53 mutations and overexpression has been extensively studied in NSCLC with conflicting results. In one study of 156 patients, tumors that stained 50% or more cells with p53 were associated with significantly longer survivals than those with low or negative staining (65 months vs. 26 months for low staining and 33 months for negative staining, $P=0.002$) [31]. Since the presence of a p53 mutation and overexpression do not necessarily correlate, other studies have attempted to evaluate the prognostic effect of p53 with respect to both mutations and overexpression [32]. Eighty-five patients with NSCLC who had undergone curative resection as part of the Lung Cancer Study Group (LCSG) study 871 were evaluated for p53 using IHC for overexpression as well as single-strand conformation polymorphism analysis and DNA sequencing for p53 mutational analysis. Of the studied patients, 64% showed p53 overexpression and 51% had mutant p53 sequences, but there was only 67% concordance. When looking specifically at p53 mutations, there was no significant difference in survival in comparison to patients with wild-type p53. With respect to IHC, there was a trend towards shortened survival for those patients with positive staining by IHC ($P=0.057$). Following stepwise multivariate analysis, neither p53 mutations nor IHC expression was independently predictive of survival. Likewise, Schiller et al. evaluated 197 tumors from patients who had undergone either adjuvant radiation or chemoradiation for stage II or IIIa NSCLC [33]. They found similar incidences of p53 mutations (45%) and IHC overexpression (55%), but no correlation could be made between p53 expression or p53 mutation status and prognosis.

At least two studies commented specifically on stage I NSCLC patients who had undergone curative resection and found a statistically significant difference in survival with respect to p53. Tomizawa et al. evaluated p53 mutations of exons 2–11 and overexpression via IHC [34]. Similar to other studies, p53 mutations were found in 49/103 (48%) of tumors. Overexpression by IHC was found in 41/103 (40%) and concordance between p53 mutations and expression was found in 69%. They found that p53 mutations but not overexpression were associated with poor prognosis ($P<0.001$) and that missense mutations rather than null mutations were associated with poor prognosis ($P<0.001$ for missense and $P=0.243$ for null mutations). In another study by Ahrendt et al., the effect of p53 mutations on patients with stage I–IIIA NSCLC was evaluated [35]. They found a statistically significant prognostic effect of p53 mutation that was limited to patients with stage I NSCLC (HR for death 2.8, 95% CI = 1.4–5.6). Four-year survival for those patients with stage I NSCLC with wild-type p53 was 78% versus 52% for mutant p53 (26% difference in survival, 95% CI = 6–46%, $P=0.009$).

More recently, Tsao et al. have evaluated 253 patients who had participated in the NCI Canada JBR.10 trial, which assigned patients with resected stage IB and II NSCLC to adjuvant cisplatin/vinorelbine or observation [36]. Tumors were assessed for p53 by IHC with those showing at least 15% staining designated as overexpressing p53. Samples were also evaluated for p53 mutations via PCR. p53 overexpression was 52% and more frequent in males and squamous cell carcinomas. Patients with p53 overexpression had significantly shorter survival in the observation arm than those with p53-negative tumors (HR = 1.89, 95% CI: 1.07–3.34; $P=0.03$) and was maintained even after multivariate adjustment ($P=0.02$). However, the presence of a p53 mutation did not appear to have any prognostic value in the observation arm (HR for mutant vs. wild type = 1.15; 95% CI: 0.75–1.77, $P=0.45$).

Other studies of the value of p53 in evaluating the prognosis of lung cancer include two meta-analyses. In a meta-analysis by Mitsudomi looking at both p53 mutations and overexpression in surgically resected patients [37], the group found that both the 3-year and 5-year survivals for patients with adenocarcinomas were decreased similarly by 21.8% ($P<0.001$) in tumors overexpressing p53 by IHC versus tumors with normal expression. When analyzing p53 by DNA mutation studies, the differences in patients with adenocarcinomas were more striking with a decrease in 3-year and 5-year survival of 41.0% ($P<0.001$) and 48.0% ($P<0.001$) respectively for those with mutations. However, in their analysis of squamous cell carcinomas, although there were trends towards shorter survival, these values were not statistically significant. In another meta-analysis by Steels published in 2001, the analysis was applied to NSCLC at various stages, but looked at combined mutations and overexpression data [38]. In any stage the HR was 1.44 (95% CI: 1.20–1.72), stage I–II 1.50 (95% CI: 1.32–1.70), stage III–IV 1.68 (95% CI: 1.30–2.18). When the data was subdivided by overexpression and p53 mutational analysis, the results remained statistically significant.

Although the majority of prior studies appear to show that p53 mutations correlate with poor overall survival in NSCLC, there are conflicting results perhaps reflecting the methodology of detection, effects of different mutations, and retrospective nature of the majority of the studies.

Thyroid Transcription Factor-1

Thyroid transcription factor-1 (TTF-1), also known as Nkx2.1 or thyroid-specific enhancer-binding protein, has long been used as a marker for NSCLC. TTF-1, located on chromosome 14q13, plays a crucial role in normal lung function and morphogenesis. It is a homeodomain-containing transcription factor that regulates tissue-specific expression of various surfactant proteins and is initiated at a very early stage of lung development [39, 40]. Expression of TTF-1 has been found in higher frequency in both small-cell lung cancer and adenocarcinoma as compared to squamous cell lung cancer [41]. In a study evaluating normal fetal and adult lung tissue along with lung adenocarcinomas, TTF-1 was expressed consistently in both the fetal and adult stages of lung development and uniformly in pneumocytes and epithelium of small-sized bronchioles. [42]. In adenocarcinomas, >50% TTF-1 expression was found in 46/64 cases (72%). Adenocarcinomas positive for TTF-1 were also noted to have a statistically significant prevalence of females, nonsmokers, and negative p53 staining.

As a prognostic marker, Perner et al. retrospectively evaluated a cohort of 538 patients with NSCLC who underwent curative resection using IHC for TTF-1 expression and FISH for assessment of TTF-1 amplification [43]. Amplification by FISH was found in 29 adenocarcinomas (12.9%) and 23 squamous cell carcinomas (9.4%) with no amplification found in adjacent normal lung tissue. However, there was no correlation found between stage, grade, or survival. For adenocarcinomas, although TTF-1 amplification was not associated with any specific patient or tumor characteristics, high TTF-1 expression by IHC was associated with female gender, smaller tumor size, and lower pathological tumor stage. When adenocarcinomas were stratified by quartiles based on the level of TTF-1 protein expression, patients with tumors in the highest quartile showed a significantly improved survival (82 months vs. 28 months; $P=0.002$). On multivariate analysis, high TTF-1 expression was shown to be an independent predictor of favorable prognosis among adenocarcinomas (HR 0.56; 95% CI=0.38–0.83; $P=0.008$). Amplification of TTF-1 also demonstrated a trend toward improved survival in adenocarcinomas, but this was not statistically significant (63 months vs. 43 months; $P=0.15$). None of the clinical correlations for TTF-1 overexpression and amplification in the adenocarcinomas were found in the squamous cell carcinoma cohort. Additionally, squamous cell carcinomas were found to have decreased levels of TTF-1 expression in comparison to the adenocarcinomas.

A meta-analysis was performed in 2006 by Berghmans et al. identifying 10 publications between 1999 and 2005 [44]. Out of the 10 publications, 4 found a statistically significant improvement in survival with those patients with TTF-1 positive tumors and 1 with a significant decrease in survival. The remaining publications did not find a statistically different outcome in favor or against TTF-1 positive tumors. This effect was demonstrated in the subset of patients with adenocarcinomas, but the lack of data in other histologies precluded the drawing of definite conclusions. Additionally, there was significant variability in methodology such as the cutoff for TTF-1 positivity.

Overall, TTF-1 expression appears to correlate with improved survival, specifically in adenocarcinomas. However, varying methodologies and small sample sizes make a combined interpretation of the data difficult and would require further validation in prospective studies.

K-ras Mutations/P21 Overexpression

Ras mutations appear to play vital roles in the oncogenesis of a variety of cancers. K-ras is one of a few well-characterized human ras genes, including H-ras and N-ras that were initially discovered in the 1960s as the main components in rat sarcomas viruses that drove carcinogenesis. They belong to a superfamily of genes coding for highly homologous small monomeric GTP-binding proteins ($p21^{ras}$). K-ras mutations have gained recent attention secondary to their effect as a potential predictive marker in both NSCLC and colon cancer for the use of EGFR targeted agents. Prior studies show that k-ras oncogene mutations can be found in about 30% of adenocarcinomas of the lung. The K-ras gene encodes a protein that binds guanine nucleotides and is involved in signal transduction [45]. Eighty percent of K-ras mutations occur in codon 12, with a smaller percentage in codons 13 and 61 [46].

The prognostic effect of K-ras mutations and p21 overexpression is controversial, much like many other of the single molecular prognostic markers. However, there have been many studies showing that K-ras mutations are associated with a poor prognosis. Mascaux et al. performed a meta-analysis regarding the prognostic indication of having a mutant K-ras gene or $p21^{ras}$ overexpression in NSCLC [47]. Overall RAS mutation was associated with a worse survival (HR 1.30; 95% CI: 1.20–1.49, $P=0.01$). In a subgroup analysis, RAS/p21 was not a statistically significant prognostic factor for survival in SCCA, but was for adenocarcinoma with a HR of 1.59 (CI 95%: 1.26–2.02, $P=0.02$). When evaluating by stage, RAS mutations/p21 overexpression did not show any significant impact on survival. Additionally, the group attempted to ascertain whether using different methods of detecting the abnormalities in K-ras expression had an effect on results. When looking at those studies that utilized IHC for p21 overexpression, the HR for overexpression was 1.08 with a CI 95% of 0.86–1.34. In contrast, studies utilizing PCR to detect K-ras mutations, had a HR of 1.40; CI 95% of 1.18–1.65. Huncharek et al. performed another separate meta-analysis evaluating eight published studies looking specifically at the K-ras mutation (not overexpression) in NSCLC [48]. Stage of the patients involved in the various studies included stages I–IV, but the majority of patients had prior resection. All of the studies utilized PCR for the detection of K-ras mutations. In total, 881 tumor samples were analyzed, with 217 positive for K-ras mutations (25%). 4/8 studies evaluated K-ras mutation outside of codon 12 (codons 13 and 61). Although the majority of studies included in the meta-analysis specified the various K-ras mutations evaluated, survival data for each mutation was generally not performed. In combination, the RR of death at 2 years is 2.35 with a 95% CI of 1.61–3.22. However, a great deal of heterogeneity in the effect of the

K-ras mutation existed. Four of the 8 studies had confidence intervals including the null value, whereas 3 studies had CIs exceeding 20. They noted that grouping studies that only evaluated mutations in similar codons or similar histologic subtypes decreased the heterogeneity. Additional causes for heterogeneity include the method of sampling, the specific mutation evaluated, and the variation in the stages included in the different studies.

Despite this data supporting a negative correlation with K-ras mutations, more recent data utilizing data from patients who participated in the JBR.10 trial did not show a prognostic effect of either Kras mutations or p21 overexpression [17]. This trial included resected stage IB and II NSCLC who were randomized to chemotherapy with cisplatin/navelbine versus observation alone. RAS gene mutation analysis was successfully performed via PCR in 450 samples looking for mutations on codons 12, 13, and 61 of H-ras, K-ras, and N-ras. One hundred and nineteen mutations were identified in 117 out of 450 patients (26%). More mutations were found in adenocarcinomas and in tumors from female patients. The RAS mutation was not found to be a significant prognostic marker for survival in univariate or multivariate analyses. In the observation arm, the HR for death was 1.23 in favor of the RAS mutant tumors with a 95% CI of 0.76–1.97, $P=0.40$. The primary difference in survival between RAS mutant and RAS wild-type tumors occurred in the chemotherapy arm, where only those with wild type RAS had an improvement of survival. However, on univariate and multivariate analysis, this difference was not significant. These results were similar to results reported previously by Schiller in another prospective study involving patients with stage II and IIIA NSCLC who had received XRT with and without chemotherapy [33].

Thus, despite many reports of RAS mutations being a poor prognostic factor, there is still considerable doubt. Comparison of results between groups is confounded by the different techniques used for detection, the different mutations detected, and the heterogeneous population.

β(beta) Tubulin

Microtubules are important for a number of important cellular functions such as chemotaxis and migration. Composed of heterodimers of alpha and β(beta)-tubulin, they are the cellular targets for taxane chemotherapeutic agents. In addition to being a possible mechanism for tumor resistance to taxane chemotherapy, overexpression of β(beta)-tubulin has been shown to be a individual prognostic marker for patients with NSCLC.

Seve et al. evaluated the effect of class III β(beta)-tubulin (bTubIII) overexpression on the prognosis of patients with NSCLC involved in the JBR.10 clinical trial [49]. JBR.10 was a North American Intergroup trial that accrued 482 patients with stage IB and II NSCLC who had undergone curative surgical resection and randomized them to observation versus adjuvant treatment with vinorelbine/cisplatin. Evaluation of the expression of bTubIII by IHC for 265 of the 482 study patients was performed. The characteristics of the patients with tubulin data were similar to the overall study group except for a higher percentage of patients with T2 tumors and a lower percentage of N1 disease. In comparing those patients with tumors having high tubulin expression there was a statistically higher number of females, fewer with squamous histology, and a trend toward older patients and worse performance status. In assessing prognosis, the combined data for both observation and chemotherapy arms demonstrated a statistically significant shortening in recurrence free survival (RFS) for patients with high tubulin expression (HR 1.52; 95% CI: 1.05–2.22; $P=0.03$) and a trend for shortened survival (HR 1.39; 95% CI: 0.96–2.01; $P=0.08$). However, in analyzing each arm separately, the difference in RFS and OS was significant only in the observation arm (RFS: HR 1.92; 95% CI: 1.16–3.18; $P=0.01$; OS: HR 1.72; 95% CI: 1.02–2.88; $P=0.04$). High tubulin expression in the patients who had received chemotherapy did not correlate with a significant difference in survival in comparison to those with low expression (RFS: HR 1.10; 95% CI: 0.62–1.95; $P=0.75$; OS: HR 1.11; 95% CI: 0.65–1.88; $P=0.7$). Corroborating this data was an analysis showing that patients with low tubulin expression did not appear to gain benefit in survival with the use of adjuvant chemotherapy whereas those patients with high expression had a significant increase in RFS with the use of adjuvant chemotherapy (HR 0.45; 95% CI: 0.27–0.75; $P=0.002$). This benefit, however, did not persist following Cox regression analysis. These findings suggest that high tubulin III expression in resected NSCLCs is associated with poorer survival, but adjuvant chemotherapy may overcome the adverse biology of these tumors (Fig. 8.5).

In the advanced setting, bTubIII has demonstrated a similar correlation with prognosis. Two studies by the same group evaluating the effect of bTubIII expression on response to chemotherapy targeting microtubules noted that high levels of bTubIII was associated with a poorer prognosis [50, 51]. In the first study, two groups of patients were analyzed using IHC on tumor biopsy specimens. The first group contained 47 patients who had received paclitaxel-based regimens and the second group contained 44 patients who had received gemcitabine-based regimens. Although no difference in overall survival between patients with high expressing tumors and patients with low expression tumors was found in those treated with gemcitabine-based chemotherapy, there was a significant difference in overall survival in those patients treated with paclitaxel-based chemotherapy (median OS 525 days in patients with low level of bTubIII vs. 206 days, $P=0.0023$). It is important to note that there did appear to be a higher response rate to paclitaxel-based chemotherapy in the patients with low bTubIII expressing tumors, which may account for the difference in survival. In the second study, 93 patients treated with navelbine-based chemotherapy were assessed in similar fashion to the prior study. Although no statistically significant difference was found in response rates, the percentage of progression on therapy was significantly higher in the patients with high bTubIII expression and correspondingly had a worse PFS and OS (OS: 162 days vs. 306 days, $P=0.001$).

Thus, bTubIII expression appears to be a prognostic marker in both early and late stage NSCLC. Whether the prognostic effect in the advanced setting is in large part due to its predictive effect of chemotherapy effecting microtubule function remains to be determined.

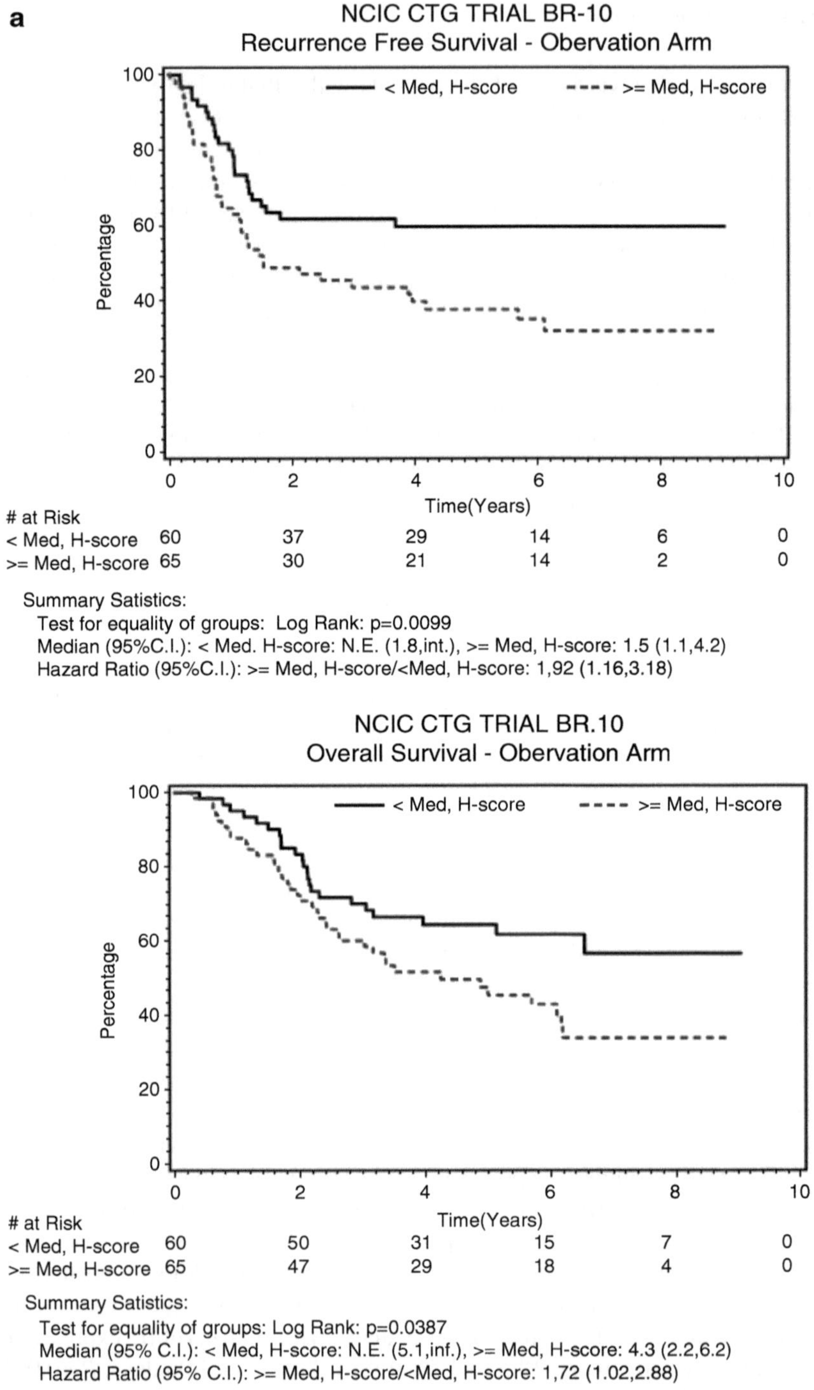

Fig. 8.5 The RFS and OS curves for patients assigned to observation alone according to bTubIII expression. (Reprinted from Sève P, Lai R, Ding K et al. Class III β-tubulin expression and benefit from adjuvant cisplatin/vinorelbine chemotherapy in operable non-small-cell lung cancer: analysis of NCIC JBR.10. Clin Cancer Res 2007;13:994–999. With permission from the American Association for Cancer Research)

EGFR

EGFR, also known as ErbB-1 and HER-1, is a 170 kDa tyrosine kinase receptor that signals multiple downstream pathways including Ras/Raf/MAPK, JAK-STAT, and PI3K/AKT pathways [52]. The importance of the EGFR pathway in NSCLC has been highlighted in the recent IPASS trial that demonstrated patients with EGFR mutations have higher response rates to both EGFR tyrosine kinase inhibitors and chemotherapy [53].

EGFR Overexpression

To evaluate the importance of the EGFR pathway, Jeon et al. assessed 262 Korean NSCLC patients for the prevalence of EGFR overexpression by both FISH and IHC and its effect on prognosis [54]. All of the study patients had surgically resected NSCLC and none had received treatment with an EGFR inhibitor. EGFR overexpression by IHC was observed in 53% of cases and 66% of squamous cell carcinomas and 38% of adenocarcinomas. FISH positivity was found in about 30% of the total studied patients. These numbers appear concordant with the rates found in studies evaluating Western populations. A high EGFR gene copy number was significantly more common in nonsmokers. There was a trend for patients with NSCLC and a high EGFR gene copy number to have a poorer prognosis. However, this did not reach statistical significance except for those patients with SCC, specifically stage I patients.

A meta-analysis was performed to evaluate the prognostic implications of EGFR overexpression by Nakamura et al. [55]. They evaluated studies published between 1990 and 2004 that had evaluated EGFR expression in NSCLC by either quantification of protein or mRNA expression. Eighteen studies were included in total with 15 studies including stages I–IIIB and 3 studies including stage IV disease. Only 50 patients out of a total of 2,972 patients were treated with gefinitib. Of the 18 studies, 6 studies had found a significant negative association (shorter survival) between EGFR expression and survival while 2 studies found a positive association. Overall, the combined HR for all 18 studies was 1.14 (95% CI: 0.97–1.34, $P=0.103$). When evaluating those studies using IHC only, the HR was 1.08 (95% CI: 0.92–1.28, $P=0.356$). Separating the studies by those dealing mostly with squamous cell carcinomas (>50%), the combined HR was 1.40 (95% CI: 0.98–2, $P=0.07$) while those with mostly adenocarcinomas had a HR of 0.90 (95% CI: 0.63–1.28, $P=0.55$).

EGFR Mutations

The TRIBUTE trial was a phase III randomized trial with 1,079 chemotherapy-naïve patients with stage IIIB or IV NSCLC who were randomized to chemotherapy (carboplatin/taxol) with or without erlotinib as first line therapy. As part of the trial, the effect of mutations in the EGFR gene in regards to patient outcome was determined [56]. Exons 18 through 21 of the EGFR gene were evaluated for 228 patients and 29 mutations found (12.7%, 95% CI: 8–17%). Although 17% of the patients with EGFR mutations were never smokers compared to 8% of wild-type patients, the majority of patients had a prior smoking history and the overall differences in smoking histories was not statistically significant. However, there was a correlation between EGFR mutations and younger age (median age 59 and 64 years for patients with mutant versus wild-type tumors respectively, $P<0.1$). When looking at the survival curves published, it appears that the EGFR mutant patients, regardless of treatment, had improved overall survival in comparison to the EGFR wild-type patients. It was also noted that ORR and TTP were also significantly better in the patients with EGFR mutations in comparison to those patients with EGFR wild-type (Fig. 8.6). These findings were similar to findings seen in an analysis of the INTACT trial published simultaneously, which had evaluated chemotherapy with and without gefitinib [57]. In this study, overall survival was not affected by the addition of gefitinib to chemotherapy in patients with EGFR mutations (HR 1.77; 95% CI: 0.50–6.23). However, EGFR-mutant patients treated with chemotherapy alone had a better OS compared with mutation negative patients (Median OS 19.4 months vs. 9.2 months; HR 0.48; 95% CI: 0.29–0.82). Improved survival was also seen with amplification of EGFR as well. Finally, in the IPASS trial, which had assessed the use of gefinitib versus carboplatin/taxol in first line unresectable NSCLC in non-smoking Asians, both chemotherapy and gefinitib arms displayed higher response rates with EGFR mutant tumors. It is unclear whether this improved response translated into an improved overall survival in these patients and whether any differences in survival could be associated with a prognostic effect of EGFR mutations or solely from the predictive nature of EGFR mutations to response to treatment.

Thus, it is still unclear as to the prognostic affect of both EGFR overexpression and EGFR mutations. Improved survival in this group of patients may be reflective of its predictive value of treatment from both chemotherapy and EGFR-targeted agents.

Thymidylate Synthase

Thymidylate synthase (TS) catalyzes the conversion of deoxyuridine monophosphate (dUMP) to deoxythmidine monophosphate (dTMP). Following phosphorylation dTMP produces TTP, which is required for multiple cell functions including DNA synthesis and repair. Both older agents such as 5-fluorouracil and newer agents such as pemetrexed target TMP synthesis to inhibit rapidly dividing cells. High expression of TS in squamous cell lung cancers is one of the proposed mechanisms by which these cancers have resistance to these drugs. Supporting this mechanism is data from Ceppi et al. showing that expression of TS is significantly higher in squamous cell carcinomas, which show an inherent resistance to pemetrexed, as opposed to adenocarcinomas of the lung [58].

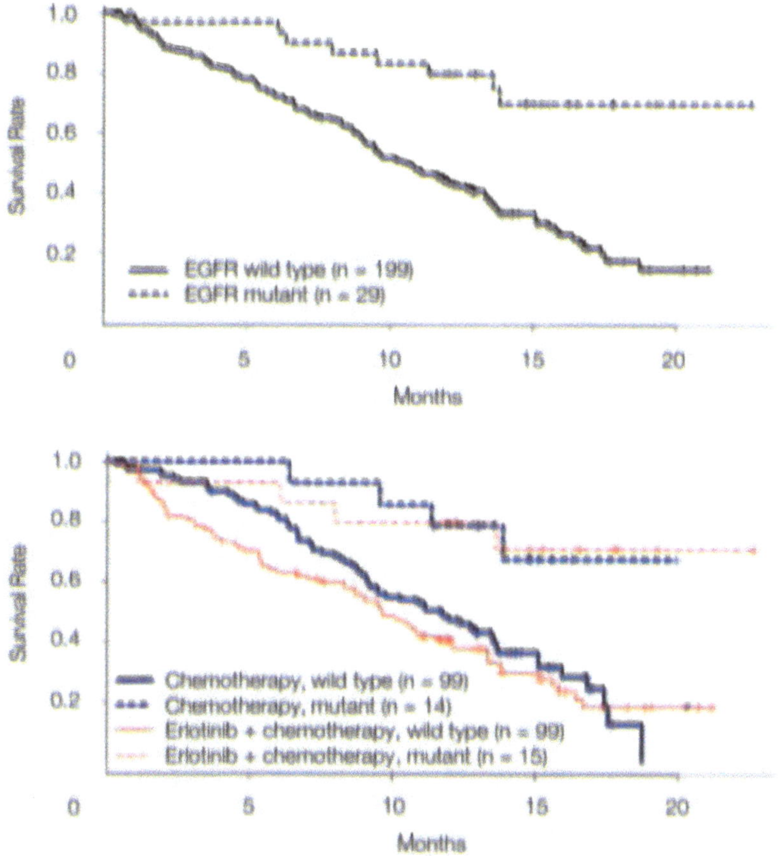

Fig. 8.6 Kaplan–Meier curves by epidermal growth factor receptor (EGFR) mutation status. *P* values refer to log-rank tests. (*Top*) Survival, by EGFR mutation status. The *P* value for patients with EGFR-mutant versus wild-type tumors is <0.001. (*Bottom*) Survival by treatment received and EGFR mutation status. There was no statistically significant difference between treatment arms for either wild type or mutant EGFR status. (Reprinted from Eberhand DA, Johnson BE, Amler LC et al. Mutations in the epidermal growth factor receptor and in KRAS are predictive and prognostic indicators in patients with non-small-cell lung cancer treated with chemotherapy alone and in combination with erlotinib. J Clin Oncol 2005;23:5900–5909. With permission from American Society of Clinical Oncology)

Independent of its predictive effect on treatment, however, TS may also serve as a marker of prognosis. Zheng et al. [59] evaluated patients with completely resected stage I NSCLC of various histologies that did not receive adjuvant chemotherapy or radiation. Cytoplasmic TS was determined by IHC and automated in situ protein quantification (AQUA) in the tumors of 160 patients and by quantitative reverse-transcriptase polymerase chain reaction (RT-PCR) in the tumors of 85 patients. There were 32 patients that overlapped between the two datasets. The authors found

Table 8.1 Overview of Prognostic Markers in Lung Cancer

Marker	Function/Pathway	Correlation	References
ERCC1	DNA excision repair	Higher expression correlates with longer survival in early stage NSCLC.	[15–19]
RRM1	Regulatory subunit of ribonucleotide reductase	Higher expression correlates with longer survival in early stage NSCLC.	[27, 28]
TTF-1	Lung morphogenesis	High TTF-1 expression correlates with improved survival, especially in adenocarcinomas.	[43, 44]
P53	Apoptotic and cell cycle check points, DNA repair	Presence of mutations correlates with shorter survival. High protein expression shows conflicting data.	[31–38]
BRCA1	DNA strand break repair, cell cycle check points	Higher expression correlates with shorter survival.	[17]
B-Tubulin	Subunits for microtubule formation	High expression has correlated to worse prognosis in both early and advanced disease in a few studies.	[50–52]
Thymidylate Synthase	Catalyzes the conversion of dUMP to dTMP for DNA synthesis and repair	High expression correlates with improved survival.	[60]
Kras	GTP-binding protein involved in signaling pathways	Conflicting results. Variable techniques and methodology confound results.	[17, 47–49]
EGFR	Receptor tyrosine kinase with multiple down-stream targets	Data still unclear as to prognostic effect of both mutations and overexpression. Some data links mutations with improved survival.	[55–58]

that high TS expression as detected by AQUA correlated with an increased overall survival (81.3 months vs. 51.7 months for those with low TS expression, $P=0.0013$). In the final multivariate model, which included TS protein expression and tumor stage, TS remained significantly associated with OS ($P=0.0013$, adjusted $P=0.032$). The HR for death for high versus low TS protein expression was 0.45. Additionally, TS expression was not found to be correlated with either RRM1 or ERCC1 expression, indicating that it may act as an independent prognostic factor from these molecular markers. Finally, the authors did not find any correlation between TS expression by IHC and TS mRNA quantitation, although there was only a small sample of patients that had data for both datasets.

Thus, TS shows some promise both as a predictive marker and prognostic marker in NSCLC, but will need to be evaluated further in larger prospective studies (Table 8.1).

Gene Expression Profiling

With advancing technology and improved analytical modeling, one of the most actively studied areas in the prognostication of lung cancer has been the development of gene signatures. Gene signatures refer to a specific pattern of gene expression that confers a specific behavior or phenotype to a tumor. By using newer technologies, a vast number of genes can be analyzed relatively quickly and associations with individual clinical outcomes or phenotypes can be predicted. Since the first gene expression profiling papers on NSCLC appeared in 2001, a number of studies have been published [60, 61]. These studies have underscored the immense genetic heterogeneity that exists in lung cancer, thus partly explaining the variability in how different tumors behave and respond to chemotherapy. The potential uses of these gene expression profiles in the literature have been numerous, including improved classification of lung cancer, creation of prognostic gene signatures, and the identification of new genes molecular pathways important in lung cancer.

Despite the vast potential for gene profiling as a prognostic tool, there remain a number of questions and obstacles. First, is the enormous genetic heterogeneity that exists in each tumor. Underscoring this fact is the lack of overlap between the various published studies in the genes selected for profiling. In theory, this heterogeneity would require thousands of samples to be analyzed to produce robust and reproducible datasets [62]. Furthermore, the creation of these gene datasets requires complicated analytical processes that are still being evaluated. There is still question as to whether its use can offer significantly more information than already established methods such as IHC and whether the analysis of a multitude of genes is significantly better than analyzing a few key markers. Finally, the practicality in terms of cost, accuracy, and reproducibility of utilizing this technology in the community will need to be evaluated.

Subclassifying Lung Cancer

One of the possible utilities of gene expression profiling is creating subclasses of lung cancer that better predicts their behavior and thus the prognosis of the patients. In a study by Bhattacharjee et al. the group evaluated the RNA of 186 lung cancer and 17 normal lung specimens in order to molecularly classify the tumors into various subtypes. The dataset included adenocarcinomas ($n=127$), squamous cell lung carcinomas ($n=21$), pulmonary carcinoids ($n=20$), SCLC ($n=6$), and adenocarcinomas suspected to be metastatic from other sites ($n=12$). After applying hierarchical clustering using the most variably expressed transcripts, they generated clusters to capture the distinctions between the established histologic classes. Concentrating only on the adenocarcinomas, four subclasses were distinguished based on gene expression clusters, noting that some adenocarcinomas shared characteristic gene expression with neuroendocrine and squamous cell lung cancers. In correlating with patient outcome, the neuroendocrine-like adenocarcinomas were associated with a less favorable survival outcome with a median survival of 21 months versus 40.5 months ($P=0.00476$). The difference was more pronounced with stage I tumors where median survival was 20 months compared with 47.8 months ($P=0.0753$). On the other side of the spectrum, the subclass of tumors that shared gene characteristics with bronchioalveolar tumors had a more favorable survival of 49.7 months versus 33.2 months ($P=0.049$). Another study published simultaneously by Garber et al. similarly used gene expression analysis to generate subclassification of adenocarcinomas in 67 patients. Similar to the Bhattacharjee group, they found that the different subclassifications were associated with significant differences in survival.

Further studies attempted to build on prior work by utilizing three different cohorts to generate the subclassifications of adenocarcinoma: bronchioid, squamoid, and magnoid [63]. Each subtype was correlated with not only a specific overall prognosis, but was also associated with stage-specific mortality and different metastatic patterns. Bronchioid tumors were associated with improved survival in early-stage disease, but squamoid tumors were associated with better survival in advanced disease. In terms of metastatic patterns, the bronchioid tumors tended to metastasize to the bones, whereas both squamoid and magnoid subtypes had a predilection for brain metastasis. Finally, in further analyzing the genetic signatures of each subtype, bronchioid tumors were noted to have a correlation with biologic pathways dominated by genes associated with growth, differentiation and development, squamoid tumors with genes involved with angiogenesis, and magnoid tumors with genes associated with inflammation, cytoskeleton, metabolism, and proliferation.

Gene Expression Signatures

Chen et al. developed a 5 gene signature model to determine prognosis by utilizing both microarray analysis and RT-PCR in 125 surgically removed NSCLC specimens [64]. Although 16 genes were found to correlate with survival after initial analysis, the five genes with the highest correlation with prognosis were selected to be included in the signature (DUSP6, MMD, STAT1, ERBB3, LCK). The five gene signature was validated in an independent cohort of 60 patients and another set of published microarray from 86 patients. In the validation cohort, patients with stage I disease and a low-risk gene signature had a longer overall survival than those with a high-risk gene signature ($P=0.02$). Although overall survival in patients with stage II did not differ significantly, this was attributed to the small number of patients. In multivariate cox regression analysis, the high-risk five gene signature was found to have statistically significant hazard ratios in all three cohorts studied (range 2.82–4.36)

Likewise, the results of a 15-gene expression signature study using patients enrolled in the JBR.10 adjuvant trial was has been presented [65]. Gene expression profiling was performed on RNA from frozen specimens of 62 patients in the observation only arm of the study resulting in a 15-gene expression signature separating high risk versus low risk for death. The signature included various genes previously implicated in other cancers, but few previously studied in NSCLC. In the training set, those patients with high risk as defined by the gene signature had a HR for death of 15.02 (95% CI: 5.12–44.04, $P<0.0001$). This separation was seen in both stage IB and stage II patients. The signature was then applied to 71 patients on the adjuvant chemotherapy arm and further validated in stage I and II patients of five independent public gene expression datasets that were used in prior studies (Director's Challenge Consortium study, Duke microarray study, University of Michigan squamous-cell microarray study). Following multivariate analysis, the gene signature was found to be statistically significant independent predictor of survival in all the datasets except the Duke dataset. Interestingly, in addition to the prognostic value of the 15 gene expression profile, they were also able to show that the high-risk patients showed benefit from chemotherapy in comparison to the low-risk patients.

Progressing Towards Clinical Application

Although the advances in prognostic models based on gene expression have been significant there remain a number obstacles and unanswered questions that need to be addressed prior to regular clinical use. Prior studies have utilized small numbers of subjects with heterogeneous tumor types, variable sample processing, and often lacked validation using multiple datasets. In an attempt to address some of the concerns, a retrospective, multicenter, blinded study was performed to not only validate some of the prior models used but also create a large microarray database of NSCLC samples using a common protocol [66]. Four hundred and forty-two lung adenocarcinoma samples and relevant clinical data were collected using cohorts from six lung-cancer treatment sites with gene expression data generated using a common protocol. Four datasets were created with two serving as a training set and the remaining two as validation sets. The authors then utilized eight different methods of calculating risk based on prior methods reported in the literature such as gene clustering, univariate testing, and on a mechanistic basis. In this study, use of gene clustering appeared to be the most consistently predictive of prognosis, whereas the majority of the other methods showed good performance in one setting that was offset by poor performance in a different setting. One of the other findings was that the use of clinical predictors in addition to gene expression data improved outcome prediction in most instances.

Although use of prognostic markers to determine the use of chemotherapy is steadily progressing towards practical use, further evaluation in large randomized clinical trials are still ongoing. The Southwest Oncology Group study 0720 will evaluate patients with surgically resected stage I NSCLC and administer adjuvant chemotherapy with gemcitabine and cisplatin based on ERCC1 or RRM1 expression determined at a central laboratory. Those patients with tumors expressing low levels of either ERCC1 or RRM1 will receive adjuvant chemotherapy, whereas patients with tumors expressing high levels of both markers will undergo active monitoring only. This trial utilizes a couple of concepts previously studied. The first is that high tumor expression of both ERCC1 and RRM1 portends a good prognosis in these

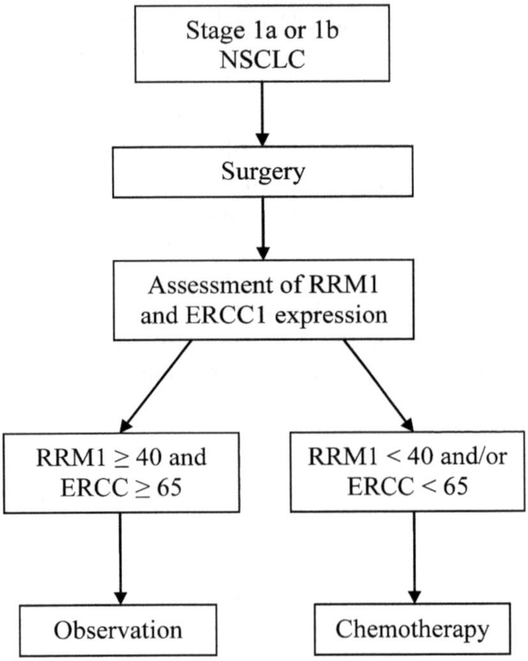

Fig. 8.7 Schema of SWOG 0720. Study utilizes ERCC1 and RRM1 expression to risk stratify patients into high-risk and low-risk categories with high-risk patients receiving adjuvant chemotherapy

patients. Additionally, it utilizes the previous finding that tumors with high expression of these molecules have a tendency towards decreased responsiveness to gemcitabine and platinum agents. This trial will thus combine both the prognostic and predictive values of these two molecular markers in making clinical decisions (Fig. 8.7).

References

1. Jemal A, Siegel R, Ward E, et al. Cancer statistics, 2009. CA Cancer J Clin. 2009;59:225–49.
2. Nesbitt JC, Putnam JB, Walsh GL, Roth JA, Mountain CF. Survival in early-stage non-small cell lung cancer. Ann Thorc Surg. 1995;60:466–72.
3. Mountain CF. Revisions in the International System for Staging Lung Cancer. Chest. 1997; 111:1710–7.
4. Scagliotti GV, Parikh P, von Pawel J, et al. Phase III study comparing cisplatin plus gemcitabine with cisplatin plus pemetrexed in chemotherapy-naïve patients with advanced-stage non-small-cell lung cancer. J Clin Oncol. 2008;26:3543–51.
5. Sandler A, Gray R, Perry MC, et al. Paclitaxel-carboplatin alone or with bevacizumab for non-small-cell lung cancer. N Engl J Med. 2006;355:2542–50.
6. Douillard J-Y, Rosell R, DeLena M, et al. Adjuvant vinorelbine plus cisplatin versus observation in patients with completely resected stage IB-IIIA non-small-cell lung cancer (Adjuvant Navelbine Internaional Trialist Association [ANITA]: a randomized controlled trial. Lancet Oncol. 2006;7:719–27.
7. Winton T, Livingston R, Johnson D, et al. Vinorelbine plus cisplatin vs. observation in resected non-small-cell lung cancer. N Engl J Med. 2005;352:2589–97.

8. Arriagada R, Bergman B, Dunant A, et al. Cisplatin-based adjuvant chemotherapy in patients with completely resected non-small-cell lung cancer. N Engl J Med. 2004;350:351–60.
9. Waller D, Peake MD, Stephens RJ, et al. Chemotherapy for patients with non-small cell lung cancer: the surgical setting of the Big Lung Trial. Eur J Cardiothorac Surg. 2004;26:173–82.
10. Reed E. Platinum-DNA adduct, nucleotide excision repair and platinum based anti-cancer chemotherapy. Cancer Treatment Rev. 1998;24:331–44.
11. Van Duin M, de Wit J, Odijk H, et al. Molecular characterization of the human excision repair gene ERCC-1: cDNA cloning and amino acid homology with yeast DNA repair gene RAD10. Cell. 1986;44:913–23.
12. Lee KB, Parker RJ, Bohr VA, et al. Cisplatin sensitivity/resistance in UV-repair deficient Chinese hamster ovary cells of complementation groups 1 and 3. Carcinogenesis. 1993; 14:2177–80.
13. Ceppi P, Volante M, Novello S, et al. ERCC1 and RRM1 gene expressions but not EFGR are predictive of shorter survival in advanced non-small-cell lung cancer treated with cisplatin and gemcitabine. Ann of Oncol. 2006;17:1818–25.
14. Coco M, Isla D, Massuri B, et al. Customizing cisplatin based on quantitative excision repair cross-complementing 1 mRNA expression: a phase III trial in non-small-cell lung cancer. J Clin Oncol. 2007;25:2747–54.
15. Olaussen KA, Dunant A, Fouret P, et al. DNA repair by ERCC1 in non-small-cell lung cancer and cisplatin-based adjuvant chemotherapy. N Engl J Med. 2006;355:983–91.
16. Simon GR, Sharma S, Cantor A, et al. ERCC1 expression is a predictor of survival in resected patients with non-small cell lung cancer. Chest. 2005;127:978–83.
17. Rosell R, Skrzypski M, Jassem E, et al. BRCA1: a novel prognostic factor in resected non-small-cell lung cancer. PLoS ONE. 2007;2:e1129.
18. Lord RV, Brabender J, Gandara J, et al. Low ERCC1 expression correlates with prolonged survival after cisplatin plus gemcitabine chemotherapy in non-small cell lung cancer. Clin Cancer Res. 2002;8:2286–91.
19. Wachters FM, Wong LSM, Timens W, et al. ERCC1, hRad51, and BRCA1 protein expression in relation to tumour response and survival of stage III/IV NSCLC patients treated with chemotherapy. Lung Cancer. 2005;50:211–9.
20. Shiraishi M, Morinaga S, Noguchi M, et al. Loss of genes on the short arm of chromosome 11 in human lung carcinomas. Jpn J Cancer Res. 1987;78:1302–8.
21. Bepler G, Fong KM, Johnson BE, et al. Cancer Detect Prev. 1998;22:14–9.
22. Engström Y, Francke U. Assignment of the structural gene for subunit M1 of human ribonucleotide reductase to the short arm of chromosome 11. Exp Cell Res. 1985;158:477–83.
23. Engström Y, Eriksson S, Jildevik I, et al. Cell cycle-dependent expression of mammalian ribonucleotide reductase. J Biol Chem. 1985;260:9114–6.
24. Fan H, Villegas C, Wright JA. Ribonucleotide reductase R2 component is novel malignancy determinant that cooperates with activated oncogenes to determine transformation and malignant potential. PNAS. 1996;93:14036–40.
25. Fan H, Huang A, Villegas C, et al. The R1 component of mamalian ribonucleotide reductase has malignancy-suppressing activity as demonstrated by gene transfer experiments. PNAS. 1997;94:13181–6.
26. Gautam A, Li Z, Bepler G. RRM1-induced metastasis suppression through PTEN-regulated pathways. Oncogene. 2003;22:2135–42.
27. Bepler G, Sharma S, Cantor A, et al. RRM1 and PTEN as prognostic parameters for overall and disease-free survival in patients with non-small-cell lung cancer. J Clin Oncol. 2004;22:1878–85.
28. Zheng Z, Chen T, Li X, et al. DNA synthesis and repair genes RRM1 and ERCC1 in lung cancer. N Engl J Med. 2007;356:800–8.
29. Deng C, Wang R. Roles of BRCA1 in DNA damage repair: a link between development and cancer. Human Mol Genetics. 2003;12:R113–23.
30. Bennett WP, Hussain P, Vahakangas KH, et al. Molecular epidemiology of human cancer risk: gene-environment interactions and p53 mutation spectrum in human lung cancer. J Pathol. 1999;187:8–18.

31. Lee J, Yoon A, Kalapurakal S, et al. Expression of p53 oncoprotein in non-small-cell lung cancer: a favorable prognostic factor. J Clin Oncol. 1995;13:1893–903.
32. Carbone DP, Mitsudomi T, Chiba I, et al. p53 immunostaining positivity is associated with reduced survival and is imperfectly correlated with gene mutations in resected non-small cell lung cancer. Chest. 1994;106:377S–81.
33. Schiller JH, Adak S, Feins R, et al. Lack of prognostic significance of p53 and K-ras mutations in primary resected non-small-cell lung cancer on E4592: a laboratory ancillary study on an Eastern Cooperative Group prospective randomized trial of postoperative adjuvant therapy. J Clin Oncol. 2001;19:448–57.
34. Tomizawa Y, Kohno T, Fujita T, et al. Correlation between status of the p53 gene and survival in patients with stage I non-small cell lung carcinoma. Oncogene. 1999;18:1007–14.
35. Ahrendt SA, Hu Y, Buta M, et al. p53 mutations and survival in stage I non-small-cell lung cancer: results of a prospective study. J Natl Cancer Inst. 2003;95:961–70.
36. Tsao M, Aviel-Ronen S, Ding K, et al. Prognostic and predictive importance of p53 and RAS for adjuvant chemotherapy in non-small-cell lung cancer. J Clin Oncol. 2007;25:5240–7.
37. Mitsudomi T, Hamajima N, Ogawa M, et al. Prognostic significance of p53 alterations in patients with non-small cell lung cancer: a meta-analysis. Clin Cancer Res. 2000;6:4055–63.
38. Steels E, Paesmans M, Berghmans T, et al. Role of p53 as a prognostic factor for survival in lung cancer: a systematic review of the literature with a meta-analysis. Eur Respir J. 2001; 18:705–19.
39. Lazzaro D, Price M, de Felice M, et al. The transcription factor TTF-1 is expressed at the onset of thyroid and lung morphogenesis and in restricted regions of the fetal brain. Development. 1991;113:1093–104.
40. Mendelson CR. Role of transcription factors in fetal lung development and surfactant protein gene expression. Annu Rev Physiol. 2000;62:875–915.
41. Di Loreto C, Di Lauro V, Puglisi F, et al. Immunocytochemical expression of tissue specific transcription factor-1 in lung carcinoma. J Clin Pathol. 1997;50:30–2.
42. Yatabe Y, Mitsudomi T, Takahashi T. TTF-1 expression in pulmonary adenocarcinomas. Am J Surg Path. 2002;26:767–73.
43. Perner S, Wagner PL, Soltermann A, et al. TTF1 expression in non-small cell lung carcinoma: association with TTF1 gene amplification and improved survival. J Pathol. 2009;217:65–72.
44. Berghmans T, Paesmans M, Mascaaux C, et al. Thyroid transcription factor 1- a new prognostic factor in lung cancer: a meta-analysis. Ann Oncol. 2006;17:1673–6.
45. Rodenhuis S. Ras in human tumors. Semin Cancer Biol. 1992;3:241–50.
46. Rodenhuis S, Slebos RJ. The ras oncogenes in human lung cancer. Am Rev Respir Dis. 1990;142:S27–30.
47. Mascaux C, Iannino N, Martin B, et al. The role of RAS oncogene in survival of patients with lung cancer: a systemic review of the literature with meta-analysis. Br J Cancer. 2005;92:131–9.
48. Huncharek M, Muscat J, Geschwind JF. K-ras oncogene mutation as a prognostic marker in non-small cell lung cancer: a combined analysis of 881 cases. Carcinogenesis. 1999;20:1507–10.
49. Sève P, Lai R, Ding K, et al. Class III β-tubulin expression and benefit from adjuvant cisplatin/vinorelbine chemotherapy in operable non-small cell lung cancer: analysis of NCIC JBR.10. Clin Cancer Res. 2007;13:994–9.
50. Sève P, Mackey J, Isaac S, et al. Class III β(beta)-tubulin expression in tumor cells predicts response and outcome in patients with non-small cell lung cancer receiving paclitaxel. Mol Cancer Ther. 2005;4:2001–7.
51. Sève P, Issac S, Trèdan O, et al. Expression of class III β(beta)-tubulin is predictive of patient outcome in patients with non-small cell lung cancer receiving vinorelbine-based chemotherapy. Clin Cancer Res. 2005;11:5481–6.
52. Normanno N, Luca AD, Bianco C, et al. Epidermal growth factor receptor (EGFR) signaling in cancer. Gene. 2006;366:2–16.
53. Mok TS, Wu YL, Thongprasert S, et al. Gefitinib or carboplatin-paclitaxel in pulmonary adenocarcinoma. N Engl J Med. 2009;361:947–57.

54. Jeon YK, Sung SW, Chung JH, et al. Clinicopathologic features and prognostic implications of epidermal growth factor receptor (EGFR) gene copy number and protein expression in non-small cell lung cancer. Lung Cancer. 2006;54:387–98.
55. Nakamura H, Kawasaki N, Taguchi M, et al. Survival of epidermal growth factor receptor overexpression in patients with non-small cell lung cancer: a meta-analysis. Thorax. 2006;61:140–5.
56. Eberhard DA, Johnson BE, Amler LC, et al. Mutations in the epidermal growth factor receptor and in KRAS are predictive and prognostic indicators in patients with non-small-cell lung cancer treated with chemotherapy alone and in combination with erlotinib. J Clin Onc. 2005;23:5900–9.
57. Bell DW, Lynch TJ, Haserlat SM, et al. Epidermal growth factor receptor mutations and gene amplification in non-small-cell lung cancer: molecular analysis of the IDEAL/INTACT gefitinib trials. J Clin Oncol. 2005;23:8081–92.
58. Ceppi P, Volante M, Saviozzi S, et al. Squamous cell carcinoma of the lung compared with other histotypes shows higher messenger RNA and protein levels for thymidylate synthase. Cancer. 2006;107:1589–96.
59. Zheng Z, Li X, Schell MJ, et al. Thymidylate synthase in situ protein expression and survival in stage I nonsmall-cell lung cancer. Cancer. 2008;112:2765–73.
60. Bhattacharjee A, Richards WG, Staunton J, et al. Classification of human lung carcinomas by mRNA expression profiling reveals distinct adenocarcinoma subclasses. PNAS. 2001;98: 13790–5.
61. Garber ME, Troyanskaya OG, Schluens K, et al. Diversity of gene expression in adenocarcinoma of the lung. PNAS. 2001;98:13784–9.
62. Ein-Dor L, Zuk O, Domany E. Thousands of samples are needed to generate a robust gene list for predicting outcome in cancer. PNAS. 2006;103:5923–8.
63. Hayes DN, Monti S, Parmigiani G, et al. Gene expression profiling reveals reproducible human lung adenocarcinoma subtypes in multiple independent patient cohorts. J Clin Oncol. 2006;24:5079–90.
64. Chen HY, Yu SL, Chen CH, et al. A five-gene signature and clinical outcome in non-small-cell lung cancer. N Engl J Med. 2007;356:11–20.
65. Tsao MS, Zhu C, Ding K, et al. A 15-gene expression signature prognostic for survival and predictive for adjuvant chemotherapy benefit in JBR.10 patients. J Clin Oncol. 2008;26(May 20 suppl);abstr 7510.
66. Shedden K, Taylor JMG, Enkemann SA, et al. Gene expression-based survival prediction in lung adenocarcinomas: a multi-site, blinded validation study. Nature Med. 2008;14:822–7.

Chapter 9
Molecular Markers of Prostate Cancer Outcome

David Ian Quinn and Gregory P. Swanson

The molecular biology of prostate cancer and its progression is characterized by aberrant activity of multiple regulatory pathways both within the prostate cells and in the surrounding milieu. These pathways can be broadly grouped into: apoptosis, androgen receptor signaling, signal transduction, cell cycle regulation, cell adhesion and cohesion, and angiogenesis (see Table 9.1). Variations at the DNA, RNA, and/or protein levels of molecules involved in these pathways are all potential candidate markers of prognosis and therapeutic response. Detailed cohort studies have delineated the clinical and pathological factors that predict outcome for men diagnosed with prostate cancer on biopsy and after a variety of treatments for clinically localized disease. On this basis, any new prognostic marker must be measured in the context of established predictors of prostate cancer recurrence and death. These are clinical or pathological disease stage, surgical margin involvement, Gleason score or grade, and serum PSA concentration at diagnosis [1–10]. For a prognostic marker to be of utility it must provide value additional to and possibly independent of that provided by these factors. However, molecular markers are not only important because of potential relationships with outcome; rather they provide putative targets for molecular based intervention in the cancer type concerned. From this perspective, while an association with adverse outcome might suggest a key role for a given molecule in the disease state, it does not mean that markers that are not prognostic are of no utility. For example, a marker that is present in a large number of prostate cancers and might be therapeutically targeted is likely to be of considerable interest and utility, even if it is not prognostically significant. Unfortunately, to date, targeting a

D.I. Quinn, M.B.B.S. (Hons), Ph.D., F.R.A.C.P., F.A.C.P. (✉)
Department of Oncology, Norris Comprehensive Cancer Center, Keck School of Medicine, University of Southern California, 1441 Eastlake Avenue, Suite 3440, Los Angeles, CA 90033, USA
e-mail: diquinn@med.usc.edu

G.P. Swanson, M.D.
Department of Radiation Oncology, Radiology and Urology, University of Texas Health Science Center San Antonio, 7703 Floyd Curl Drive MC 7889, San Antonio, TX 78229, USA

H.-J. Lenz (ed.), *Biomarkers in Oncology: Prediction and Prognosis*,
DOI 10.1007/978-1-4419-9755-5_9, © Springer Science+Business Media New York 2013

Table 9.1 Summary of molecular aberration in prostate cancer

Process	Key molecules/markers	Selected references
Apoptosis	p53, Bcl-2	[144–149, 190]
Androgen receptor signaling	AR, possible alternate signal transduction pathways	[211, 216, 222, 238, 253, 254, 260, 423]
Signal transduction	Epidermal growth factor receptor family	[285, 286]
Cell cycle regulation	C-myc, $p16^{INK4A}$, $p27^{KIP1}$, pRb, apoptotic index, Ki67	[55, 60, 61, 67, 132, 135]
Cell adhesion and cohesion	E-cadherin, α(alpha)-catenin, metallo-proteinase, chondroitin sulfate	[335–337, 339, 368, 369, 382, 424–428]
Angiogenesis	VEGF, VEGF receptors, nitric oxide	[155, 157, 373, 374, 377]

single marker or pathway is only modestly successful, and it will be the identification of multiple pathways that can be targeted that likely will yield the greatest success. This review focuses on molecular markers of outcome for largely clinically localized prostate cancer and presents data predominantly from series of patients treated with radical prostatectomy with supplemental data from series involving patients treated with other modalities and with advanced disease where relevant.

In taking a translational research approach to study cancer outcome, one can take a candidate gene approach in which known genes of putative importance in a particular cancer are assessed in a series of tumor samples and compared with clinicopathological factors including outcome. Alternatively, one can use a variety of techniques in an attempt to discover new genes that may be important in the cancer concerned. Techniques designed to detect chromosomal abnormalities in prostate cancer have identified a number of potential candidate molecules for evaluation in prostate cancer (Tables 9.2 and 9.3). More recently the ability to assay tumor tissue using cDNA and oligonucleotide arrays with identified sequences for many thousands of molecules has expanded the scope and number of such markers inestimably [11, 12]. Candidate molecules identified in these ways can then be evaluated in tumor samples. The construction of tumor tissue microarrays in which cores of multiple different cancers are assembled in one paraffin block and can be stained for protein expression on a single slide allows rapid assessment and validation of these markers [13]. In addition, selection of overexpressed molecules by cellular localization and function can lead to the development of new markers for cancer in blood and other body fluids [14]. The search for prognostic tissue markers is not an end itself because apart from providing information on outcome they may also lead to advances in diagnostic methods, delineate therapeutic targets and identify other related molecules important in cancer development and progression.

Cellular Proliferation and Death in Prostate Cancer

The essential elements in the progression of any hormone-dependent cancer are deregulated proliferation, avoidance of apoptosis, resistance to hormonal control and metastasis. Each of these important biological events has important clinical correlates (see Table 9.4).

Table 9.2 Summary of chromosomal abnormalities described in prostate cancer selected for prevalence and prognostic potential

Chromosomal locus	Possible product	Percentage	Disease stage	Therapeutic status: hormonal therapy	References
1q gain		52	Metastases	Androgen independent	[130]
2q14 gain	Bin 1	40	Metastases	Naive	[429, 430]
5q loss		39	Metastases	Androgen independent	[130]
6q14–21 loss		25	Localized	Untreated	[431]
6q loss		39	Metastases	Androgen independent	[130]
7p gain	EGF—Receptor	8	Localized	Untreated	[432]
8p loss	Undefined tumor suppressor genes	80	Metastases	Androgen independent	[130]
8p loss		33	Localized	Untreated	[433, 434]
		65	Locally recurrent	Untreated	
		83	LN metastases	Untreated	
8p12-12 LOH		63	PIN		[435, 436]
		90.6	Localized	Untreated	
8p22 loss		62	Localized T3N0M0	Untreated	[132]
8p22 loss		63	Metastases	Untreated and androgen independent	[437–440]
8p 21.2 loss	Loss of NKX3-1		Localized T3N0M0	Untreated	[441, 442]
8q gain	c-myc	33–54	Localized T3N0M0	Untreated	[132, 434, 443–447]
8q24.3	Gain of MIR 151		Localized T3N0M0	Untreated	[441]
8q gain		57–85	Metastases	Untreated and androgen independent	[129, 130, 444]
9q21 point mutations	$p16I^{NK4A}$ $p15^{INK4B}$ $p19^{ARF}$	0	Localized	Untreated	[78]
9q21 LOH			Localized		[448]
		15	T2N0M0	Untreated	
		46	T3N0M0	Untreated	
9q21 LOH		20	Localized	Untreated	[78]
		46	Metastases	Untreated	

(continued)

Table 9.2 (continued)

Chromosomal locus	Possible product	Percentage	Disease stage	Therapeutic status: hormonal therapy	References
9q21 methylation		13	Localized	Untreated	[78]
		8	Metastases	Untreated	
10p15 loss	Kruppel-like factor 6 (KLF6 or Zf9)	15–77	Localized	Untreated	[449, 450]
10q loss		30	Localized	Untreated	[451, 452]
10q21 LOH	ANX7	35	Localized	Untreated	[453]
10q23 loss	PTEN	50	Metastases	Untreated and androgen independent	[130, 442, 454]
10q23.3 LOH	PTEN	14	Localized	Untreated	[130, 455]
		43	T2-3,N+	Untreated	
		63	Metastases	Androgen independent	
10q24 LOH	LAPSER1	55	Localized	Untreated	[439, 452]
11p gain	H-ras, Kai-1	52	Metastases	Androgen independent	[130]
13q14.2 loss	pRb or chromosome condensation 1-like (CHC1-L)	33	Localized	Untreated	[63, 456]
13q loss		75	Metastases	Untreated and androgen independent	[64, 130]
16q loss	E-cadherin	30	Localized	Untreated	[451]
16q23.1–24 loss	E-cadherin	55	Metastases	Untreated and androgen independent	[130, 439, 442, 457]
17q11–12 gain	HER-2/neu, erbB2	30	Metastases	Untreated and androgen independent	[130, 444]
17p loss	p53	18	Localized	Untreated	[173, 447]
17p13.1 loss	p53	50	Metastases	Untreated and androgen independent	[130]
17p 21 loss	BRCA1	14	Localized	Untreated	[458]
Xq11–13	Androgen receptor	22–36	Metastases	Androgen independent	[131, 136, 219, 444]

Table 9.3 Summary of selected transmembrane serine protease 2 (TMPRSs2):E26 transformation specific (ETS) family fusion studies

Specific translocation	Treatment	Cohort size	Stage	Translocation present (%)	Effect on prostate cancer outcome summary: possibly prognostic	Special notes	References
TMPRSS2:ERG	RP	54	T1-3,N0	59	Poorer relapse-free survival	RT PCR	[272]
TMPRSS2:ERG	RP	114	T1-3,N0	63	Poorer relapse-free survival	RT PCR; Independent with Gleason score	[262]
TMPRSS2:ERG	RP	165	Clinically localized	49	Poorer relapse-free survival: independent	FISH; Prognostic across all subgroups for Gleason score and stage	[273]
TMPRSS2:ERG and other variants	RP	54	Clinically localized	60 for TMPRSS2:ERG, 26 for other variants	Nil	RT PCR	[459]
TMPRSS2:ERG	RP	150	T1-3,N0	33	Poorer relapse-free survival	FISH; Prognostic across all subgroups for Gleason score and stage	[275]
TMPRSS2:ERG	RP	125	T1-3,N0-1	48	Poorer relapse-free survival	FISH; Not independent. Additive effect with PTEN loss	[276]
TMPRSS2:ERG	RP, population based cohort	214	Clinical localized	35.5	Nil	Multiple fusion copies associated with poorer prostate cancer specific survival	[271]
TMPRSS2:ERG	RP	521	T1-3,N0-1	42	*Nil*	FISH, copy number increased associated with stage, Gleason score and aneuploidy	[277]
TMPRSS2:ERG	RP	235	T1-3,N0-1	48.5	Not reported	FISH	[266]

(continued)

Table 9.3 (continued)

Specific translocation	Treatment	Cohort size	Stage	Translocation present (%)	Effect on prostate cancer outcome summary: possibly prognostic	Special notes	References
TMPRSS2:ERG	Watchful waiting	117	Clinically localized	15	Associated with prostate cancer specific mortality	RT-PCR	[274]
TMPRSS2:ERG	RP	540	T1-3,N0-1	47	Not reported	FISH	[460]
SLC45A3:ERG	RP	540	T1-3,N0-1	9	Not reported	FISH, concurrent SLC45A3 and TMPRSS2 fusion in 11 % with ERG fusions	[460]
ERG, ETV1 rearrangements	Prostate cancer managed conservatively	308	Tx, N1, M1	46	ERG/ETV1 rearrangements stratify for survival in patients with PTEN loss	Strong association between ERG/ETV1 and PTEN loss	[461]
TMPRSS2:ERG	Prostate biopsies, androgen deprivation treated patients	178	N1, M1	34	*Nil*	Fusion associated with high Ki-67, lower age, high tumor volume but not Gleason score, stage or recurrence	[278]
TMPRSS2:ETV4	RP	98	T1-3,N0-1	2	Not reported	RT PCR, FISH	[267, 462]
TMPRSS2:ETV1	RP	429	T1-3,N0-1	1.9	Not associated	FISH; Associated with increased PSA, clinical stage, Gleason score	[463]

TMPRSS2:ETV1	RP	96	T1-3,N0-1	2			FISH	[462]
TMPRSS2:ERG	Familial prostate cancer	75		59		Not reported	Linkage analysis suggests homogeneity within families for fusion type	[280]
TMPRSS2:ERG	Castrate resistant, autopsy series, non-osseous metastases	30 patients, 97 sites	M1			NA	FISH; Multiple sites from an individual case harbored the same gene fusion molecular subtype suggesting clonal expansion of disease	[279]

Table 9.4 Summary of sequential proliferative and apoptotic changes in prostate carcinogenesis and prostate cancer progression

Normal prostate tissue	500	NA	NA
Low grade prostatic intraepithelial neoplasia	150	Increased	Unchanged
High grade prostatic intraepithelial neoplasia	56	Increased	Increased
Localized prostate cancer	50	No changed	Decreased
Metastatic prostate cancer: lymph nodes	33	Increased	Increased
Metastatic prostate cancer: bone	54	Increased	Increased
Hormone responsive prostate cancer	NA	Decreased	Increased
Prostate cancer—at onset of hormone resistance	NA	No change compared to untreated but increased compared to hormone responsive	Increased compared to untreated but decreased[a] compared to hormone responsive
Prostate cancer—hormone resistant—agonal	NA	No change	Decreased[a]

[a]Decrease may relate to local or general nutrient delivery
Based on data from refs. [121, 464–466]

Increased proliferation index, whether measured by Ki67 (MIB1), PCNA (proliferating cell nuclear antigen), S phase fraction on flow cytometry, thymidine labeling, or bromo-deoxyuridine incorporation, correlates with the presence of advanced stage disease [15, 16] or increased tumor grade [16–18]. Ki67 index is independently predictive of outcome in patients with clinically localized disease treated with radical prostatectomy [16, 17, 19–22] with radiation therapy (RT) [23] and in patients being observed [24]. Recurrent tumors have Ki67 indices approximately double that of the primary tumor [25, 26] Recent work suggests that a high Ki67 index predicts relapse in patients classified as low risk by other parameters and that neuroendocrine differentiation (as measured by tissue chromogranin expression) and mini chromosomal maintenance protein 7 (MCM-7) overexpression may add to risk in high Ki67 tumors [27–29]. MCM-7 is a DNA replication licensing gene, which when amplified and overexpressed is associated with increased proliferation and size of xenograft tumors in preclinical models and with biochemical relapse in one RP series [30]. In several series increased expression of the polycomb cell cycle regulatory molecule, enhancer of zeste homolog 2 (EZH2), which is a histone methyltransferase regulated by microRNA 101, is associated with increased proliferation, decreased survival and castrate resistant phenotype as well as clinical castrate resistance [29, 31–33]. Subsequent work has shown that the global level of histone modification (acetylation or methylation) in tumor tissue is prognostic in a number of tumors including prostate cancer [34]. As with the marker panels used in breast cancer [35], most of the predictive markers in the panels under development for prostate cancer are proliferative markers. In a recent series, a 31-gene panel of proliferative markers (called cell cycle progression or CCP signature) was one of the most significant variables on multivariate analysis for failure after radical prostatectomy. Although only 12 patients died of cancer, the panel was predictive of death. In a separate cohort of patients that had undergone TURP and were followed, 35 % died of cancer and the CCP was more informative than any other variable in predicting prostate cancer death [36].

Several studies [37–39] have identified increased apoptotic index, (ApI), a measure of the number of apoptosing cells within a PC, as adversely prognostic. Counter intuitively, one study found increased ApI was independently predictive of outcome following RP whereas in the same set p53 and bcl-2 were not [39]. Unfortunately, these studies have been undertaken in relatively small groups making the wider application of reported results problematic but nonetheless pointing to the potential importance of apoptosis in PC.

Cell Cycle Regulation

Genetic aberrations in the control of G_1 to S phase progression in the cell cycle are present in virtually all human cancers (see Fig. 9.1). Progression through the G_1/S phase checkpoint is controlled by the sequential transcriptional activation of cyclin genes, and the consequent transient accumulation and activation of a sequence of cyclin/cyclin-dependent kinases (CDK) complexes resulting in hyperphosphorylation of the retinoblastoma gene product pRb [40] (Fig. 9.1). There have been significant recent advances in knowledge of the molecular basis of cell cycle control due to the discovery and functional analysis of the cell cycle regulatory cyclins, CDKs and CDK inhibitors [41, 42]. A number of endogenous inhibitors of CDK catalytic activity (CDIs) exist with varying but overlapping specificities [42–44]. $p27^{Kip1}$ inhibits cyclin E/Cdk-2 activity but also binds to D-type cyclins. $p21^{WAF1/CIP1}$ is, in part, p53-regulated, and binds to a range of cyclin/CDK complexes including those with cyclins D1 and E and acts as an inhibitor in some settings but also act as an adaptor protein for cyclin/cdk assembly in others [45–47]. $p16^{INK4A}$ inhibits Cdk-4 and Cdk-6 catalytic activity [48, 49]. c-Myc has stimulatory effects on cell cycle progression at least in part through interaction with components of the $p27^{Kip1}$/cyclin E/Cdk-2 complex [50]. A series of molecules regulate the physiological effect of c-Myc: Mad, Max and Mxi1, which through heterodimer interaction regulates the transcription and cell cycle regulatory activity of c-Myc [51]. Interestingly, c-Myc and Mad interact to regulate AR-mediated transcription [52, 53].

These CDIs and the functionally associated pRb genes are all tumor suppressor genes of potential significance in PC. Each of the cyclins as well as c-myc is a potential oncogene in PC.

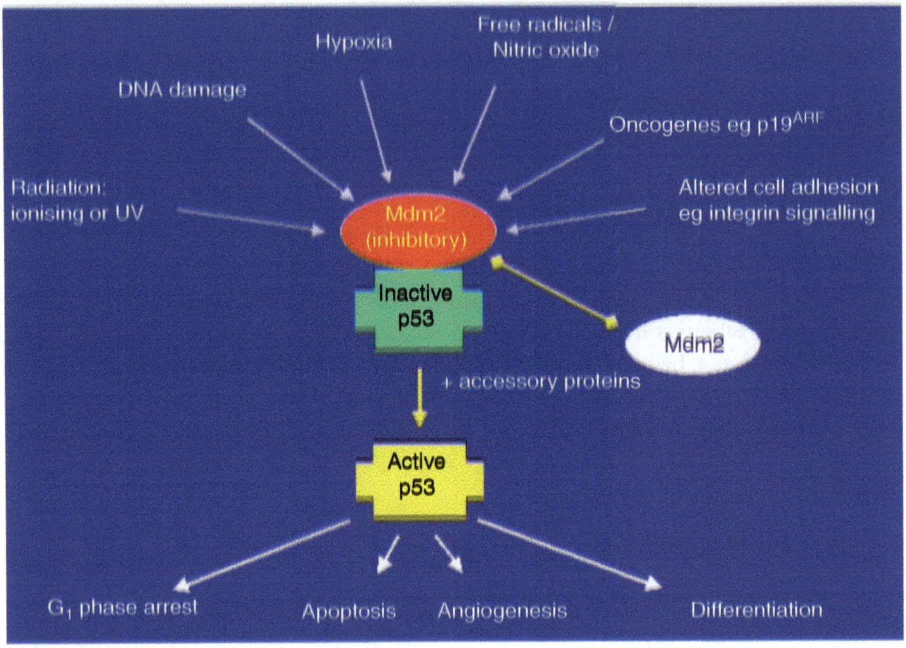

Fig. 9.1 Summary diagram of p53 interaction and function. P53 can be activated by a number of genotoxic and epigenetic stimuli and in turn inhibits cell cycle progression, apoptosis and angiogenesis and induce differentiation

Retinoblastoma Protein

When retinoblastoma protein (pRb), is present in a hypophosphorylated form during G_0 and G_1 phases it serves to inhibit cell cycle progression into S-phase [40]. Phosphorylation of pRB by cyclin D/CDK complexes in G_1 phase inactivates pRb and is essential for progression through the cell cycle. Hence, pRb has a central role in cell cycle regulation (see Fig. 9.1.).

Retinoblastoma gene mutations correlate closely with loss of retinoblastoma protein expression as measured by immunohistochemistry [54–56]. Loss of pRb expression as measured by immunohistochemistry is prognostic in endometrial, non-small-cell lung and bladder cancer [57–59]. Despite this there are few sizeable series of PC in which role of pRb expression as a prognostic indicator has been examined. Loss of pRb expression has been reported in as many as 100 % and as few as 1 % of PC while loss of at least one *Rb* allele is reported in between 20 and 60 % of tumors [54, 60–64]. Generally, there is progressive loss of pRb expression with increasing prostate cancer grade and stage. Localized PCs show loss of pRb expression in 1–45 % of cases [60, 62, 65] while the number rises to 20–60 % in advanced prostate cancer [62, 66]. Whether pRb expression portents relapse and predicts survival is a matter of debate (see Table 9.5). Data from the St. Vincent's Campus Prostate Cancer Group suggests pRb expression has limited prognostic value but may warrant further study [67].

Cyclins

The D-type cyclins include three known variants (D1, D2 and D3) with 57 % total homology and 78 % homology in the functional region known as the "cyclin box" [68]. Despite this close homology, each is encoded by distinct genes: *CCND1*: 11q13, *CCND2*: 12p13 and *CCND3*: 6q21 [68]. Functionally, the three subtypes of D cyclin behave similarly. Cyclin D1 overexpression is a common molecular aberration in many human cancers. However, in localized PC the presence of CCND1 amplification and cyclin D1 overexpression is reported as being rare and probably occurs in less than 5 % of cases ([69], Henshall et al., unpublished data). However, several authors have reported a higher rate of cyclin D1 or overall cyclin D expression in localized PC with apparent prognostic effect [70] (see Table 9.5). There are currently no reported studies of cyclin D2 or D3 expression and outcome in PC in the literature. Two studies have addressed cyclin A overexpression with one finding it to have independent prognostic effect [70, 71] (see Table 9.5). Cyclin E overexpression is prognostic in a number of tumors either in concert with decreased p27 expression or alone [47, 72, 73]. Work on cyclin E expression in PC is very limited with a single reported study in the literature [74] (see Table 9.5). Further study of cyclin expression as a prognostic parameter in PC is warranted.

$p16^{INK4A}$

The tumor suppressor gene INK4A located at 9q21 is frequently inactivated in human cancers, including melanoma, pancreatic cancer and squamous cell carcinoma of the head and neck [49]. The product of INK4A was first identified as a 16 kDa molecule that *in*hibited the effect of CD*K4* and hence the designation $p16^{INK4A}$ [75]. By inhibiting CDK4, it at least partially prevents the phosphorylation of pRb (see Fig. 9.1.). The two most common mechanisms for loss of $p16^{INK4A}$ function are homozygous deletion and loss of transcription due to hypermethylation of the $p16^{INK4A}$ promoter [76]. Hypermethylation of $p16^{INK4A}$ was detected in the androgen-independent PC cell line PC-3 [76], and biallelic inactivation of $p16^{INK4A}$ by a combination of gene deletion and methylation have been reported in a small subset of tumors [77–80]. Others studies have failed to detect $p16^{INK4A}$ gene mutations in small series of primary PCs [81–83]. Mechanistically, $p16^{INK4A}$overexpression should result in enhanced cell cycle regulation by limiting the phosphorylation of pRb.

The available data on INK4A gene status and/or $p16^{INK4A}$ expression in relation to PC outcome are limited to three studies, which despite some methodological

Table 9.5 Cell cycle markers and prostate cancer outcome

Molecule	Treatment	Cohort size	Stage	Dichotomizing level for marker expression	Effect on prostate cancer outcome	Special notes	References
Retinoblastoma protein					Summary: inconclusive		
Decrease or loss	RP	71	T1-2,N0	NA	Poorer survival		[467]
	RP	118	T1-2,N0	NA	Nil		[65]
Cyclins					Summary: inconclusive		
Increase cyclin D1	RP	140	T1-3,N0-1	>5 % nuclear accumulation	Nil		[71]
Increased cyclin D	RP	213	T1-3,N0-1		Prognostic but loses significance with other factors	Antibody cocktail for all cyclin Ds	[70]
Increased cyclin A	RP	213	T1-3,N0-1		Independently prognostic		[70]
Increased cyclin A	RP	28	T1-2,N0	Index with Ki67	Nil		[74]
Increased cyclin B	RP	28	T1-2,N0	Index with Ki67	Nil		[74]
Increased cyclin E	RP	28	T1-2,N0	Index with Ki67	Nil		[74]
$p16^{INK4A}$					Summary: Prognostic		
Increased $p16^{INK4A}$	RP	88	T1-3,N0-1	>5 % nuclear accumulation	Prognostic	Immunohistochemistry confirmed by in situ hybridization	[84]
	RP	104	T1-3,N0-1	NA, fluorescence index	Independently prognostic	CDK4 not elevated. Ploidy and S-phase fraction not prognostic	[85]
	RP	206	T1-3,N0-1	>1 % nuclear accumulation	Independently prognostic	Elevation in HGPIN also prognostic	[67]
Increased $p21^{WAF1/CIP1}$					Summary: probably prognostic		

	RP	213	T1-3,N0-1	>5 % nuclear accumulation	Independently prognostic	Independent of p53	[468]
	RP	88	T1-3,N0-1	>5 % nuclear accumulation	Prognostic	Independent of p53	[92]
	RP	60		>5 % nuclear accumulation	Independently prognostic	Independent of p53	[469]
	RP	86	T1-4,N0-1	>10 % nuclear accumulation	Nil		[128]
Decreased p27^{Kip1}					Summary: probably prognostic		
	RP	113	T1-3,N0-1	<25 % nuclear accumulation	Independently prognostic	Effect greatest in patients treated with neoadjuvant hormonal therapy	[123]
	RP	96	T3, N0-1	10, 50 %	Prognostic	Low p27^{Kip1} associated with high Gleason score	[124]
	RP	86	T1-3,N0-1		Independently prognostic with stage	Low p27^{Kip1} associated with high Gleason score	[126]
	RP	95	T1-4,N0-1	<10 % nuclear accumulation	Independently prognostic for recurrence		[127]
	RP	138	T1-3,N0-1	<50 % nuclear accumulation	Nil		[470]
	RP	73	T1-3,N0-1	Variety	Nil		[471]
	RP	104	T1-3,N0-1	Median 64 % nuclear accumulation	Nil		[326]
	RP	161	T1-3,N0-1	<45 % nuclear accumulation	Prognostic in organ confined only		[472]

(continued)

Table 9.5 (continued)

Molecule	Treatment	Cohort size	Stage	Dichotomizing level for marker expression	Effect on prostate cancer outcome	Special notes	References
C-myc amplification					Summary: probably prognostic		
	RP	114	T3	C-myc copy number by FISH	Prognostic	Limited by technical requirements for analysis using FISH	[132]
	RP	52	T2-3,N1-3	C-myc copy number by FISH	Prognostic		[189]

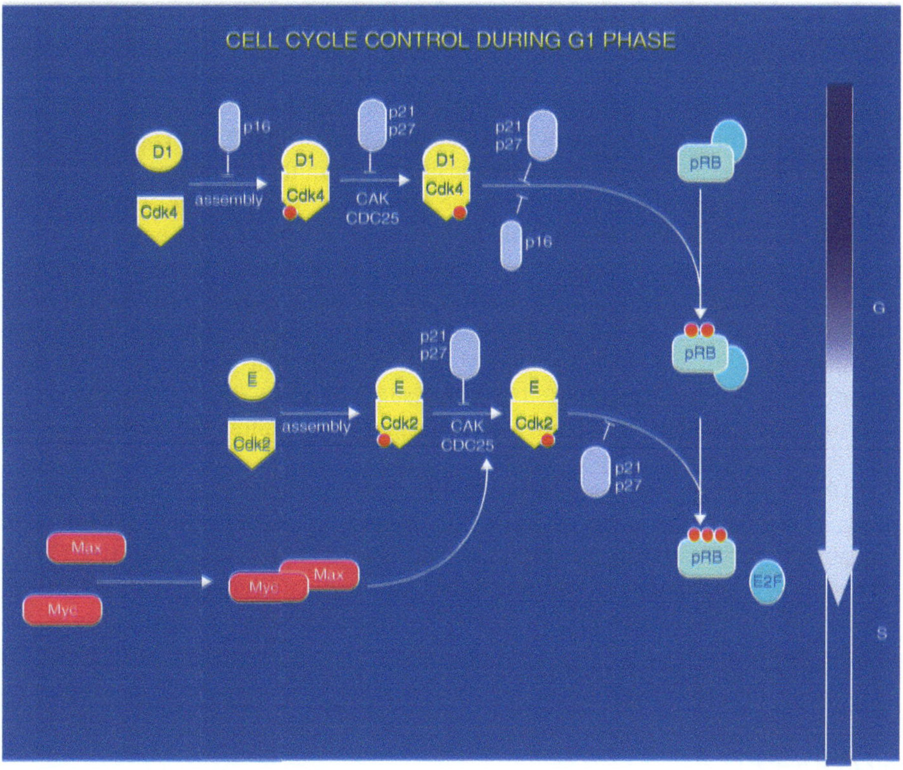

Fig. 9.2 Summary diagram of cell cycle progression during G_1 phase. A simplified model of interactions between some of the molecules involved in G_1 phase of the cell cycle. Progression through G_1 phase of the cell cycle requires the activity of cyclin D1 and cyclin E and their catalytic partners cyclin dependent kinase subunits, Cdk-4/6 and Cdk-2 respectively. The active cyclin-Cdk complexes bind to and phosphorylate pRb. In its unphosphorylated form pRb sequesters transcription factors of the E2F family and pRb phosphorylation releases E2F. This allows transcription of essential E2F responsive genes and cell cycle progression from G_1 to S phase. The cell cycle is further regulated by two families of cyclin dependent kinase inhibitors, the INK4 family (such as $p16^{INK4A}$) and the Cip/Kip family ($p21^{WAF1/CIP1}$, $p27^{Kip1}$). C-myc exerts a positive effect on cell cycle progression through cyclin E and p27

differences deliver the same conclusion: $p16^{INK4A}$ overexpression is adversely prognostic. These case series are summarized in Table 9.5 [67, 84, 85]. The studies to find $p16^{INK4A}$ overexpression adversely prognostic in PC have done so in the presence of elevated INK4A exon 1α transcripts [84], in the absence of a concurrent elevation of CDK4 expression in transition from benign to malignant prostate tissue [85] and without correlation with loss in retinoblastoma protein expression [67] (Fig. 9.2). Overexpression of $p16^{INK4A}$ in these tumors may indicate the presence of an inactive pRB as in several other human cancers [48] and elevated INK4A exon 1α(alpha) transcript expression is consistent with a downstream feedback effect on $p16^{INK4A}$ gene transcription [86]. The question as to how prostate cancer cells escape the effects of increased p16^{INK4A} expression in braking cell cycle progression is important. In vitro studies suggest increased levels of p16^{INK4A} are important in inducing prostate epithelial cell senescence and that abrogation of the p16^{INK4A}/Rb pathway is required for these cells to bypass senescence and undergo immortalization as part of tumourigenesis [87]. Hence, elevation of p16^{INK4A} expression as the result of pRb loss is an attractive hypothesis to explain this. However, if this is correct then one might expect pRb loss to be prognostic by itself (see above) and the apparent loss of a defined relationship between p16^{INK4A} and CDK4 between benign and malignant prostate tissue is left unexplained. In a PC xenograft model, examining cell cycle changes with androgen withdrawal and development of androgen independence, p16^{INK4A} expression increased progressively after androgen withdrawal and plateaued but was then unchanged with development of androgen independence. These fluctuations occurred in the presence of easily detectable pRb expression suggesting that the development of resistance to the inhibitory effect of p16^{INK4A} may occur independent of pRb status.

p16^{INK4A} overexpression appears to be prognostic in PC treated with RP but this needs confirmation in other cohorts and, ideally, in patients treated with other modalities apart from surgery. The status of other components of the p16^{INK4A}/Rb pathway, particularly pRb expression, needs to be evaluated concurrently so that the underlying mechanisms that result in p16^{INK4A} overexpression being prognostic can be understood.

p21$^{WAF1/CIP1}$

The use of p21$^{WAF1/CIP1}$ as prognostic biomarker in a range of tumors has yielded conflicting results with studies reporting that reduced or increased expression of p21$^{WAF1/CIP1}$ can be adversely prognostic within the same tumor type, breast cancer being the prime example [88]. One would expect that it would act as a tumor suppressor though the inhibition of CDKs 2 and 4 (see Fig. 9.1.). The causes of variation of p21$^{WAF1/CIP1}$ expression in tumors are still to be fully elucidated. p21$^{WAF1/CIP1}$ is rarely mutated in human cancers although several PCs containing point mutations have been reported [89]. Reduced p21$^{WAF1/CIP1}$ expression might be expected in the presence of p53 dysfunction given the original proposal that it was a primary regulator by which p53 asserts cell cycle inhibition (p21$^{WAF1/CIP1}$/p53 concordance). However, it has subsequently become clear that p21$^{WAF1/CIP1}$ is also regulated by other factors and can exert inhibitory effects on the cell cycle and apoptosis independent of p53 effect in both settings of development and cancer [45, 90, 91]. Several investigators have demonstrated that p21$^{WAF1/CIP1}$ expression does not correlate with p53 status in a variety of cancer types [88, 92]. The reasons for this are complex but include alternative regulation of p21$^{WAF1/CIP1}$ by other molecules particularly those involved in cell cycle regulation, altered degradation or p53 mutation that alters its effect on apoptosis but not on p21$^{WAF1/CIP1}$ and the cell cycle [90, 93]. One further possible explanation in PC, is that androgens may directly stimulate p21$^{WAF1/CIP1}$

transcription [94]. It is likely that $p21^{WAF1/CIP1}$ expression is the result of an epigenetic response to several cellular regulators and that either reduced or increased expression could be prognostic in certain environments. Generally, clinical studies suggest that increased $p21^{WAF1/CIP1}$ expression is adversely prognostic in patients treated with radical prostatectomy (see Table 9.5). Recent work suggests that $p21^{WAF1/CIP1}$ overexpression may predict resistance to radiation therapy for local recurrence after RP [95] and with the development of hormone-refractory prostate cancer [96].

Hence, $p21^{WAF1/CIP1}$ overexpression is prognostic in localized PC independent of p53 status. Its interrelationship with other cell cycle regulators and various p53 alterations in predicting outcome requires further evaluation.

p27^Kip1

$p27^{Kip1}$ is encoded by a gene at 12p12-12p13.1 [97]. $p27^{Kip1}$ null are characterized by diffuse hyperplasia or hypertrophy of glandular organs including the prostate [98, 99]. $p27^{Kip1}$ acts as a tumor suppressor by inhibiting some of the CDK complexes (see Fig. 9.1). Despite the fact that no or reduced $p27^{Kip1}$ expression is adversely prognostic in several cancers [72, 88, 100–106], mutation is a rare event in early human tumors [97, 107, 108]. An interesting recent finding is that homozygous deletion at 12p12-12p13.1 was present in 47 % of patients dying of metastatic PC[109], suggesting that this genetic change might be a significant late event in the progression of PC [109]. Reduction in $p27^{Kip1}$ expression in localized tumors comes about through post-transcriptional regulation, predominantly through a proteasome-associated ubiquitin-mediated degradation mechanism [99, 105, 110–112]. In transition from benign prostate to prostate cancer, as well as other tumors, this degradation mechanism is turned on without compensatory increase in protein production [99, 113]. There are also examples of $p27^{Kip1}$ overexpression being adversely prognostic [114], presumably as an epigenetic regulatory response to other cell cycle molecular aberrations [103]. $p27^{Kip1}$ function and expression is complementary to that of cyclin E in some systems while its inhibitory effect may also be abrogated by c-Myc overexpression [115–118]. Studies of in vitro and xenograft systems show that the expression and cell cycle inhibitory effect of $p27^{Kip1}$ are reduced by androgen stimulation [119–121]. Castration or androgen depletion results in an increase in $p27^{Kip1}$ expression with concurrent cell cycle arrest. Reintroduction of androgen or the development of androgen independence results in reduced $p27^{Kip1}$ expression to levels lower than before castration. The implication from this work is that $p27^{Kip1}$ plays an important role in maintenance of cell cycle arrest in androgen dependent tumors and that reduced expression, particularly in the setting of androgen deprivation, may indicate the presence of androgen-independent prostate cancer cells [120, 121].

Several studies have examined the relationship between $p27^{Kip1}$ expression and clinical outcome and found that low or undetectable $p27^{Kip1}$ protein is associated with increased tumor grade and stage and remains an independent predictor of treatment failure after prostatectomy defined by PSA and/or clinical recurrence (see Table 9.5) [99, 122–128]. $p27^{Kip1}$ expression appears not to correlate with preoperative serum PSA [124]. Different studies use different percentages of cancer nuclei staining ranging from 10 to 50 % to dichotomize cohorts. In one of these studies, neoadjuvant hormonal therapy (NHT) was administered preoperatively to 24 of 113 patients in a variable manner [123]. Tumors from patients who received NHT tended to express higher levels of $p27^{Kip1}$ than did those from untreated patients. Patients whose tumor $p27^{Kip1}$ remained low after NHT had a shorter relapse-free survival. Together this suggests that $p27^{Kip1}$ is a key molecule in prostate cancer cell response to androgen.

Hence, reduced $p27^{Kip1}$ expression predicts a shorter disease free survival in patients with localized prostate cancer in most reported series. The predictive importance of $p27^{Kip1}$ in patients treated with NHT requires evaluation in other cohorts. The interrelation of $p27^{Kip1}$ with other components of the cell cycle and the predictive potential of $p27^{Kip1}$ in prostate biopsies and with treatment modalities apart from surgery should also bear further investigation.

c-Myc

Chromosome 8 is often subject to alteration in PC with loss on 8p and gain on 8q being common (see Tables 9.2 and 9.3) [129–131]. While a series of potential tumor suppressor genes are postulated in the region commonly lost at 8q21-22, amplification at the 8q24 locus which includes *C-MYC* has attracted more attention because of its prognostic utility in PC [132]. C-Myc serves as a transcription factor, the upregulation of which results in cell proliferation. A series of investigators report that *C-MYC* amplification is present in up to 50 % of HGPIN and 73 % of primary PC [133–135] and that *C-MYC* amplification increases with transition through PIN to localized PC to metastases [135, 136] and with increasing Gleason score [137, 138]. In a report on 144 patients with high-grade, locally advanced (pT3) PC, Sato et al. [132] found that increased copy number for *C-MYC* using fluorescence in situ hybridization strongly predicted systemic progression and patient death. In addition, aberrations elsewhere on chromosome 8 appear to occur in sequence with *C-MYC* amplification and influence outcome in a cumulative manner that requires further study.

C-MYC amplification is a feature of increasing grade and stage in PC and predicts adverse outcome in locally advanced disease. The technical demands of FISH make it difficult to apply in routine practice. While some studies report a good correlation between amplification on FISH and c-Myc overexpression by IHC, this has not been universal and furthermore c-Myc overexpression detected by IHC has not been demonstrated to be of prognostic significance [139]. A recent report using RNA expression controlled for by matching with benign epithelium for c-myc demonstrates that overexpression is associated with recurrence [140], a result described by other investigators with novel antibodies to c-myc [141]. *C-MYC* is an important oncogene in PC but more research is required to determine its relationship with other biomarkers and its prognostic role in subsets of PC patients.

Apoptosis (Programmed Cell Death)

The major apoptotic regulators, p53 [142] and Bcl-2 [143] both demonstrate abnormal function and expression as prostate cancer progresses and are mechanistically implicated in hormone resistance [144–149]. Following therapy with androgen ablation, p53 and Bcl-2 expression as well as the apoptotic index increases in a large proportion of cases [150]. Failure of apoptotic response as measured by the apoptotic index correlates with relapse [150]. In addition, the mean increase in Bcl-2 expression is greater in cases that do not respond to hormone therapy or progress early after its commencement [150]. In vitro and animal tumor xenograft experiments demonstrate resistance to spontaneous as well as androgen deprivation-, radiation- or chemotherapy-induced apoptosis mediated, at least in part, by Bcl-2 overexpression [145, 151].

p53

p53 functions by regulating the transcription of genes involved in G_1-phase growth arrest of cells in response to DNA damage (see Fig. 9.2). In normal cells, in response to cellular stress, p53 is upregulated. p53 also has roles in the regulation of the spindle checkpoint, centrosome homeostasis and G_2-M phase transition [152]. p53 regulates apoptosis [142, 152, 153] and tumor angiogenesis in benign and malignant cells [142, 154–157]. Hence, the effects of p53 related to cancer can be summarized into three processes: cell cycle regulation, apoptosis and angiogenesis/metastasis.

Nuclear accumulation of p53 detected by immunohistochemistry (IHC) typically indicates the presence of p53 gene mutations [158, 159] although the correlation between nuclear accumulation of p53 and the presence of p53 gene mutation can vary [160]. Lack of p53 accumulation may occur in the presence of p53 mutations particularly nonsense mutations with truncated p53, single-base mutations not causing any change in the amino acid sequence and mutations outside of exons 5 to 8 [161, 162]. Mutations that limit the ability of p53 to interact with regulatory proteins such as Mdm-2 may cause p53 nuclear accumulation but that such mechanisms are dependent on other cellular factors such as DNA integrity [163]. Regardless of the mechanisms involved, nuclear accumulation of p53 is a prognostic indicator in several human cancers including breast [155, 164, 165], lung [166] and colorectal carcinoma [167]. Mutations can cause accumulation of poorly functioning p53 or the loss of p53, either of which results in a loss of p53 function and a potentially poorer outcome [168] (see below).

The value of p53 nuclear accumulation as a prognostic factor in localized prostate cancer has been debated. A number of studies have shown that p53 nuclear accumulation detected by IHC is prognostic at a variety of dichotomizing cut off points based on number of p53-positive nuclei. These studies either describe a poor prognosis group of patients with ≥20 % p53-positive nuclei [92, 144, 169, 170] or a group of patients with lower percentages of positive cells in a heterogeneous, focal staining pattern where either the presence of any nuclear accumulation or the presence of clusters of cells showing nuclear accumulation is adversely prognostic [146, 171, 172]. However, other studies comparing p53 nuclear accumulation with assessment of p53 gene mutations have failed to provide conclusive evidence for the importance of p53 in localized prostate cancer or a strong correlation between nuclear accumulation and p53 gene mutation [173–176]. In studying other cancers, several authors have suggested that assessment of p53 gene mutation and p53 expression in combination may more accurately define prognostically important p53 dysfunction [160, 177, 178].

Comparison of prostate cancer metastases with primary prostate cancers in the same patients suggest that foci with p53 mutations are clonally expanded in metastases [148, 179–181], perhaps explaining the high frequency of IHC positivity and presence of gene mutations in hormone refractory and metastatic prostate cancer [26, 174–176, 182–185]. Two studies have demonstrated significant heterogeneity in the distribution of *p53* mutations between and within foci of carcinoma in the same prostate [186, 187]. Other studies document heterogeneity for other genes and suggest that clones responsible for metastases do not always originate from within the dominant tumor focus [135, 188, 189]. Recent work demonstrates the focal presence of p53 mutations within areas of p53 protein accumulation detected by immunohistochemistry [168]. The likelihood exists that in localized prostate cancer, p53 overexpression and mutation as well as other genetic aberrations may be limited to subgroups of prognostically important malignant cells. These studies add to others that demonstrate increased p53 nuclear accumulation in metastatic, recurrent and/or androgen insensitive prostate cancer compared to clinically localized disease [26, 174–176, 183–185]. Borre et al. reported on a population observed with no treatment after prostate diagnosis and found p53 nuclear accumulation to be predictive of prostate cancer related death [190]. In work done at the Garvan Institute, Quinn et al. demonstrated the increasingly adverse prognostic effect of an increased percentage of cell with p53 nuclear accumulation that was independent of PSA, Gleason score and pathological stage [149] (Fig. 9.3). Interestingly, at low levels of p53 expression, the presence of clusters of 12 or more p53 positive cells was adversely prognostic (Fig. 9.2) [149]. Taken together, these studies suggest that prostate tumor cells harboring p53 mutations and perhaps other genetic aberrations are clonally expanded in metastases.

There are more than one hundred studies reporting series of patients with PC evaluated for p53 nuclear accumulation. No attempt will be made to recapitulate this expansive literature here. Essentially this literature demonstrates increasing p53 expression with increasing grade and stage with a prognostic effect that may or may not be independent of these two variables. However, several studies examine the issue of clinical utility of p53 in pretreatment biopsy material in particular therapeutic settings that deserve further scrutiny and are summarized in Table 9.6. p53 is a prognostic marker in prostate cancer, however, because of the heterogeneity of aberration on localized disease and a surfeit in therapeutic agents with potential to abrogate its effect. it has practical and clinical limitations.

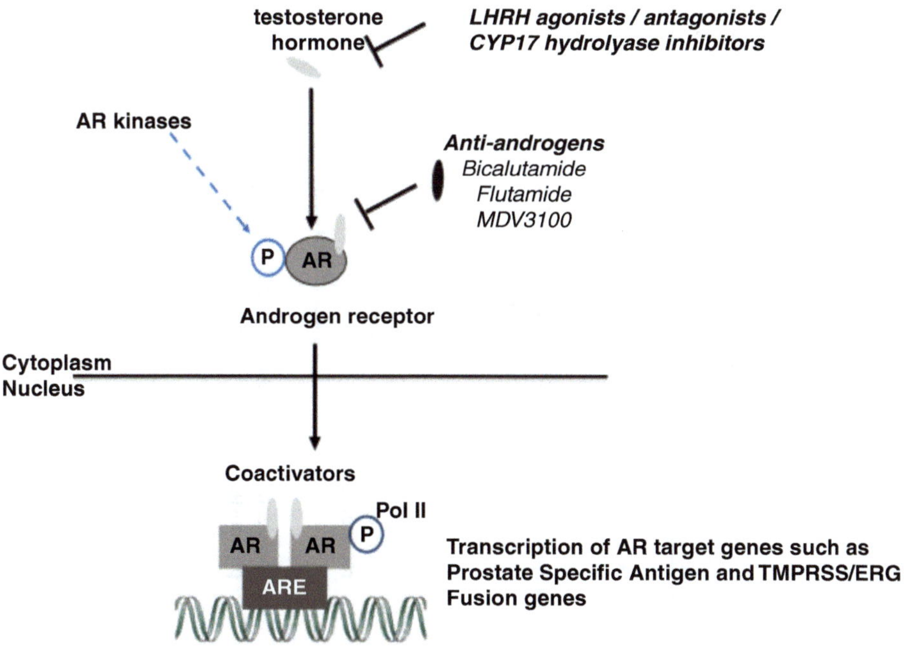

Fig. 9.3 Androgen receptor signaling including prostate specific antigen and TMPRSS/ERG products

Bcl-2

The bcl-2 gene was initially identified as the proto-oncogene Tran located to the immunoglobulin (Ig) heavy-chain locus in follicular B-cell lymphoma. It is the prototype of a novel class of oncogenes that inhibit apoptosis or programmed cell death [191, 192]. Therefore, an increase in Bcl-2 can result in increased cell survival. Bcl-2 is part of an expanding family of apoptosis-regulatory molecules, which may act as either death antagonists (Bcl-2, Bcl-xL, and Mcl-1) or death agonists (Bax, Bak, Bcl-xS, Bad, and Bid). The selective and competitive dimerization between pairs of antagonists and agonists determines how a cell will respond to a given signal [143].

Within the prostate, bcl-2 expression is commonly seen in the basal layer of benign glands, PIN and some cancer, whereas expression in epithelial cells is abnormal. Several studies [145–147, 193–196] demonstrate that increased expression of Bcl-2 in PC confers androgen resistance, particularly in advanced disease, and may facilitate progression to androgen independence. Stattin et al. studied bcl-2 expression in two similar sets of patients treated with castration for locally advanced PC and found that bcl-2 increased in both responders and nonresponders but that the increase was far greater in responders and correlated with apoptotic index [150]. Recent work suggests that Bcl-2 overexpression has a role in resistance to RT in PC [197].

Table 9.6 Selected studies on the apoptotic markers, p53 and Bcl-2, and outcome in prostate cancer

Molecule	Treatment	Cohort size	Stage	Dichotomizing level for marker expression	Effect on prostate cancer outcome	Special notes	References
p53	Observation-cohort	221	Unrestricted at presentation	>50 % nuclear accumulation—biopsy	Independently prognostic—predicted overall survival	Hormonal therapy at clinical progression	[190, 473, 474]
	External beam radiation therapy with hormone therapy—RTOG 8610	129	Clinically localized, T1-3, N0	>20 % nuclear accumulation—biopsy	Independently prognostic—distant metastases	P53 status predicted from patient given RT+Hormones but not those given RT alone	[169]
	RP	263	Clinically localized, T1-3,N0-1	Variety: Cluster of 12 cells, >5, 20 % nuclear accumulation—prostatectomy	Independently prognostic—PSA recurrence.	>20 % nuclear accumulation predicted prostate cancer related death	[3, 4, 149]
	RP	175	Clinically localized, T1-3,N0-1	>0 % nuclear accumulation—prostatectomy	Independently prognostic—PSA recurrence	Also found Bcl2 overexpression prognostic	[146, 171]
	RP	129	Clinically localized, T1-3,N0-1	>0 % nuclear accumulation—biopsy	Not prognostic in biopsy		[146, 171, 475]
	RP	76	Clinically localized, T1-3,N0-1	>0 % nuclear accumulation—biopsy and prostatectomy	Prognostic in both—PSA recurrence		[352]

Bcl-2							
	RP	175	Clinically localized, T1-3,N0-1	>0 % nuclear accumulation—prostatectomy	Independently prognostic—PSA recurrence	Also found p53 overexpression prognostic	[146, 171]
	RP	129	Clinically localized, T1-3,N0-1	>0 % nuclear accumulation—biopsy	Not prognostic in biopsy		[146, 171, 475]
	RP	76	Clinically localized, T1-3,N0-1	>0 % nuclear accumulation—biopsy and prostatectomy	Prognostic in prostatectomy but not in biopsy—PSA recurrence		[352]
	External beam radiation	52	Clinically localized	>0 % nuclear accumulation—biopsy	Prognostic		[476]

A number of studies have proposed that increased Bcl-2 expression is adversely prognostic in localized prostate cancer and a selection of these is presented in Table 9.6.

These studies suggest that bcl-2 expression increases with grade and stage. For this reason, bcl-2 overexpression may be useful prognostically in relatively more advanced tumors such as those selected to have RT or hormonal therapy rather than RP. This is one potential reason that bcl-2 expression on biopsy may be independently prognostic in RT cohorts and not those treated with RP. Another is that patients with bcl-2 overexpression do better with RT because the cells are more sensitive to its effects. A prospective trial of RT with cases stratified for normal against bcl-2 overexpression in PC on biopsy and matched for clinical stage and Gleason score could test this hypothesis in a clinical setting.

Androgen Receptor Signaling

The expression of the steroid hormone receptors is prognostic in a number of hormone-dependent tumors. The best example is the estrogen receptor (ER) in breast cancer where loss of expression of ER predicts a more aggressive disease course independent of treatment given and resistance to hormonal therapies such as tamoxifen. While estrogen receptor expression is altered with PC progression [198], AR expression represents a more obvious potential marker of prognosis and hormonal responsiveness in prostate cancer (see Fig. 9.3). Early studies or AR expression provided conflicting results and only served to demonstrate that heterogeneity markedly increases with progression from benign through PIN to localized PC and metastases [199–206]. In examining tumor material from 30 patients with prostate cancer, Tilley et al. used anti-peptide antibodies to the amino- and carboxyl-termini of the AR and demonstrated differential expression as the disease progressed from early stage to bone metastases [207]. More advanced disease had increased expression of amino-terminus epitopes. The prognostic significance of carboxy-terminus epitope expression remains to be determined but it has been suggested that differential expression between amino and carboxy epitopes may correlate with AR mutation and/or amplification [208]. Recent studies using commercially available antibodies directed at either the amino-terminus or the whole AR molecule [209] suggest that AR overexpression is a feature of progression, recurrence, LN metastases and/or anti-androgen resistance in human prostate cancer [207, 210–216]. A recent study failed to find an association between AR expression in the primary PC and outcome but did find that AR expression in >70 % of LN metastases predicted for a poorer cancer specific survival in the subset of patients with LN involvement after controlling for Gleason score and preoperative PSA in multivariate analysis [216, 217].

The relationship between AR expression and mutation or amplification of the AR gene is poorly understood. However, several studies suggest that overexpression may correlate with mutation and/or amplification and with androgen resistance [218–220]. High-level AR amplification has been described in more than 30 % of

PC recurring after androgen ablation [219, 221]. A report linked AR overexpression in prostate cancer epithelial cells in combination with reduced AR expression in the surrounding stromal cells with increasing tumor grade [214]. Further work at the Garvan Institute demonstrated that the combination of high AR expression in the epithelium and reduced expression in the adjacent stroma is adversely prognostic. This suggested the presence of aberrant stromal signaling through a paracrine mechanism [222] and provides supporting evidence for paracrine stromal-epithelial regulation of AR expression as PC progresses [220]. Work from other investigators has confirmed this finding [223]. It is possible that overexpression of AR results in part from lack of response to homeostatic degradation mechanisms [224] in cells with a mutated or amplified AR gene while adjacent stromal cells have normal AR which is downregulated. Recent work has demonstrated an association between the level of AR expression in the malignant epithelial nuclei of diagnostic biopsy or prostatectomy specimens and prostate cancer specific mortality from castrate-resistant cancer [225].

In addition, a number of growth factors have been implicated in PC stromal-epithelial interaction including TGFβ(beta) [226, 227], yet to be identified TGF analogues [228], the FGF family including keratinocyte growth factor (KGF, FGF7) and FGF10 [229–232], MCM7 [233] and a variety of cytokines including IL-6 [234]. TGFβ(beta) is progressively overexpressed in epithelial cells with prostate cancer progression with corresponding loss of TGFβ(beta) cell cycle inhibition [227]. In prostate stromal cell models, TGFβ(beta) blocks androgen-induced proliferation and results in redistribution of AR from the nucleus to the cytoplasm [235, 236]. Recent work demonstrates that increased preoperative serum TGFβ(beta) levels predict relapse after radical prostatectomy [237].

A complex picture has emerged with the evaluation of recurrent or metastatic PC for AR mutation and amplification. In evaluating material from ten bone marrow metastases from clinically hormone-independent prostate cancers, Taplin et al. found that AR was highly expressed [238]. Fifty percent (5/10) of these PCs contained AR mutations associated with promiscuous receptor stimulation by a variety of hormones including progesterone, adrenal androgens and estrogen as well as paradoxical stimulation by the antiandrogen, hydroxy-flutamide. Subsequent studies by the same group and others [210–219, 239–244] demonstrated a high propensity for mutation at a single site (codon 877) in patients treated with flutamide and for these mutations to predict flutamide withdrawal response in androgen-insensitive disease. It has since become evident that biclutamide therapy is associated with AR mutation and amplification in metastases suggesting that the effect is at least class specific to nonsteroidal antiandrogens [244, 245]. Tilley et al. identified a series of different androgen receptor point mutations in 44 % of 25 hormonally naïve patients with the incidence of mutation increasing with disease stage [246]. Individual AR mutants had differential binding affinity for different hormones and different downstream effects [244, 246–252]. It has been suggested that pathways downstream of the AR can be stimulated by aberrant activation of the erbB2 (HER-2/neu receptor tyrosine kinase) pathway [253]. The cellular model used in this system also suggests that activation of the AR pathway can be synergistically mediated through effect of both erbB2 and AR [253, 254]. There is experimental and human PC tissue evidence for retinoblastoma protein, c-Myc, interleukin-4 and 6, ETS gene and p53 regulation of AR expression [52, 255–259].

Hence, it is possible that in selected prostate cancer cells, AR may be amplified, overexpressed through epigenetic regulation and/or contain mutations that allow stimulation by a range of hormones and anti-androgens [260]. It is likely that therapy, particularly with nonsteroidal antiandrogens, may provide selective pressure that leads to preferential expression of cells with AR mutations or amplification. In addition, autocrine or paracrine mechanisms may, in lieu of, or in concert with AR, activate pathways to produce downstream AR responses [260]. Determining which mechanisms are active at various stages of prostate cancer progression and how they might interact with other molecular markers of PC virulence is clearly important.

5-α Reductase

The expression of 5-α (alpha) reductase is increased in high grade and androgen insensitive PC [261]. There may also be a cancer progression related shift in localization of 5-α reductase from the nucleus to the cytoplasm [261]. The prognostic implications of these observed changes require further evaluation.

Signal Transduction

Transmembrane Serine Protease 2: Erythoblastosis Virus E26 Transformation Specific Family Fusion

Recent work has identified fusion between the 5′-untranslated regions of transmembrane serine protease 2 (TMPRSS2) (Chromosome 21q22.3) with the erythoblastosis virus E26 transformation specific (ETS) transcription factor family members as an early event in prostate cancer tumorigenesis [262–266] (Table 9.2). The ETS family member involved can be either ERG (21q22.2), ETV1 (7p21.2), or ETV4 (17q21), suggests a mechanism for overexpression of the ETS genes in a large number of prostate cancers [263, 267–269]. The fusion most often results in the placing of ERG transcriptional activity under the androgen-regulated transcriptional control of TMPRSS2 and is present in between 35 and 65 % of invasive prostate cancers [270, 271] (see Fig. 9.3). The presence of this gene as measured by FISH or RT-PCR has been associated with clinical and pathological factors associated with progression and early progression in some series but not others [271–278]. Whether the differences in prognostic effect of TMPRSS2:ETS fusion in different cohorts reflects variation in biology, hereditary, treatment or other factors such as aneuploidy or interstitial deletion is not clear [271, 274, 277, 279, 280]. The presence of TMPRSS2:ERG fusion is more common in Caucasian men [281, 282]. ETS-related gene expression in urine or prostatic massage fluid from men undergoing prostate biopsy was associated with cancer in the biopsy specimen especially in men with a screening serum PSA less than 4 ng/ml [283, 284].

Epidermal Growth Factor Receptor Family

Aberrant expression of the epidermal growth factor receptor (EGFr) family is common in prostate cancer [285–287] although the extent and prevalence of this varies depending upon techniques used to demonstrate it and the population studied. Convergent signaling between androgen regulated processes and the pathway by which signal is transduced from cell surface receptor through Raf-1, MEK, MAP kinase and p27KIP1 have been mechanistically delineated in cell culture models, although the clinical relevance of these findings is still unclear [288]. A recent study has demonstrated overexpression of EGFr in 18 % of prostate cancer patients with increased EGFr gene copy number in 3.3 %, with each of these associated with higher Gleason grade and stage and, in the case of EGFr expression, PSA recurrence [289].

HER-2/neu is a candidate marker for predicting prostate cancer progression. Varying rates of HER-2/neu overexpression ranging from 9 to 64 % of PCs has been reported depending on the investigative method employed and the specificity of reagents used [290–296]. Overexpression of HER-2/neu correlated with increasing grade and increasing stage in separate series [285, 290]. Fox et al. found that overexpression of HER-2/neu by IHC predicted outcome in T1A PCs [292]. HER-2/neu amplification assessed by FISH was associated with disease recurrence in a series of 106 primary tumors [293]. Within the California Cancer Consortium, patients were screened prospectively for shed serum Her2 antigen, immunohistochemistry and FISH but demonstrated a very low rate of abnormal expression and no response to trastuzumab, a therapeutic monoclonal antibody directed at Her2/neu [297]. Activation specific antibodies for HER-2/neu may permit the delineation of a group of PC patients with functional over activity as distinct from overexpression. Other members of the erbB family including EGF-R, c-erbB3, and c-erbB4 may warrant evaluation as prognostic markers [298–300].

Ras

C-RAS was one of the first oncogenes identified and point mutations that correlate with increased ex vivo activity were an important part of models of prostate cancer in rodents [226, 301, 302]. Early studies in human tumors showed that activated Ras was increasingly evident as the disease progressed into the metastases [303]. However, detection of activating mutations of C-RAS in localized tumors proved variable and it soon became clear that their measurement was not likely to be of important prognostic significance [304–306]. Studies using antibodies to Ras peptide sequence have failed to demonstrate a relationship with clinicopathological or outcome parameters [307]. Most of the studies undertaken on Ras have occurred in North American Caucasians populations. There is significant racial variation in C-RAS point mutation type and frequency and therefore Ras activity and expression may warrant further investigation as a prognostic marker in other racial groups [308, 309]. Recent work shows that ETS gene fusion involves several elements of the ras/raf-signaling pathway including BRAF and RAF1, although the importance of these uncommon fusions for therapy in selected patients is unclear [310].

Phosphoinositide 3-Kinase/Akt Pathway

The phosphoinositide 3-kinase (PI3K)/Akt pathway is an important signal transduction pathway in many cell types and influences cycle kinetics via $p27^{Kip1}$ regulation [311–314]. Within this pathway there are several molecules that demonstrate altered expression in a variety of cancers [315]. In murine prostate carcinogenesis models, prostate-specific deletion of PTEN (phosphatase and tensin homologue), which modulates the PI3K/Akt pathway, resulted in metastatic prostate cancer while AKT activation saw the development of PIN [316, 317]. PTEN is a tumor suppressor phosphatase that is commonly altered in lethal metastatic prostate cancer [181, 318–322]. In vitro work shows that reconstitution of PTEN suppresses androgen receptor transcription and increases sensitivity to cytotoxic drugs [323, 324]. This may have clinical relevance since the PI3K/Akt and MAP kinase pathways becomes hyperactive with development of androgen independence in paired tumor samples [325]. While loss of PTEN expression correlates with increased Gleason score and increased pathological stage in patients with clinically localized PC, evidence of an effect on outcome has been lacking [322, 326]. However, recent data from a Japanese cohort does suggest that the presence of a deletion in PTEN is associated with PSA recurrence after controlling for other factors [327], while data from a US cohort suggests that an index incorporating PTEN and Akt expression may have potential [328]. Similarly, increased Akt expression is reported to correlate with increased Gleason score and pretherapy PSA concentration >10 ng/ml in localized prostate cancer but a link to outcome has not been delineated [329, 330].

Cellular Adhesion/Cohesion

E-Cadherin and Related Molecules

E-cadherin is involved the regulation of cell-cell adhesion and cell morphology [331, 332]. Functionally, cadherins form a complex with other molecules of importance in this process, particularly catenins [333, 334]. Reduced expression of one or more component of this complex has generally been associated with a more aggressive cancer phenotype, as measured by a number of parameters, as well as a poorer outcome in a number of cancers including prostate cancer [335–339]. Downregulation of E-cadherin expression in localized prostate cancer is associated with increased expression of other cadherin family members, particularly N-cadherin [340]. It has been suggested that while E-cadherin promotes epithelial cell–epithelial cell adhesion, N-cadherin promotes epithelial cell–stromal cell adhesion [341]. In an apparent paradox, E-cadherin is overexpressed in metastases [342, 343]. This suggests that E-cadherin expression is transiently turned off through an epigenetic mechanism during invasion and diapedesis into vessel walls only to be reactivated at the site of established metastases [342]. Other cadherins may play a role in this switching. "Reexpression" of E-cadherin has also recently been described in the transition from primary to metastases in breast cancer [344]. Recent work has focused on interaction of the cadherins with other molecules that modulate their function by truncation of the cadherin protein or stoichiometrically [345–350]. The impact of these modulators on clinical prognostication and therapeutics requires further delineation.

There are several studies evaluating E-cadherin expression and prostate cancer outcome. These are summarized in Table 9.7. Overall, they suggest a significant prognostic effect for E-Cadherin expression in prostate cancer. Clinical utility of E-cadherin expression is limited by heterogeneous expression in prostate cancer so that biopsy results may not be predictive [351, 352]. In addition, this area is further complicated by the observation that there is a switch in expression from E-cadherin to N-cadherin as part of epithelial–mesenchymal transition (EMT) as prostate cancer progresses and that EMT and this switch specifically is associated with outcome [353]. Hence, E-cadherin and related molecules have potential as prognostic markers in prostate cancer but require further testing in large cohorts to determine whether they are independent markers of outcome and if the effects are related to specific subgroups.

The Wnt signaling pathway mediates a variety of cellular functions including cell polarity, tissue patterning, control of cellular proliferation, and development of neoplasia [354–356]. This pathway is initially activated by a Wnt ligand binding to a Frizzled receptor which subsequently transduces a signal through activation of β(beta)-catenin [356]. Although expression of Wnt ligands [357, 358], Frizzled receptors [358, 359] and β(beta)-catenin [360–362] in prostate cancer has been established for many years, recent studies have demonstrated that Wnt-1 [362], nuclear β(beta)-catenin [363] and the Wnt-pathway inhibitor, secreted frizzled-related protein 4 (sFRP4) [364], have an association with prostate cancer outcome. Increased Wnt-1 expression correlates with increased Gleason score and serum PSA levels which is consistent with its role as an oncogene [362]. Conversely, increased expression of sFRP4 in a membranous pattern of immunostaining in >20 % of malignant epithelial cells independently predicts for a longer biochemical relapse-free survival in patients with localized prostate cancer ($p=0.02$) [364]. Interestingly, loss of β(beta)-catenin expression in the nucleus of malignant epithelial cells is associated with both prostate cancer progression and an increased risk of relapse in localized prostate cancer in particular in the low-risk subgroup of

Table 9.7 Selected studies of cellular adhesion and cohesion molecules

Molecule	Treatment	Cohort size	Stage	Dichotomizing level for marker expression	Effect on Prostate cancer outcome summary prognostic	Special notes	References
Reduced E-cadherin	RP/TURP	89 (42/47)	Clinically localized/ locally advanced, T1-4,N0-1	Nil expression or aberrant location (non-basal layer expression)	Prognostic		[424]
	RP	67	T1-4,N0-1	Low expression	Prognostic for disease-free survival		[477]
	RP	72	Clinically localized, T1-3,N0-1	Aberrant expression	Prognostic for disease-free survival—PSA recurrence	Biopsy expression nonprognostic	[352]
	RP	56	T1-4,N0-1	Low expression	Prognostic for early development of clinical metastases		[478]
	RP	104	Clinically localized, T1-4,N0-1	Low expression; switch from E- to N-cadherin as epithelial-mesenchymal transition marker	Low E-cadherin associated with short biochemical and clinical FS. High N- to E-ratio & EMT with cancer specific survival	P cadherin expression in basal cells associated with metastases	[353]
	TURP	99	T1-4,N0-1, M1	Low expression	Independently prognostic for overall survival relative to Gleason score but not presence of metastases		[336]
Increased chondroitin sulfate	RP	157	T1-4,N0-1	Absorbance cut point above 7.0	Independently prognostic for PSA recurrence	May be most useful in patients with PSA <10 ng/ml	[368–370]

patients with preoperative PSA levels <10 ng/ml [363]. In vitro studies suggest that β(beta)-catenin signaling in the nucleus can promote or repress tumor growth and development depending on the cofactors present [360, 365–367], and it may be the balance of these effects towards tumor repression in prostate cancer that accounts for higher levels of nuclear β(beta)-catenin predicting for a better prognosis.

Altered expression of molecules in the prostatic stroma including chondroitin sulfate [368–370] and hevin [371] as well as cell surface markers such as CD44 [293, 372] also have prognostic impact and represent potential therapeutic targets.

Angiogenesis

Neoangiogenesis is essential for the growth and metastatic propagation of cancer. Increased micro vessel formation is a feature of many cancers including prostate cancer where quantification of micro vessel density correlates with disease stage and outcome [155, 157, 373–377]. Aberrant blood vessel formation is associated with anomalies in pathways involved in apoptosis, androgen receptor signaling, signal transduction, cytokine function, and cellular adhesion [156, 256, 378–381]. Blood vessel formation is regulated by molecules involved in adhesion as well as vascular endothelial growth factor (VEGF) [382], nitric oxide, and cyclooxygenases. VEGF is crucial for the development of tumor masses exceeding a diameter of 3–5 mm [383].

Preclinical data with prostate cancer cell lines demonstrate that VEGF is a potentially important factor in stimulating cell proliferation as well as angiogenesis and lymphagenesis [380]. In experimental prostate cancer models, VEGF expression is upregulated in prostate and prostate cancer tissue by androgens and castration results in an initial fall in VEGF [384–386]. The expression and effect of VEGF is regulated by a series of heterogeneous molecules. These include necropolis, activator protein 2α(alpha), angiopoietins, ephrins, and interleukin 6 and 8 [387–391].

VEGF is highly expressed in most prostate cancers [373, 377, 392]. The distribution of VEGF within prostate cancers is interesting. As expected, there are significant levels in endothelial cells and in the cytoplasm of cancer cells, with parallel increase with Gleason grade [393]. Neuroendocrine cells are highly expressive of VEGF isoform A and, in contradistinction to endothelial and adenocarcinoma cells where levels are androgen dependent, there is no fall in expression with androgen blockade [377, 393–396]. This finding may have therapeutic implications for hormone resistant disease and VEGF targeting. Higher VEGF tissue expression predicts biochemical PSA relapse following prostatectomy in one series [378] and death from prostate cancer in a cohort that underwent observation for clinically localized disease [377] and two other cohorts with castrate-resistant PC [397, 398]. Others, however, have found tissue VEGF expression not to be predictive of recurrence [22]. In patients undergoing radical prostatectomy, elevated preoperative serum or urine VEGF levels are predictive of earlier disease progression [399, 400]. Serum VEGF falls after prostatectomy [401]. Patients with metastatic prostate cancer have serum

VEGF concentrations significantly higher than normal populations [402, 403]. There are at least four isoforms of VEGF (A, B, C and D) each with different roles and receptor affinities, but without clear differential prognostic or predictive ability at this time [404, 405]. A recent study using prostate cancer specimens from a variety of disease states found that vascular proliferation was predictive of prostate cancer specific survival in localized, hormone naïve and castrate-resistant disease, even though VEGF expression was not prognostic [406]. Interestingly, castrate-resistant PC was characterized by decreased VEGF-A and increased hypoxia inducible factor alpha expression [406].

VEGF receptor expression occurs diffusely through prostate carcinoma [407]. Each of the receptors has different physiological roles [404]. VEGFR1 (Flt-1) promotes vessel sprouting and branching while inhibiting tubular elongation possibly through release of soluble component that negatively modulates VEGF and VEGFR2 (Flk-1/KDR) [408, 409]. VEGFR2 promotes tubular elongation of blood vessels while VEGFR3 (Flt-4) is directed at lymphangiogenesis and possibly lymph node metastasis [410]. VEGFR2 signaling is responsible for increased prostate cancer cellular proliferation as well as neoangiogenesis [411, 412]. In prostate cancer progressive disease is associated with decreased VEGFR1 and increased VEGFR2 [413]. Recent work suggests that VEGF and VEGFR2 may have a role in the development of osteoblastic bone metastases that are characteristic of advanced prostate cancer [414]. The mechanism postulated for this involves preferential expression of integrins on the cell surface. Higher VEGF receptor 3 expression predicts early tumor progression after RP [415]. Increased VEGFR3 expression in lymphatic endothelial cells predicts increasing disease stage and particularly lymph node involvement at RP [416].

Hence, VEGF expression is prognostic in PC while varied expression of VEGFR2 and VEGFR3 may have respective roles in bone and lymph node metastases.

Gene Expression Profiling to Delineate Markers of Outcome

A contemporary approach to discover new genes of prognostic significance is to utilize microarray analysis to define gene expression profiles that cosegregate with poor clinical outcome [12, 417–420]. The most advanced published data on the utility of such an assay is currently in breast cancer where the Netherlands Cancer Institute and Antoni van Leewenhoek Hospital have pioneered the use of microarray profile analysis based on 70 genes, in conjunction with conventional prognostic tests to determine which women will receive adjuvant treatment after surgery [418, 419]. The use of a microarray-based prognostic tool in the treatment of prostate cancer remains in development. Three prostate cancer gene expression datasets have utilized primary prostate cancers with outcome data in an attempt to define gene expression profiles associated with prostate cancer recurrence [12, 420, 421] (Table 9.8). While a comprehensive meta-analysis of these data is still to be performed, commonalities do exist. Lapointe et al. reported that while there was no overlap between the 23 genes associated with early recurrence in their cohort and

Table 9.8 Selected studies of expression profiling of prostate cancers to delineate markers of poor prognosis

Cohort with recurrence data	Cohort follow-up	Array platform	Definition of recurrence	Key findings	References
N=21 8 recurrences	13 relapse-free patients >4 years post RP	U95Av2 Affymetrix oligonucleotide array (~10,000 genes)	Two successive PSA >0.2 ng/ml	No single gene was statistically associated with recurrence; a 5 gene outcome prediction model was used to predict recurrence[a].	[420]
N=72 17 recurrences	28.25 months median follow-up	Customized Affymetrix oligonucleotide array (~46,000 unique sequences)	Two successive PSA >0.3 ng/ml +/– clinical recurrence	~200 probesets showed strong correlation with relapse with additional predictive value relative to preoperative serum PSA.	[12]
N=259	57 months median follow up	Tissue microarray for 14 molecules	Two successive PSA >0.2 ng/ml	EZH2 increased and E-cadherin decreased predicted recurrence.	[350]
N=100	70 months median follow up	cDNA array (12,625 genes)	3 rising PSA values	218 genes up or downregulated associated with outcome. Gene set validated with discrimination over Kattan postoperative nomogram.	[479]
N=29 7 recurrences	11.5 months median relapse-free survival	cDNA array (26,260 genes)	PSA >0.07 ng/ml or occurrence of clinical metastasis	4 genes positively, 19 genes negatively associated with early recurrence; validated MUC1 and AZGP1 as prognostic. AZGP1 validated and confirmed by another group.	[421, 480]
N=79		cDNA array	Two successive PSA >0.2 ng/ml	5–8 gene signature to distinguish recurrence or not. Improved prediction from clinical parameters from ROC AUC 0.75 to 0.89	[481]

(continued)

Table 9.8 (continued)

Cohort with recurrence data	Cohort follow-up	Array platform	Definition of recurrence	Key findings	References
N=639		cDNA array (22,283 genes)	Two successive PSA >0.2 ng/ml	17 gene signature distinguished between PSA recurrence by 5-years or not. Improved prediction from clinical parameters from ROC AUC 0.75 to 0.85	[482]
N=442	9.5 years	Selected 31 gene panel of cell progression cycle genes to produce a CCP index	RP cohort: Two successive PSA >0.2 ng/ml; Locally advanced TURP cohort: death	CCP index predicted recurrence in RP cohort and death in the TURP cohort independent of any clinical or pathological parameter.	[36]

[a]The top 5 genes used in over half of the models included chromogranin A, platelet-derived growth factor receptor β(beta), HOXC6, inositol triphosphate receptor 3 (IPTR3) and sialyltransferase-1

Table 9.9 Selected studies of validated prognostic markers identified by gene expression profiling of prostate cancers

Molecule	Treatment	Cohort size	Effect on prostate cancer outcome	Special notes	References
Hepsin	RP	78	Absent or low expression is prognostic		[483, 484]
PIM1	RP	78	Decreased expression is prognostic		[484]
EZH2	RP	64	Moderate to strong expression is prognostic	Increased expression in metastatic PC[a]	[31, 350]
MTA1	RP	108	Decreased expression is prognostic	Increased expression in metastatic PC[a]	[485]
MUC1	RP	225	Increased expression is prognostic		[421]
AZGP1	RP	225	Decreased expression is prognostic		[421]

[a]Relative to localized prostate cancer and benign prostate [31, 485]

those identified by Singh et al., their set of genes predicted recurrence for patients included in the latter study. Similarly, none of the probesets identified by Henshall et al. overlapped with the probesets selected by Singh et al. However, a potential functional link was noted between the TRP channel trp-p8 and calnexin, both predictors of outcome in the Henshall et al. study, and chromogranin A and inositol triphosphate receptor identified by Singh et al., because TRP ion channels are linked to the phosphatidylinositol signal transduction pathway. Importantly, the data from all three studies provide strong evidence for a gene expression profile of poor prognosis in localized prostate cancer. The critical next steps in developing a clinically useful gene expression panel for prostate cancer is to assure the fidelity of sample preparation (e.g., laser captured populations of malignant epithelial cells), adapt a widely-available array platform, and translate the approach for application to fixed tissues to enable analysis of larger cohorts of patients with longer follow-up.

An increasing number of potential prognostic markers identified by gene expression profiling are being validated using immunohistochemistry on tissue microarrays comprised of large cohorts of patients treated for localized disease with radical prostatectomy (Table 9.9). The clinical utility of these molecules in identifying patients with aggressive prostate cancer will ultimately need to be analyzed for their ability to improve preoperative prediction of prostate cancer recurrence [5].

Conclusion

A limited number of molecular markers in prostate cancer tissue are of clinical utility in predicting outcome or response to therapy. Current markers with potential include p53, Bcl-2, $p16^{INK4A}$, $p27^{Kip1}$. c-myc, androgen receptor, E-cadherin and

VEGF. Recent techniques for high volume assessment of gene expression will accelerate the discovery of new predictive and prognostic molecules. The test of these and other markers of outcome will be not only their predictive potential but also their ability to change the natural history of prostate cancer through directed intervention.

To find a useful marker or signature in prostate cancer, we have many challenges. Our current classification of prostate cancer even at the very rudimentary molecular level is lacking. The estrogen, progesterone and Her2-neu receptor status of breast cancer has allowed stratification of a complex disease for clinical trials and as a paradigm for molecular signature generation. To date this has not been possible in prostate cancer, although recent work suggests the imprinting of the TMPRSS2-ERG, PTEN and androgen receptor configurational status may be important [422]. Similarly, basic molecular predictors of outcome in the adjuvant, hormone naïve and castrate resistant settings have been slow to develop in a disease that at its most aggressive evolves over a decade. Finally, predictors of response to standard therapies have been difficult to characterize in the absence of a single dominant gene or the ability to sub-segment the disease. To move forward, markers or gene signatures will need to have strong biological base, be linked to a therapeutic intervention and have enough strength to add to the formidable triad of stage, Gleason score and serum PSA in prostate cancer.

References

1. Kattan MW, Eastham JA, Stapleton AM, Wheeler TM, Scardino PT. A preoperative nomogram for disease recurrence following radical prostatectomy for prostate cancer. J Natl Cancer Inst. 1998;90:766–71.
2. Kattan MW, Wheeler TM, Scardino PT. Postoperative nomogram for disease recurrence after radical prostatectomy for prostate cancer. J Clin Oncol. 1999;17:1499–507.
3. Quinn DI, Henshall SM, Haynes A-M, et al. Prognostic significance of pathologic features in localized prostate cancer treated with radical prostatectomy: implications for staging systems and predictive models. J Clin Oncol. 2001;19:3692–705.
4. Quinn DI, Henshall SM, Brenner PC, et al. Prognostic significance of preoperative factors in localized prostate carcinoma treated with radical prostatectomy. Cancer. 2003;97:1884–93.
5. Kattan MW, Zelefsky MJ, Kupelian PA, et al. Pretreatment nomogram that predicts 5-year probability of metastasis following three-dimensional conformal radiation therapy for localized prostate cancer. J Clin Oncol. 2003;21:4568–71.
6. Graefen M, Karakiewicz PI, Cagiannos I, et al. Validation study of the accuracy of a postoperative nomogram for recurrence after radical prostatectomy for localized prostate cancer. J Clin Oncol. 2002;20:951–6.
7. Graefen M, Karakiewicz PI, Cagiannos I, et al. International validation of a preoperative nomogram for prostate cancer recurrence after radical prostatectomy. J Clin Oncol. 2002;20:3206–12.
8. Bostwick DG, Grignon DJ, Hammond ME, et al. Prognostic factors in prostate cancer. College of American Pathologists Consensus Statement 1999. Arch Pathol Lab Med. 2000;124:995–1000.
9. Stephenson AJ, Scardino PT, Eastham JA, et al. Postoperative nomogram predicting the 10-year probability of prostate cancer recurrence after radical prostatectomy. J Clin Oncol. 2005;23:7005–12.

10. Swanson GP, Basler JW. Prognostic factors for failure after prostatectomy. J Cancer. 2010;2:1–19.
11. Henshall SM, Afar DE, Rasiah KK, et al. Expression of the zinc transporter ZnT4 is decreased in the progression from early prostate disease to invasive prostate cancer (small star, filled). Oncogene. 2003;22:6005–12.
12. Henshall SM, Afar DE, Hiller J, et al. Survival analysis of genome-wide gene expression profiles of prostate cancers identifies new prognostic targets of disease relapse. Cancer Res. 2003;63:4196–203.
13. Horvath L, Henshall S. The application of tissue microarrays to cancer research. Pathology. 2001;33:125–9.
14. Welsh JB, Sapinoso LM, Kern SG, et al. Large-scale delineation of secreted protein biomarkers overexpressed in cancer tissue and serum. Proc Natl Acad Sci U S A. 2003;100:3410–5.
15. Cher ML, Chew K, Rosenau W, Carroll PR. Cellular proliferation in prostatic adenocarcinoma as assessed by bromodeoxyuridine uptake and Ki-67 and PCNA expression. Prostate. 1995;26:87–93.
16. Keshgegian AA, Johnston E, Cnaan A. Bcl-2 oncoprotein positivity and high MIB-1 (Ki-67) proliferative rate are independent predictive markers for recurrence in prostate carcinoma. Am J Clin Pathol. 1998;110:443–9.
17. Harper ME, Glynne-Jones E, Goddard L, et al. Relationship of proliferating cell nuclear antigen (PCNA) in prostatic carcinomas to various clinical parameters. Prostate. 1992;20:243–53.
18. Nemoto R, Kawamura H, Miyakawa I, et al. Immunohistochemical detection of proliferating cell nuclear antigen (PCNA)/cyclin in human prostate adenocarcinoma. J Urol. 1993;149:165–9.
19. Bubendorf L, Sauter G, Moch H, et al. Ki67 labelling index: an independent predictor of progression in prostate cancer treated by radical prostatectomy. J Pathol. 1996;178:437–41.
20. Cher ML, Stephenson RA, James BC, Carroll PR. Cellular proliferative fraction of metastatic lymph nodes predicts survival in stage D1 (TxN+M0) prostate cancer [see comments]. J Urol. 1996;155:1674–7.
21. Cheng L, Pisansky TM, Sebo TJ, et al. Cell proliferation in prostate cancer patients with lymph node metastasis: a marker for progression. Clin Cancer Res. 1999;5:2820–3.
22. Miyake H, Muramaki M, Kurahashi T, Takenaka A, Fujisawa M. Expression of potential molecular markers in prostate cancer: correlation with clinicopathological outcomes in patients undergoing radical prostatectomy. Urol Oncol. 2010;28:145–51.
23. Khoo VS, Pollack A, Cowen D, et al. Relationship of Ki-67 labeling index to DNA-ploidy, S-phase fraction, and outcome in prostate cancer treated with radiotherapy. Prostate. 1999;41:166–72.
24. Bubendorf L, Tapia C, Gasser TC, et al. Ki67 labeling index in core needle biopsies independently predicts tumor-specific survival in prostate cancer. Hum Pathol. 1998;29:949–54.
25. Oomens EH, van Steenbrugge GJ, van der Kwast TH, Schroder FH. Application of the monoclonal antibody Ki-67 on prostate biopsies to assess the fraction of human prostatic carcinoma. J Urol. 1991;145:81–5.
26. Grossfeld GD, Olumi AF, Connolly JA, et al. Locally recurrent prostate tumors following either radiation therapy or radical prostatectomy have changes in Ki-67 labeling index, p53 and bcl-2 immunoreactivity. J Urol. 1998;159:1437–43.
27. Khatami A, Hugosson J, Wang W, Damber JE. Ki-67 in screen-detected, low-grade, low-stage prostate cancer, relation to prostate-specific antigen doubling time, Gleason score and prostate-specific antigen relapse after radical prostatectomy. Scand J Urol Nephrol. 2009;43:12–8.
28. May M, Siegsmund M, Hammermann F, Loy V, Gunia S. Prognostic significance of proliferation activity and neuroendocrine differentiation to predict treatment failure after radical prostatectomy. Scand J Urol Nephrol. 2007;41:375–81.
29. Laitinen S, Martikainen PM, Tolonen T, Isola J, Tammela TL, Visakorpi T. EZH2, Ki-67 and MCM7 are prognostic markers in prostatectomy treated patients. Int J Cancer. 2008;122:595–602.

30. Ren B, Yu G, Tseng GC, et al. MCM7 amplification and overexpression are associated with prostate cancer progression. Oncogene. 2006;25:1090–8.
31. Varambally S, Dhanasekaran SM, Zhou M, et al. The polycomb group protein EZH2 is involved in progression of prostate cancer. Nature. 2002;419:624–9.
32. Bachmann IM, Halvorsen OJ, Collett K, et al. EZH2 expression is associated with high proliferation rate and aggressive tumor subgroups in cutaneous melanoma and cancers of the endometrium, prostate, and breast. J Clin Oncol. 2006;24:268–73.
33. Varambally S, Cao Q, Mani RS, et al. Genomic loss of microRNA-101 leads to overexpression of histone methyltransferase EZH2 in cancer. Science. 2008;322:1695–9.
34. Seligson DB, Horvath S, Shi T, et al. Global histone modification patterns predict risk of prostate cancer recurrence. Nature. 2005;435:1262–6.
35. Paik S, Shak S, Tang G, et al. A multigene assay to predict recurrence of tamoxifen-treated, node-negative breast cancer. N Engl J Med. 2004;351:2817–26.
36. Cuzick J, Swanson GP, Fisher G, et al. Prognostic value of an RNA expression signature derived from cell cycle proliferation genes for recurrence and death from prostate cancer: a retrospective study in two cohorts. Lancet Oncol. 2011;12(3):245–55.
37. Wheeler TM, Rogers E, Aihara M, Scardino PT, Thompson TC. Apoptotic index as a biomarker in prostatic intraepithelial neoplasia (PIN) and prostate cancer. J Cell Biochem Suppl. 1994;19:202–7.
38. Aihara M, Scardino PT, Truong LD, et al. The frequency of apoptosis correlates with the prognosis of Gleason Grade 3 adenocarcinoma of the prostate. Cancer. 1995;75:522–9.
39. Stapleton AM, Zbell P, Kattan MW, et al. Assessment of the biologic markers p53, Ki-67, and apoptotic index as predictive indicators of prostate carcinoma recurrence after surgery. Cancer. 1998;82:168–75.
40. Weinberg RA. The retinoblastoma protein and cell cycle control. Cell. 1995;81:323–30.
41. Sherr CJ, Roberts JM. Inhibitors of mammalian G1 cyclin-dependent kinases. Genes Dev. 1995;9:1149–63.
42. Sherr CJ. Cancer cell cycles. Science. 1996;274:1672–7.
43. Toyoshima H, Hunter T. p27, a novel inhibitor of G1 cyclin-Cdk protein kinase activity, is related to p21. Cell. 1994;78:67–74.
44. Hall M, Bates S, Peters G. Evidence for different modes of action of cyclin-dependent kinase inhibitors: p15 and p16 bind to kinases, p21 and p27 bind to cyclins. Oncogene. 1995;11: 1581–8.
45. Macleod KF, Sherry N, Hannon G, et al. p53-dependent and independent expression of p21 during cell growth, differentiation, and DNA damage. Genes Dev. 1995;9:935–44.
46. LaBaer J, Garrett MD, Stevenson LF, et al. New functional activities for the p21 family of CDK inhibitors. Genes Dev. 1997;11:847–62.
47. Sutherland RL, Musgrove EA. Cyclin E and prognosis in patients with breast cancer. N Engl J Med. 2002;347:1546–7.
48. Ruas M, Peters G. The p16^{INK4a}/CDKN2A tumor suppressor and its relatives. Biochim Biophys Acta. 1998;1378:F115–77.
49. Liggett WH, Sidransky D. Role of the p16 tumor suppressor gene in cancer. J Clin Oncol. 1998;16:1197–206.
50. Prall OW, Rogan EM, Musgrove EA, Watts CK, Sutherland RL. c-Myc or cyclin D1 mimics estrogen effects on cyclin E-Cdk2 activation and cell cycle reentry. Mol Cell Biol. 1998;18:4499–508.
51. Amati B, Land H. Myc-Max-Mad: a transcription factor network controlling cell cycle progression, differentiation and death. Curr Opin Genet Dev. 1994;4:102–8.
52. Grad JM, Dai JL, Wu S, Burnstein KL. Multiple androgen response elements and a Myc consensus site in the androgen receptor (AR) coding region are involved in androgen-mediated up-regulation of AR messenger RNA. Mol Endocrinol. 1999;13:1896–911.
53. Kokontis J, Takakura K, Hay N, Liao S. Increased androgen receptor activity and altered c-myc expression in prostate cancer cells after long-term androgen deprivation. Cancer Res. 1994;54:1566–73.

54. Bookstein R, Rio P, Madreperla SA, et al. Promoter deletion and loss of retinoblastoma gene expression in human prostate carcinoma. Proc Natl Acad Sci U S A. 1990;87:7762–6.
55. Geradts J, Hu SX, Lincoln CE, Benedict WF, Xu HJ. Aberrant RB gene expression in routinely processed, archival tumor tissues determined by three different anti-RB antibodies. Int J Cancer. 1994;58:161–7.
56. Geradts J, Wilson PA. High frequency of aberrant p16(INK4A) expression in human breast cancer. Am J Pathol. 1996;149:15–20.
57. Susini T, Baldi F, Howard C, et al. Expression of the retinoblastoma-related gene Rb2/p130 correlates with clinical outcome in endometrial cancer. J Clin Oncol. 1998;16:1085–93.
58. Caputi M, Groeger AM, Esposito V, et al. Loss of pRb2/p130 expression is associated with unfavorable clinical outcome in lung cancer. Clin Cancer Res. 2002;8:3850–6.
59. Cote RJ, Dunn MD, Chatterjee SJ, et al. Elevated and absent pRb expression is associated with bladder cancer progression and has cooperative effects with p53. Cancer Res. 1998;58: 1090–4.
60. Ittmann MM, Wieczorek R. Alterations of the retinoblastoma gene in clinically localized, stage B prostate adenocarcinomas. Hum Pathol. 1996;27:28–34.
61. Brooks JD, Bova GS, Isaacs WB. Allelic loss of the retinoblastoma gene in primary human prostatic adenocarcinomas. Prostate. 1995;26:35–9.
62. Phillips SM, Barton CM, Lee SJ, et al. Loss of the retinoblastoma susceptibility gene (RB1) is a frequent and early event in prostatic tumorigenesis. Br J Cancer. 1994;70:1252–7.
63. Cooney KA, Wetzel JC, Merajver SD, Macoska JA, Singleton TP, Wojno KJ. Distinct regions of allelic loss on 13q in prostate cancer. Cancer Res. 1996;56:1142–5.
64. Melamed J, Einhorn JM, Ittman MM. Allelic loss on chromosome 13q in human prostate carcinoma. Clin Cancer Res. 1997;3:1867–72.
65. Vesalainen S, Lipponen P. Expression of retinoblastoma gene (Rb) protein in T1-2 M0 prostatic adenocarcinoma. J Cancer Res Clin Oncol. 1995;121:429–33.
66. Cordon-Cardo C. Mutations of cell cycle regulators. Biological and clinical implications for human neoplasia. Am J Pathol. 1995;147:545–60.
67. Henshall SM, Quinn DI, Lee CS, et al. Overexpression of the cell cycle inhibitor p16INK4A in high-grade prostatic intraepithelial neoplasia predicts early relapse in prostate cancer patients. Clin Cancer Res. 2001;7:544–50.
68. Xiong Y, Menninger J, Beach D, Ward DC. Molecular cloning and chromosomal mapping of CCND genes encoding human D-type cyclins. Genomics. 1992;13:575–84.
69. Gumbiner LM, Gumerlock PH, Mack PC, et al. Overexpression of cyclin D1 is rare in human prostate carcinoma. Prostate. 1999;38:40–5.
70. Aaltomaa S, Eskelinen M, Lipponen P. Expression of cyclin A and D proteins in prostate cancer and their relation to clinopathological variables and patient survival. Prostate. 1999;38: 175–82.
71. Kallakury BV, Sheehan CE, Ambros RA, Fisher HA, Kaufman Jr RP, Ross JS. The prognostic significance of p34cdc2 and cyclin D1 protein expression in prostate adenocarcinoma. Cancer. 1997;80:753–63.
72. Porter PL, Malone KE, Heagerty PJ, et al. Expression of cell-cycle regulators p27Kip1 and cyclin E, alone and in combination, correlate with survival in young breast cancer patients. Nat Med. 1997;3:222–5.
73. Iida H, Towatari M, Tanimoto M, Morishita Y, Kodera Y, Saito H. Overexpression of cyclin E in acute myelogenous leukemia. Blood. 1997;90:3707–13.
74. Mashal RD, Lester S, Corless C, et al. Expression of cell cycle-regulated proteins in prostate cancer. Cancer Res. 1996;56:4159–63.
75. Serrano M, Hannon GJ, Beach D. A new regulatory motif in cell-cycle control causing specific inhibition of cyclin D/CDK4. Nature. 1993;366:704–7.
76. Herman JG, Merlo A, Mao L, et al. Inactivation of the CDKN2/p16/MTS1 gene is frequently associated with aberrant DNA methylation in all human cancers. Cancer Res. 1995;55: 4525–30.

77. Komiya A, Suzuki H, Aida S, Yatani R, Shimazaki J. Mutational analysis of CDKN2 (CDK4I/MTS1) gene in tissues and cell lines of human prostate cancer. Jpn J Cancer Res. 1995; 86:622–5.
78. Jarrard DF, Bova GS, Ewing CM, et al. Deletional, mutational, and methylation analyses of CDKN2 (p16/MTS1) in primary and metastatic prostate cancer. Genes Chromosomes Cancer. 1997;19:90–6.
79. Cairns P, Polascik TJ, Eby Y, et al. Frequency of homozygous deletion at p16/CDKN2 in primary human tumours. Nat Genet. 1995;11:210–2.
80. Tamimi Y, Bringuier PP, Smit F, van Bokhoven A, Debruyne FM, Schalken JA. p16 mutations/deletions are not frequent events in prostate cancer. Br J Cancer. 1996;74:120–2.
81. Gaddipati JP, McLeod DG, Sesterhenn IA, et al. Mutations of the p16 gene product are rare in prostate cancer. Prostate. 1997;30:188–94.
82. Chen W, Weghorst CM, Sabourin CLK, et al. Absence of *p16/MTS1* gene mutations in human prostate cancer. Carcinogenesis. 1996;17:2603–7.
83. Park DJ, Wilczynski SP, Pham EY, Miller CW, Koeffler HP. Molecular analysis of the INK4 family of genes in prostate carcinomas. J Urol. 1997;157:1995–9.
84. Lee CT, Capodieci P, Osman I, et al. Overexpression of the cyclin-dependent kinase inhibitor p16 is associated with tumor recurrence in human prostate cancer. Clin Cancer Res. 1999;5:977–83.
85. Halvorsen OJ, Hostmark J, Haukaas S, Hoisaeter PA, Akslen LA. Prognostic significance of p16 and CDK4 proteins in localized prostate carcinoma. Cancer. 2000;88:416–24.
86. Li Y, Nichols MA, Shay JW, Xiong Y. Transcriptional repression of the D-type cyclin-dependent kinase inhibitor p16 by the retinoblastoma susceptibility gene product pRb. Cancer Res. 1994;54:6078–82.
87. Jarrard DF, Sarkar S, Shi Y, et al. p16/pRb pathway alterations are required for bypassing senescence in human prostate epithelial cells. Cancer Res. 1999;59:2957–64.
88. Tsihlias J, Kapusta L, Slingerland J. The prognostic significance of altered cyclin-dependent kinase inhibitors in human cancer. Annu Rev Med. 1999;50:401–23.
89. Gao X, Chen YQ, Wu N, et al. Somatic mutations of the WAF1/CIP1 gene in primary prostate cancer. Oncogene. 1995;11:1395–8.
90. Rowan S, Ludwig RL, Haupt Y, et al. Specific loss of apoptotic but not cell-cycle arrest function in a human tumor derived p53 mutant. EMBO J. 1996;15:827–38.
91. Wang J, Walsh K. Resistance to apoptosis conferred by Cdk inhibitors during myocyte differentiation. Science. 1996;273:359–61.
92. Osman I, Drobnjak M, Fazzari M, Ferrara J, Scher HI, Cordon-Cardo C. Inactivation of the p53 pathway in prostate cancer: impact on tumor progression. Clin Cancer Res. 1999;5:2082–8.
93. Russell A, Hendley J, Germain D. Inhibitory effect of p21 in MCF-7 cells is overcome by its coordinated stabilization with D-type cyclins. Oncogene. 1999;18:6454–9.
94. Lu S, Liu M, Epner DE, Tsai SY, Tsai MJ. Androgen regulation of the cyclin-dependent kinase inhibitor p21 gene through an androgen response element in the proximal promoter. Mol Endocrinol. 1999;13:376–84.
95. Rigaud J, Tiguert R, Decobert M, et al. Expression of p21 cell cycle protein is an independent predictor of response to salvage radiotherapy after radical prostatectomy. Prostate. 2004;58: 269–76.
96. Fizazi K, Martinez LA, Sikes CR, et al. The association of p21((WAF-1/CIP1)) with progression to androgen-independent prostate cancer. Clin Cancer Res. 2002;8:775–81.
97. Ponce-Castaneda MV, Lee MH, Latres E, et al. p27Kip1: chromosomal mapping to 12p12-12p13.1 and absence of mutations in human tumors. Cancer Res. 1995;55:1211–4.
98. Fero ML, Rivkin M, Tasch M, et al. A syndrome of multiorgan hyperplasia with features of gigantism, tumorigenesis, and female sterility in p27(Kip1)-deficient mice. Cell. 1996;85: 733–44.
99. Cordon-Cardo C, Koff A, Drobnjak M, et al. Distinct altered patterns of p27KIP1 gene expression in benign prostatic hyperplasia and prostatic carcinoma. J Natl Cancer Inst. 1998;90: 1284–91.

100. Catzavelos C, Bhattacharya N, Ung YC, et al. Decreased levels of the cell-cycle inhibitor p27Kip1 protein: prognostic implications in primary breast cancer. Nat Med. 1997;3: 227–30.
101. Lloyd RV, Jin L, Qian X, Kulig E. Aberrant p27kip1 expression in endocrine and other tumors. Am J Pathol. 1997;150:401–7.
102. Tan P, Cady B, Wanner M, et al. The cell cycle inhibitor p27 is an independent prognostic marker in small (T1a, b) invasive breast carcinomas. Cancer Res. 1997;57:1259–63.
103. Fredersdorf S, Burns J, Milne AM, et al. High level expression of p27(kip1) and cyclin D1 in some human breast cancer cells: Inverse correlation between the expression of p27(kip1) and degree of malignancy in human breast and colorectal cancers. Proc Natl Acad Sci U S A. 1997;94:6380–5.
104. Esposito V, Baldi A, De Luca A, et al. Prognostic role of the cyclin-dependent kinase inhibitor p27 in non-small cell lung cancer. Cancer Res. 1997;57:3381–5.
105. Loda M, Cukor B, Tam SW, et al. Increased proteasome-dependent degradation of the cyclin-dependent kinase inhibitor p27 in aggressive colorectal carcinomas. Nat Med. 1997;3:231–4.
106. Singh SP, Lipman J, Goldman H, et al. Loss or altered subcellular localization of p27 in Barrett's associated adenocarcinoma. Cancer Res. 1998;58:1730–5.
107. Kawamata N, Morosetti R, Miller CW, et al. Molecular analysis of the cyclin-dependent kinase inhibitor gene p27/Kip1 in human malignancies. Cancer Res. 1995;55:2266–9.
108. Spirin KS, Simpson JF, Takeuchi S, Kawamata N, Miller CW, Koeffler HP. p27/Kip1 mutation found in breast cancer. Cancer Res. 1996;56:2400–4.
109. Kibel AS, Freije D, Isaacs WB, Bova GS. Deletion mapping at 12p12-13 in metastatic prostate cancer. Genes Chromosomes Cancer. 1999;25:270–6.
110. Pagano M, Tam SW, Theodoras AM, et al. Role of the ubiquitin-proteasome pathway in regulating abundance of the cyclin-dependent kinase inhibitor p27. Science. 1995;269:682–5.
111. Millard SS, Yan JS, Nguyen H, Pagano M, Kiyokawa H, Koff A. Enhanced ribosomal association of p27(Kip1) mRNA is a mechanism contributing to accumulation during growth arrest. J Biol Chem. 1997;272:7093–8.
112. Vlach J, Hennecke S, Amati B. Phosphorylation-dependent degradation of the cyclin-dependent kinase inhibitor p27. EMBO J. 1997;16:5334–44.
113. Jin L, Qian X, Kulig E, et al. Transforming growth factor-beta, transforming growth factor-beta receptor II, and p27Kip1 expression in nontumorous and neoplastic human pituitaries. Am J Pathol. 1997;151:509–19.
114. Vrhovac R, Delmer A, Tang R, Marie JP, Zittoun R, Ajchenbaum-Cymbalista F. Prognostic significance of the cell cycle inhibitor p27Kip1 in chronic B-cell lymphocytic leukemia. Blood. 1998;91:4694–700.
115. Vlach J, Hennecke S, Alevizopoulos K, Conti D, Amati B. Growth arrest by the cyclin-dependent kinase inhibitor p27Kip1 is abrogated by c-Myc. EMBO J. 1996;15:6595–604.
116. Perez-Roger I, Solomon DL, Sewing A, Land H. Myc activation of cyclin E/Cdk2 kinase involves induction of cyclin E gene transcription and inhibition of p27(Kip1) binding to newly formed complexes. Oncogene. 1997;14:2373–81.
117. Muller D, Bouchard C, Rudolph B, et al. Cdk2-dependent phosphorylation of p27 facilitates its Myc-induced release from cyclin E/cdk2 complexes. Oncogene. 1997;15:2561–76.
118. Sheaff RJ, Groudine M, Gordon M, Roberts JM, Clurman BE. Cyclin E-CDK2 is a regulator of p27Kip1. Genes Dev. 1997;11:1464–78.
119. Kokontis JM, Hay N, Liao S. Progression of LNCaP prostate tumor cells during androgen deprivation: hormone-independent growth, repression of proliferation by androgen, and role for p27Kip1 in androgen-induced cell cycle arrest. Mol Endocrinol. 1998;12:941–53.
120. Myers RB, Oelschlager DK, Coan PN, et al. Changes in cyclin dependent kinase inhibitors p21 and p27 during the castration induced regression of the CWR22 model of prostatic adenocarcinoma. J Urol. 1999;161:945–9.
121. Agus DB, Cordon-Cardo C, Fox W, et al. Prostate cancer cell cycle regulators: response to androgen withdrawal and development of androgen independence. J Natl Cancer Inst. 1999;91:1869–76.

122. Guo Y, Sklar GN, Borkowski A, Kyprianou N. Loss of the cyclin-dependent kinase inhibitor p27Kip1 protein in human prostate cancer correlates with tumor grade. Clin Cancer Res. 1997;3:2269–74.
123. Tsihlias J, Kapusta LR, DeBoer G, et al. Loss of cyclin-dependent kinase inhibitor p27Kip1 is a novel prognostic factor in localized human prostate adenocarcinoma. Cancer Res. 1998;58:542–8.
124. Cote RJ, Shi Y, Groshen S, et al. Association of p27Kip1 levels with recurrence and survival in patients with stage C prostate carcinoma. J Natl Cancer Inst. 1998;90:916–20.
125. De Marzo AM, Meeker AK, Epstein JI, Coffey DS. Prostate stem cell compartments: expression of the cell cycle inhibitor p27Kip1 in normal, hyperplastic, and neoplastic cells. Am J Pathol. 1998;153:911–9.
126. Yang RM, Naitoh J, Murphy M, et al. Low p27 expression predicts poor disease-free survival in patients with prostate cancer. J Urol. 1998;159:941–5.
127. Kuczyk M, Machtens S, Hradil K, et al. Predictive value of decreased p27Kip1 protein expression for the recurrence-free and long-term survival of prostate cancer patients. Br J Cancer. 1999;81:1052–8.
128. Kuczyk MA, Bokemeyer C, Hartmann J, et al. Predictive value of altered p27Kip1 and p21WAF/Cip1 protein expression for the clinical prognosis of patients with localized prostate cancer. Oncol Rep. 2001;8:1401–7.
129. Cher ML, MacGrogan D, Bookstein R, Brown JA, Jenkins RB, Jensen RH. Comparative genomic hybridization, allelic imbalance, and fluorescence in situ hybridization on chromosome 8 in prostate cancer. Genes Chromosomes Cancer. 1994;11:153–62.
130. Cher ML, Bova GS, Moore DH, et al. Genetic alterations in untreated metastases and androgen-independent prostate cancer detected by comparative genomic hybridization and allelotyping. Cancer Res. 1996;56:3091–102.
131. Nupponen NN, Kakkola L, Koivisto P, Visakorpi T. Genetic alterations in hormone-refractory recurrent prostate carcinomas. Am J Pathol. 1998;153:141–8.
132. Sato K, Qian J, Slezak JM, et al. Clinical significance of alterations of chromosome 8 in high-grade, advanced, nonmetastatic prostate carcinoma. J Natl Cancer Inst. 1999;91:1574–80.
133. Qian J, Jenkins RB, Bostwick DG. Detection of chromosomal anomalies and c-myc gene amplification in the cribriform pattern of prostatic intraepithelial neoplasia and carcinoma by fluorescence in situ hybridization. Mod Pathol. 1997;10:1113–9.
134. Fox SB, Persad RA, Royds J, Kore RN, Silcocks PB, Collins CC. p53 and c-myc expression in stage A1 prostatic adenocarcinoma: useful prognostic determinants? J Urol. 1993; 150:490–4.
135. Jenkins RB, Qian J, Lieber MM, Bostwick DG. Detection of c-myc oncogene amplification and chromosomal anomalies in metastatic prostatic carcinoma by fluorescence in situ hybridization. Cancer Res. 1997;57:524–31.
136. Bubendorf L, Kononen J, Koivisto P, et al. Survey of gene amplifications during prostate cancer progression by high-throughout fluorescence in situ hybridization on tissue microarrays. Cancer Res. 1999;59:803–6 [published erratum appears in *Cancer Res* 1999;59(6):1388].
137. Buttyan R, Sawczuk IS, Benson MC, Siegal JD, Olsson CA. Enhanced expression of the c-myc protooncogene in high-grade human prostate cancers. Prostate. 1987;11:327–37.
138. Fleming WH, Hamel A, MacDonald R, et al. Expression of the c-myc protooncogene in human prostatic carcinoma and benign prostatic hyperplasia. Cancer Res. 1986;46:1535–8.
139. Gurel B, Iwata T, Koh CM, et al. Nuclear MYC protein overexpression is an early alteration in human prostate carcinogenesis. Mod Pathol. 2008;21:1156–67.
140. Hawksworth D, Ravindranath L, Chen Y, et al. Overexpression of C-MYC oncogene in prostate cancer predicts biochemical recurrence. Prostate Cancer Prostatic Dis. 2010;13:311–5.
141. Yang G, Timme TL, Frolov A, Wheeler TM, Thompson TC. Combined c-Myc and caveolin-1 expression in human prostate carcinoma predicts prostate carcinoma progression. Cancer. 2005;103:1186–94.
142. Kirsch DG, Kastan MB. Tumor-suppressor p53: implications for tumor development and prognosis. J Clin Oncol. 1998;16:3158–68.

143. Reed JC. Bcl-2 and the regulation of programmed cell death. J Cell Biol. 1994;124:1–6.
144. Visakorpi T, Kallioniemi OP, Heikkinen A, Koivula T, Isola J. Small subgroup of aggressive, highly proliferative prostatic carcinomas defined by p53 accumulation. J Natl Cancer Inst. 1992;84:883–7.
145. Raffo AJ, Perlman H, Chen MW, Day ML, Streitman JS, Buttyan R. Overexpression of bcl-2 protects prostate cancer cells from apoptosis in vitro and confers resistance to androgen depletion in vivo. Cancer Res. 1995;55:4438–45.
146. Bauer JJ, Sesterhenn IA, Mostofi FK, McLeod DG, Srivastava S, Moul JW. Elevated levels of apoptosis regulator proteins p53 and bcl-2 are independent prognostic biomarkers in surgically treated clinically localized prostate cancer. J Urol. 1996;156:1511–6.
147. Apakama I, Robinson MC, Walter NM, et al. bcl-2 overexpression combined with p53 protein accumulation correlates with hormone-refractory prostate cancer. Br J Cancer. 1996;74:1258–62.
148. Meyers FJ, Gumerlock PH, Chi SG, Borchers H, Deitch AD, deVere White RW. Very frequent p53 mutations in metastatic prostate carcinoma and in matched primary tumors. Cancer. 1998;83:2534–9.
149. Quinn DI, Henshall SM, Head DR, et al. Prognostic significance of p53 nuclear accumulation in localized prostate cancer treated with radical prostatectomy. Cancer Res. 2000;60:1585–94.
150. Stattin P, Westin P, Damber JE, Bergh A. Short-term cellular effects induced by castration therapy in relation to clinical outcome in prostate cancer. Br J Cancer. 1998;77:670–5.
151. Rokhlin OW, Guseva N, Tagiyev A, Knudson CM, Cohen MB. Bcl-2 oncoprotein protects the human prostatic carcinoma cell line PC3 from TRAIL-mediated apoptosis. Oncogene. 2001; 20:2836–43.
152. Agarwal ML, Taylor WR, Chernov MV, Chernova OB, Stark GR. The p53 network. J Biol Chem. 1998;273:1–4.
153. Liebermann DA, Hoffman B, Steinman RA. Molecular controls of growth arrest and apoptosis: p53-dependent and independent markers. Oncogene. 1995;11:199–210.
154. Dameron KM, Volpert OV, Tainsky MA, Bouck N. Control of angiogenesis in fibroblasts by p53 regulation of thrombospondin-1. Science. 1994;265:1582–4.
155. Gasparini G, Weidner N, Bevilacqua P, et al. Tumor microvessel density, p53 expression, tumor size, and peritumoral lymphatic vessel invasion are relevant prognostic markers in node-negative breast carcinoma. J Clin Oncol. 1994;12:454–66.
156. Yu ED, Yu E, Meyer GE, Brawer MK. The relation of p53 protein nuclear accumulation and angiogenesis in human prostate cancer. Prostate Cancer Prostatic Dis. 1997;1:39–44.
157. Mydlo JH, Kral JG, Volpe M, Axotis C, Macchia RJ, Pertschuk LP. An analysis of microvessel density, androgen receptor, p53 and HER-2/neu expression and Gleason score in prostate cancer. Preliminary results and therapeutic implications. Eur Urol. 1998;34:426–32.
158. Finlay CA, Hinds PW, Tan TH, Eliyahn D, Oren M, Levine AJ. Activating mutations for transformation by p53 produce a gene product that forms an *hsc70-p53* complex withan altered half-life. Mol Cell Biol. 1988;8:531–9.
159. Bartek J, Iggo R, Gannon J, Lane DP. Genetic and immunochemical analysis of mutant p53 in human breast cancer cell lines. Oncogene. 1990;5:893–9.
160. Casey G, Lopez ME, Ramos JC, et al. DNA sequence analysis of exons 2 through 11 and immunohistochemical staining are required to detect all known p53 alterations in human malignancies. Oncogene. 1996;13:1971–81.
161. Bodner SM, Minna JD, Jensen SM, et al. Expression of mutant p53 proteins in lung cancer correlates with the class of p53 gene mutation. Oncogene. 1992;7:743–9.
162. Melhem MF, Law JC, el-Ashmawy L, et al. Assessment of sensitivity and specificity of immunohistochemical staining of p53 in lung and head and neck cancers. Am J Pathol. 1995;146:1170–7.
163. Midgley CA, Lane DP. p53 protein stability in tumour cells is not determined by mutation but is dependent on Mdm2 binding. Oncogene. 1997;15:1179–89.
164. Thor AD, Moore DH, Edgerton SM, et al. Accumulation of p53 tumor suppressor gene protein: an independent marker of prognosis in breast cancers. J Natl Cancer Inst. 1992;84:845–55.

165. Elledge RM, Clark GM, Fuqua SA, Yu YY, Allred DC. p53 protein accumulation detected by five different antibodies: relationship to prognosis and heat shock protein 70 in breast cancer. Cancer Res. 1994;54:3752–7.
166. Xu H-J, Cagle PT, Hu S-X, Li J, Benedict WF. Altered retinoblastoma amd p53 protein status in non-small cell carcinoma of the lung: potential synergistic effects on prognosis. Clin Cancer Res. 1996;2:1169–76.
167. Goh H-S, Yao J, Smith DR. p53 point mutation and survival in colorectal cancer patients. Cancer Res. 1995;55:5217–21.
168. Griewe GL, Dean RC, Zhang W, et al. p53 Immunostaining guided laser capture microdissection (p53-LCM) defines the presence of p53 gene mutations in focal regions of primary prostate cancer positive for p53 protein. Prostate Cancer Prostatic Dis. 2003;6:281–5.
169. Grignon DJ, Caplan R, Sarkar FH, et al. p53 status and prognosis of locally advanced prostatic adenocarcinoma: a study based on RTOG 8610. J Natl Cancer Inst. 1997; 89:158–65.
170. Kuczyk MA, Serth J, Bokemeyer C, et al. The prognostic value of p53 for long-term and recurrence-free survival following radical prostatectomy. Eur J Cancer. 1998;34:679–86.
171. Bauer JJ, Sesterhenn IA, Mostofi KF, McLeod DG, Srivastava S, Moul JW. p53 nuclear protein expression is an independent prognostic marker in clinically localised prostate cancer patients undergoing radical prostatectomy. Clin Cancer Res. 1995;1:1295–300.
172. Yang G, Stapleton AMF, Wheeler TM, et al. Clustered p53 immunostaining: a novel pattern associated with prostate cancer progression. Clin Cancer Res. 1996;2:399–401.
173. Brooks JD, Bova GS, Ewing CM, et al. An uncertain role for p53 gene alterations in human prostate cancers. Cancer Res. 1996;56:3814–22.
174. Navone NM, Troncoso P, Pisters LL, et al. p53 protein accumulation and gene mutation in the progression of human prostate carcinoma. J Natl Cancer Inst. 1993;85:1657–69.
175. Bookstein R, MacGrogan D, Hilsenbeck SG, Sharkey F, Allred DC. p53 is mutated in a subset of advanced-stage prostate cancers. Cancer Res. 1993;53:3369–73.
176. Dinjens WN, van der Weiden MM, Schroeder FH, Bosman FT, Trapman J. Frequency and characterization of p53 mutations in primary and metastatic human prostate cancer. Int J Cancer. 1994;56:630–3.
177. Chi SG. deVere White RW, Meyers FJ, Siders DB, Lee F, Gumerlock PH. p53 in prostate cancer: frequent expressed transition mutations. J Natl Cancer Inst. 1994;86:926–33.
178. Gumerlock PH, Chi SG, Shi XB, et al. p53 abnormalities in primary prostate cancer: single-strand conformation polymorphism analysis of complementary DNA in comparison with genomic DNA. The cooperative prostate network. J Natl Cancer Inst. 1997;89:66–71.
179. Stapleton AMF, Timme TL, Gousse AE, et al. Primary human prostate cancer cells harboring p53 mutations are clonally expanded in metastases. Clin Cancer Res. 1997;3:1389–97.
180. Bova GS. Molecular genetics of hormone refractory prostate cancer metastasis. In: Haslam SZ, Barrack E, editors. Keystone symposia: breast and prostate cancer; 21–26 Feb 1998. Copper Mountain, CO; 1998.
181. Suzuki H, Freije D, Nusskern DR, et al. Interfocal heterogeneity of PTEN/MMAC1 gene alterations in multiple metastatic prostate cancer tissues. Cancer Res. 1998;58:204–9.
182. Hughes JH, Cohen MB, Robinson RA. p53 immunoreactivity in primary and metastatic prostatic adenocarcinoma. Mod Pathol. 1995;8:462–6.
183. Eastham JA, Stapleton AMF, Gousse AE, et al. Association of p53 mutations with metastatic prostate cancer. Clin Cancer Res. 1995;1:1111–8.
184. Rakozy C, Grignon DJ, Sarkar FH, Sakr WA, Littrup P, Forman J. Expression of bcl-2, p53, and p21 in benign and malignant prostatic tissue before and after radiation therapy. Mod Pathol. 1998;11:892–9.
185. Prendergast NJ, Atkins MR, Schatte EC, Paulson DF, Walther PJ. p53 immunohistochemical and genetic alterations are associated at high incidence with post-irradiated locally persistent prostate carcinoma. J Urol. 1996;155:1685–92.
186. Mirchandani D, Zheng J, Miller GJ, et al. Heterogeneity in intratumor distribution of p53 mutations in human prostate cancer. Am J Pathol. 1995;147:92–101.

187. Konishi N, Hiasa Y, Matsuda H, et al. Intratumor cellular heterogeneity and alterations in ras oncogene and p53 tumor suppressor gene in human prostate carcinoma. Am J Pathol. 1995;147:1112–22.
188. Geburek BM, Kollmorgen TA, Qian J, D'Souza-Gburek SM, Lieber MM, Jenkins RB. Chromosomal anomalies in stage D1 prostate adenocarcinoma primary tumors and lymph node metastases detected by fluorescence in situ hybridization. J Urol. 1997;157:223–7.
189. Qian J, Hirasawa K, Bostwick DG, et al. Loss of p53 and c-myc overrepresentation in stage T(2-3)N(1-3)M(0) prostate cancer are potential markers for cancer progression. Mod Pathol. 2002;15:35–44.
190. Borre M, Stausbol-Gron B, Overgaard J. p53 accumulation associated with bcl-2, the proliferation marker MIB-1 and survival in patients with prostate cancer subjected to watchful waiting. J Urol. 2000;164:716–21.
191. Haldar S, Beatty C, Tsujimoto Y, Croce CM. The bcl-2 gene encodes a novel G protein. Nature. 1989;342:195–8.
192. Tsujimoto Y, Croce CM. Analysis of the structure, transcripts, and protein products of bcl-2, the gene involved in human follicular lymphoma. Proc Natl Acad Sci U S A. 1986;83: 5214–8.
193. McDonnell TJ, Troncoso P, Brisbay SM, et al. Expression of the protooncogene bcl-2 in the prostate and its association with emergence of androgen-independent prostate cancer. Cancer Res. 1992;52:6940–4.
194. Colombel M, Symmans F, Gil S, et al. Detection of the apoptosis-suppressing oncoprotein bcl-2 in hormone-refractory human prostate cancers. Am J Pathol. 1993;143:390–400.
195. Berchem GJ, Bosseler M, Sugars LY, Voeller HJ, Zeitlin S, Gelmann EP. Androgens induce resistance to bcl-2-mediated apoptosis in LNCaP prostate cancer cells. Cancer Res. 1995;55:735–8.
196. McConkey DJ, Greene G, Pettaway CA. Apoptosis resistance increases with metastatic potential in cells of the human LNCaP prostate carcinoma line. Cancer Res. 1996;56: 5594–9.
197. Rosser CJ, Reyes AO, Vakar-Lopez F, et al. Bcl-2 is significantly overexpressed in localized radio-recurrent prostate carcinoma, compared with localized radio-naive prostate carcinoma. Int J Radiat Oncol Biol Phys. 2003;56:1–6.
198. Horvath LG, Henshall SM, Lee CS, et al. Frequent loss of estrogen receptor-beta expression in prostate cancer. Cancer Res. 2001;61:5331–5.
199. Gorelic LS, Lamm DL, Ramzy I, Radwin HM, Shain SA. Androgen receptors in biopsy specimens of prostate adenocarcinoma. Heterogeneity of distribution and relation to prognostic significance of receptor measurements for survival of advanced cancer patients. Cancer. 1987;60:211–9.
200. de Winter JA, Trapman J, Brinkmann AO, et al. Androgen receptor heterogeneity in human prostatic carcinomas visualized by immunohistochemistry. J Pathol. 1990;160:329–32.
201. Sadi MV, Barrack ER. Androgen receptors and growth fraction in metastatic prostate cancer as predictors of time to tumour progression after hormonal therapy. Cancer Surv. 1991;11:195–215.
202. van der Kwast TH, Schalken J, Ruizeveld de Winter JA, et al. Androgen receptors in endocrine-therapy-resistant human prostate cancer. Int J Cancer. 1991;48:189–93.
203. Chodak GW, Kranc DM, Puy LA, Takeda H, Johnson K, Chang C. Nuclear localization of androgen receptor in heterogeneous samples of normal, hyperplastic and neoplastic human prostate. J Urol. 1992;147:798–803.
204. Miyamoto KK, McSherry SA, Dent GA, et al. Immunohistochemistry of the androgen receptor in human benign and malignant prostate tissue. J Urol. 1993;149:1015–9.
205. Ruizeveld de Winter JA, Janssen PJ, Sleddens HM, et al. Androgen receptor status in localized and locally progressive hormone refractory human prostate cancer. Am J Pathol. 1994;144:735–46.
206. Magi-Galluzzi C, Xu X, Hlatky L, et al. Heterogeneity of androgen receptor content in advanced prostate cancer. Mod Pathol. 1997;10:839–45.

207. Tilley WD, Lim-Tio SS, Horsfall DJ, Aspinall JO, Marshall VR, Skinner JM. Detection of discrete androgen receptor epitopes in prostate cancer by immunostaining: measurement by color video image analysis. Cancer Res. 1994;54:4096–102.
208. Peterziel H, Culig Z, Stober J, et al. Mutant androgen receptors in prostatic tumors distinguish between amino-acid-sequence requirements for transactivation and ligand binding. Int J Cancer. 1995;63:544–50.
209. Loda M, Fogt F, French FS, et al. Androgen receptor immunohistochemistry on paraffin-embedded tissue. Mod Pathol. 1994;7:388–91.
210. Hobisch A, Culig Z, Radmayr C, Bartsch G, Klocker H, Hittmair A. Distant metastases from prostatic carcinoma express androgen receptor protein. Cancer Res. 1995;55:3068–72.
211. Prins GS, Sklarew RJ, Pertschuk LP. Image analysis of androgen receptor immunostaining in prostate cancer accurately predict response to hormonal therapy. J Urol. 1998;159:641–9.
212. Koivisto P, Kononen J, Palmberg C, et al. Androgen receptor gene amplification: a possible molecular mechanism for androgen deprivation therapy failure in prostate cancer. Cancer Res. 1997;57:314–9.
213. Koivisto P, Kolmer M, Visakorpi T, Kallioniemi O-P. Androgen receptor gene and hormonal therapy failure of prostate cancer. Am J Pathol. 1998;152:1–9.
214. Olapade-Olaopa EO, MacKay EH, Taub NA, Sandhu DP, Terry TR, Habib FK. Malignant transformation of human prostatic epithelium is associated with the loss of androgen receptor immunoreactivity in the surrounding stroma. Clin Cancer Res. 1999;5:569–76.
215. Takeda H, Akakura K, Masai M, Akimoto S, Yatani R, Shimazaki S. Androgen receptor content of prostate carcinoma cells estimated by immunohistochemistry is related to prognosis of patients with stage D2 prostate carcinoma. Cancer. 1996;77:934–40.
216. Sweat SD, Pacelli A, Bergstralh EJ, Slezak JM, Cheng L, Bostwick DG. Androgen receptor expression in prostate cancer lymph node metastases is predictive of outcome after surgery. J Urol. 1999;161:1233–7.
217. Sweat SD, Pacelli A, Bergstralh EJ, Slezak JM, Bostwick DG. Androgen receptor expression in prostatic intraepithelial neoplasia and cancer. J Urol. 1999;161:1229–32.
218. Wilson CM, Griffin JE, Wilson JD, Marcelli M, Zoppi S, McPhaul MJ. Immunoreactive androgen receptor expression in subjects with androgen resistance. J Clin Endocrinol Metab. 1992;75:1474–8.
219. Visakorpi T, Hyytinen E, Koivisto P, et al. In vivo amplification of the androgen receptor gene and progression of human prostate cancer. Nat Genet. 1995;9:401–6.
220. Olumi AF, Grossfeld GD, Hayward SW, Carroll PR, Tlsty TD, Cunha GR. Carcinoma-associated fibroblasts direct tumor progression of initiated human prostatic epithelium. Cancer Res. 1999;59:5002–11.
221. Koivisto P, Hyytinen E, Palmberg C, et al. Analysis of genetic changes underlying local recurrence of prostate carcinoma during androgen deprivation therapy. Am J Pathol. 1995;147:1608–14.
222. Henshall SM, Quinn DI, Lee CS, et al. Altered expression of androgen receptor in the malignant epithelium and adjacent stroma is associated with early relapse in prostate cancer. Cancer Res. 2001;61:423–7.
223. Rosner IL, Ravindranath L, Furusato B, et al. Higher tumor to benign ratio of the androgen receptor mRNA expression associates with prostate cancer progression after radical prostatectomy. Urology. 2007;70:1225–9.
224. Wolf DA, Herzinger T, Hermeking H, Blaschke D, Horz W. Transcriptional and posttranscriptional regulation of human androgen receptor expression by androgen. Mol Endocrinol. 1993;7:924–36.
225. Donovan MJ, Osman I, Khan FM, et al. Androgen receptor expression is associated with prostate cancer-specific survival in castrate patients with metastatic disease. BJU Int. 2009;105:462–7.
226. Thompson TC, Timme TL, Kadmon D, Park SH, Egawa S, Yoshida K. Genetic predisposition and mesenchymal-epithelial interactions in ras + myc-induced carcinogenesis in reconstituted mouse prostate. Mol Carcinog. 1993;7:165–79.

227. Lee C, Sintich SM, Mathews EP, et al. Transforming growth factor-beta in benign and malignant prostate. Prostate. 1999;39:285–90.
228. Kooistra A, Romijn JC, Schroder FH. Stromal inhibition of epithelial cell growth in the prostate; overview of an experimental study. Urol Res. 1997;25 Suppl 2:S97–105.
229. Gleave M, Hsieh JT, Gao CA, von Eschenbach AC, Chung LW. Acceleration of human prostate cancer growth in vivo by factors produced by prostate and bone fibroblasts. Cancer Res. 1991;51:3753–61.
230. Planz B, Wang Q, Kirley SD, Lin CW, McDougal WS. Androgen responsiveness of stromal cells of the human prostate: regulation of cell proliferation and keratinocyte growth factor by androgen. J Urol. 1998;160:1850–5.
231. Lu W, Luo Y, Kan M, McKeehan WL. Fibroblast growth factor-10. A second candidate stromal to epithelial cell andromedin in prostate. J Biol Chem. 1999;274:12827–34 [published erratum appears in *J Biol Chem* 1999;274(39):28058].
232. Memarzadeh S, Xin L, Mulholland DJ, et al. Enhanced paracrine FGF10 expression promotes formation of multifocal prostate adenocarcinoma and an increase in epithelial androgen receptor. Cancer Cell. 2007;12:572–85.
233. Shi YK, Yu YP, Zhu ZH, et al. MCM7 interacts with androgen receptor. Am J Pathol. 2008;173:1758–67.
234. Hobisch A, Eder IE, Putz T, et al. Interleukin-6 regulates prostate-specific protein expression in prostate carcinoma cells by activation of the androgen receptor. Cancer Res. 1998;58:4640–5.
235. Gerdes MJ, Dang TD, Larsen M, Rowley DR. Transforming growth factor-beta1 induces nuclear to cytoplasmic distribution of androgen receptor and inhibits androgen response in prostate smooth muscle cells. Endocrinology. 1998;139:3569–77.
236. Leung HY, Mehta P, Gray LB, Collins AT, Robson CN, Neal DE. Keratinocyte growth factor expression in hormone insensitive prostate cancer. Oncogene. 1997;15:1115–20.
237. Kattan MW, Shariat SF, Andrews B, et al. The addition of interleukin-6 soluble receptor and transforming growth factor beta1 improves a preoperative nomogram for predicting biochemical progression in patients with clinically localized prostate cancer. J Clin Oncol. 2003;21:3573–9.
238. Taplin ME, Bubley GJ, Shuster TD, et al. Mutation of the androgen-receptor gene in metastatic androgen-independent prostate cancer. N Engl J Med. 1995;332:1393–8.
239. Veldscholte J, Ris-Stalpers C, Kuiper GG, et al. A mutation in the ligand binding domain of the androgen receptor of human LNCaP cells affects steroid binding characteristics and response to anti-androgens. Biochem Biophys Res Commun. 1990;173:534–40.
240. Veldscholte J, Berrevoets CA, Ris-Stalpers C, et al. The androgen receptor in LNCaP cells contains a mutation in the ligand binding domain which affects steroid binding characteristics and response to antiandrogens. J Steroid Biochem Mol Biol. 1992;41:665–9.
241. Suzuki H, Akakura K, Komiya A, Aida S, Akimoto S, Shimazaki J. Codon 877 mutation in the androgen receptor gene in advanced prostate cancer: relation to antiandrogen withdrawal syndrome. Prostate. 1996;29:153–8.
242. Fenton MA, Shuster TD, Fertig AM, et al. Functional characterization of mutant androgen receptors from androgen-independent prostate cancer. Clin Cancer Res. 1997;3:1383–8.
243. Taplin ME, Bubley GJ, Ko YJ, et al. Selection for androgen receptor mutations in prostate cancers treated with androgen antagonist. Cancer Res. 1999;59:2511–5.
244. Steinkamp MP, O'Mahony OA, Brogley M, et al. Treatment-dependent androgen receptor mutations in prostate cancer exploit multiple mechanisms to evade therapy. Cancer Res. 2009;69:4434–42.
245. Palmberg C, Koivisto P, Hyytinen E, et al. Androgen receptor gene amplification in a recurrent prostate cancer after monotherapy with the nonsteroidal potent antiandrogen Casodex (bicalutamide) with a subsequent favorable response to maximal androgen blockade. Eur Urol. 1997;31:216–9.
246. Tilley WD, Buchanan G, Hickey TE, Bentel JM. Mutations in the androgen receptor gene are associated with progression of human prostate cancer to androgen independence. Clin Cancer Res. 1996;2:277–86.

247. Culig Z, Hobisch A, Cronauer MV, et al. Mutant androgen receptor detected in an advanced-stage prostatic carcinoma is activated by adrenal androgens and progesterone. Mol Endocrinol. 1993;7:1541–50.
248. Gaddipati JP, McLeod DG, Heidenberg HB, et al. Frequent detection of codon 877 mutation in the androgen receptor gene in advanced prostate cancers. Cancer Res. 1994;54:2861–4.
249. Elo JP, Kvist L, Leinonen K, et al. Mutated human androgen receptor gene detected in a prostatic cancer patient is also activated by estradiol. J Clin Endocrinol Metab. 1995;80:3494–500.
250. Bentel JM, Tilley WD. Androgen receptors in prostate cancer. J Endocrinol. 1996;151:1–11.
251. Choong CS, Sturm MJ, Strophair JA, et al. Partial androgen insensitivity caused by an androgen receptor mutation at amino acid 907 (Gly->Arg) that results in decreased ligand binding affinity and reduced androgen receptor messenger ribonucleic acid levels. J Clin Endocrinol Metabol. 1996;81:236–43.
252. Tan J, Sharief Y, Hamil KG, et al. Dehydroepiandrosterone activates mutant androgen receptors expressed in the androgen-dependent human prostate cancer xenograft CWR22 and LNCaP cells. Mol Endocrinol. 1997;11:450–9.
253. Craft N, Shostak Y, Carey M, Sawyers CL. A mechanism for hormone-independent prostate cancer through modulation of androgen receptor signaling by the HER-2/neu tyrosine kinase. Nat Med. 1999;5:280–5.
254. Yeh S, Lin HK, Kang HY, Thin TH, Lin MF, Chang C. From HER2/Neu signal cascade to androgen receptor and its coactivators: a novel pathway by induction of androgen target genes through MAP kinase in prostate cancer cells. Proc Natl Acad Sci U S A. 1999;96:5458–63.
255. Lu J, Danielsen M. Differential regulation of androgen and glucocorticoid receptors by retinoblastoma protein. J Biol Chem. 1998;273:31528–33.
256. Koivisto PA, Rantala I. Amplification of the androgen receptor gene is associated with P53 mutation in hormone-refractory recurrent prostate cancer. J Pathol. 1999;187:237–41.
257. Jiang Z, Iczkowski KA, Woda BA, Tretiakova M, Yang XJ. P504S immunostaining boosts diagnostic resolution of "suspicious" foci in prostatic needle biopsy specimens. Am J Clin Pathol. 2004;121:99–107.
258. Lee SO, Lou W, Hou M, Onate SA, Gao AC. Interleukin-4 enhances prostate-specific antigen expression by activation of the androgen receptor and Akt pathway. Oncogene. 2003;22:7981–8.
259. Bernard D, Pourtier-Manzanedo A, Gil J, Beach DH. Myc confers androgen-independent prostate cancer cell growth. J Clin Invest. 2003;112:1724–31.
260. Jenster G. The role of the androgen receptor in the development and progression of prostate cancer. Semin Oncol. 1999;26:407–21.
261. Bonkhoff H, Stein U, Aumuller G, Remberger K. Differential expression of 5 alpha-reductase isoenzymes in the human prostate and prostatic carcinomas. Prostate. 1996;29:261–7.
262. Petrovics G, Liu A, Shaheduzzaman S, et al. Frequent overexpression of ETS-related gene-1 (ERG1) in prostate cancer transcriptome. Oncogene. 2005;24:3847–52.
263. Perner S, Demichelis F, Beroukhim R, et al. TMPRSS2:ERG fusion-associated deletions provide insight into the heterogeneity of prostate cancer. Cancer Res. 2006;66:8337–41.
264. Furusato B, Gao CL, Ravindranath L, et al. Mapping of TMPRSS2-ERG fusions in the context of multi-focal prostate cancer. Mod Pathol. 2008;21:67–75.
265. Mosquera JM, Perner S, Genega EM, et al. Characterization of TMPRSS2-ERG fusion high-grade prostatic intraepithelial neoplasia and potential clinical implications. Clin Cancer Res. 2008;14:3380–5.
266. Perner S, Mosquera JM, Demichelis F, et al. TMPRSS2-ERG fusion prostate cancer: an early molecular event associated with invasion. Am J Surg Pathol. 2007;31:882–8.
267. Tomlins SA, Mehra R, Rhodes DR, et al. TMPRSS2:ETV4 gene fusions define a third molecular subtype of prostate cancer. Cancer Res. 2006;66:3396–400.
268. Tomlins SA, Laxman B, Dhanasekaran SM, et al. Distinct classes of chromosomal rearrangements create oncogenic ETS gene fusions in prostate cancer. Nature. 2007;448:595–9.

269. Wang J, Cai Y, Yu W, Ren C, Spencer DM, Ittmann M. Pleiotropic biological activities of alternatively spliced TMPRSS2/ERG fusion gene transcripts. Cancer Res. 2008;68: 8516–24.
270. Tomlins SA, Rhodes DR, Perner S, et al. Recurrent fusion of TMPRSS2 and ETS transcription factor genes in prostate cancer. Science. 2005;310:644–8.
271. FitzGerald LM, Agalliu I, Johnson K, et al. Association of TMPRSS2-ERG gene fusion with clinical characteristics and outcomes: results from a population-based study of prostate cancer. BMC Cancer. 2008;8:230.
272. Wang J, Cai Y, Ren C, Ittmann M. Expression of variant TMPRSS2/ERG fusion messenger RNAs is associated with aggressive prostate cancer. Cancer Res. 2006;66:8347–51.
273. Nam RK, Sugar L, Yang W, et al. Expression of the TMPRSS2:ERG fusion gene predicts cancer recurrence after surgery for localised prostate cancer. Br J Cancer. 2007;97:1690–5.
274. Demichelis F, Fall K, Perner S, et al. TMPRSS2:ERG gene fusion associated with lethal prostate cancer in a watchful waiting cohort. Oncogene. 2007;26:4596–9.
275. Saramaki OR, Harjula AE, Martikainen PM, Vessella RL, Tammela TL, Visakorpi T. TMPRSS2:ERG fusion identifies a subgroup of prostate cancers with a favorable prognosis. Clin Cancer Res. 2008;14:3395–400.
276. Yoshimoto M, Joshua AM, Cunha IW, et al. Absence of TMPRSS2:ERG fusions and PTEN losses in prostate cancer is associated with a favorable outcome. Mod Pathol. 2008;21: 1451–60.
277. Gopalan A, Leversha MA, Satagopan JM, et al. TMPRSS2-ERG gene fusion is not associated with outcome in patients treated by prostatectomy. Cancer Res. 2009;69:1400–6.
278. Leinonen KA, Tolonen TT, Bracken H, et al. Association of SPINK1 expression and TMPRSS2:ERG fusion with prognosis in endocrine-treated prostate cancer. Clin Cancer Res. 2010;16:2845–51.
279. Mehra R, Tomlins SA, Yu J, et al. Characterization of TMPRSS2-ETS gene aberrations in androgen-independent metastatic prostate cancer. Cancer Res. 2008;68:3584–90.
280. Hofer MD, Kuefer R, Maier C, et al. Genome-wide linkage analysis of TMPRSS2-ERG fusion in familial prostate cancer. Cancer Res. 2009;69:640–6.
281. Mosquera JM, Mehra R, Regan MM, et al. Prevalence of TMPRSS2-ERG fusion prostate cancer among men undergoing prostate biopsy in the United States. Clin Cancer Res. 2009;15:4706–11.
282. Magi-Galluzzi C, Tsusuki T, Elson P, et al. TMPRSS2-ERG gene fusion prevalence and class are significantly different in prostate cancer of Caucasian, African-American and Japanese patients. Prostate. 2011;71(5):489–97.
283. Clark JP, Munson KW, Gu JW, et al. Performance of a single assay for both type III and type VI TMPRSS2:ERG fusions in noninvasive prediction of prostate biopsy outcome. Clin Chem. 2008;54:2007–17.
284. Rice KR, Chen Y, Ali A, et al. Evaluation of the ETS-related gene mRNA in urine for the detection of prostate cancer. Clin Cancer Res. 2010;16:1572–6.
285. Myers RB, Srivastava S, Oelschlager DK, Grizzle WE. Expression of p160erbB-3 and p185erbB-2 in prostatic intraepithelial neoplasia and prostatic adenocarcinoma. J Natl Cancer Inst. 1994;86:1140–5.
286. Myers RB, Brown D, Oelschlager DK, et al. Elevated serum levels of p105(erbB-2) in patients with advanced-stage prostatic adenocarcinoma. Int J Cancer. 1996;69:398–402.
287. Scher HI, Sarkis A, Reuter V, et al. Changing pattern of expression of the epidermal growth factor receptor and transforming growth factor alpha in the progression of prostatic neoplasms. Clin Cancer Res. 1995;1:545–50.
288. Ye D, Mendelsohn J, Fan Z. Androgen and epidermal growth factor down-regulate cyclin-dependent kinase inhibitor p27Kip1 and costimulate proliferation of MDA PCa 2a and MDA PCa 2b prostate cancer cells. Clin Cancer Res. 1999;5:2171–7.
289. Schlomm T, Kirstein P, Iwers L, et al. Clinical significance of epidermal growth factor receptor protein overexpression and gene copy number gains in prostate cancer. Clin Cancer Res. 2007;13:6579–84.

290. Ross JS, Nazeer T, Church K, et al. Contribution of HER-2/neu oncogene expression to tumor grade and DNA content analysis in the prediction of prostatic carcinoma metastasis. Cancer. 1993;72:3020–8.
291. Kuhn EJ, Kurnot RA, Sesterhenn IA, Chang EH, Moul JW. Expression of the c-erbB-2 (HER-2/neu) oncoprotein in human prostatic carcinoma. J Urol. 1993;150:1427–33.
292. Fox SB, Persad RA, Coleman N, Day CA, Silcocks PB, Collins CC. Prognostic value of c-erbB-2 and epidermal growth factor receptor in stage A1 (T1a) prostatic adenocarcinoma. Br J Urol. 1994;74:214–20.
293. Kallakury BV, Sheehan CE, Ambros RA, et al. Correlation of p34cdc2 cyclin-dependent kinase overexpression, CD44s downregulation, and HER-2/neu oncogene amplification with recurrence in prostatic adenocarcinomas. J Clin Oncol. 1998;16:1302–9.
294. Visakorpi T. New pieces to the prostate puzzle. Nat Med. 1999;5:264–5.
295. Mark HF, Feldman D, Das S, et al. Fluorescence in situ hybridization study of HER-2/neu oncogene amplification in prostate cancer. Exp Mol Pathol. 1999;66:170–8.
296. Morote J, de Torres I, Caceres C, Vallejo C, Schwartz Jr S, Reventos J. Prognostic value of immunohistochemical expression of the c-erbB-2 oncoprotein in metastasic prostate cancer. Int J Cancer. 1999;84:421–5.
297. Lara Jr PN, Chee KG, Longmate J, et al. Trastuzumab plus docetaxel in HER-2/neu-positive prostate carcinoma: final results from the California Cancer Consortium Screening and Phase II Trial. Cancer. 2004;100:2125–31.
298. Visakorpi T, Kallioniemi OP, Koivula T, Harvey J, Isola J. Expression of epidermal growth factor receptor and ERBB2 (HER-2/Neu) oncoprotein in prostatic carcinomas. Mod Pathol. 1992;5:643–8.
299. Mellon K, Thompson S, Charlton RG, et al. p53, c-erbB-2 and the epidermal growth factor receptor in the benign and malignant prostate. J Urol. 1992;147:496–9.
300. Robinson D, He F, Pretlow T, Kung HJ. A tyrosine kinase profile of prostate carcinoma. Proc Natl Acad Sci U S A. 1996;93:5958–62.
301. Lu X, Park SH, Thompson TC, Lane DP. Ras-induced hyperplasia occurs with mutation of p53, but activated ras and myc together can induce carcinoma without p53 mutation. Cell. 1992;70:153–61.
302. Thompson TC, Park SH, Timme TL, et al. Loss of p53 function leads to metastasis in ras+myc-initiated mouse prostate cancer. Oncogene. 1995;10:869–79.
303. Fan K. Heterogeneous subpopulations of human prostatic adenocarcinoma cells: potential usefulness of P21 protein as a predictor for bone metastasis. J Urol. 1988;139:318–22.
304. Peehl DM, Wehner N, Stamey TA. Activated Ki-ras oncogene in human prostatic adenocarcinoma. Prostate. 1987;10:281–9.
305. Moul JW, Friedrichs PA, Lance RS, Theune SM, Chang EH. Infrequent RAS oncogene mutations in human prostate cancer. Prostate. 1992;20:327–38.
306. Watanabe M, Shiraishi T, Yatani R, Nomura AM, Stemmermann GN. International comparison on ras gene mutations in latent prostate carcinoma. Int J Cancer. 1994;58:174–8.
307. Bushman EC, Nayak RN, Bushman W. Immunohistochemical staining of ras p21: staining in benign and malignant prostate tissue. J Urol. 1995;153:233–7.
308. Konishi N, Hiasa Y, Tsuzuki T, Tao M, Enomoto T, Miller GJ. Comparison of ras activation in prostate carcinoma in Japanese and American men. Prostate. 1997;30:53–7.
309. Shiraishi T, Muneyuki T, Fukutome K, et al. Mutations of ras genes are relatively frequent in Japanese prostate cancers: pointing to genetic differences between populations. Anticancer Res. 1998;18:2789–92.
310. Palanisamy N, Ateeq B, Kalyana-Sundaram S, et al. Rearrangements of the RAF kinase pathway in prostate cancer, gastric cancer and melanoma. Nat Med. 2010;16:793–8.
311. Ramaswamy S, Nakamura N, Vazquez F, et al. Regulation of G1 progression by the PTEN tumor suppressor protein is linked to inhibition of the phosphatidylinositol 3-kinase/Akt pathway. Proc Natl Acad Sci U S A. 1999;96:2110–5.
312. Graff JR, Konicek BW, McNulty AM, et al. Increased AKT activity contributes to prostate cancer progression by dramatically accelerating prostate tumor growth and diminishing p27Kip1 expression. J Biol Chem. 2000;275:24500–5.

313. Liang J, Zubovitz J, Petrocelli T, et al. PKB/Akt phosphorylates p27, impairs nuclear import of p27 and opposes p27-mediated G1 arrest. Nat Med. 2002;8:1153–60.
314. Radu A, Neubauer V, Akagi T, Hanafusa H, Georgescu MM. PTEN induces cell cycle arrest by decreasing the level and nuclear localization of cyclin D1. Mol Cell Biol. 2003;23:6139–49.
315. Tolcher AW. Novel therapeutic molecular targets for prostate cancer: the mTOR signaling pathway and epidermal growth factor receptor. J Urol. 2004;171:S41–3. discussion S4.
316. Majumder PK, Yeh JJ, George DJ, et al. Prostate intraepithelial neoplasia induced by prostate restricted Akt activation: the MPAKT model. Proc Natl Acad Sci U S A. 2003;100:7841–6.
317. Wang S, Gao J, Lei Q, et al. Prostate-specific deletion of the murine Pten tumor suppressor gene leads to metastatic prostate cancer. Cancer Cell. 2003;4:209–21.
318. Li J, Yen C, Liaw D, et al. PTEN, a putative protein tyrosine phosphatase gene mutated in human brain, breast, and prostate cancer. Science. 1997;275:1943–7.
319. Cairns P, Okami K, Halachmi S, et al. Frequent inactivation of PTEN/MMAC1 in primary prostate cancer. Cancer Res. 1997;57:4997–5000.
320. Whang YE, Wu X, Suzuki H, et al. Inactivation of the tumor suppressor PTEN/MMAC1 in advanced human prostate cancer through loss of expression. Proc Natl Acad Sci U S A. 1998;95:5246–50.
321. Wu X, Senechal K, Neshat MS, Whang YE, Sawyers CL. The PTEN/MMAC1 tumor suppressor phosphatase functions as a negative regulator of the phosphoinositide 3-kinase/Akt pathway. Proc Natl Acad Sci U S A. 1998;95:15587–91.
322. McMenamin ME, Soung P, Perera S, Kaplan I, Loda M, Sellers WR. Loss of PTEN expression in paraffin-embedded primary prostate cancer correlates with high Gleason score and advanced stage. Cancer Res. 1999;59:4291–6.
323. Huang H, Cheville JC, Pan Y, Roche PC, Schmidt LJ, Tindall DJ. PTEN induces chemosensitivity in pten-mutated prostate cancer cells by suppression of bcl-2 expression. J Biol Chem. 2001;276:38830–6.
324. Nan B, Snabboon T, Unni E, Yuan XJ, Whang YE, Marcelli M. The PTEN tumor suppressor is a negative modulator of androgen receptor transcriptional activity. J Mol Endocrinol. 2003;31:169–83.
325. Edwards J, Krishna NS, Witton CJ, Bartlett JM. Gene amplifications associated with the development of hormone-resistant prostate cancer. Clin Cancer Res. 2003;9:5271–81.
326. Halvorsen OJ, Haukaas SA, Akslen LA. Combined loss of PTEN and p27 expression is associated with tumor cell proliferation by Ki-67 and increased risk of recurrent disease in localized prostate cancer. Clin Cancer Res. 2003;9:1474–9.
327. Yoshimoto M, Cunha IW, Coudry RA, et al. FISH analysis of 107 prostate cancers shows that PTEN genomic deletion is associated with poor clinical outcome. Br J Cancer. 2007;97:678–85.
328. Bedolla R, Prihoda TJ, Kreisberg JI, et al. Determining risk of biochemical recurrence in prostate cancer by immunohistochemical detection of PTEN expression and Akt activation. Clin Cancer Res. 2007;13:3860–7.
329. Liao Y, Grobholz R, Abel U, et al. Increase of AKT/PKB expression correlates with gleason pattern in human prostate cancer. Int J Cancer. 2003;107:676–80.
330. Malik SN, Brattain M, Ghosh PM, et al. Immunohistochemical demonstration of phospho-Akt in high Gleason grade prostate cancer. Clin Cancer Res. 2002;8:1168–71.
331. Takeichi M. Cadherin cell adhesion receptors as a morphogenetic regulator. Science. 1991;251:1451–5.
332. Steinberg MS, Takeichi M. Experimental specification of cell sorting, tissue spreading, and specific spatial patterning by quantitative differences in cadherin expression. Proc Natl Acad Sci U S A. 1994;91:206–9.
333. Shimoyama Y, Nagafuchi A, Fujita S, et al. Cadherin dysfunction in a human cancer cell line: possible involvement of loss of alpha-catenin expression in reduced cell-cell adhesiveness. Cancer Res. 1992;52:5770–4.

334. Hirano S, Kimoto N, Shimoyama Y, Hirohashi S, Takeichi M. Identification of a neural alpha-catenin as a key regulator of cadherin function and multicellular organization. Cell. 1992;70:293–301.
335. Umbas R, Schalken JA, Aalders TW, et al. Expression of the cellular adhesion molecule E-cadherin is reduced or absent in high-grade prostate cancer. Cancer Res. 1992;52:5104–9.
336. Richmond PJ, Karayiannakis AJ, Nagafuchi A, Kaisary AV, Pignatelli M. Aberrant E-cadherin and alpha-catenin expression in prostate cancer: correlation with patient survival. Cancer Res. 1997;57:3189–93.
337. Aaltomaa S, Lipponen P, Ala-Opas M, Eskelinen M, Kosma VM. Alpha-catenin expression has prognostic value in local and locally advanced prostate cancer. Br J Cancer. 1999;80:477–82.
338. Umbas R, Isaacs WB, Bringuier PP, Xue Y, Debruyne FM, Schalken JA. Relation between aberrant alpha-catenin expression and loss of E-cadherin function in prostate cancer. Int J Cancer. 1997;74:374–7.
339. Cheng L, Nagabhushan M, Pretlow TP, Amini SB, Pretlow TG. Expression of E-cadherin in primary and metastatic prostate cancer. Am J Pathol. 1996;148:1375–80.
340. Tomita K, van Bokhoven A, van Leenders GJ, et al. Cadherin switching in human prostate cancer progression. Cancer Res. 2000;60:3650–4.
341. Bussemakers MJ, Van Bokhoven A, Tomita K, Jansen CF, Schalken JA. Complex cadherin expression in human prostate cancer cells. Int J Cancer. 2000;85:446–50.
342. De Marzo AM, Knudsen B, Chan-Tack K, Epstein JI. E-cadherin expression as a marker of tumor aggressiveness in routinely processed radical prostatectomy specimens. Urology. 1999;53:707–13.
343. Bryden AA, Freemont AJ, Clarke NW, George NJ. Paradoxical expression of E-cadherin in prostatic bone metastases. BJU Int. 1999;84:1032–4.
344. Bukholm IK, Nesland JM, Borresen-Dale AL. Re-expression of E-cadherin, alpha-catenin and beta-catenin, but not of gamma-catenin, in metastatic tissue from breast cancer patients. J Pathol. 2000;190:15–9.
345. Kuniyasu H, Ukai R, Johnston D, Troncoso P, Fidler IJ, Pettaway CA. The relative mRNA expression levels of matrix metalloproteinase to E-cadherin in prostate biopsy specimens distinguishes organ-confined from advanced prostate cancer at radical prostatectomy. Clin Cancer Res. 2003;9:2185–94.
346. Kuefer R, Hofer MD, Gschwend JE, et al. The role of an 80 kDa fragment of E-cadherin in the metastatic progression of prostate cancer. Clin Cancer Res. 2003;9:6447–52.
347. Rashid MG, Sanda MG, Vallorosi CJ, Rios-Doria J, Rubin MA, Day ML. Posttranslational truncation and inactivation of human E-cadherin distinguishes prostate cancer from matched normal prostate. Cancer Res. 2001;61:489–92.
348. Sasaki CY, Lin H, Morin PJ, Longo DL. Truncation of the extracellular region abrogrates cell contact but retains the growth-suppressive activity of E-cadherin. Cancer Res. 2000;60:7057–65.
349. Rios-Doria J, Day KC, Kuefer R, et al. The role of calpain in the proteolytic cleavage of E-cadherin in prostate and mammary epithelial cells. J Biol Chem. 2003;278:1372–9.
350. Rhodes DR, Sanda MG, Otte AP, Chinnaiyan AM, Rubin MA. Multiplex biomarker approach for determining risk of prostate-specific antigen-defined recurrence of prostate cancer. J Natl Cancer Inst. 2003;95:661–8.
351. Ruijter E, van de Kaa C, Aalders T, et al. Heterogeneous expression of E-cadherin and p53 in prostate cancer: clinical implications. BIOMED-II Markers for Prostate Cancer Study Group. Mod Pathol. 1998;11:276–81.
352. Brewster SF, Oxley JD, Trivella M, Abbott CD, Gillatt DA. Preoperative p53, bcl-2, CD44 and E-cadherin immunohistochemistry as predictors of biochemical relapse after radical prostatectomy. J Urol. 1999;161:1238–43.
353. Gravdal K, Halvorsen OJ, Haukaas SA, Akslen LA. A switch from E-cadherin to N-cadherin expression indicates epithelial to mesenchymal transition and is of strong and independent importance for the progress of prostate cancer. Clin Cancer Res. 2007;13:7003–11.

354. Nusse R, Varmus HE. Wnt genes. Cell. 1992;69:1073–87.
355. Logan CY, Nusse R. The Wnt signaling pathway in development and disease. Annu Rev Cell Dev Biol. 2004;20:781–810.
356. Miller JR. The Wnts. Genome Biol. 2002;3:reviews 3001.
357. Iozzo RV, Eichstetter I, Danielson KG. Aberrant expression of the growth factor Wnt-5A in human malignancy. Cancer Res. 1995;55:3495–9.
358. Wissmann C, Wild PJ, Kaiser S, et al. WIF1, a component of the Wnt pathway, is down-regulated in prostate, breast, lung, and bladder cancer. J Pathol. 2003;201:204–12.
359. Sagara N, Toda G, Hirai M, Terada M, Katoh M. Molecular cloning, differential expression, and chromosomal localization of human frizzled-1, frizzled-2, and frizzled-7. Biochem Biophys Res Commun. 1998;252:117–22.
360. Chesire DR, Ewing CM, Gage WR, Isaacs WB. In vitro evidence for complex modes of nuclear beta-catenin signaling during prostate growth and tumorigenesis. Oncogene. 2002;21:2679–94.
361. de la Taille A, Rubin MA, Chen MW, et al. Beta-catenin-related anomalies in apoptosis-resistant and hormone-refractory prostate cancer cells. Clin Cancer Res. 2003;9:1801–7.
362. Chen G, Shukeir N, Potti A, et al. Up-regulation of Wnt-1 and beta-catenin production in patients with advanced metastatic prostate carcinoma: potential pathogenetic and prognostic implications. Cancer. 2004;101:1345–56.
363. Horvath LG, Henshall SM, Lee CS, et al. Lower levels of nuclear beta-catenin predict for a poorer prognosis in localized prostate cancer. Int J Cancer. 2005;113(3):415–22.
364. Horvath LG, Henshall SM, Kench JG, et al. Membranous expression of secreted frizzled-related protein 4 predicts for good prognosis in localized prostate cancer and inhibits PC3 cellular proliferation in vitro. Clin Cancer Res. 2004;10:615–25.
365. Mulholland DJ, Read JT, Rennie PS, Cox ME, Nelson CC. Functional localization and competition between the androgen receptor and T-cell factor for nuclear beta-catenin: a means for inhibition of the Tcf signaling axis. Oncogene. 2003;22:5602–13.
366. Damalas A, Ben-Ze'ev A, Simcha I, et al. Excess beta-catenin promotes accumulation of transcriptionally active p53. EMBO J. 1999;18:3054–63.
367. Sasaki T, Suzuki H, Yagi K, et al. Lymphoid enhancer factor 1 makes cells resistant to transforming growth factor beta-induced repression of c-myc. Cancer Res. 2003;63:801–6.
368. Ricciardelli C, Quinn DI, Raymond WA, et al. Elevated levels of peritumoral chondroitin sulfate are predictive of poor prognosis in patients treated by radical prostatectomy for early-stage prostate cancer. Cancer Res. 1999;59:2324–8232.
369. Ricciardelli C, Mayne K, Sykes PJ, et al. Elevated levels of versican but not decorin predict disease progression in early-stage prostate cancer. Clin Cancer Res. 1998;4:963–71.
370. Ricciardelli C, Mayne K, Sykes PJ, et al. Elevated stromal chondroitin sulfate glycoaminoglycan predicts progression in early stage prostate cancer. Clin Cancer Res. 1997;3:983–92.
371. Nelson PS, Plymate SR, Wang K, et al. Hevin, an antiadhesive extracellular matrix protein, is down-regulated in metastatic prostate adenocarcinoma. Cancer Res. 1998;58:232–6.
372. Noordzij MA, van Steenbrugge GJ, Schroder FH, Van der Kwast TH. Decreased expression of CD44 in metastatic prostate cancer. Int J Cancer. 1999;84:478–83.
373. Jackson MW, Bentel JM, Tilley WD. Vascular endothelial growth factor (VEGF) expression in prostate cancer and benign prostatic hyperplasia. J Urol. 1997;157:2323–8.
374. Silberman MA, Partin AW, Veltri RW, Epstein JI. Tumor angiogenesis correlates with progression after radical prostatectomy but not with pathologic stage in Gleason sum 5 to 7 adenocarcinoma of the prostate. Cancer. 1997;79:772–9.
375. Weidner N, Carroll PR, Flax J, Blumenfeld W, Folkman J. Tumor angiogenesis correlates with metastasis in invasive prostate carcinoma. Am J Pathol. 1993;143:401–9.
376. Borre M, Offersen BV, Nerstrom B, Overgaard J. Microvessel density predicts survival in prostate cancer patients subjected to watchful waiting. Br J Cancer. 1998;78:940–4.
377. Borre M, Nerstrom B, Overgaard J. Association between immunohistochemical expression of vascular endothelial growth factor (VEGF), VEGF-expressing neuroendocrine-differentiated tumor cells, and outcome in prostate cancer patients subjected to watchful waiting. Clin Cancer Res. 2000;6:1882–90.

378. Strohmeyer D, Rossing C, Bauerfeind A, et al. Vascular endothelial growth factor and its correlation with angiogenesis and p53 expression in prostate cancer. Prostate. 2000; 45:216–24.
379. Fernandez A, Udagawa T, Schwesinger C, et al. Angiogenic potential of prostate carcinoma cells overexpressing bcl-2. J Natl Cancer Inst. 2001;93:208–13.
380. Ferrer FA, Miller LJ, Andrawis RI, et al. Angiogenesis and prostate cancer: in vivo and in vitro expression of angiogenesis factors by prostate cancer cells. Urology. 1998;51:161–7.
381. Mabjeesh NJ, Willard MT, Frederickson CE, Zhong H, Simons JW. Androgens stimulate hypoxia-inducible factor 1 activation via autocrine loop of tyrosine kinase receptor/phosphatidylinositol 3′-kinase/protein kinase B in prostate cancer cells. Clin Cancer Res. 2003;9:2416–25.
382. Kuniyasu H, Troncoso P, Johnston D, et al. Relative expression of type IV collagenae, E-cadherin, and vascular endothelial growth factor/vascular permeability factor in prostatectomy specimens distinguishes organ-confined from pathologically advanced prostate cancers. Clin Cancer Res. 2000;6:2295–308.
383. Kim KJ, Li B, Winer J, et al. Inhibition of vascular endothelial growth factor-induced angiogenesis suppresses tumour growth in vivo. Nature. 1993;362:841–4.
384. Joseph IB, Nelson JB, Denmeade SR, Isaacs JT. Androgens regulate vascular endothelial growth factor content in normal and malignant prostatic tissue. Clin Cancer Res. 1997; 3:2507–11.
385. Stewart RJ, Panigrahy D, Flynn E, Folkman J. Vascular endothelial growth factor expression and tumor angiogenesis are regulated by androgens in hormone responsive human prostate carcinoma: evidence for androgen dependent destabilization of vascular endothelial growth factor transcripts. J Urol. 2001;165:688–93.
386. Sordello S, Bertrand N, Plouet J. Vascular endothelial growth factor is up-regulated in vitro and in vivo by androgens. Biochem Biophys Res Commun. 1998;251:287–90.
387. Miao HQ, Lee P, Lin H, Soker S, Klagsbrun M. Neuropilin-1 expression by tumor cells promotes tumor angiogenesis and progression. FASEB J. 2000;14:2532–9.
388. Richard C, Kim G, Koikawa Y, et al. Androgens modulate the balance between VEGF and angiopoietin expression in prostate epithelial and smooth muscle cells. Prostate. 2002; 50:83–91.
389. Gagnon ML, Bielenberg DR, Gechtman Z, et al. Identification of a natural soluble neuropilin-1 that binds vascular endothelial growth factor: in vivo expression and antitumor activity. Proc Natl Acad Sci U S A. 2000;97:2573–8.
390. Ruiz M, Pettaway C, Song R, Stoeltzing O, Ellis L, Bar-Eli M. Activator protein 2a inhibits tumorigenicity and represses vascular endothelial growth factor transcription in prostate cancer cells. Cancer Res. 2004;64:631–8.
391. Levine L, Lucci 3rd JA, Pazdrak B, et al. Bombesin stimulates nuclear factor kappa B activation and expression of proangiogenic factors in prostate cancer cells. Cancer Res. 2003;63:3495–502.
392. Ferrer FA, Miller LJ, Andrawis RI, et al. Vascular endothelial growth factor (VEGF) expression in human prostate cancer: in situ and in vitro expression of VEGF by human prostate cancer cells. J Urol. 1997;157:2329–33.
393. Mazzucchelli R, Montironi R, Santinelli A, Lucarini G, Pugnaloni A, Biagini G. Vascular endothelial growth factor expression and capillary architecture in high-grade PIN and prostate cancer in untreated and androgen-ablated patients. Prostate. 2000;45:72–9.
394. Chevalier S, Defoy I, Lacoste J, et al. Vascular endothelial growth factor and signaling in the prostate: more than angiogenesis. Mol Cell Endocrinol. 2002;189:169–79.
395. Harper ME, Glynne-Jones E, Goddard L, Thurston VJ, Griffiths K. Vascular endothelial growth factor (VEGF) expression in prostatic tumours and its relationship to neuroendocrine cells. Br J Cancer. 1996;74:910–6.
396. Ismail AH, Altaweel W, Chevalier S, Kassouf W, Aprikian AG. Expression of vascular endothelial growth factor-A in human lymph node metastases of prostate cancer. Can J Urol. 2004;11:2146–50.

397. George DJ, Halabi S, Shepard TF, et al. Prognostic significance of plasma vascular endothelial growth factor levels in patients with hormone-refractory prostate cancer treated on Cancer and Leukemia Group B 9480. Clin Cancer Res. 2001;7:1932–6.
398. Small EJ, Meyer M, Marshall ME, et al. Suramin therapy for patients with symptomatic hormone-refractory prostate cancer: results of a randomized phase III trial comparing suramin plus hydrocortisone to placebo plus hydrocortisone. J Clin Oncol. 2000;18:1440–50.
399. Chan LW, Moses MA, Goley E, et al. Urinary VEGF and MMP levels as predictive markers of 1-year progression-free survival in cancer patients treated with radiation therapy: a longitudinal study of protein kinetics throughout tumor progression and therapy. J Clin Oncol. 2004;22:499–506.
400. Shariat SF, Anwuri VA, Lamb DJ, Shah NV, Wheeler TM, Slawin KM. Association of preoperative plasma levels of vascular endothelial growth factor and soluble vascular cell adhesion molecule-1 with lymph node status and biochemical progression after radical prostatectomy. J Clin Oncol. 2004;22:1655–16563.
401. George DJ, Regan MM, Oh WK, et al. Radical prostatectomy lowers plasma vascular endothelial growth factor levels in patients with prostate cancer. Urology. 2004;63:327–32.
402. Kohli M, Kaushal V, Spencer HJ, Mehta P. Prospective study of circulating angiogenic markers in prostate-specific antigen (PSA)-stable and PSA-progressive hormone-sensitive advanced prostate cancer. Urology. 2003;61:765–9.
403. Figg WD, Kruger EA, Price DK, Kim S, Dahut WD. Inhibition of angiogenesis: treatment options for patients with metastatic prostate cancer. Invest New Drugs. 2002;20:183–94.
404. Ferrara N. Vascular endothelial growth factor: basic science and clinical progress. Endocr Rev. 2004;25:581–611.
405. Rinaldo F, Li J, Wang E, Muders M, Datta K. RalA regulates vascular endothelial growth factor-C (VEGF-C) synthesis in prostate cancer cells during androgen ablation. Oncogene. 2007;26:1731–8.
406. Gravdal K, Halvorsen OJ, Haukaas SA, Akslen LA. Proliferation of immature tumor vessels is a novel marker of clinical progression in prostate cancer. Cancer Res. 2009;69:4708–15.
407. Kollermann J, Helpap B. Expression of vascular endothelial growth factor (VEGF) and VEGF receptor Flk-1 in benign, premalignant, and malignant prostate tissue. Am J Clin Pathol. 2001;116:115–21.
408. Kearney JB, Kappas NC, Ellerstrom C, DiPaola FW, Bautch VL. The VEGF receptor flt-1 (VEGFR-1) is a positive modulator of vascular sprout formation and branching morphogenesis. Blood. 2004;103:4527–35.
409. Elkin M, Orgel A, Kleinman HK. An angiogenic switch in breast cancer involves estrogen and soluble vascular endothelial growth factor receptor 1. J Natl Cancer Inst. 2004; 96:875–8.
410. Shimizu K, Kubo H, Yamaguchi K, et al. Suppression of VEGFR-3 signaling inhibits lymph node metastasis in gastric cancer. Cancer Sci. 2004;95:328–33.
411. Jackson MW, Roberts JS, Heckford SE, et al. A potential autocrine role for vascular endothelial growth factor in prostate cancer. Cancer Res. 2002;62:854–9.
412. Sweeney P, Karashima T, Kim SJ, et al. Anti-vascular endothelial growth factor receptor 2 antibody reduces tumorigenicity and metastasis in orthotopic prostate cancer xenografts via induction of endothelial cell apoptosis and reduction of endothelial cell matrix metalloproteinase type 9 production. Clin Cancer Res. 2002;8:2714–24.
413. Huss WJ, Hanrahan CF, Barrios RJ, Simons JW, Greenberg NM. Angiogenesis and prostate cancer: identification of a molecular progression switch. Cancer Res. 2001;61:2736–43.
414. Dai J, Kitagawa Y, Zhang J, et al. Vascular endothelial growth factor contributes to the prostate cancer-induced osteoblast differentiation mediated by bone morphogenetic protein. Cancer Res. 2004;64:994–9.
415. Li R, Younes M, Wheeler TM, et al. Expression of vascular endothelial growth factor receptor-3 (VEGFR-3) in human prostate. Prostate. 2004;58:193–9.
416. Zeng Y, Opeskin K, Baldwin ME, et al. Expression of vascular endothelial growth factor receptor-3 by lymphatic endothelial cells is associated with lymph node metastasis in prostate cancer. Clin Cancer Res. 2004;10:5137–44.

417. Sorlie T, Perou CM, Tibshirani R, et al. Gene expression patterns of breast carcinomas distinguish tumor subclasses with clinical implications. Proc Natl Acad Sci U S A. 2001; 98:10869–74.
418. van't Veer LJ, Dai H, van de Vijver MJ, et al. Gene expression profiling predicts clinical outcome of breast cancer. Nature. 2002;415:530–6.
419. van de Vijver MJ, He YD, van't Veer LJ, et al. A gene-expression signature as a predictor of survival in breast cancer. N Engl J Med. 2002;347:1999–2009.
420. Singh D, Febbo PG, Ross K, et al. Gene expression correlates of clinical prostate cancer behavior. Cancer Cell. 2002;1:203–9.
421. Lapointe J, Li C, Higgins JP, et al. Gene expression profiling identifies clinically relevant subtypes of prostate cancer. Proc Natl Acad Sci U S A. 2004;101:811–6.
422. Tomlins SA, Mehra R, Rhodes DR, et al. Integrative molecular concept modeling of prostate cancer progression. Nat Genet. 2007;39:41–51.
423. Kirdani RY, Emrich LJ, Pontes EJ, Priore RL, Murphy GP. A comparison of estrogen and androgen receptor levels in human prostatic tissue from patients with non-metastatic and metastatic carcinoma and benign prostatic hyperplasia. J Steroid Biochem. 1985;22:569–75.
424. Umbas R, Isaacs WB, Bringuier PP, et al. Decreased E-cadherin expression is associated with poor prognosis in patients with prostate cancer. Cancer Res. 1994;54:3929–33.
425. Morita N, Uemura H, Tsumatani K, et al. E-cadherin and alpha-, beta- and gamma-catenin expression in prostate cancers: correlation with tumour invasion. Br J Cancer. 1999;79: 1879–83.
426. Wood M, Fudge K, Mohler JL, et al. In situ hybridization studies of metalloproteinases 2 and 9 and TIMP-1 and TIMP-2 expression in human prostate cancer. Clin Exp Metastasis. 1997;15:246–58.
427. Luo J, Lubaroff DM, Hendrix MJ. Suppression of prostate cancer invasive potential and matrix metalloproteinase activity by E-cadherin transfection. Cancer Res. 1999;59:3552–6.
428. Sanchez-Sweatman OH, Orr FW, Singh G. Human metastatic prostate PC3 cell lines degrade bone using matrix metalloproteinases. Invasion Metastasis. 1998;18:297–305.
429. Ge K, Minhas F, Duhadaway J, et al. Loss of heterozygosity and tumor suppressor activity of Bin1 in prostate carcinoma. Int J Cancer. 2000;86:155–61.
430. Devaney J, Stirzaker C, Qu W, et al. Epigenetic deregulation across 2q14.2 differentiates normal from prostate cancer and provides a regional panel of novel DNA methylation cancer biomarkers. Cancer Epidemiol Biomarkers Prev. 2011;20:148.
431. Cooney KA, Wetzel JC, Consolino CM, Wojno KJ. Identification and characterization of proximal 6q deletions in prostate cancer. Cancer Res. 1996;56:4150–3.
432. Alers JC, Krijtenburg PJ, Vissers KJ, Bosman FT, van der Kwast TH, van Dekken H. Interphase cytogenetics of prostatic adenocarcinoma and precursor lesions: analysis of 25 radical prostatectomies and 17 adjacent prostatic intraepithelial neoplasias. Genes Chromosomes Cancer. 1995;12:241–50.
433. Trapman J, Sleddens HF, van der Weiden MM, et al. Loss of heterozygosity of chromosome 8 microsatellite loci implicates a candidate tumor suppressor gene between the loci D8S87 and D8S133 in human prostate cancer. Cancer Res. 1994;54:6061–4.
434. El Gammal AT, Bruchmann M, Zustin J, et al. Chromosome 8p deletions and 8q gains are associated with tumor progression and poor prognosis in prostate cancer. Clin Cancer Res. 2009;16:56–64.
435. Emmert-Buck MR, Vocke CD, Pozzatti RO, et al. Allelic loss on chromosome 8p12-21 in microdissected prostatic intraepithelial neoplasia. Cancer Res. 1995;55:2959–62.
436. Vocke CD, Pozzatti RO, Bostwick DG, et al. Analysis of 99 microdissected prostate carcinomas reveals a high frequency of allelic loss on chromosome 8p12-21. Cancer Res. 1996;56:2411–6.
437. Bova GS, MacGrogan D, Levy A, Pin SS, Bookstein R, Isaacs WB. Physical mapping of chromosome 8p22 markers and their homozygous deletion in a metastatic prostate cancer. Genomics. 1996;35:46–54.

438. Bova GS, Carter BS, Bussemakers MJ, et al. Homozygous deletion and frequent allelic loss of chromosome 8p22 loci in human prostate cancer. Cancer Res. 1993;53:3869–73.
439. Cabeza-Arvelaiz Y, Thompson TC, Sepulveda JL, Chinault AC. LAPSER1: a novel candidate tumor suppressor gene from 10q24.3. Oncogene. 2001;20:6707–17.
440. Ishii H, Baffa R, Numata SI, et al. The FEZ1 gene at chromosome 8p22 encodes a leucine-zipper protein, and its expression is altered in multiple human tumors. Proc Natl Acad Sci U S A. 1999;96:3928–33.
441. Barnabas N, Xu L, Savera A, Hou Z, Barrack ER. Chromosome 8 markers of metastatic prostate cancer in African American men: gain of the MIR151 gene and loss of the NKX3-1 gene. Prostate. 2010;71(8):857–71.
442. Lapointe J, Li C, Giacomini CP, et al. Genomic profiling reveals alternative genetic pathways of prostate tumorigenesis. Cancer Res. 2007;67:8504–10.
443. Tsuchiya N, Kondo Y, Takahashi A, et al. Mapping and gene expression profile of the minimally overrepresented 8q24 region in prostate cancer. Am J Pathol. 2002;160:1799–806.
444. Kaltz-Wittmer C, Klenk U, Glaessgen A, et al. FISH analysis of gene aberrations (MYC, CCND1, ERBB2, RB, and AR) in advanced prostatic carcinomas before and after androgen deprivation therapy. Lab Invest. 2000;80:1455–64.
445. Gurel B, Ali TZ, Montgomery EA, et al. NKX3.1 as a marker of prostatic origin in metastatic tumors. Am J Surg Pathol. 2010;34:1097–105.
446. Lin D, Watahiki A, Bayani J, et al. ASAP1, a gene at 8q24, is associated with prostate cancer metastasis. Cancer Res. 2008;68:4352–9.
447. Penney KL, Salinas CA, Pomerantz M, et al. Evaluation of 8q24 and 17q risk loci and prostate cancer mortality. Clin Cancer Res. 2009;15:3223–30.
448. Perinchery G, Bukurov N, Nakajima K, Chang J, Li LC, Dahiya R. High frequency of deletion on chromosome 9p21 may harbor several tumor- suppressor genes in human prostate cancer. Int J Cancer. 1999;83:610–4.
449. Narla G, Heath KE, Reeves HL, et al. KLF6, a candidate tumor suppressor gene mutated in prostate cancer. Science. 2001;294:2563–6.
450. Fukuhara H, Maruyama T, Nomura S, et al. Functional evidence for the presence of tumor suppressor gene on chromosome 10p15 in human prostate cancers. Oncogene. 2001;20:314–9.
451. Carter BS, Ewing CM, Ward WS, et al. Allelic loss of chromosomes 16q and 10q in human prostate cancer. Proc Natl Acad Sci U S A. 1990;87:8751–5.
452. Matsuyama H, Pan Y, Yoshihiro S, et al. Clinical significance of chromosome 8p, 10q, and 16q deletions in prostate cancer. Prostate. 2003;54:103–11.
453. Srivastava M, Bubendorf L, Srikantan V, et al. ANX7, a candidate tumor suppressor gene for prostate cancer. Proc Natl Acad Sci U S A. 2001;98:4575–80.
454. Feilotter HE, Nagai MA, Boag AH, Eng C, Mulligan LM. Analysis of PTEN and the 10q23 region in primary prostate carcinomas. Oncogene. 1998;16:1743–8.
455. Rubin MA, Gerstein A, Reid K, et al. 10q23.3 loss of heterozygosity is higher in lymph node-positive (pT2–3, N+) versus lymph node-negative (pT2–3, N0) prostate cancer. Hum Pathol. 2000;31:504–8.
456. Latil A, Morant P, Fournier G, Mangin P, Berthon P, Cussenot O. CHC1-L, a candidate gene for prostate carcinogenesis at 13q14.2, is frequently affected by loss of heterozygosity and underexpressed in human prostate cancer. Int J Cancer. 2002;99:689–96.
457. Cher ML, Ito T, Weidner N, Carroll PR, Jensen RH. Mapping of regions of physical deletion on chromosome 16q in prostate cancer cells by fluorescence in situ hybridization (FISH). J Urol. 1995;153:249–54.
458. Bednarz N, Eltze E, Semjonow A, et al. BRCA1 loss preexisting in small subpopulations of prostate cancer is associated with advanced disease and metastatic spread to lymph nodes and peripheral blood. Clin Cancer Res. 2010;16:3340–8.
459. Lapointe J, Kim YH, Miller MA, et al. A variant TMPRSS2 isoform and ERG fusion product in prostate cancer with implications for molecular diagnosis. Mod Pathol. 2007;20:467–73.

460. Esgueva R, Perner S, J LaFargue C, et al. Prevalence of TMPRSS2-ERG and SLC45A3-ERG gene fusions in a large prostatectomy cohort. Mod Pathol. 2010;23:539–46.
461. Reid AH, Attard G, Ambroisine L, et al. Molecular characterisation of ERG, ETV1 and PTEN gene loci identifies patients at low and high risk of death from prostate cancer. Br J Cancer. 2010;102:678–84.
462. Mehra R, Tomlins SA, Shen R, et al. Comprehensive assessment of TMPRSS2 and ETS family gene aberrations in clinically localized prostate cancer. Mod Pathol. 2007;20:538–44.
463. Attard G, Clark J, Ambroisine L, et al. Heterogeneity and clinical significance of ETV1 translocations in human prostate cancer. Br J Cancer. 2008;99:314–20.
464. Berges RR, Vukanovic J, Epstein JI, et al. Implication of cell kinetic changes during the progression of human prostatic cancer. Clin Cancer Res. 1995;1:473–80.
465. Matsushima H, Goto T, Hosaka Y, Kitamura T, Kawabe K. Correlation between proliferation, apoptosis, and angiogenesis in prostate carcinoma and their relation to androgen ablation. Cancer. 1999;85:1822–7.
466. Westin P, Stattin P, Damber JE, Bergh A. Castration therapy rapidly induces apoptosis in a minority and decreases cell proliferation in a majority of human prostatic tumors. Am J Pathol. 1995;146:1368–75.
467. Theodorescu D, Broder SR, Boyd JC, Mills SE, Frierson Jr HF. p53, bcl-2 and retinoblastoma proteins as long-term prognostic markers in localized carcinoma of the prostate. J Urol. 1997;158:131–7.
468. Aaltomaa S, Lipponen P, Eskelinen M, Ala-Opas M, Kosma VM. Prognostic value and expression of p21(waf1/cip1) protein in prostate cancer. Prostate. 1999;39:8–15.
469. Matsushima H, Sasaki T, Goto T, et al. Immunohistochemical study of p21WAF1 and p53 proteins in prostatic cancer and their prognostic significance. Hum Pathol. 1998;29:778–83.
470. Cheville JC, Lloyd RV, Sebo TJ, et al. Expression of p27kip1 in prostatic adenocarcinoma. Mod Pathol. 1998;11:324–8.
471. Erdamar S, Yang G, Harper JW, et al. Levels of expression of p27KIP1 protein in human prostate and prostate cancer: an immunohistochemical analysis. Mod Pathol. 1999;12:751–5.
472. Freedland SJ, de Gregorio F, Sacoolidge JC, et al. Predicting biochemical recurrence after radical prostatectomy for patients with organ-confined disease using p27 expression. Urology. 2003;61:1187–92.
473. Borre M, Stausbol-Gron B, Nerstrom B, Overgaard J. Immunohistochemical BCL-2 and Ki-67 expression predict survival in prostate cancer patients followed expectantly. Prostate Cancer Prostatic Dis. 1998;1:268–75.
474. Borre M, Nerstrom B, Overgaard J. The natural history of prostate carcinoma based on a Danish population treated with no intent to cure. Cancer. 1997;80:917–28.
475. Stackhouse GB, Sesterhenn IA, Bauer JJ, et al. p53 and bcl-2 immunohistochemistry in pretreatment prostate needle biopsies to predict recurrence of prostate cancer after radical prostatectomy. J Urol. 1999;162:2040–5.
476. Scherr DS, Vaughan Jr ED, Wei J, et al. BCL-2 and p53 expression in clinically localized prostate cancer predicts response to external beam radiotherapy. J Urol. 1999;162:12–6 [published erratum appears in *J Urol* 1999;162(2):503].
477. Kuczyk M, Serth J, Machtens S, et al. Expression of E-cadherin in primary prostate cancer: correlation with clinical features. Br J Urol. 1998;81:406–12.
478. Ross JS, Figge HL, Bui HX, et al. E-cadherin expression in prostatic carcinoma biopsies: correlation with tumor grade, DNA content, pathologic stage, and clinical outcome. Mod Pathol. 1994;7:835–41.
479. Glinsky GV, Glinskii AB, Stephenson AJ, Hoffman RM, Gerald WL. Gene expression profiling predicts clinical outcome of prostate cancer. J Clin Invest. 2004;113:913–23.
480. Henshall SM, Horvath LG, Quinn DI, et al. Zinc-alpha2-glycoprotein expression as a predictor of metastatic prostate cancer following radical prostatectomy. J Natl Cancer Inst. 2006;98:1420–4.

481. Stephenson AJ, Smith A, Kattan MW, et al. Integration of gene expression profiling and clinical variables to predict prostate carcinoma recurrence after radical prostatectomy. Cancer. 2005;104:290–8.
482. Nakagawa T, Kollmeyer TM, Morlan BW, et al. A tissue biomarker panel predicting systemic progression after PSA recurrence post-definitive prostate cancer therapy. PLoS One. 2008;3:e2318.
483. Magee JA, Araki T, Patil S, et al. Expression profiling reveals hepsin overexpression in prostate cancer. Cancer Res. 2001;61:5692–6.
484. Dhanasekaran SM, Barrette TR, Ghosh D, et al. Delineation of prognostic biomarkers in prostate cancer. Nature. 2001;412:822–6.
485. Hofer MD, Kuefer R, Varambally S, et al. The role of metastasis-associated protein 1 in prostate cancer progression. Cancer Res. 2004;64:825–9.

180. Stephenson AJ, Smith A, Kattan MW, et al. Integration of gene expression profiling and [illegible]

[illegible]

Chapter 10
Prediction of Chemotherapy Toxicities

Pierre Laurent-Puig, Thierry Lecomte, Marie-Anne Loriot, Valerie Boige, and Helene Blons

Introduction

Predicting responses to a medicinal product (therapeutic response or toxic effect) is becoming an increasingly important issue in patient care. The response to drugs varies from one individual to another, and this has important consequences for drug efficacy and drug toxicity [1]. Genetic factors affecting the metabolism and transport of drugs account for some of this interindividual variability; pharmacogenetics is the study of the influence of differences in DNA sequences on the response to drugs (European Medicines Agency, EMEA), and its ultimate goal is to optimize medicinal treatments in terms of efficacy and safety of use. Pharmacogenetics is a rapidly expanding field because it makes possible to predict, inexpensively and using relatively simple tools, the potential efficacy and/or the risk of toxicity of a drug in any particular patient.

Identifying markers that predict responses to chemotherapy is an important challenge in oncology [2]. By definition, the drugs used to treat cancer are toxic and, in view of the seriousness of the illness being treated, some degree of toxicity is acceptable. This means that these drugs have a narrow therapeutic window. Therefore, it is essential to identify the factors that can alter drug response and

P. Laurent-Puig, M.D., Ph.D. (✉)
Department of Biochemestry, Hôpital Europèen Georges-Pompidou,
20 rue Leblanc, Paris 75015, France
e-mail: Pierre.laurent-puig@parisdescartes.fr

T. Lecomte, M.D., Ph.D.
Department of Hepato-Gastroenterology, CHRU of Tours, CHU Trousseau,
Chambray-lès-Tours, France

M.-A. Loriot, M.D., Ph.D. • H. Blons, M.D., Ph.D.
Department of Biology, Hôpital Europèen Georges-Pompidou, Paris, France

V. Boige, M.D., Ph.D.
Department of Medicine, Institut Gustave Roussy, Villejuif, France

H.-J. Lenz (ed.), *Biomarkers in Oncology: Prediction and Prognosis*,
DOI 10.1007/978-1-4419-9755-5_10, © Springer Science+Business Media New York 2013

modify the efficacy/toxicity equilibrium. Because a variety of different effective agents may now be available for any given type of cancer, deciding which treatment regimen is likely to be the most appropriate—in other words, the least toxic and the most effective—is more complicated than ever, and characterizing factors that are predictive of toxicity and efficacy could lead to significant improvement in both the quality of treatment and outcomes. At least two different classes of markers to predict efficacy and toxicity can be studied: those related to the target and those related to metabolic pathways involve chemotherapeutic agents. Such markers can be analyzed at either the somatic level (i.e., in the tumor cells themselves) or at the constitutional level. In the former case, the markers identified would tend to be predictive of responsiveness, whereas in the latter, they would likely be predictive of toxicity as well as efficacy.

Drugs are for most xenobiotics, i.e., chemicals foreign to the body. They are usually lipophilic molecules that must be metabolized to hydrophilic compounds to increase their solubility to be more easily eliminated in bile and/or urine.

Xenobiotics are often hydrophobic and/or chemically reactive. The body has to render them hydrophilic and/or neutralize the reactive chemical functions [3]. This means that the body needs an armory of enzymes capable of carrying out these functions against compounds whose the chemical structure is, a priori, unknown. In addition, these xenobiotics must be transported by membrane proteins to penetrate into the body, and then to be distributed within it and eliminated [4].

The first step in the metabolism of a drug (called phase "0" metabolism) administered, for example, orally is crossing the intestinal barrier to enter the vascular compartment. At the intestinal barrier, there are carriers (efflux transporters) intended to expel them, represented, for example, by P-glycoprotein (P-gp), codes by MDR1 or ABCB1 gene. The various steps of drug metabolism are mainly hepatic and then divided into two groups: the reactions of phase I and phase II [5]. The phase I reactions are functionalization reactions catalyzed mainly by enzymes of the superfamily of cytochrome P450 monooxygenases (CYP). Other phase I enzymes include dehydrogenases, reductases, and hydrolases. The phase II reactions are for the most part conjugation reactions that make the metabolites generated by phase I reactions even more hydrophilic. Among the enzymes of phase II reactions, we find the N-acetlytransferases (NAT), glutathione S-transferase (GST) or sulfotransferases (SULT), and UDP-glucuronosyltransferases (UGT).

Finally, to be removed from the cell, these conjugated metabolites must be transported across the membrane proteins (phase III), which belong to the same family as the P-gp: the ABC protein (ATP-binding cassette, e.g., ABCC1 or MRP1 in the old nomenclature, ABCC2, etc.).

Some enzyme and transport proteins belong to the same functional class corresponding to superfamilies (e.g., CYP, NATs) with many isoforms encoded by different genes but with a strong homology in their amino acid sequences. Within a single superfamily, the isoforms have an overlapping substrate specificity. The expression or activity of proteins involved in transport, metabolism and pharmacodynamics of drugs varies depending on physiopathological, environmental and genetic (polymorphisms) factors. These variations can have significant impact on the effect of drugs (efficacy and/or tolerance).

As with all body proteins, the expression and activity of enzymes that catalyze reactions of biotransformation of drugs depend predominantly on the information carried by genes. Sequence of these genes can be altered by point mutations or SNPs (Single Nucleotide Polymorphism), partial or total deletions, or duplications or amplifications. These different versions of gene sequences define alleles and each individual has two allelic versions of the same gene, identical or different identifying a genotype. A genetic polymorphism is defined by the existence of at least two different alleles for a given gene (one allele is considered as the reference allele), present at a frequency of at least 1% in a population [6]. The threshold of 1% is arbitrary. The number of alleles varies greatly from one gene to another one (from 2 to over 50) and variants whose frequency is less than 1% are numerous. Furthermore, the frequency and nature of the variants are variable according to the ethnicity. Genetic polymorphisms can be responsible for variations in gene expression and/or activity of proteins they encode; however, the functional significance of numerous allelic variants is still unknown. A large number of xenobiotic metabolism enzymes (XME) of phase I and II, as well as targets and drug transporters have polymorphic genes [7, 8]. In the case of drug enzyme metabolism, allelic variants of their genes cause a decrease or an increase in activity or a complete absence of the enzyme protein [7, 8]. The genetic polymorphisms of enzymes of drug metabolism are expressed in the general population in the form of distinct metabolic phenotypes, defining, in the most general case, two groups of individuals called poor metabolizers (lack of enzyme activity) and fast metabolizers (normal enzyme activity). The existence of so-called ultrarapid metabolizers (increased enzyme activity) or intermediate (partial deficient activity) is also known for some polymorphic enzymes [7, 8].

Family studies have shown that the poor metabolizer phenotype is usually transmitted as an autosomal recessive trait, poor metabolizers, are homozygous or compound heterozygous for nonfunctional alleles. The frequency of these phenotypes varies in the population according to the polymorphism and, for the same enzyme, varies according to ethnic or geographic origins of populations studied [9]. For example, there are currently more than 70 allelic variants of the gene that codes for cytochrome P450 2D6 (CYP2D6) with 20 known as nonfunctional and responsible for a lack of enzyme activity. The mutations that characterize these nonfunctional alleles are diverse (nonsense, missense, frameshift or reading frameshift microdeletion, or insertion mutations affecting the consensus splice sites). In addition to these, microlesions were also described as macrolesions—complete gene deletions, causing a complete lack of activity of CYP2D6, or gene amplifications (from 2 to 13 copies of the gene), causing overexpression of the CYP2D6 gene associated with an ultrafast phenotype.

The methods to be implemented to determine the metabolic capacity of an enzyme are based either on the determination of phenotype (direct measurement of enzyme activity or indirectly based on the administration of a test substrate followed by a measurement of residual amounts of substrates and their metabolites), or the genotype-based identification of genetic polymorphisms at the origin of the variability of expression and activity of the enzyme studied.

In this chapter we focus on five different enzymes: thiopurine *S*-methyltransferase (TPMT) because it is one of the first example anticancer agents toxicity prediction;

dihydropyrimidine dehydrogenase (DYPD), thymidylate syntase (TYMS), and methylenetetrahydrofolate reductase (MTHFR) because of their potential implications in the adverse effect prediction of the most widely anticancer agent used (i.e., 5-Fluorouracil 5-FU); UDP glucuronosyltransferase 1 family, polypeptide A1 because of the recommendation of the FDA to genotype UGT1A1 before to treat patients with irinotecan and finally two targets of new anticancer agents vascular endothelial growth factor (VEGF) and epidermal growth factor receptor (EGFR) for illustrate the role of polymorphism in the target of new anticancer agents in prediction of their toxicity.

Thiopurine *S*-Methyltransferase

The 6-mercaptopurine (6MP) and its prodrug, azathioprine (AZA) belong to the family of drugs known as the thiopurines, in use for decades either as immunosuppressive or anticancer drugs. The metabolism of these drugs is schematized in Fig. 10.1. The active metabolites are the 6-thioguanine nucleotides (6TGNs), but they may also be toxic at high concentrations [10–13]. The principal cytotoxic mechanism of these agents is generally considered to be mediated via

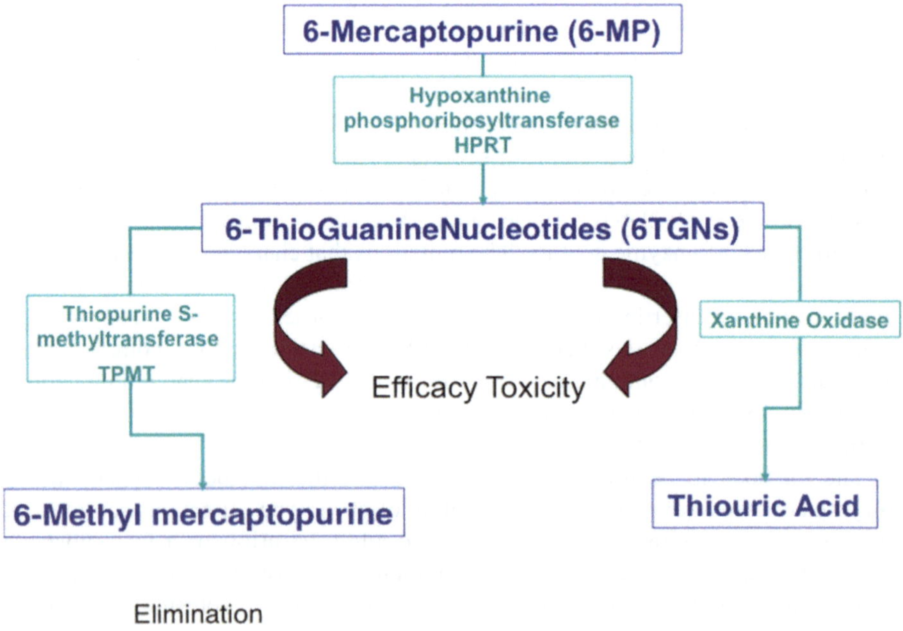

Fig. 10.1 Metabolism of thiopurine *S*-methyltransferase

incorporation of TGN into DNA and RNA. These metabolites are formed by a multistep pathway that is initiated by hypoxanthine phosphoribosyltransferase. Alternatively, these agents can undergo S-methylation catalyzed by the thiopurine *S*-methyl transferase (TPMT) or oxidation into thiouric acid via xanthine oxidase (Fig. 10.1). Metabolism via either xanthine oxidase or TPMT reduces formation of active TGN. Interindividual differences in TGN accumulation have been shown to be a significant determinant of hematotoxicity and antileukemic or immunomodulator effects of thiopurines [14, 15]. Indeed, the cellular accumulation of TGN is inversely related to TPMT activity. This enzyme was shown to be genetically polymorphic many years ago [16–19]. The molecular basis for altered TPMT activity has now been defined for the majority of the patients. To date, the most frequent deficient alleles, including TPMT*2, TPMT*3A, and TPMT*3C alleles, account for 80–95% of intermediate or low enzyme activity cases [20]. Of the total population, 89% have a normal level of enzyme activity (homozygous wild-type TPMT), 10.7% have intermediate (heterozygous), and 0.3% (1/300) have low or no enzyme activity (homozygous mutant TPMT) [21]. The a priori knowledge of an individual's TPMT activity can identify those patients prone to early leukopenic events when treated with standard doses of thiopurines as a result of intermediate or low TPMT activity. The consequences of TPMT variations are important for the toxicity of the thiopurines as well as for their efficacy. Indeed, these drugs were shown to be myelotoxic, at therapeutic doses, in some patients. Although not all of the myelotoxic effect could be explained by the TPMT defect [22, 23], a close relation between TPMT activity, 6TGN erythrocyte concentration, and myelotoxicity was clearly proven [13, 24, 25]. Among intolerant patients developing dose-limiting hematopoietic toxicity from therapy containing thiopurines, the prevalence of TPMT deficient and heterozygous individuals was sixfold higher when compared with the general population [26]. However, with appropriate dosage adjustments, TPMT deficient patients can be treated with thiopurines without acute limiting toxicity. Moreover, it has also been shown that the variations in TPMT activity could be responsible for variations in the efficacy of 6MP. Among acute leukemia children, a high activity of TPMT is associated with a lower therapeutic efficacy [27–29]; TPMT pharmacogenetics highlights the potential clinical importance of the translation of pharmacogenetics from bench to bedside. The determination of either the TPMT phenotype by determining its activity in erythrocytes [16, 30, 31] or the TPMT genotype [17, 18, 32] is quite easy and will be helpful to adjust drug dosage [33–35]. Prior knowledge of TPMT status avoids exposure of individuals with no TPMT activity to potentially fatal treatment with AZA or 6-MP and provides one of the best examples of predictive pharmacogenetics in therapeutics. Finally, a cost-effectiveness study of TMPT genotyping, prior to thiopurine treatment in children with acute lymphoblastic leukemia, indicated that TPMT genotyping should be seriously considered as an integral part of healthcare prior to the initiation of therapy with thiopurine drugs [35].

Dihydropyrimidine Dehydrogenase

5-Fluorouracil (5-FU) and orally available 5-FU prodrugs are prescribed for the treatment of many cancers such as colorectal cancer and breast cancer. The cytosolic enzyme dihydropyrimidine dehydrogenase DPD plays an important role in 5-FU degradation [36]. It catalyses the first step in the degradation pathway of 5-fluorouracil to 5-fluoro-dihydrouracil, which is degraded further to fluoroalanine and fluoroacetate (Fig. 10.2). Extensive degradation of 5-FU may limit its metabolism to active metabolites, such as FdUMP, which may result in clinical resistance to 5-FU [36]. There is an association between the DPD activity in lymphocytes, which is subject to a wide variability in human population mainly due to genetic polymorphism, and the systemic clearance of 5-FU [37]. A weak DPD activity leads to a decrease of 5-FU catabolism associated with an increase of 5-FU active metabolites and an increase risk of severe toxicities, which can ultimately lead to death. DPD is found in nearly every organ but is mostly expressed in the liver, kidney, and lungs [38]. The role of DPD is an important factor of availability of 5-FU and the DPD activity was show to be inversely related to the plasma concentration of 5-FU in cancer patients receiving continuous infusion of 5-FU [39]. DPD activity shows a wide range of individual variation (up to 20-fold differences) among individuals [40, 41]. Complete or near-complete enzyme deficiency occurs in one patient out of 10,000, and it is associated with potentially life-threatening toxicity after administration of 5-FU or related drug [42]. Although total DPD deficiency is rare, 3–5%

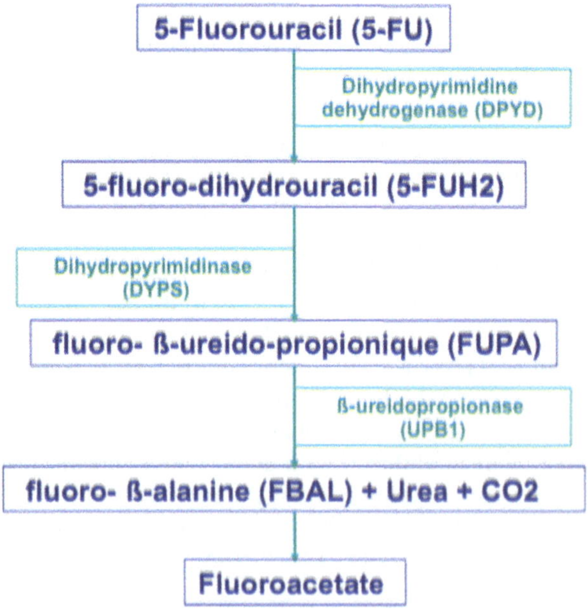

Fig. 10.2 Catabolism of 5-fluorouracil

of the population has low enzyme activity that is associated with an increased risk of toxicity in patient treated with pyrimidine-based antimetabolite analogues, such as 5-FU and capecitabine [43–46]. Patients who had from partial to complete loss of DPD activity are exposed to excessive accumulation of active 5-FU metabolites following treatment with 5-FU and related drug and, consequently, exhibit significantly greater risk of hematopoietic, neurological, and gastrointestinal 5-FU-induced toxicity, which can be fatal [47]. Approximately, a decreased DPD activity has been detected in half of patients suffering from severe 5-FU toxicity [42, 48–50], and patients with a partial DPD deficiency have a 3.4-fold higher risk of developing grade IV neutropenia than patients with a normal DPD activity [49]. Furthermore, the occurrence of toxicity is twice as fast in patients with low DPD activity compared with patient with normal DPD activity [37, 51]. The clinical presentation of DPD deficiency is similar to that of an accidental overdose of 5-FU. Estimating this frequency of patients harboring at least a partial DPD deficiency, the pretherapeutic detection of this metabolic dysfunction could prevent severe and unwanted side effects due to fluoropyrimidine drugs.

The human gene coding for DPD (DPYD) is located on chromosome 1 at position 1p22 and comprises 23 exons. Families studies with DPD-deficient subjects (absence of DPD activity in fibroblasts) were used to characterize many DPYD gene variants associated with decreased activity of DPD. To date, more than 30 genetic polymorphisms in the DPYD gene have been reported [52]. Of these, more than half might be associated with decreased activity of DPD [48, 49, 53]. In the Western population, the frequency of all these variants associated with a decreased activity of DPYD was approximately 3% in the heterozygous and 0.1% in the homozygous state [41, 54, 55]. Among these, the most common polymorphism, accounting for 40–50% of all DPYD variants, is the splice site variant of exon 14 (IVS14 +1G>A, DPYD allele * 2A), resulting in the total excision of exon 14 [56] and the deletion of a segment of 165 amino acids corresponding to the binding site of pyrimidine substrate [57]. Homozygous patients for this polymorphism have a null DPD activity, and heterozygous patients have a strong reduced DPD activity [54]. The clinical relevance of DPYD gene single nucleotide polymorphism on 5-FU tolerance was recently evaluated on a prospective series. A set of nine DPYD SNPs was prospectively determined by pyrosequencing on 487 patients, among them the presence of the one of the three following polymorphisms (IVS14 +1G>A, 2846A>T or 1679T>G) was associated with severe toxicity. These three polymorphisms were studied in an extended population of 1,200 patients receiving 5-FU and the presence of one of them was highly correlated with severe toxicity ($P=2.8\times10^{-10}$) [54]. Sensitivity, specificity, and positive and negative predictive values of the detection of these three polymorphism as predictive factors for toxic side effects were 0.31, 0.98, 0.62, 0.94 respectively. Another study that included 683 patients with various types of cancers treated prospectively by several 5-FU regimen has shown that detection of the IVS14 +1G>A polymorphism had a sensitivity of 0.055 and a predictive positive value of 0.46 for predicting severe toxicity. The inclusion of additional DPYD variants improved prediction only marginally. The toxicities significantly associated with mutants were mucositis and leucopenia. Surprisingly, an interaction between IVS14 +1G>A polymorphism and sex was highlighted as the prediction of toxicity for this polymorphism was higher among men than in women (odds ratio of 39.9 for men and 0.62 in women) [58]. The impact of determination of DYPD deficiency in terms of cost effectiveness should be studied, in order to convince the oncologists to use the different tools available to measure it.

Methylenetetrahydrofolate Reductase

The 5–10 methylenetetrahydrofolate reductase (MTHFR) catalyzes the irreversible conversion of the 5,10 methylenetetrahydrofolate, required for purine and thymidine synthesis, to 5-methyltetrahydrofolate the primary methyl donor for the remethylation of homocysteine to methionine, which is indispensable for nucleic acid methylation [59] (Fig. 10.3). Reduced enzyme activity is associated with elevated homocysteine, an established risk factor for occlusive heart disease [60], and low serum folate [61]. Two nonsynonymous C677T (A222V) (NM_005957.3:c.665C>T; NP_005948.3:p.Ala222Val; in former nomenclature this variant is numbered C677T, we kept this former nomenclature to be coherent with the literature) and A1298C (E429A) (NM_005957.3:c.1286A>C; NP_005948.3:p.Glu429Ala; in former

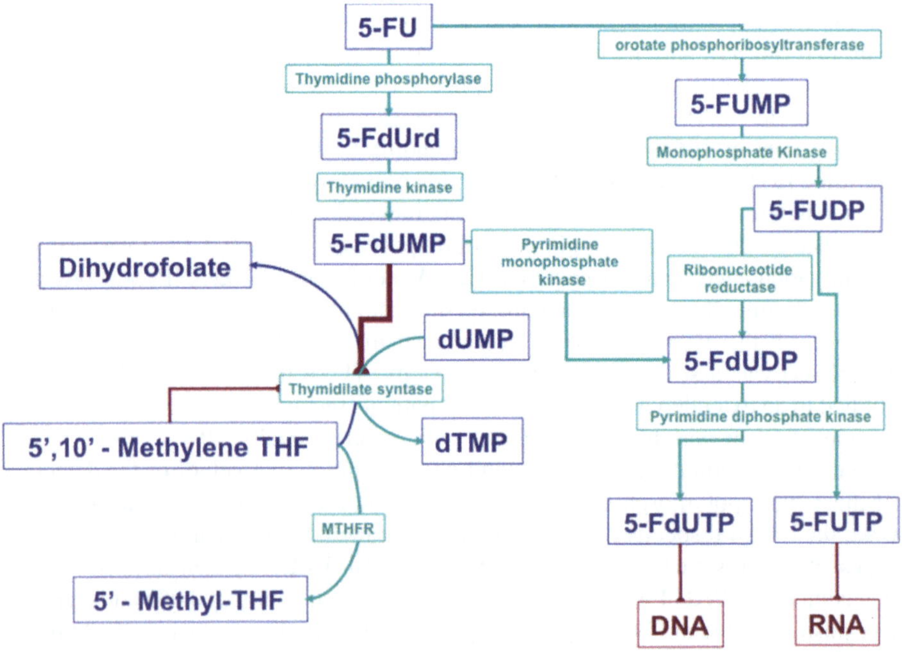

Fig. 10.3 Metabolism of 5-fluorouracil

nomenclature this variant is numbered A1298C, we kept this former nomenclature be coherent with the literature) variants have been shown to modify the activity of MTHFR enzyme. The variants have been associated with a reduced activity of MTHFR, more important for the C677T than for the A1298C, an increased plasma level of homocyteine and an altered distribution of folates mainly for the C677T allele [62–66]. Haplotype analyses showed a strong linkage disequilibrium between the two variants (*D′* estimate of –0.95; personal data) suggesting functional interference between these two polymorphisms [67, 68]. The haplotype 665T/1286C is very rare and patients homozygous for both variants are even not present in different studies suggesting that such genotypes could result in severe deficient phenotype. Moreover the functional impact of C665T and A1286T polymorphism is affected by folates status [67, 69]. Some cancer drugs antifolates and fluoropyrimidine, methotrexate (MTX), 5-FU and raltitrexed (RTX), interfere with folate metabolism, and drug efficacies are dependent of the folate pool in cancer cells [70]. Therefore it has been suggested that MTHFR polymorphism could play a role in toxicity and efficacy of these compounds. Numerous studies try to explore a possible association between C665T, A1286V or the combination of two by haplotype analysis and a toxic effect of MTX both in cancer and in anti-inflammatory treatment. At least 35 studies explore this association in different human population (Caucasian, Japanese, Asian, Indian, African-American, Jewish, and Hispanic) in different association of treatment (MTX alone or in combination with anticancer agents or with immunosuppressive drug) (for review see [66]). The side effects investigated were heterogeneous from one series to another. A positive association between 677T allele and adverse effect of MTX has been found in approximately half of the series, in one series a lower rate of haematologic toxicity was observed in patients carrying 677T allele [71], and no correlation was found in the remaining series [66]. The effect of the A1298C allele was less studied, but the results are even more discordant with positive and negative association between 1286C allele and adverse effect of MTX. Therefore, no clinical conclusion can be drawn from these series, and we need a large prospective series to measure the clinical impact of the determination these polymorphisms in predicting side effects of MTX.

The pharmacological target of 5-FU is the thymidilate synthase (TS), and the drug exerts its effect by forming a ternary complex between its active compound the 5-fluoro-2 deoxyuridine-5 monophosphate (5FUMP), thymidylate synthase, and 5–10 methylene tetrahydrofolate (CH2FH4) thereby inhibiting TS activity [72]. Since a loss in MTHFR enzymatic activity may favor an increase in intracellular CH2FH4 concentrations stabilizing the binding of 5-fluorodeoxyuridine monophosphate to TS, it can be hypothesized that tumors exhibiting mutated MTHFR genotypes may be more sensitive to 5-FU cytotoxicity (adverse side effects or tumor response) [73, 74]. If the 677T allele has been reported initially associated with efficacy of 5-FU in patient treated in monotherapy in advanced colorectal cancer [75–77], the more recent published series failed to confirm such association when the 5-FU is associated with irinotecan or oxaliplatin [78–80]. Concerning the association between the MTHFR polymorphism and 5-FU toxicity, Table 10.1

Table 10.1 Relation between polymorphism of MTHFR gene and 5-FU toxicity and efficacy

Type of study/chemotherapy regimen	Type of cancer and number of patients studied (*n*)	Polymorphisms studied	Results	References
Prospective study/5-FU ± folic acid or levamizole	Solid Cancer (683)	C677T, A1298C	No association with toxicity in univariate analysis Very moderate reduced risk of toxicity for 677 alleleT in multivariate analysis	[58]
Prospective study/FOLFIRI	Metastatic colorectal cancer (146)	C677T, A1298C	No association with toxicity	[82]
Prospective/FOLFOX-4	Metastatic colorectal cancer (166)	C677T, A1298C	No association with toxicity	[78]
Retrospective study/LV5FU2 or FUFOL	Advanced colorectal cancer (76); Most of them treated in first line	C677T A1298C	No association with toxicity CC genotype associated with toxicity	[81]
Prospective study/ Fluoropyrimidine based chemotherapy mainly FUFOL regimen	Advanced colorectal cancer (43)	C677T	No association with toxicity	[77]
Prospective study/ Capecitabine	metastatic or locally advanced colorectal cancer (54)	C677T, A1298C	Genotypes and diplotypes predicted for grade 2/3 toxicities A1298C polymorphism is an ind ependent predictor of toxicity in multivariate analysis	[83]

summarizes the different results observed [58, 77, 78, 81–83]. Based on the different series published up to now and also taking into account the largest prospective study [58], the impact of MTHFR polymorphisms on severe FU related toxicity seems to be negligible [58].

The quinazoline antifolate Raltitrexed is a potent and specific inhibitor of TS. This compound is polyglutamated by folylpolyglutamate synthase into cells; the increased availability of 5,10-methylentetrahydrofolate, as a result of impaired MTHFR activity, could compete with Raltitrexed for polyglutamation and binding to TS and therefore interfering Raltitrexed cytotoxicity (adverse side effect or tumor response). Only one series reported that homozygotes for the MTHFR 677 TT polymorphism incurred significantly less Raltitrexed-associated toxicity than those with either wild-type or heterozygous genotypes [84].

Thymidylate Synthase

Thymidylate synthase (TS) is the main intracellular target of fluoropyrimidines [85]. The uracil analogue 5-FU is a prodrug, which is metabolized to 5-fluoro-2-deoxyuridine monophosphate (5-FdUMP) (Fig. 10.3). This active metabolite inhibits the thymidylate synthase that is a crucial enzyme for de novo synthesis of pyrimidine, required DNA synthesis. 5-FdUMP forms stable complexes with TS and folate as a cofactor, thus blocking the conversion of dUMP to dTMP.

The interpatient variability in TS expression is a factor influencing pharmacodynamic effects of fluoropyrimidines. Several studies have underlined the relationship between intratumoral TS protein expression and response to 5-FU-based chemotherapy. Patients with low TS levels have better clinical outcome than those with high TS levels [86–89]. TS protein expression is affected by different underlying functional polymorphisms [90–94].

The TYMS gene is located on the short arm of chromosome 18. The TYMS promoter enhancer region is polymorphic, and several polymorphisms influence the translation efficiency of TYMS mRNA [90, 95, 96]. TYMS promoter comprises a 28-bp sequence, usually presented as a double-tandem repeat (TSER*2 allele) or a triple-tandem repeat (TSER*3 allele), and it was demonstrated that homozygous TSER*3/TSER*3 cells over-expressed *TYMS* mRNA compared with homozygous TSER*2/TSER*2 cells [90, 96]. A single nucleotide polymorphism G>C has been described at the twelfth nucleotide of the second repeat of the TSER*3 allele, leading to a tri-allelic locus (TSER*2, TSER*3G, and TSER*3C). This polymorphism changes a critical residue in the USF E-box consensus element. The TSER*3C allele showed transcriptional activity that was similar to that of the TSER*2 allele [92]. More recently, a novel nucleotide G>C change in the first tandem repeat of the TSER*2 allele has been reported [97, 98]. The discovery of this novel polymorphism raises the possibility of nucleotide change occurring in other tandem repeats. Furthermore, a common polymorphism in the 3′-untranslated region (3′-UTR) of the TYMS gene has been identified, usually presented as a deletion of 6 bp at position 1,494 [94]. A significant association between the 6-bp deletion and low TYMS mRNA expression in colorectal tumor tissue has been described [99].

A combined analysis of functional polymorphisms affecting TS activity has been reported. Patients possessing genetic changes in the 5′-UTR and 3′-UTR associated with low TS activity were the most likely to respond to chemotherapy [100]. Interestingly, a linkage disequilibrium was observed between the number of tandem repeats and insertion/deletion polymorphisms [99].

Ethnic variations of the TS genotypes have been reported in the literature. The number of tandem repeats differs widely according to patients' ethnicity. Indeed the frequency of homozygous TSER*3/TSER*3 genotype varies from 40% in Caucasians to 70% in Chinese population [101, 102]. The four and nine repeat alleles are found at higher frequencies in Africans (2–7%) compared to Caucasians or Asians (0–1%) [103].

Controversial data have been reported concerning the relation between polymorphisms of *TYMS* gene alleles and tumor response or survival of patients treated by fluoropyrimidines. In one hand, homozygous TSER*3/TSER*3 genotype has been shown to be associated with higher TS expression, leading to lower fluorouracil efficacy, while homozygous double repeat genotype (TSER*2/TSER*2) has been associated with preferable clinical outcomes after 5-FU-based chemotherapy [100, 104–106].

In another hand, survival or response to 5-FU treatment in patients with TSER*3/TSER*3 genotype was better than or equal to that with TSER*2/TSER*2 genotype [75, 107, 108]. These results suggest that the whole transcriptional activity of TYMS is not only dependent of the number of tandem repeats. The single nucleotide polymorphisms in the tandem repeats, which modify the transcriptional activity of TYMS, can possibly explain these inconclusive data. Moreover, the 6-bp insertion/deletion polymorphism was shown to be associated with survival in colorectal cancer patients treated with adjuvant 5-FU [109].

As with fluoropyrimidines efficacy, TYMS polymorphisms have been evaluated in pharmacogenetic studies examining fluoropyrimidines toxicity. The low TYMS mRNA expression level in normal tissue is supposed to be associated with a higher risk of the cytotoxic effects of 5-FU. The decrease in TYMS mRNA expression in normal tissue of TSER*2/TSER*2 patients is supposed to sensitize the normal cells against damage by 5-FU-based chemotherapy.

Several studies on TYMS polymorphisms showed a significant inverse association between the number of 28-bp tandem repeats in the TYMS promoter region and the severity of 5-FU toxicity [58, 104, 110–112]. In the first reported study, which included 50 colorectal patients who received 5-FU chemotherapy, patients homozygous and heterozygous for TSER*3 allele experienced a significant lower incidence of severe 5-FU toxicity than patient homozygous for TSER*3 (27% and 32% versus 63%; $p=0.008$) [104]. In our own published study, patients with TSER*2/TSER*2 genotype were 20 times more likely to have severe toxicity to 5-FU compared with TSER*3/TSER*3 carriers [111]. However, this association was not constantly

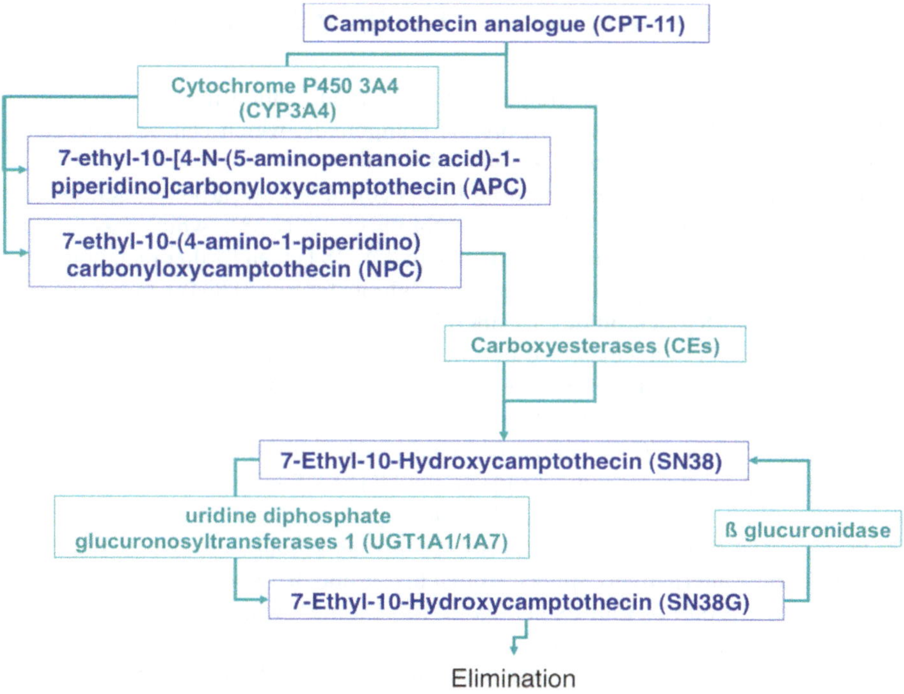

Fig. 10.4 Metabolism of SN-38

found [83, 113, 114]. Consideration of the G>C SNP in the TSER*3 allele is not a better determinant of toxicity during 5-FU-based treatment [83]. The polymorphism 3′UTR indel of *TYMS* has not been as extensively studied as TSER polymorphism and no relation was observed in two series [83–111].

Therefore, the value of TYMS polymorphisms in predicting toxicity to 5-FU-based therapy is not clearly established and requires further investigation. These apparent contradictory data illustrate the complexity and difficulty to demonstrate the utility of the pharmacogenetic concept into routine clinical practice. Heterogeneity in clinical features in patients treated with 5-FU-based chemotherapy may represent a major limitation for observing actual pharmacogenetic effects of functional germ-line polymorphisms. Despite the large number of studies attempting to identify useful molecular predictors of response to 5-FU in terms of efficacy and toxicity, no reliable TYMS polymorphisms of 5-FU toxicity have been validated to permit their use as a standard of care for the management of patients with cancer treated with 5-FU-based chemotherapy.

Combining polymorphisms of DPYD, MTHFR, and TYMS with the mode of administration of 5-FU bolus versus infusional, the supplementation by folinic acid and the gender, Schwab et al. [58] have proposed a nomogram based on the multifactorial model, for estimating individual 5-FU toxicity risk. (Fig. 10.4)

UDP Glucuronosyltransferase 1 Family, Polypeptide A1

Glucuronidation are the most frequent phase II modification in drug metabolism. These reactions lead to more hydrophilic compounds, which can be more easily excreted in biological effluents like bile [115, 116].

For example Irinotecan is a prodrug that is converted by carboxylesterase to an active metabolite 7-ethyl-10-hydroxycamptothecin (SN-38), which has a 100–1,000-fold higher cytotoxicity than irinotecan. SN-38 is then further metabolized in the liver by uridine diphosphateglucuronosyltransferases (UGTs) to an inactive metabolite, SN-38 glucuronide (SN-38G) [117, 118].

Among the UGT enzymes, two families have been identified UGT1 and UGT2, which are divided into three subgroups, UGT1A, UGT2A and UGT2B [116, 119]. Altogether 17 human enzymes have been identified thus far [120]. Contrary to observations for the UGT2 family, for which each isoform is coded by a specific gene clustered on chromosome 4 (4q13), the UGT1A family is coded by a unique gene located on chromosome 2 (2q37) encompassing a 290 kilobase region. The N-terminal end of UGT1A isoforms is the substrate-binding site and is coded by a specific exon 1 alternatively spliced from a first group of 13 potential exons located upstream to a group of four exons (exon 2 to exon 5), which are common to the different isoforms [120–122]. UGT1A1 is responsible for the glucuronidation of bilirubin, and serum level of total bilirubin. Several polymorphisms have been identified in the promoter region and in the coding sequences of UGT1A family. Some of them are associated with a UGT1A1 deficiency leading to three syndromes of unconjugated hyperbilirubinemia Crigler–Najjar type I and type II and the Gilbert syndrome [123–126]. The latter one is owing to a polymorphism located in the TATA box. The number of TA repeats (5, 6, 7, or 8) in the TATA box is indeed inversely correlated with gene transcriptional efficiency. In Gilbert's syndrome, patients are homozygous for seven TA repeats (*28 allele). Several cases of irinotecan severe toxicity were reported in such patients leading to hypothesize the role of UGT1A1 in the glucuronidation of SN-38 [127]. The suspected role of UGT1A1 was also reinforced by pharmacokinetic results demonstrating that SN-38 is glucuronidated primarily by UGT1A1 [117, 128–131] and that the *28 allele affected, in vitro, the SN-38 glucuronidation rate in human livers [130]. The rate of SN-38 glucuronidation decreased by 50% in patients homozygous for the *28 allele, and by 25% for heterozygous patients [130]. Several studies have shown a significant association between UGT1A1 *28 polymorphism and the occurrence of severe neutropenia occurring usually within 2 months after initiation of treatment [132–135]. These first results led the US Food and Drug Administration (FDA) to advise Pfizer Pharmaceuticals, the manufacturer of irinotecan, to amend the product information for the drug to include the association between the UGT1A1*28 genotype and hematologic toxicity and to recommend that patients with the UGT1A1*28/*28 genotype receive a lower starting dose of irinotecan. From that date some series do not confirm these initial reported results [136–138]. A recent meta-analysis [139] compiling data from nine studies, including 821 patients treated with different regimens of irinotecan, was performed. The results showed that the risk of hematologic toxicity between patients with a UGT1A1*28/*28 genotype and those with a UGT1A1*1/*1 or UGT1A1*1/*28 genotype increased statistically significantly as irinotecan dose increased (slope = 0.012; $P = .028$) (Fig. 10.4) and was significant from an irinotecan dose of 150 mg/m^2. This meta-analysis also confirmed the absence of a link between this allele and the occurrence of severe diarrhea [139]. Recently, 1,405 patients included in the European trial comparing 3 PETACC in the adjuvant chemotherapy with 5-FU chemotherapy with 5-FU and irinotecan according to the scheme FOLFIRI in CRC stage II and III, the risk of severe or febrile neutropenia was significantly increased in patients homozygous for UGT1A1*28 allele. However, in multivariate analysis, female gender was more discriminating than the genotype to predict the risk of neutropenia in the FOLFIRI experimental arm [140].

Two other variants alleles (UGT1A1 - 3156G>A and UGT1A1 - 3279G>T) located in the promoter region of UGT1A1 gene, in linkage disequilibrium with UGT1A1*28 allele, modify the capacity of SN-38 glucuronidation by UGT1A [141, 142]. Innocenti et al. reported that the SNP -3156G>A was also associated with neutropenia induced by irinotecan [132]. Based on the bilirubin level of individual patients, the authors concluded that this variant -3156G>A would explain in part why patients with the same genotype at the TATA box may present different toxicities. The -3156G/A or A/A genotypes, would increase the deficit in glucuronidation compared to G/G genotype. In a recent study, we investigated the relationship between polymorphisms UGT1A1*28 and UGT1A1 - 3156G>A and the risk of toxicity of the association of 5-FU and irinotecan in adjuvant setting in 93 patients with colon cancer stage III [143]. The occurrence of neutropenia grade 3 or 4 was significantly more frequent in patients with UGT1A1*28/*28 genotype compared to patients with *1/*28 or *1/*1 genotypes (50% versus 23% versus 14% respectively, $p = 0.035$). A significant difference was also observed according to UGT1A1 polymorphism -3156G>A (57% neutropenia grade 3 or 4 in case of A/A genotype versus 28% for G/A genotype and 10% for G/G genotype, $p = 0.008$). For the authors, the -3156G>A polymorphism seems to be a better predictor than the UGT1A1 TA repeats polymorphism to predict the occurrence of severe neutropenia due to irinotecan treatment. A link between the severity of the toxicity induced by irinotecan and UGT1A1 polymorphism -3279T>G has also been reported [144]. The sequencing of UGT1A1 gene among 195 Japanese patients, 85 had been treated with chemotherapy based on irinotecan for CRC, has confirmed the existence of linkage disequilibrium between different UGT1A1 promoter polymorphisms, including the frequent association of -3156A, 7TA and -3279G allele [145]. A pharmacokinetic study in the 85 patients treated with irinotecan has shown that the ratio SN-38G/AUC AUC SN-38 varied depending on different haplotypes. Two other UGT1A family members, the UGT1A7 and UGT1A9, could play a role in the glucuronidation of SN-38.

The two most common variant alleles of UGT1A7 gene (UGT1A7*2 and UGT1A7*3) exhibited much lower SN-38 glucuronidation activities compared with UGT1A7*1 allele [146–148] suggesting that these variants could play a role in the occurrence irinotecan toxicity. A fraction of SN-38G excreted into the bile and into the digestive tract, is deglucuronided in SN-38 under the action of bacterial β(beta)-glucuronidase, probably contributing to the occurrence irinotecan-delayed induced diarrhea [149]. It is possible that UGT1A7, expressed mainly in the digestive tract converts SN-38 into SN-38G. This could explain why the occurrence of diarrhea was more frequently observed in carriers of variant UGT1A7*2 and UGT1A7*3 in a series of 81 patients receiving the association of irinotecan and cispaltin for lung cancer [150] However, this relation was not retrieved in another Asian series of Ando et al. [146], and even an inverse relation was observed in a third series [136]. Genotypes UGT1A7*2/UGT1A7*2 and UGT1A7*3/UGT1A7*3 were associated with a lower risk of diarrhea and improved effectiveness of chemotherapy.

Another polymorphism of UGT1A9 gene, corresponding to a thymidine insertion in the promoter region at position −118 $(T)_{10}$ allele or UGT1A9*22 allele is associated with a 2.6-fold higher transcriptional activity compared with the −118 $(T)_9$ allele, based on in vitro transcriptional reporter assays [151]. An association between UGT1A9*22 allele and an unanticipated higher risk of toxic side effect had been reported including diarrhea [136].

These unexpected results between individual genotypes and toxicity of irinotecan-based chemotherapy could be due to the existence of strong linkage disequilibrium occurring between all these polymorphisms. The most common haplotype, corresponding to the combination of UGT1A1*1, UGT1A6*1, UGT1A7*1 and UGT1A9*22 alleles, appears to be associated with a lower response rate and a higher risk gastro-intestinal toxicity when treated with irinotecan [136].

From all these studies, the clinical relevance of the prediction of irinotecan side effect remains to be clearly determined. The polymorphism corresponding to the variant allele UGT1A1*28 is associated, in dose dependant manner, with irinotecan-induced neutropenia. However, the results of ongoing clinical trials taking into account the genotype of UGT1A1 to determine the dose of irinotecan administered to patients are impatiently awaited to confirm or not the interest of the systematic genotyping before the initiation of treatment.

Targets of New Therapies

With increasing success of targeted anticancer agents including monoclonal antibody therapeutics and inhibitor tyrosine kinase, it is important to evaluate the impact of pharmacogenetics on toxicity of these new therapies. Genetic polymorphism could not only influence efficacy of this new agent as monoclonal antibody but may also contribute to toxicity. We will focus on two targets vascular endothelial growth factor and epidermal growth factor receptor.

With the use of bevacizumab, a monoclonal antibody against vascular endothelial growth factor (VEGF), evaluation of VEGF genotype has been recently evaluated as a predictive biomarker candidate of effects of bevacizumab-based chemotherapy. In patients with metastatic breast cancer receiving bevacizumab-based chemotherapy, two genotypes, VEGF-634 CC and VEGF-1498 TT, were associated with significantly less grade 3 or 4 hypertension when compared with the combined alternate genotypes [152]. Although the level of circulating VEGF as a biomarker remains unclear, baseline plasma levels of VEGF were not available in this study, the polymorphisms could not be compared with the circulating level of VEGF in these patients.

The hypothesis that polymorphisms of EGFR gene are associated with adverse effects of EGFR inhibitors in particular skin toxicity, which is most frequent adverse effect, has been evaluated. The EGFR gene, in intron 1, contains a highly polymorphic sequence which affects transcription efficiency of the gene [153]. It consists of a variable number of CA dinucleotide repeats ranging from 9 to 21. Two others functional EGFR variants associated with EGFR regulation have been reported: a G>A *SNP* in codon 497 (extracellular subdomain IV) and the -216G>T EGFR promoter SNP within the Sp-1 binding site [154, 155].

The intron 1 CA repeat polymorphism of EGFR gene has been evaluated in pharmacogenetic studies examining anti-EGFR drugs and related skin toxicity. In several clinical studies with patient who received EGFR inhibitor tyrosine kinase as erlotinib or gefitinib, the occurrence of skin toxicity was found to be associated with the presence of the EGFR intron-1 short (CA)n allele [156]. Furthermore, the homozygous EGFR intron-1 short (CA)n allele is associated with increased grade 2–3 skin toxicity in colorectal cancer patients who received cetuximab [157]. Gefitinib and erlotinib are substrates for the efflux transporter *ABCG2* [158]. One study suggests that patients with reduced ABCG2 activity due to a common genetic variant (ABCG2 421C>A) are at increased risk for gefitinib-induced diarrhea [159]. In another study correlation between ABCG2 polymorphisms and high concentration of gefitinib in patients treated with gefitinib was reported [156]. Investigations in the pharmacogenetics area will likely have an impact on attempts to further optimize and individualize treatment regimens involving new therapies.

References

1. Lazarou J, Pomeranz BH, Corey PN. Incidence of adverse drug reactions in hospitalized patients: a meta-analysis of prospective studies. JAMA. 1998;279:1200–5.
2. Ulrich CM, Robien K, McLeod HL. Cancer pharmacogenetics: polymorphisms, pathways and beyond. Nat Rev Cancer. 2003;3:912–20.
3. Guengerich FP. Mechanisms of cytochrome P450 substrate oxidation: mini review. J Biochem Mol Toxicol. 2007;21:163–8.
4. Borst P, Elferink RO. Mammalian ABC transporters in health and disease. Annu Rev Biochem. 2002;71:537–92.
5. Testa B, Kramer SD. The biochemistry of drug metabolism–an introduction: part 1. principles and overview. Chem Biodivers. 2006;3:1053–101.
6. Meyer UA. Genotype or phenotype: the definition of a pharmacogenetic polymorphism. Pharmacogenetics. 1991;1:66–7.
7. Guttmacher AE, Collins FS. Welcome to the genomic era. N Engl J Med. 2003;349:996–8.
8. Evans WE, McLeod HL. Pharmacogenomics—drug disposition, drug targets, and side effects. N Engl J Med. 2003;348:538–49.

9. Gaedigk A. Interethnic differences of drug-metabolizing enzymes. Int J Clin Pharmacol Ther. 2000;38:61–8.
10. Rowland K, Lennard L, Lilleyman JS. High-performance liquid chromatographic assay of methylthioguanine nucleotide. J Chromatogr B Biomed Sci Appl. 1998;705:29–37.
11. Soria-Royer C, Legendre C, Mircheva J, Premel S, Beaune P, Kreis H. Thiopurine-methyltransferase activity to assess azathioprine myelotoxicity in renal transplant recipients. Lancet. 1993;341:1593–4.
12. Chan GL, Erdmann GR, Gruber SA, Matas AJ, Canafax DM. Azathioprine metabolism: pharmacokinetics of 6-mercaptopurine, 6-thiouric acid and 6-thioguanine nucleotides in renal transplant patients. J Clin Pharmacol. 1990;30:358–63.
13. Ben Ari Z, Mehta A, Lennard L, Burroughs AK. Azathioprine-induced myelosuppression due to thiopurine methyltransferase deficiency in a patient with autoimmune hepatitis. J Hepatol. 1995;23:351–4.
14. Lennard L, Lilleyman JS, Van Loon J, Weinshilboum RM. Genetic variation in response to 6-mercaptopurine for childhood acute lymphoblastic leukaemia. Lancet. 1990;336:225–9.
15. Yates CR, Krynetski EY, Loennechen T, et al. Molecular diagnosis of thiopurine S-methyltransferase deficiency: genetic basis for azathioprine and mercaptopurine intolerance. Ann Intern Med. 1997;126:608–14.
16. Weinshilboum RM, Raymond FA, Pazmino PA. Human erythrocyte thiopurine methyltransferase: radiochemical microassay and biochemical properties. Clin Chim Acta. 1978;85:323–33.
17. Otterness D, Szumlanski C, Lennard L, et al. Human thiopurine methyltransferase pharmacogenetics: gene sequence polymorphisms. Clin Pharmacol Ther. 1997;62:60–73.
18. Szumlanski C, Otterness D, Her C, et al. Thiopurine methyltransferase pharmacogenetics: human gene cloning and characterization of a common polymorphism. DNA Cell Biol. 1996;15:17–30.
19. Spire-Vayron de la Moureyre C, Debuysere H, Mastain B, et al. Genotypic and phenotypic analysis of the polymorphic thiopurine S-methyltransferase gene (TPMT) in a European population. Br J Pharmacol. 1998;125:879–87.
20. McLeod HL, Krynetski EY, Relling MV, Evans WE. Genetic polymorphism of thiopurine methyltransferase and its clinical relevance for childhood acute lymphoblastic leukemia. Leukemia. 2000;14:567–72.
21. Weinshilboum RM, Sladek SL. Mercaptopurine pharmacogenetics: monogenic inheritance of erythrocyte thiopurine methyltransferase activity. Am J Hum Genet. 1980;32:651–62.
22. Naughton MA, Battaglia E, O'Brien S, Walport MJ, Botto M. Identification of thiopurine methyltransferase (TPMT) polymorphisms cannot predict myelosuppression in systemic lupus erythematosus patients taking azathioprine. Rheumatology. 1999;38:640–4.
23. Colombel JF, Ferrari N, Debuysere H, et al. Genotypic analysis of thiopurine S-methyltransferase in patients with Crohn's disease and severe myelosuppression during azathioprine therapy. Gastroenterology. 2000;118:1025–30.
24. Lennard L, Gibson BE, Nicole T, Lilleyman JS. Congenital thiopurine methyltransferase deficiency and 6-mercaptopurine toxicity during treatment for acute lymphoblastic leukaemia. Arch Dis Child. 1993;69:577–9.
25. Relling MV, Hancock ML, Rivera GK, et al. Mercaptopurine therapy intolerance and heterozygosity at the thiopurine S-methyltransferase gene locus. J Natl Cancer Inst. 1999;91:2001–8.
26. Evans WE, Hon YY, Bomgaars L, et al. Preponderance of thiopurine S-methyltransferase deficiency and heterozygosity among patients intolerant to mercaptopurine or azathioprine. J Clin Oncol. 2001;19:2293–301.
27. Anstey A, Lennard L. The role of genetic variation in thiopurine methyltransferase activity and efficacy and/or side effects of azathioprine therapy in dermatologic patients. Arch Dermatol. 1995;131:1087–8.
28. Lilleyman JS, Lennard L. Mercaptopurine metabolism and risk of relapse in childhood lymphoblastic leukaemia. Lancet. 1994;343:1188–90.

29. Evans WE, Relling MV. Pharmacogenomics: translating functional genomics into rational therapeutics. Science. 1999;286:487–91.
30. Lennard L, Singleton HJ. High-performance liquid chromatographic assay of human red blood cell thiopurine methyltransferase activity. J Chromatogr B Biomed Appl. 1994;661:25–33.
31. Jacqz-Aigrain E, Bessa E, Medard Y, Mircheva Y, Vilmer E. Thiopurine methyltransferase activity in a French population: h.p.l.c. assay conditions and effects of drugs and inhibitors. Br J Clin Pharmacol. 1994;38:1–8.
32. Krynetski EY, Tai HL, Yates CR, et al. Genetic polymorphism of thiopurine S-methyltransferase: clinical importance and molecular mechanisms. Pharmacogenetics. 1996;6:279–90.
33. Lennard L. Clinical implications of thiopurine methyltransferase—optimization of drug dosage and potential drug interactions. Ther Drug Monit. 1998;20:527–31.
34. Lennard L. Therapeutic drug monitoring of antimetabolic cytotoxic drugs. Br J Clin Pharmacol. 1999;47:131–43.
35. Krynetski E, Evans WE. Drug methylation in cancer therapy: lessons from the TPMT polymorphism. Oncogene. 2003;22:7403–13.
36. Heggie GD, Sommadossi JP, Cross DS, Huster WJ, Diasio RB. Clinical pharmacokinetics of 5-fluorouracil and its metabolites in plasma, urine, and bile. Cancer Res. 1987;47:2203–6.
37. Fleming RA, Milano G, Thyss A, et al. Correlation between dihydropyrimidine dehydrogenase activity in peripheral mononuclear cells and systemic clearance of fluorouracil in cancer patients. Cancer Res. 1992;52:2899–902.
38. Diasio RB, Harris BE. Clinical pharmacology of 5-fluorouracil. Clin Pharm. 1989;16:215–37.
39. Harris BE, Song R, Soong SJ, Diasio RB. Relationship between dihydropyrimidine dehydrogenase activity and plasma 5-fluorouracil levels with evidence for circadian variation of enzyme activity and plasma drug levels in cancer patients receiving 5-fluorouracil by protracted continuous infusion. Cancer Res. 1990;50:197–201.
40. Etienne MC, Lagrange JL, Dassonville O, et al. Population study of dihydropyrimidine dehydrogenase in cancer patients. J Clin Oncol. 1994;12:2248–53.
41. Lu Z, Zhang R, Diasio RB. Dihydropyrimidine dehydrogenase activity in human peripheral blood mononuclear cells and liver: population characteristics, newly identified deficient patients, and clinical implication in 5-fluorouracil chemotherapy. Cancer Res. 1993;53:5433–8.
42. Milano G, Etienne MC, Pierrefite V, Barberi-Heyob M, Deporte-Fety R, Renee N. Dihydropyrimidine dehydrogenase deficiency and fluorouracil-related toxicity. Br J Cancer. 1999;79:627–30.
43. Saeki H, Ito S, Futatsugi M, Kimura Y, Ohga T, Sugimachi K. Role of dihydropyrimidine dehydrogenase activity in patients with esophageal cancer. Anticancer Res. 2002;22:3789–92.
44. Raida M, Schwabe W, Hausler P, et al. Prevalence of a common point mutation in the dihydropyrimidine dehydrogenase (DPD) gene within the 5′-splice donor site of intron 14 in patients with severe 5-fluorouracil (5-FU)- related toxicity compared with controls. Clin Cancer Res. 2001;7:2832–9.
45. Salgueiro N, Veiga I, Fragoso M, et al. Mutations in exon 14 of dihydropyrimidine dehydrogenase and 5-Fluorouracil toxicity in Portuguese colorectal cancer patients. Genet Med. 2004;6:102–7.
46. van Kuilenburg AB, De Abreu RA, van Gennip AH. Pharmacogenetic and clinical aspects of dihydropyrimidine dehydrogenase deficiency. Ann Clin Biochem. 2003;40:41–5.
47. van Kuilenburg AB, Muller EW, Haasjes J, et al. Lethal outcome of a patient with a complete dihydropyrimidine dehydrogenase (DPD) deficiency after administration of 5-fluorouracil: frequency of the common IVS14+1G>A mutation causing DPD deficiency. Clin Cancer Res. 2001;7:1149–53.
48. van Kuilenburg AB, Haasjes J, Richel DJ, et al. Clinical implications of dihydropyrimidine dehydrogenase (DPD) deficiency in patients with severe 5-fluorouracil-associated toxicity: identification of new mutations in the DPD gene. Clin Cancer Res. 2000;6:4705–12.

49. Van Kuilenburg AB, Meinsma R, Zoetekouw L, Van Gennip AH. Increased risk of grade IV neutropenia after administration of 5-fluorouracil due to a dihydropyrimidine dehydrogenase deficiency: high prevalence of the IVS14+1g>a mutation. Int J Cancer. 2002;101:253–8.
50. Johnson MR, Diasio RB. Importance of dihydropyrimidine dehydrogenase (DPD) deficiency in patients exhibiting toxicity following treatment with 5-fluorouracil. Adv Enzyme Regul. 2001;41:151–7.
51. Diasio RB, Beavers TL, Carpenter JT. Familial deficiency of dihydropyrimidine dehydrogenase. Biochemical basis for familial pyrimidinemia and severe 5-fluorouracil-induced toxicity. J Clin Invest. 1988;81:47–51.
52. Mattison LK, Soong R, Diasio RB. Implications of dihydropyrimidine dehydrogenase on 5-fluorouracil pharmacogenetics and pharmacogenomics. Pharmacogenomics. 2002;3: 485–92.
53. McLeod HL, Collie-Duguid ES, Vreken P, et al. Nomenclature for human DPYD alleles. Pharmacogenetics. 1998;8:455–9.
54. Morel A, Boisdron-Celle M, Fey L, et al. Clinical relevance of different dihydropyrimidine dehydrogenase gene single nucleotide polymorphisms on 5-fluorouracil tolerance. Mol Cancer Ther. 2006;5:2895–904.
55. van Kuilenburg AB. Dihydropyrimidine dehydrogenase and the efficacy and toxicity of 5-fluorouracil. Eur J Cancer. 2004;40:939–50.
56. Van Kuilenburg AB, Meinsma R, Zoetekouw L, Van Gennip AH. High prevalence of the IVS14 + 1G>A mutation in the dihydropyrimidine dehydrogenase gene of patients with severe 5-fluorouracil-associated toxicity. Pharmacogenetics. 2002;12:555–8.
57. Vreken P, Van Kuilenburg AB, Meinsma R, et al. A point mutation in an invariant splice donor site leads to exon skipping in two unrelated Dutch patients with dihydropyrimidine dehydrogenase deficiency. J Inherit Metab Dis. 1996;19:645–54.
58. Schwab M, Zanger UM, Marx C, et al. Role of genetic and nongenetic factors for fluorouracil treatment-related severe toxicity: a prospective clinical trial by the German 5-FU Toxicity Study Group. J Clin Oncol. 2008;26:2131–8.
59. Rosenblatt DS. Methylenetetrahydrofolate reductase. Clin Invest Med. 2001;24:56–9.
60. Lewis SJ, Ebrahim S, Davey Smith G. Meta-analysis of MTHFR 677C->T polymorphism and coronary heart disease: does totality of evidence support causal role for homocysteine and preventive potential of folate? BMJ. 2005;331:1053.
61. Ueland PM, Hustad S, Schneede J, Refsum H, Vollset SE. Biological and clinical implications of the MTHFR C677T polymorphism. Trends Pharmacol Sci. 2001;22:195–201.
62. Weisberg I, Tran P, Christensen B, Sibani S, Rozen R. A second genetic polymorphism in methylenetetrahydrofolate reductase (MTHFR) associated with decreased enzyme activity. Mol Genet Metab. 1998;64:169–72.
63. Brattstrom L, Wilcken DE, Ohrvik J, Brudin L. Common methylenetetrahydrofolate reductase gene mutation leads to hyperhomocysteinemia but not to vascular disease: the result of a meta-analysis. Circulation. 1998;98:2520–6.
64. Bagley PJ, Selhub J. A common mutation in the methylenetetrahydrofolate reductase gene is associated with an accumulation of formylated tetrahydrofolates in red blood cells. Proc Natl Acad Sci U S A. 1998;95:13217–20.
65. Bottiger AK, Hurtig-Wennlof A, Sjostrom M, Yngve A, Nilsson TK. Association of total plasma homocysteine with methylenetetrahydrofolate reductase genotypes 677C>T, 1298A>C, and 1793G>A and the corresponding haplotypes in Swedish children and adolescents. Int J Mol Med. 2007;19:659–65.
66. De Mattia E, Toffoli G. C677T and A1298C MTHFR polymorphisms, a challenge for antifolate and fluoropyrimidine-based therapy personalisation. Eur J Cancer. 2009;45:1333–51.
67. Ulvik A, Ueland PM, Fredriksen A, et al. Functional inference of the methylenetetrahydrofolate reductase 677C>T and 1298A>C polymorphisms from a large-scale epidemiological study. Hum Genet. 2007;121:57–64.
68. Ogino S, Wilson RB. Genotype and haplotype distributions of MTHFR677C>T and 1298A>C single nucleotide polymorphisms: a meta-analysis. J Hum Genet. 2003;48:1–7.

69. Bailey LB, Gregory 3rd JF. Polymorphisms of methylenetetrahydrofolate reductase and other enzymes: metabolic significance, risks and impact on folate requirement. J Nutr. 1999;129:919–22.
70. Kawakami K, Omura K, Kanehira E, Watanabe G. Methylenetetrahydrofolate reductase polymorphism is associated with folate pool in gastrointestinal cancer tissue. Anticancer Res. 2001;21:285–9.
71. Costea I, Moghrabi A, Laverdiere C, Graziani A, Krajinovic M. Folate cycle gene variants and chemotherapy toxicity in pediatric patients with acute lymphoblastic leukemia. Haematologica. 2006;91:1113–6.
72. Longley DB, Harkin DP, Johnston PG. 5-fluorouracil: mechanisms of action and clinical strategies. Nat Rev Cancer. 2003;3:330–8.
73. Kuhn JG. Fluorouracil and the new oral fluorinated pyrimidines. Ann Pharmacother. 2001;35:217–27.
74. Sohn KJ, Croxford R, Yates Z, Lucock M, Kim YI. Effect of the methylenetetrahydrofolate reductase C677T polymorphism on chemosensitivity of colon and breast cancer cells to 5-fluorouracil and methotrexate. J Natl Cancer Inst. 2004;96:134–44.
75. Jakobsen A, Nielsen JN, Gyldenkerne N, Lindeberg J. Thymidylate synthase and methylenetetrahydrofolate reductase gene polymorphism in normal tissue as predictors of fluorouracil sensitivity. J Clin Oncol. 2005;23:1365–9.
76. Etienne MC, Formento JL, Chazal M, et al. Methylenetetrahydrofolate reductase gene polymorphisms and response to fluorouracil-based treatment in advanced colorectal cancer patients. Pharmacogenetics. 2004;14:785–92.
77. Cohen V, Panet-Raymond V, Sabbaghian N, Morin I, Batist G, Rozen R. Methylenetetrahydrofolate reductase polymorphism in advanced colorectal cancer: a novel genomic predictor of clinical response to fluoropyrimidine-based chemotherapy. Clin Cancer Res. 2003;9:1611–5.
78. Ruzzo A, Graziano F, Loupakis F, et al. Pharmacogenetic profiling in patients with advanced colorectal cancer treated with first-line FOLFOX-4 chemotherapy. J Clin Oncol. 2007;25:1247–54.
79. Suh KW, Kim JH, Kim do Y, Kim YB, Lee C, Choi S. Which gene is a dominant predictor of response during FOLFOX chemotherapy for the treatment of metastatic colorectal cancer, the MTHFR or XRCC1 gene? Ann Surg Oncol. 2006;13:1379–85.
80. Marcuello E, Altes A, Menoyo A, Rio ED, Baiget M. Methylenetetrahydrofolate reductase gene polymorphisms: genomic predictors of clinical response to fluoropyrimidine-based chemotherapy? Cancer Chemother Pharmacol. 2006;57:835–40.
81. Capitain O, Boisdron-Celle M, Poirier AL, Abadie-Lacourtoisie S, Morel A, Gamelin E. The influence of fluorouracil outcome parameters on tolerance and efficacy in patients with advanced colorectal cancer. Pharmacogenomics J. 2008;8:256–67.
82. Ruzzo A, Graziano F, Loupakis F, et al. Pharmacogenetic profiling in patients with advanced colorectal cancer treated with first-line FOLFIRI chemotherapy. Pharmacogenomics J. 2008;8:278–88.
83. Sharma R, Hoskins JM, Rivory LP, et al. Thymidylate synthase and methylenetetrahydrofolate reductase gene polymorphisms and toxicity to capecitabine in advanced colorectal cancer patients. Clin Cancer Res. 2008;14:817–25.
84. Stevenson JP, Redlinger M, Kluijtmans LA, et al. Phase I clinical and pharmacogenetic trial of irinotecan and raltitrexed administered every 21 days to patients with cancer. J Clin Oncol. 2001;19:4081–7.
85. Danenberg PV. Thymidylate synthetase—a target enzyme in cancer chemotherapy. Biochim Biophys Acta. 1977;473:73–92.
86. Johnston PG, Lenz HJ, Leichman CG, et al. Thymidylate synthase gene and protein expression correlate and are associated with response to 5-fluorouracil in human colorectal and gastric tumors. Cancer Res. 1995;55:1407–12.
87. Aschele C, Debernardis D, Casazza S, et al. Immunohistochemical quantitation of thymidylate synthase expression in colorectal cancer metastases predicts for clinical outcome to fluorouracil-based chemotherapy. J Clin Oncol. 1999;17:1760–70.

88. Popat S, Matakidou A, Houlston RS. Thymidylate synthase expression and prognosis in colorectal cancer: a systematic review and meta-analysis. J Clin Oncol. 2004;22:529–36.
89. Miyoshi T, Kondo K, Toba H, et al. Predictive value of thymidylate synthase and dihydropyrimidine dehydrogenase expression in tumor tissue, regarding the efficacy of postoperatively administered UFT (tegafur+uracil) in patients with non-small cell lung cancer. Anticancer Res. 2007;27:2641–8.
90. Horie N, Aiba H, Oguro K, Hojo H, Takeishi K. Functional analysis and DNA polymorphism of the tandemly repeated sequences in the 5′-terminal regulatory region of the human gene for thymidylate synthase. Cell Struct Funct. 1995;20:191–7.
91. Kawakami K, Ruszkiewicz A, Bennett G, Moore J, Watanabe G, Iacopetta B. The folate pool in colorectal cancers is associated with DNA hypermethylation and with a polymorphism in methylenetetrahydrofolate reductase. Clin Cancer Res. 2003;9:5860–5.
92. Mandola MV, Stoehlmacher J, Muller-Weeks S, et al. A novel single nucleotide polymorphism within the 5′ tandem repeat polymorphism of the thymidylate synthase gene abolishes USF-1 binding and alters transcriptional activity. Cancer Res. 2003;63:2898–904.
93. Morganti M, Ciantelli M, Giglioni B, et al. Relationships between promoter polymorphisms in the thymidylate synthase gene and mRNA levels in colorectal cancers. Eur J Cancer. 2005;41:2176–83.
94. Ulrich CM, Bigler J, Velicer CM, Greene EA, Farin FM, Potter JD. Searching expressed sequence tag databases: discovery and confirmation of a common polymorphism in the thymidylate synthase gene. Cancer Epidemiol Biomarkers Prev. 2000;9:1381–5.
95. Kaneda S, Takeishi K, Ayusawa D, Shimizu K, Seno T, Altman S. Role in translation of a triple tandemly repeated sequence in the 5′-untranslated region of human thymidylate synthase mRNA. Nucleic Acids Res. 1987;15:1259–70.
96. Kawakami K, Salonga D, Park JM, et al. Different lengths of a polymorphic repeat sequence in the thymidylate synthase gene affect translational efficiency but not its gene expression. Clin Cancer Res. 2001;7:4096–101.
97. Gusella M, Bolzonella C, Crepaldi G, Ferrazzi E, Padrini R. A novel G/C single-nucleotide polymorphism in the double 28-bp repeat thymidylate synthase allele. Pharmacogenomics J. 2006;6:421–4.
98. Lincz LF, Scorgie FE, Garg MB, Ackland SP. Identification of a novel single nucleotide polymorphism in the first tandem repeat sequence of the thymidylate synthase 2R allele. Int J Cancer. 2007;120:1930–4.
99. Mandola MV, Stoehlmacher J, Zhang W, et al. A 6 bp polymorphism in the thymidylate synthase gene causes message instability and is associated with decreased intratumoral TS mRNA levels. Pharmacogenetics. 2004;14:319–27.
100. Kawakami K, Graziano F, Watanabe G, et al. Prognostic role of thymidylate synthase polymorphisms in gastric cancer patients treated with surgery and adjuvant chemotherapy. Clin Cancer Res. 2005;11:3778–83.
101. Marsh S, McKay JA, Cassidy J, McLeod HL. Polymorphism in the thymidylate synthase promoter enhancer region in colorectal cancer. Int J Oncol. 2001;19:383–6.
102. Marsh S, Collie-Duguid ES, Li T, Liu X, McLeod HL. Ethnic variation in the thymidylate synthase enhancer region polymorphism among caucasian and asian populations. Genomics. 1999;58:310–2.
103. Marsh S, Ameyaw MM, Githang'a J, Indalo A, Ofori-Adjei D, McLeod HL. Novel thymidylate synthase enhancer region alleles in African populations. Hum Mutat. 2000;16:528.
104. Pullarkat ST, Stoehlmacher J, Ghaderi V, et al. Thymidylate synthase gene polymorphism determines response and toxicity of 5-FU chemotherapy. Pharmacogenomics J. 2001;1:65–70.
105. Villafranca E, Okruzhnov Y, Dominguez MA, et al. Polymorphisms of the repeated sequences in the enhancer region of the thymidylate synthase gene promoter may predict downstaging after preoperative chemoradiation in rectal cancer. J Clin Oncol. 2001;19:1779–86.
106. Gosens MJ, Moerland E, Lemmens VP, Rutten HT, Tan-Go I, van den Brule AJ. Thymidylate synthase genotyping is more predictive for therapy response than immunohistochemistry in patients with colon cancer. Int J Cancer. 2008;123:1941–9.

107. Hitre E, Budai B, Adleff V, et al. Influence of thymidylate synthase gene polymorphisms on the survival of colorectal cancer patients receiving adjuvant 5-fluorouracil. Pharmacogenet Genomics. 2005;15:723–30.
108. Tsuji T, Hidaka S, Sawai T, et al. Polymorphism in the thymidylate synthase promoter enhancer region is not an efficacious marker for tumor sensitivity to 5-fluorouracil-based oral adjuvant chemotherapy in colorectal cancer. Clin Cancer Res. 2003;9:3700–4.
109. Dotor E, Cuatrecases M, Martinez-Iniesta M, et al. Tumor thymidylate synthase 1494del6 genotype as a prognostic factor in colorectal cancer patients receiving fluorouracil-based adjuvant treatment. J Clin Oncol. 2006;24:1603–11.
110. Ichikawa W, Takahashi T, Suto K, Sasaki Y, Hirayama R. Orotate phosphoribosyltransferase gene polymorphism predicts toxicity in patients treated with bolus 5-fluorouracil regimen. Clin Cancer Res. 2006;12:3928–34.
111. Lecomte T, Ferraz JM, Zinzindohoue F, et al. Thymidylate synthase gene polymorphism predicts toxicity in colorectal cancer patients receiving 5-fluorouracil-based chemotherapy. Clin Cancer Res. 2004;10:5880–8.
112. Seo BG, Kwon HC, Oh SY, et al. Comprehensive analysis of excision repair complementation group 1, glutathione S-transferase, thymidylate synthase and uridine diphosphate glucuronosyl transferase 1A1 polymorphisms predictive for treatment outcome in patients with advanced gastric cancer treated with FOLFOX or FOLFIRI. Oncol Rep. 2009;22: 127–36.
113. Park DJ, Stoehlmacher J, Zhang W, Tsao-Wei D, Groshen S, Lenz HJ. Thymidylate synthase gene polymorphism predicts response to capecitabine in advanced colorectal cancer. Int J Colorectal Dis. 2002;17:46–9.
114. Gusella M, Frigo AC, Bolzonella C, et al. Predictors of survival and toxicity in patients on adjuvant therapy with 5-fluorouracil for colorectal cancer. Br J Cancer. 2009;100:1549–57.
115. Ouzzine M, Barre L, Netter P, Magdalou J, Fournel-Gigleux S. The human UDP-glucuronosyltransferases: structural aspects and drug glucuronidation. Drug Metab Rev. 2003;35:287–303.
116. Kiang TK, Ensom MH, Chang TK. UDP-glucuronosyltransferases and clinical drug-drug interactions. Pharmacol Ther. 2005;106:97–132.
117. Mathijssen RH, Marsh S, Karlsson MO, et al. Irinotecan pathway genotype analysis to predict pharmacokinetics. Clin Cancer Res. 2003;9:3246–53.
118. Mathijssen RH, van Alphen RJ, Verweij J, et al. Clinical pharmacokinetics and metabolism of irinotecan (CPT-11). Clin Cancer Res. 2001;7:2182–94.
119. Guillemette C. Pharmacogenomics of human UDP-glucuronosyltransferase enzymes. Pharmacogenomics J. 2003;3:136–58.
120. Innocenti F, Ratain MJ. "Irinogenetics" and UGT1A: from genotypes to haplotypes. Clin Pharmacol Ther. 2004;75:495–500.
121. van Es HH, Bout A, Liu J, et al. Assignment of the human UDP glucuronosyltransferase gene (UGT1A1) to chromosome region 2q37. Cytogenet Cell Genet. 1993;63:114–6.
122. Gong QH, Cho JW, Huang T, et al. Thirteen UDPglucuronosyltransferase genes are encoded at the human UGT1 gene complex locus. Pharmacogenetics. 2001;11:357–68.
123. Bosma PJ, Chowdhury JR, Bakker C, et al. The genetic basis of the reduced expression of bilirubin UDP-glucuronosyltransferase 1 in Gilbert's syndrome. N Engl J Med. 1995;333: 1171–5.
124. Bosma PJ, Chowdhury JR, Huang TJ, et al. Mechanisms of inherited deficiencies of multiple UDP-glucuronosyltransferase isoforms in two patients with Crigler-Najjar syndrome, type I. FASEB J. 1992;6:2859–63.
125. Aono S, Yamada Y, Keino H, et al. Identification of defect in the genes for bilirubin UDP-glucuronosyl-transferase in a patient with Crigler-Najjar syndrome type II. Biochem Biophys Res Commun. 1993;197:1239–44.
126. Monaghan G, Ryan M, Seddon R, Hume R, Burchell B. Genetic variation in bilirubin UPD-glucuronosyltransferase gene promoter and Gilbert's syndrome. Lancet. 1996;347:578–81.
127. Wasserman E, Myara A, Lokiec F, et al. Severe CPT-11 toxicity in patients with Gilbert's syndrome: two case reports. Ann Oncol. 1997;8:1049–51.

128. Iyer L, King CD, Whitington PF, et al. Genetic predisposition to the metabolism of irinotecan (CPT-11). Role of uridine diphosphate glucuronosyltransferase isoform 1A1 in the glucuronidation of its active metabolite (SN-38) in human liver microsomes. J Clin Invest. 1998;101:847–54.
129. Ando Y, Ueoka H, Sugiyama T, Ichiki M, Shimokata K, Hasegawa Y. Polymorphisms of UDP-glucuronosyltransferase and pharmacokinetics of irinotecan. Ther Drug Monit. 2002;24:111–6.
130. Iyer L, Hall D, Das S, et al. Phenotype-genotype correlation of in vitro SN-38 (active metabolite of irinotecan) and bilirubin glucuronidation in human liver tissue with UGT1A1 promoter polymorphism. Clin Pharmacol Ther. 1999;65:576–82.
131. Paoluzzi L, Singh AS, Price DK, et al. Influence of genetic variants in UGT1A1 and UGT1A9 on the in vivo glucuronidation of SN-38. J Clin Pharmacol. 2004;44:854–60.
132. Innocenti F, Undevia SD, Iyer L, et al. Genetic variants in the UDP-glucuronosyltransferase 1A1 gene predict the risk of severe neutropenia of irinotecan. J Clin Oncol. 2004;22:1382–8.
133. Rouits E, Boisdron-Celle M, Dumont A, Guerin O, Morel A, Gamelin E. Relevance of different UGT1A1 polymorphisms in irinotecan-induced toxicity: a molecular and clinical study of 75 patients. Clin Cancer Res. 2004;10:5151–9.
134. Ando Y, Saka H, Ando M, et al. Polymorphisms of UDP-glucuronosyltransferase gene and irinotecan toxicity: a pharmacogenetic analysis. Cancer Res. 2000;60:6921–6.
135. Marcuello E, Altes A, Menoyo A, Del Rio E, Gomez-Pardo M, Baiget M. UGT1A1 gene variations and irinotecan treatment in patients with metastatic colorectal cancer. Br J Cancer. 2004;91:678–82.
136. Carlini LE, Meropol NJ, Bever J, et al. UGT1A7 and UGT1A9 polymorphisms predict response and toxicity in colorectal cancer patients treated with capecitabine/irinotecan. Clin Cancer Res. 2005;11:1226–36.
137. Toffoli G, Cecchin E, Corona G, et al. The role of UGT1A1*28 polymorphism in the pharmacodynamics and pharmacokinetics of irinotecan in patients with metastatic colorectal cancer. J Clin Oncol. 2006;24:3061–8.
138. Massacesi C, Terrazzino S, Marcucci F, et al. Uridine diphosphate glucuronosyl transferase 1A1 promoter polymorphism predicts the risk of gastrointestinal toxicity and fatigue induced by irinotecan-based chemotherapy. Cancer. 2006;106:1007–16.
139. Hoskins JM, Goldberg RM, Qu P, Ibrahim JG, McLeod HL. UGT1A1*28 genotype and irinotecan-induced neutropenia: dose matters. J Natl Cancer Inst. 2007;99:1290–5.
140. Roth AD, Yan P, Dietrich D, et al. Is UGT1A1*28 homozygosity the strongest predictor for severe hematotoxicity in patients treated with 5-fluorouracil (5-FU)-irinotecan (IRI)? Results of the PETACC 3 - EORTC 40993 -SAKK 60/00 trial comparing IRI/5-FU/folinic acid (FA) to 5-FU/FA in stage II- III colon cancer (COC) patients. J Clin Oncol 2008;26:187S (suppl;abstract 4036).
141. Innocenti F, Grimsley C, Das S, et al. Haplotype structure of the UDP-glucuronosyltransferase 1A1 promoter in different ethnic groups. Pharmacogenetics. 2002;12:725–33.
142. Zhou Q, Sparreboom A, Tan EH, et al. Pharmacogenetic profiling across the irinotecan pathway in Asian patients with cancer. Br J Clin Pharmacol. 2005;59:415–24.
143. Cote JF, Kirzin S, Kramar A, et al. UGT1A1 polymorphism can predict hematologic toxicity in patients treated with irinotecan. Clin Cancer Res. 2007;13:3269–75.
144. Kitagawa C, Ando M, Ando Y, et al. Genetic polymorphism in the phenobarbital-responsive enhancer module of the UDP-glucuronosyltransferase 1A1 gene and irinotecan toxicity. Pharmacogenet Genomics. 2005;15:35–41.
145. Sai K, Saeki M, Saito Y, et al. UGT1A1 haplotypes associated with reduced glucuronidation and increased serum bilirubin in irinotecan-administered Japanese patients with cancer. Clin Pharmacol Ther. 2004;75:501–15.
146. Ando M, Ando Y, Sekido Y, Shimokata K, Hasegawa Y. Genetic polymorphisms of the UDP-glucuronosyltransferase 1A7 gene and irinotecan toxicity in Japanese cancer patients. Jpn J Cancer Res. 2002;93:591–7.

147. Guillemette C, Ritter JK, Auyeung DJ, Kessler FK, Housman DE. Structural heterogeneity at the UDP-glucuronosyltransferase 1 locus: functional consequences of three novel missense mutations in the human UGT1A7 gene. Pharmacogenetics. 2000;10:629–44.
148. Villeneuve L, Girard H, Fortier LC, Gagne JF, Guillemette C. Novel functional polymorphisms in the UGT1A7 and UGT1A9 glucuronidating enzymes in Caucasian and African-American subjects and their impact on the metabolism of 7-ethyl-10-hydroxycamptothecin and flavopiridol anticancer drugs. J Pharmacol Exp Ther. 2003;307:117–28.
149. Takasuna K, Hagiwara T, Hirohashi M, et al. Involvement of beta-glucuronidase in intestinal microflora in the intestinal toxicity of the antitumor camptothecin derivative irinotecan hydrochloride (CPT-11) in rats. Cancer Res. 1996;56:3752–7.
150. Han J-Y, Lim H-S, Shin ES, et al. Comprehensive analysis of UGT1A polymorphisms predictive for pharmacokinetics and treatment outcome in patients with non-small-cell lung cancer treated with irinotecan and cisplatin. J Clin Oncol. 2006;24:2237–44.
151. Yamanaka H, Nakajima M, Katoh M, et al. A novel polymorphism in the promoter region of human UGT1A9 gene (UGT1A9*22) and its effects on the transcriptional activity. Pharmacogenetics. 2004;14:329–32.
152. Schneider BP, Wang M, Radovich M, et al. Association of vascular endothelial growth factor and vascular endothelial growth factor receptor-2 genetic polymorphisms with outcome in a trial of paclitaxel compared with paclitaxel plus bevacizumab in advanced breast cancer: ECOG 2100. J Clin Oncol. 2008;26:4672–8.
153. Chrysogelos SA. Chromatin structure of the EGFR gene suggests a role for intron 1 sequences in its regulation in breast cancer cells. Nucleic Acids Res. 1993;21:5736–41.
154. Brandt B, Meyer-Staeckling S, Schmidt H, Agelopoulos K, Buerger H. Mechanisms of egfr gene transcription modulation: relationship to cancer risk and therapy response. Clin Cancer Res. 2006;12:7252–60.
155. Liu W, Innocenti F, Wu MH, et al. A functional common polymorphism in a Sp1 recognition site of the epidermal growth factor receptor gene promoter. Cancer Res. 2005;65:46–53.
156. Rudin CM, Liu W, Desai A, et al. Pharmacogenomic and pharmacokinetic determinants of erlotinib toxicity. J Clin Oncol. 2008;26:1119–27.
157. Graziano F, Ruzzo A, Loupakis F, et al. Pharmacogenetic profiling for cetuximab plus irinotecan therapy in patients with refractory advanced colorectal cancer. J Clin Oncol. 2008;26:1427–34.
158. Li J, Cusatis G, Brahmer J, et al. Association of variant ABCG2 and the pharmacokinetics of epidermal growth factor receptor tyrosine kinase inhibitors in cancer patients. Cancer Biol Ther. 2007;6:432–8.
159. Cusatis G, Gregorc V, Li J, et al. Pharmacogenetics of ABCG2 and adverse reactions to gefitinib. J Natl Cancer Inst. 2006;98:1739–42.

Chapter 11
Surrogate Markers: The Role of Positron Emission Tomography Scanning

Derek G. Power and David H. Ilson

Introduction

Individualization of cancer treatment resulting in optimization of outcomes is a priority of modern oncology research. Cancer treatment is increasingly multidisciplinary. Trimodality therapy of surgery, radiation, and chemotherapy has resulted in better outcomes for many solid tumor malignancies. Multimodal strategies are now commonly used in gastrointestinal cancers. The use of concurrent chemotherapy and radiation is an accepted approach in localized rectal, esophagogastric, and pancreatic cancers, although the role of radiotherapy remains controversial [1–3]. There have been recent and significant developments in the understanding of cancer pathogenesis at the molecular level. Targeted therapies acting on key elements of cancer pathways have modestly improved outcomes in advanced solid tumor malignancies. Vascular endothelial growth factor inhibitors, e.g., bevacizumab, and epidermal growth factor receptor inhibitors, e.g., cetuximab, are now commonly combined with chemotherapy in the treatment of metastatic colorectal cancer [4, 5].

The identification of those patients destined to fail to respond to therapy is a challenge. There is often a wide differential in response to multimodal treatment. The timing and the decision to operate on localized disease often depend on response to preoperative treatment. The early identification of responding patients may provide reassurance as to efficacy of the current treatment, and could potentially avoid needless toxicity and expense from a presumably ineffective regimen. Much work has been done studying the genetic heterogeneity of gastrointestinal cancers in an attempt to identify biomarkers and genetic/protein signatures that predict response

D.G. Power, M.D.
Department of Medicine, Gastrointestinal Oncology Service, Memorial Sloan Kettering Cancer Center, New York, NY, USA

D.H. Ilson, M.D., Ph.D. (✉)
Department of Medical Oncology Solid Tumor GI, Memorial Sloan-Kettering Cancer Center, 1275 York Avenue, H-192, New York, NY 10065, USA
e-mail: ilsond@mskcc.org

H.-J. Lenz (ed.), *Biomarkers in Oncology: Prediction and Prognosis*,
DOI 10.1007/978-1-4419-9755-5_11,

to treatment and favorable outcome [6, 7]. To date, the lack of validation and clinical applicability of candidate biomarkers has limited their ability to predict those patients who will respond to treatment or to serve as prognostic markers for better outcome. The use of metabolic imaging with fluorodeoxyglucose (FDG)-positron emission tomography (PET) scanning has become a valuable tool in oncology and, with combined CT technology, can play an important role in diagnosis and staging of the disease. The Biomarkers Definitions Working Group includes the use of imaging techniques for detection and staging of cancer [8]. This review will focus on the role of PET as a surrogate marker in assessing tumor response to therapy and tumor control in prognosis. Gastroesophageal cancer has provided a paradigm for PET response assessment strategies. Our review will deal primarily with upper gastrointestinal cancers.

Gastroesophageal Cancer

Globally both gastric and esophageal cancers are significant health problems and account for approximately 1.4 million new cases per year with 1.1 million cancer-related deaths [9]. The last three decades have seen a dramatic epidemiologic shift in the location of both gastric and esophageal cancers as well as the histologic subtype of esophageal cancers. Tumors of the lower esophagus and proximal stomach are classified as gastro-esophageal junction (GEJ) cancers and this cancer has been increasing by 5–10% per year since the mid 1970s and is the most rapidly increasing cancer in many Western countries [10]. Distal esophageal and GEJ adenocarcinoma are now the predominant esophageal cancer subtype, and the majority of gastric cancers are now located in the proximal stomach [11]. The 5 year survival of gastro-esophageal cancers (distal esophagus, GEJ, and proximal stomach being the majority of cases) has not changed significantly over the last 25–30 years. Approximately 50–60% of patients present with distant metastatic disease and the median overall survival with systemic chemotherapy have remained at less than 1 year [12]. However, progress has been made in the treatment of localized disease. While surgery is the cornerstone of treatment for localized disease, local and distant recurrence is commonplace [13]. It is now accepted that neoadjuvant treatment with chemotherapy (including perioperative treatment) or chemoradiotherapy can improve outcome compared with surgery alone in locally advanced esophagogastric cancer [14]. Adjuvant chemoradiation [15] or adjuvant chemotherapy (in an Asian population) [16] may also play a role. Treatment is generally better tolerated prior to surgery and neoadjuvant strategies are increasingly being accepted as a standard for localized disease [3, 17–19]. Outcomes still remain poor however. The median overall survival for localized gastroesophageal cancer is 18–22 months and 5 year survival rates rarely exceed 20–40% [20].

The challenge has been to identify patients who respond to neoadjuvant therapy as it has been shown that these patients have superior outcomes. Pathologic complete response (pCR) after neoadjuvant therapy is associated with an increased chance, of long term survival, of up to 50–60% at 5 years [21]. However, only 40–50% of patients have any response (partial or complete) to therapy. Biomarkers to identify these patients have been evaluated mostly in the context of single arm, phase II studies, but without validation in controlled trials they have limited clinical applicability to date [7, 22]. Metabolic imaging with PET/CT scanning for potential response assessment is proving to be more readily applicable to the clinic, and many studies have reported promising results.

PET Scanning

A PET scan provides unique information about metabolic changes associated with disease in a noninvasive way and can visualize the whole tumor [23]. This overcomes the problem of intratumoral heterogeneity which has been a significant issue with biomarker analysis derived from tumor biopsies. FDG-PET exploits the increased use of glucose by the cancer cell. There are many molecular probes that can be labeled with positron emitters (Table 11.1), however the vast majority of clinical experience with PET scanning has been amassed using the glucose analogue, FDG, labeled with the positron emitter fluorine-18 (^{18}F). FDG accumulates markedly in the majority of human cancer cells and PET scanning using the radiolabeled tracer ^{18}F-FDG can therefore assess the preferentially high rate of glucose turnover in cancer cells. In recent years ^{18}F-FDG PET has become a valuable imaging modality in a wide variety of malignancies. The main use has been in cancer diagnosis and staging. ^{18}F-FDG PET has its limitations however. False positives are seen in infectious or inflammatory tissue [24]. This can be of particular importance if one is assessing response in irradiated tissue. A time-dependent "metabolic-flare" phenomenon due to energy dependent cellular repair mechanisms can result after

Table 11.1 PET-tracers used in oncology

Tracer	Measured effect
^{18}F-FDG	Glucose metabolism
^{18}F-FLT	DNA synthesis
^{11}C-Methionine	Protein synthesis
^{11}C-Tyrosine	Amino acid transport
^{11}C-Fluorotyrosine	Amino acid transport
^{11}C-Fluoroethyltyrosine	Amino acid transport
^{11}C-Fluorohydroxyphenylalanine	Amino acid transport Dopamine synthesis
^{11}C-Choline	Cell membrane metabolism
^{18}F-Fluorocholine	Cell membrane metabolism
^{18}F-Fluoro-17β(beta)-estradiol	Estrogen receptor status
^{18}F-Fluorodihydrotestosterone	Androgen receptor status
^{18}F-Octreotide(analogues)	Somatostatin receptor status
^{15}O-Water	Perfusion

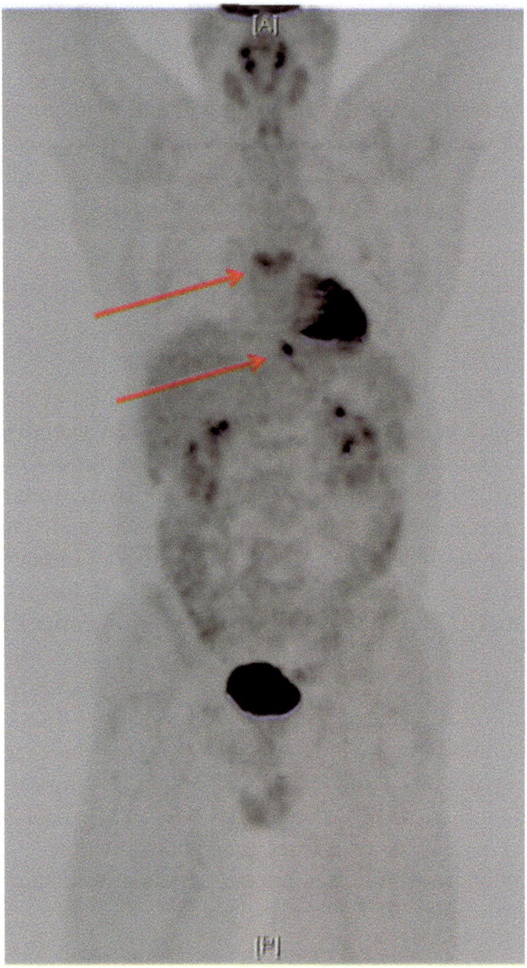

Fig. 11.1 F18-FDG PET scan showing increased FDG uptake in the distal esophagus/GEJ (SUV = 6.9) representing malignancy (*red arrow*). Another abnormal focus of FDG uptake is seen in the sternum (SUV = 6.0) representing a lytic bone metastasis (*red arrow*). The remainder of the tracer distribution is within normal limits

treatment with chemoradiation and can lead to confusing PET findings. Weaknesses of PET include the following: (1) if a tumor is sub 5 mm the resolution of ^{18}F-FDG PET is poor; (2) tumors with a low metabolic rate, e.g., gastric mucinous adenocarcinoma, may not pick up the radiolabeled tracer; and (3) if the tumor is located in a region of the body with high metabolic activity, e.g., brain, it may be missed. The latter can be of relevance if one is following up a patient with brain metastases. ^{18}F-FDG PET is now approved for use in the baseline staging of many malignancies and is included as level 2A evidence in National Comprehensive Cancer Network Guidelines (NCCN® Practice Guidelines in Oncology-v1.2009). The main role of PET in staging of solid tumor malignancies is to rule out distant metastatic disease in those cases where the staging CT scan does not show metastatic disease and a surgical strategy is being considered. Figure 11.1 shows an F18-FDG PET scan showing increased FDG uptake in the distal esophagus/GEJ (SUV = 6.9) representing malignancy (red arrow). Another abnormal focus of FDG uptake is seen in the sternum (SUV=6.0) representing a lytic bone metastasis (red arrow). The remainder of the tracer distribution is within normal limits. In recent times PET scans have been integrated with CT scans to provide concurrent fused metabolic and structural images. This allows for both the accurate localization of metabolically active lesions and an assessment of indeterminate CT masses [23, 25].

PET has been found to have a useful role in many other aspects of cancer care, including planning of radiotherapy treatment fields. PET imaging of radiolabeled anticancer drugs has been useful to noninvasively study tissue pharmacokinetics [26]. The identification of therapeutic targets and monitoring their inhibition has been studied in antiestrogen therapy and ER-positive breast cancer, antiandrogen therapy in prostate cancer, and octreotide therapy in neuroendocrine tumors [27–29]. Imaging of brain tumors has been studied by amino-acid PET and has lead to improved radiotherapy planning [30]. Monitoring cancer processes such as tumor cell proliferation, apoptosis, and perfusion using a variety of positron emitting molecular probes, e.g., ^{18}F-Thymidine, ^{15}O-Water, amino acids, and choline, have also been investigated [31].

Monitoring effectiveness of cancer treatment has highlighted a potential role for PET as an imaging biomarker that may be easily transferable to the clinical setting. Many studies have shown that a persistently abnormal ^{18}F-FDG PET scan after completion of chemotherapy or chemoradiation is directly associated with a high risk of recurrence and a poor prognosis [31]. Much of the data have been reported in malignant lymphoma, but gastrointestinal, breast, and lung cancer studies have shown similar data. Early PET imaging (within 2–4 weeks of starting treatment) compared to a baseline scan can show a favorable or unfavorable response and may warrant a change in therapy prior to surgical intervention. The rationale for this strategy is that metabolic changes, as seen on PET scan, precede structural changes seen on CT scan [32, 33]. Such a strategy is particularly attractive in localized gastroesophageal cancer as the optimal timing of major surgery is of critical importance. The post-treatment T and N stage predicts survival and therefore accurate early assessment of response to preoperative therapy, not feasible by conventional CT scan imaging, may be most useful.

Many different methods have been used to assess tumor uptake of PET tracers, e.g., Tumor to Liver Ratios (TLR) and Tumor to Non-Tumor Ratios. However, the Standardized Uptake Value (SUV) has proven to be the most reproducible [34, 35]. Attempting to extrapolate SUV data analogous to WHO and RECIST responses reported in CT imaging is likely to be suboptimal, as threshold SUV is likely to be disease specific. For optimal therapeutic response assessment, changes of the SUV relative to baseline have been shown to be the most reliable parameter [34]. Several studies have looked at methodological variations in the acquisition of PET data, which could result in nonstandardized reporting of data. These included imaging time after FDG injection, acquisition protocol, reconstruction algorithm, PET versus PET/CT, and SUV normalization. In these studies, the prediction of response to chemotherapy as assessed by SUV changes was not influenced by any of these factors, thus demonstrating the robustness of FDG-PET across institutions and protocols

[36, 37]. The European Organization of Research and Treatment of Cancer (EORTC) have endorsed changes in SUV during therapy as assessed by PET or PET/CT as a methodologically reliable and validated response parameter [34].

Gastroesophageal Cancer and PET

^{18}F-FDG PET and ^{18}F-FDG PET/CT can be used to assess response to therapy in localized gastroesophageal cancers in two different ways: early in therapy, or after completion of therapy prior to surgery. Most studies have evaluated PET response after completion of preoperative therapy. In this setting, residual ^{18}F-FDG uptake on the post-therapy scan is correlated with the initial PET/CT scan, with histopathologic response, and with survival. The hypothesis is that an FDG-avid tumor that returns to background FDG level after treatment should not contain residual cancer, and those tumors that maintain residual FDG activity contain viable tumor and will have a worse outcome.

A few studies have examined the role of ^{18}F-FDG PET and ^{18}F-FDG PET/CT earlier on in the course of therapy, prior to therapy completion, i.e., after 2–6 weeks. Changes in the pretreatment and early follow-up scan are assessed by percentage SUV drop. If this drop is above a predefined threshold, then this may reflect response to treatment, which can be used to predict final histopathologic response and ultimately patient survival. Early PET response may act as a surrogate biomarker for response to treatment and outcome prior to a major surgical intervention. Treatment could potentially be changed or surgery performed earlier in nonresponding patients.

PET Response After Completion of Therapy

There are 22 studies examining PET response after completion of preoperative therapy for gastroesophageal cancer (four of these studies also look at early response assessment) (Tables 11.2 and 11.3) [33, 38–58]. Most of the studies use combined chemoradiation prior to surgery. One of the earliest studies is by Brucher and colleagues who reported a prospective study of 27 patients with squamous cell carcinoma of the esophagus who underwent concurrent chemoradiation with 5-fluorouracil. They defined a PET response as ≥52% reduction in SUV. This threshold for response was strongly associated with median overall survival compared with PET nonresponders (22.5 months versus 8.8 months for responders and nonresponders respectively, $p=0.0001$) [40]. The threshold for response also differentiated histopathologic responders from nonresponders with a sensitivity of 100% and a specificity of 55%. Flamen and colleagues showed in 36 patients with esophageal cancer (27 cases were squamous cell carcinoma and 9 were adenocarcinoma of the GEJ) that a >80% reduction of the tumor to liver tracer uptake ratio (TLR) strongly correlated with a major response to preoperative chemoradiation. Sensitivity was 71% and specificity

Table 11.2 ^{18}F-FDG-PET and ^{18}F-FDG-PET/CT response after completion of preoperative therapy for localized gastroesophageal cancer

Study	Site	Tumor type	Design	*n*	Rx	PET response	Path response	Outcome
Brucher [40]	E	SCC	P	27	CRT	≥52%↓SUV	<10%	PET correlated with OS
Kato [45]	E	SCC	R	10	CRT	59.8%↓SUV	<1/3	Δ(delta)SUV no correlation
Flamen [44]	E/GEJ	SCC/A	P	36	CRT	≥80%↓TLR	pCR	PET correlated with OS
Arslan [38]	E	SCC/A	R	24	CRT	NR	pCR or mic disease	Δ(delta)Tumor Vol correlates with PATH
Downey [42]	E	SCC/A	P	39	CRT	≥60%↓SUV	NR	PET correlated with OS/DFS
Brink [39]	E	SCC/A	P	20	CRT	NR	NR	Δ(delta)SUV no correlation
Swisher [54]	E	SCC/A	R	83	CRT		<10%	Posttherapy SUV<4 correlates with PATH
Javeri [55]	E/GEJ	A	R	151	CRT	>52%↓SUV [dichotomized analysis]		%SUV↓ predicts OS ($p=0.01$) [continuous variable]
Melcher [49]	E	SCC/A	P	23	C	NR	<10%	Δ(delta)SUV no correlat'n with PATH
Song [53]	E	SCC	P	32	CRT	87.9%↓SUV	pCR	PET correlates with PATH if 1st SUV≥4
Cerfolio [41]	E/GEJ	SCC/A	P	48	CRT	Median%↓SUVmax	pCR	PET predicts pCR
Duong [43]	E/GEJ	SCC/A	P	53	CRT	CMR	NR	PET correlates with OS
Kim [46]	E	SCC	P	62	CRT	CMR	pCR and mic disease	CMR correlates with DFS/OS
Mamede [47]	E	SCC/A	R	25	CRT	<59.4%↓SUV	<10%	PET associated with PATH (64% accuracy)
Smithers [52]	E/GEJ	A	P	23	C	84.6%↓SUV	TRG 1–2	PET does not correlate with PATH
				23	CRT	52.1%↓SUV	TRG 1–2	
Port [50]	E	SCC/A	R	62	C	>50%↓SUV	<10%	PET correlates with DFS
McLouh [48]	E	SCC/A	R	81	CRT	CMR	pCR	CMR no correlat'n with PATH
Schmidt [51]	E	SCC/A	P	55	CRT	Correlate with Path response	<10%	Δ(delta)SUV no correlat'n with PATH or survival

A adenocarcinoma, *SCC* squamous cell carcinoma, *CRT* chemoradiotherapy, *TLR* tumor liver ratio, *NR* not reported, *pCR* pathologic complete response, *TRG* Tumor regression grade, *SUV* Standard uptake value, *CMR* Complete metabolic response, *PATH* Pathology, *E* Esophagus, *P* Prospective, *R* Randomized, *mic* microscopic, *C* Chemotherapy, *GEJ* Gastroesophageal junction

Table 11.3 ^{18}F-FDG-PET and ^{18}F-FDG-PET/CT response early and after completion of preoperative therapy for localized gastroesophageal cancer

Study	Site	Tumor type	Design	*n*	Rx	PET response	Path response	Outcome
Kroep [57]	E/GEJ	SCC/A	P	13	C	≥40%↓SUV at 6 weeks ≥60%↓SUV at complet'n	<10% <10%	PET at complet'n correlates with PATH
Wieder [33]	E	SCC	P	38	CRT	>30%↓SUV at 2 weeks >52%↓SUV at complet'n	<10% <10%	Early PET correlates with OS
Levine [58]	E	SCC/A	P	57	CRT	NR	pCR or mic disease	SUV > 15 at 2 weeks correlates with PATH
Konski [56]	E/GEJ	SCC/A	R	44	CRT	NR	pCR	No correlat'n bt early or late PET and PATH

SUV Standard uptake value, *PATH* Pathology

was 82%. The concordance between response by PET, as defined above, and histopathology was 78%. The median overall survival for PET responders compared with nonresponders was 16.3 months versus 6.4 months, respectively, $p=0.002$ [44]. Downey and colleagues from our institution enrolled 39 patients with esophageal cancer (adenocarcinoma and squamous cell carcinoma) in a prospective study assessing baseline PET, PET response after treatment with induction chemoradiation, and then surgery. PET response was defined as ≥60% reduction in SUV. Two year overall survival for responders was 89% compared with 63% for nonresponders ($p=0.088$). Disease free survival at 2 years trended towards significance (63% versus 38% respectively, $p=0.055$) [42]. Only 17 patients in this study underwent esophagectomy. Normalization of the PET scan after chemoradiation did not correlate with the achievement of a pathologic complete response.

One of the largest retrospective data series is reported by Swisher et al. The best prognosticator of survival was an SUV of <4 after completion of preoperative chemoradiation. The survival at 18 months for PET responders was 77% compared with 34% for nonresponders ($p=0.01$). Histopathologic response, with an accuracy of 76% and corresponding sensitivity and specificity of 62% and 84% respectively, was also associated with PET response ($p=0.01$) [54]. Notably, in this series PET response also could not rule out residual disease found at surgery as ^{18}F-FDG uptake in the tumor bed was the same in patients with a pCR and those with <10% viable cells. Swisher and colleagues also recently reported an updated series of 151 patients with gastroesophageal adenocarcinoma who received preoperative chemoradiation. In multivariate analysis, the percentage SUV decrease (as a continuous variable) was the only prognosticator of overall survival, OR 0.99 (95% CI 0.987–0.998), $p=0.01$. There was no significant association between pathologic complete response and percentage SUV decrease [55]. Another retrospective study of 81 patients by McLoughlin and colleagues reported that complete PET response could not differentiate pCR from those who still had residual disease. The authors recommend that all patients should still be referred for surgical resection in the absence of distant metastatic disease [48]. In a prospective study of 48 patients with adenocarcinoma (85%) or squamous carcinoma (15%) of the esophagus, Cerfolio et al. reported that ^{18}F-FDG PET/CT was more accurate than EUS/FNA and CT in predicting a pCR. The accuracy, sensitivity and specificity of PET were 88%, 87%, and 88% respectively [41]. Port et al. reported a retrospective series of 62 patients with esophageal cancer (51 cases of adenocarcinoma). Similar to the studies by Swisher and Javeri, complete PET response was not associated with pCR. However patients with a ≥50% reduction in SUV had a significantly superior disease free survival than PET nonresponders (35.5 months versus 17.9 months, respectively, $p=0.03$) [50]. A recent prospective study by Kim et al. using platinum-based chemoradiation defined complete response by ^{18}F-FDG PET as >80% reduction in SUV. On multivariate analysis complete PET response was independently associated with better disease free survival and overall survival ($p=0.006$, and $p=0.033$, respectively). At a median follow-up of 19.3 months (range, 3.9–57.1 months), median overall survival (OS) was not reached in patients with complete metabolic response, compared to 22.4 months in patients who did not achieve complete metabolic response [46].

In the majority of these studies (Tables 11.2 and 11.3), improvement in SUV levels is positively correlated with histopathologic response and better outcome (DFS and OS). However, it is difficult to draw definitive conclusions from small studies and retrospective data. Also, many of the studies assessing late PET response differ in the timing of the second PET scan after completion of chemoradiation (2–7 weeks), which results in nonstandardized reporting of the second SUV. The optimal time to obtain the posttreatment PET scan is not known with certainty [56]. It is possible that posttreatment inflammation could falsely elevate the posttreatment SUV if the scan is obtained too soon after treatment. A long interval between treatment completion and the second scan could result in a larger percent SUV reduction as seen in the Levine study [58]. As therapy is completed prior to the second PET scan, it is almost academic what this scan shows, as we will know the pathologic stage when the patient has surgery, and it is the pT and N findings which will determine overall survival. A posttherapy PET scan, therefore, may have no impact on therapeutic decision making.

Konski and colleagues were the first to report the use of PET in after chemoradiation in patients with esophageal cancer who did not undergo surgery. In a total of 81 patients, 44 underwent esophagectomy (95% adenocarcinoma). Univariate-analysis revealed posttreatment SUV predicted disease free survival in the definitive, non surgical chemoradiation group. Twenty-five of 37 patients had performance of a posttreatment PET scan. The median decrease in SUV was 65%, and a 1 unit increase in the posttreatment SUV increased disease-specific mortality by 30% ($p=0.01$). SUV, however, was not significant on multivariate analysis [56]. Thus the use of PET scans to decide whether or not esophagectomy is warranted is not validated.

Early PET Response During Therapy

There is a clear rationale to perform a PET scan earlier in the course of treatment to assess response (i.e., at 2–4 weeks). Early PET response may indicate that the current treatment is working and justifies continuing therapy. Figure 11.2, on the left-hand side shows an F18-FDG PET scan showing abnormal FDG uptake, consistent with malignancy, in the esophagus at the level of the thoracic inlet (red arrow). On the right-hand side is a negative F18-FDG PET scan showing interval resolution of disease in the proximal esophagus at the thoracic inlet after induction chemotherapy (red arrow). No new disease identified. If the PET response were not favorable, the treatment could be changed, or discontinued with earlier referral for surgery. Nine studies have looked at early PET response in localized esophageal cancer (for looking at both early and late PET response) (Table 11.4) [59–64]. Work by Weber and colleagues showed that measurement of early changes in ^{18}F-FDG uptake by the tumor was easily reproducible, and useful for predicting clinical and pathological response after neoadjuvant chemotherapy. In a prospective study of 37 patients with locally advanced adenocarcinoma of the gastroesophageal junction

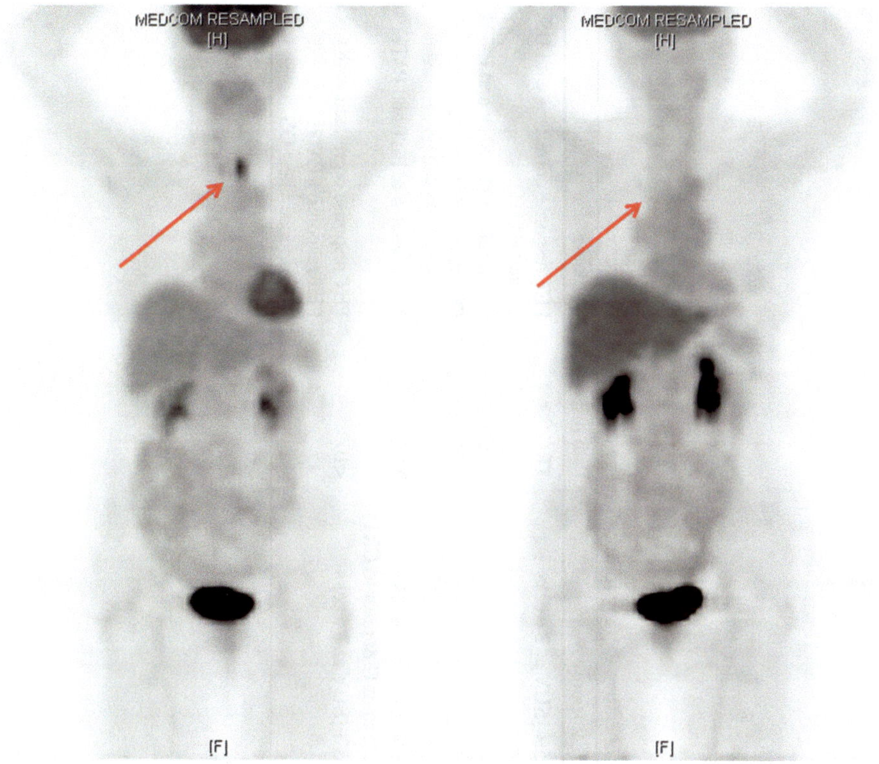

Fig. 11.2 On the left-hand side is an F18-FDG PET scan showing abnormal FDG uptake, consistent with malignancy, in the esophagus at the level of the thoracic inlet (*red arrow*). On the right-hand side is a negative F18-FDG PET scan showing interval resolution of disease in the proximal esophagus at the thoracic inlet after induction chemotherapy (*red arrow*). No new disease identified

(GEJ), ^{18}F-FDG PET was performed at baseline and repeated on day 14 after the first cycle of cisplatin-based chemotherapy. PET response was defined as >35% reduction in SUV compared with baseline. Pathologic response was defined as a Manard tumor regression grade of 1–2. PET response was significantly associated with histopathologic response ($p=0.001$). PET response also predicted clinical response with a sensitivity and specificity of 93% and 95%, respectively. Metabolic response was also significantly associated with longer time to progression and overall survival ($p=0.001$ and $p=0.04$, respectively). Wieder et al. reported a prospective study in 38 patients with squamous cell carcinoma of the esophagus assessing early and late PET response to neoadjuvant 5-FU and radiation [65]. Early PET response was defined as >30% reduction in SUV and late metabolic response was >52% reduction in SUV. Pathologic response was defined as <10% viable tumor cells. In 23 patients who underwent esophagectomy, early PET response was better able to discriminate between histopathologic response and nonresponse, and there was a strong correlation with overall survival ($p<0.011$). In contrast, a prospective

Table 11.4 ^{18}F-FDG-PET and ^{18}F-FDG-PET/CT response early during preoperative therapy for localized gastroesophageal cancer

Study	Site	Tumor type	Design	*n*	Rx	PET response	Path response	Outcome
Weber [64]	GEJ	A	P	37	C	≥35%↓SUV at 2 weeks	TRG1-2	PET response correlates with OS and PATH
Gillham [59]	E/GEJ	SCC/A	P	32	CRT	NR	TRG1-2	No correlat'n bt ΔSUV and PATH
Ott [62]	GEJ	A	P	65	C	≥35%↓SUV at 2 weeks	RTG1-2	PET response correlates with OS and PATH and recurrence
Ribi [63]	E	SCC/A	P	66	C-CRT	≥40%↓SUV at 6 weeks (end of C & prior to CRT)	TRG1-2	No correlat'n bt PET and PATH
Lordick [60]	GEJ	GEJ	P	119	C	≥35%↓SUV at 2 weeks	<10%	PET response correlated with OS PET response + PATH response = best OS

PATH Pathology

study by Gillham et al. in 32 patients reported that ^{18}F-FDG PET failed to predict histopathologic response. In this study the early PET scan was performed 1 week after cisplatin-based chemoradiation [59]. Ribi et al. reported a 66 patient study in abstract form and found that a 40% reduction in SUV was associated with a favorable histopathologic response. PET was preformed at baseline and after the second cycle of chemotherapy with docetaxel and cisplatin [63]. Treatment then continued weekly for 5 weeks with docetaxel/cisplatin and radiation.

It is important to note a number of methodological differences in some of these studies. The Weber and Ribi studies performed early PET response after chemotherapy (after 1 and 2 cycles respectively). The Ribi study then proceeded to use chemoradiation prior to surgery. The Gillham study performed an early PET response after 1 week of chemoradiation. As cited above (PET scanning section), the interpretation of PET scans in previously irradiated tissue may be difficult and may result in overestimation of glucose uptake.

The data from Weber was validated in a more recent study performed by Ott and colleagues. Ott reported a prospective study of 65 patients with untreated locally advanced GEJ adenocarcinoma [62]. Early PET response was defined, as in the Weber study, as >35% decrease in SUV compared with baseline. This threshold predicted histopathologic response with high sensitivity and specificity (80% and 78% respectively), and after a median of 42 months follow-up there was a significant difference in median survival between responders and nonresponders (not reached and 18 months respectively, $p=0.01$). In a multivariate analysis metabolic response was the only predictor for recurrence ($p<0.018$).

The pivotal study suggesting a role for early PET response in tailoring individual patient treatment was reported by the group in the MUNICON (Metabolic response evalUatioN for Individualisation of neoadjuvant Chemotherapy in oesOphageal and oesophagogastric adeNocarcinoma) study. This was the first study where a PET response resulted in a treatment change. On this prospective phase II trial, 110 patients with locally advanced adenocarcinoma of the esophagus and GEJ (Siewert I and II) received platinum and 5-FU based chemotherapy. ^{18}F-FDG PET was performed at baseline and after 2 weeks of induction treatment. Metabolic response was defined as in the Weber and Ott studies. The response rate (>35% decrease in SUV) was 49% and 104 patients underwent esophagectomy (50 in the responder group and 54 in the nonresponder group). Prior to surgery, metabolic responders continued to receive platinum-based chemotherapy for a total of 12 weeks. Nonresponders, however, proceeded to immediate surgery after only 2 weeks of chemotherapy. After a median follow-up of 2.3 years there was a significant difference in median overall survival between the responders and nonresponders (not yet reached versus 25.8 months, respectively, $p=0.015$). Median event free survival was also significantly different between the two groups (29.7 months versus 14.1 months, respectively, $p=0.002$). Major histopathologic response (<10% residual tumor) was noted in 58% of the PET responders and no histological response was noted in metabolic nonresponders. Those patients who were PET nonresponders, who terminated chemotherapy early and underwent surgery had a similar outcome compared to those patients in the prior study from this group who were metabolic nonresponders yet completed 12 weeks of preoperative chemotherapy, that is, patients proceeding to earlier surgery without completion of chemotherapy did not have an inferior outcome. Comparing the two study groups of nonresponding patients in the MUICON trial and in the prior trial, the median recurrence free period (14.1 months versus 10 months, respectively), and the median overall survival (25.8 months versus 14.1 months) were not inferior. Early discontinuation of preoperative treatment based on PET response did not negatively impact outcome in those patients who proceeded to earlier surgery [60].

Should patients who are metabolic nonresponders receive an alternate treatment prior to surgical resection? Ott, Lordick, and colleagues reported in abstract from a 32-patient study in which 13 metabolic nonresponders to induction chemotherapy alone (41%) were treated with salvage therapy, essentially adding concurrent radiotherapy while continuing the same chemotherapy. After 1 year follow-up 54% of the nonresponder group had developed distant metastatic disease compared with 37% in the responding group. Median overall survival was not reached for the responders and was 14 months for the nonresponders. The authors concluded that salvage chemoradiation continuing the same chemotherapy used during induction for PET nonresponders after induction chemotherapy provided no clear benefit [66]. Given the prior nonresponse in these patients, it is not altogether surprising that adding radiation therapy to a demonstrated inactive chemotherapy regimen had a poor outcome.

Our phase II study of cisplatin/irinotecan induction followed by cisplatin/irinotecan/radiation and then surgery for locally advanced esophageal cancer (75% adenocarcinoma) has been reported in abstract form in 53 evaluable patients [67]. Early PET response was assessed retrospectively after 6 weeks of induction therapy (cisplatin/irinotecan given for two, 3-week cycles), prior to the addition of concurrent radiotherapy to two additional cycles of cisplatin/irintoecan, followed by surgery. Metabolic response was defined as per the MUNICON trial. Time to progression was significantly superior in the PET responders and nonresponders (40.8 months versus 8.8 months, $p=0.002$). Three of four patients who had actual disease progression on PET scan after induction chemotherapy were taken off protocol, and were successfully salvaged when switched to radiation combined with either paclitaxel/5-FU or cisplatin (1 pathologic CR, 1 near pathologic CR, and 1 clinical CR—all 3 patients remain alive and without disease at more than 4 years after treatment). This strategy highlights the potential for early PET response assessment during induction chemotherapy to identify early treatment failures, and may direct patients to alternative chemotherapy during radiation.

Another significant finding in the MUNICON study is those patients who are PET responders but histopathologic nonresponders (20%) have survival outcomes similar to PET and histopathologic nonresponders (52%). Therefore, histopathologic response is still the most important prognosticator and is superior to metabolic response [60]. Reasons for the lack of histopathologic response in those patients who are metabolic responders are as yet unclear. However, it is noteworthy that PET responders can identify histopathologic responders early (after 2 weeks of induction chemotherapy) in 58% of cases (MUNICON data). Recent data have shown that serial endoscopic biopsies are unlikely to predict pathologic response in patients undergoing chemoradiation for esophageal cancer [68]. There is also much debate on SUV thresholds that are used to define PET response. The MUNICON group deemed a >35% decrease in SUV to be the most appropriate cut off. However, in squamous cell carcinoma of the esophagus and in rectal cancer different cut-offs may be more accurate [40, 69]. Baseline SUVmax was thought to predict worse outcome after chemoradiation in line with the data in surgery only studies [70]. However, recent data from our institution have not borne this out. Pretreatment SUVmax does stratify patients into high and low response groups to chemoradiation, but overall survival is similar [71]. Data from series employing surgery alone have further complicated this issue. Kato and colleagues report their retrospective experience with 184 consecutive esophageal cancer patients imaged preoperatively using ^{18}F-FDG PET. On multivariate analysis peak SUV and the number of PET-positive lymph nodes were found to be independent predictive factors for overall survival [72]. Other series have indicated that the greater number of baseline positive lesions identified on PET scan (including the primary tumor and discrete nodal sites) was an independent predictor of overall survival, $p=0.03$ [73].

Future Strategies

Based on the promising data from the MUNICON study, there now exists the possibility of tailoring multimodal treatment using PET scan as a marker of therapy response. The EUROCON study is a large randomized multicenter effort currently recruiting patients with distal esophageal and GEJ tumors. Figure 11.3 shows the algorithm for this trial. PET scan metabolic responders will continue and complete induction chemotherapy and metabolic nonresponders will be randomized to either immediate surgical resection, or salvage chemoradiation employing a different chemotherapy followed by surgery. The induction chemotherapy will be epirubicin–platinum and fluoropyrimidine, and chemoradiation in the nonresponding patients will be taxane-based. Other multicenter randomized trials are investigating the role of early PET in neoadjuvant chemoradiation strategies for localized esophageal cancer (NEOPEC—Neoadjuvant Therapy Monitoring with PET and CT in Esophageal Cancer). As yet there is no PET-guided tailored therapy for squamous cell carcinoma of the esophagus.

New molecular imaging probes are also being studied. ^{18}F-FLT PET has been compared with ^{18}F-FDG PET in the detection of esophageal cancer, but results so far have been disappointing [74]. Work is underway combining ^{18}F-FDG PET with serum and tissue biomarkers, e.g., VEGF, Ki-67, glucose transporter-1, and apoptosis markers (cleaved caspase-3) [75]. The incorporation of targeted agents, e.g., cetuximab and bevacizumab, into early PET response strategies is also being studied in metastatic and localized gastroesophageal cancers [76, 77]. Di Fabio et al. reported a metabolic response (no SUV reported) in 60% of patients with metastatic gastric and GEJ cancer after treatment with FOLFIRI+Cetuximab. Median progression free survival (11 month follow-up) was significantly longer in metabolic responders

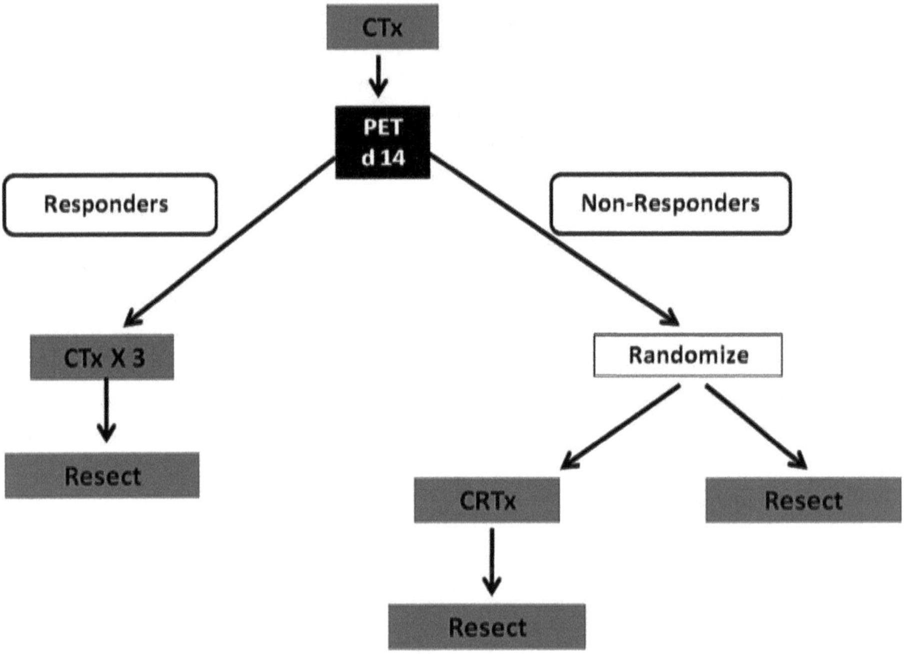

Fig. 11.3 Design of the EUROCON study. *CTx* chemotherapy, *CRTx* chemoradiotherapy, *X 3* 3 cycles, *d14* day 14

(11 months versus 5 months, $p=0.0016$) [76]. Metabolic response with targeted therapy has been studied in gastrointestinal stromal tumors (GIST) [78]. Data suggest that FDG-PET is a valuable tool in monitoring response to imatinib and has the potential to monitor response in other diseases treated with tyrosine kinase inhibitors [31].

PET and Gastric Cancer

The use of PET in true gastric cancer is not as well defined as in esophageal or GEJ cancers. Approximately one-third of gastric cancers are not ^{18}F-FDG PET avid. These tumors are usually diffuse Laurens-subtype, well differentiated, filled with mucin, and localized to the distal third of the stomach [61, 79–81]. The German group of Ott and Lordick has reported early PET response as defined by >35% reduction in SUV 2 weeks after initiation of cisplatin-based preoperative chemotherapy in gastric cancer [82]. At 2-years, median survival for metabolic responders was not reached and median survival for nonresponders was 18.9 months ($p=0.002$). Early PET response also correctly predicted histopathologic response in 10 (77%) of 13 responders, and 19 (86%) of 22 nonresponders. Histopathologic response was defined as <10% viable tumor cells in the resected specimen. Shah and colleagues from our institution, in a retrospective study of 41 patients, identified a decrease of

45% SUV when the PET scan was performed at day 35 after preoperative cisplatin/irinotecan, as the best criterion for predicting response and prognosis. Median disease free survival was not reached for the PET responders and was 14.4 months for the nonresponders [80]. SUV response was significantly associated with histopathologic response (<50% residual tumor, $p=0.07$). Ott and colleagues have reported that the prognosis of FDG nonavid gastric cancer is similar to that of FDG-avid gastric cancers that do not display an early PET response to chemotherapy [61]. Thus, PET nonavidity may be a subgroup of biologically unfavorable tumors [79]. To date other groups have not validated this finding [80]. Ott has also reported that ^{18}F-FLT PET may be more sensitive than ^{18}F-FDG PET in detecting gastric cancer. Thus, the addition of FLT-PET to FDG-PET may improve early PET evaluation of response to neoadjuvant treatment of gastric cancer [83]. There are no data as yet on early metabolic response in patients with gastric/GEJ cancer treated with preoperative chemoradiation.

PET-Guided Therapy

The early identification of patients who are responding to therapy is imperative to optimize potential benefits from therapy and minimize exposure and toxicity to potentially ineffective therapy. More importantly, a potential change to a more effective alternative therapy may be achieved. Our increased understanding of tumor biology at the molecular level has revealed the complex heterogenous nature of cancer. Molecular signatures using DNA array, which evaluates a whole spectrum of genes, and proteomic technology, which evaluates circulating polypeptide profiles, hold promise in predicting tumor behavior, prognosis, and response to treatment. However, these techniques have largely not been validated and the data reported are not easily applicable to clinical practice. In contrast, molecular imaging, primarily with ^{18}F-FDG PET, is now commonly used in clinical practice for staging of esophagogastric cancer. The potential for FDG-PET to provide a meaningful role in assessment of treatment response and tailoring of therapy has been shown in prospective and retrospective nonrandomized studies mainly in upper gastrointestinal cancers. Validation in multicenter randomized studies is now under way. The search for validated biomarkers that accurately predict tumor response to treatment and outcome is one of the main goals of modern oncology research.

References

1. Bosset JF, Collette L, Calais G, et al. Chemotherapy with preoperative radiotherapy in rectal cancer. N Engl J Med. 2006;355:1114–23.
2. Herman JM, Swartz MJ, Hsu CC, et al. Analysis of fluorouracil-based adjuvant chemotherapy and radiation after pancreaticoduodenectomy for ductal adenocarcinoma of the pancreas: results of a large, prospectively collected database at the Johns Hopkins Hospital. J Clin Oncol. 2008;26:3503–10.

3. Tepper J, Krasna MJ, Niedzwiecki D, et al. Phase III trial of trimodality therapy with cisplatin, fluorouracil, radiotherapy, and surgery compared with surgery alone for esophageal cancer: CALGB 9781. J Clin Oncol. 2008;26:1086–92.
4. Gruenberger B, Tamandl D, Schueller J, et al. Bevacizumab, capecitabine, and oxaliplatin as neoadjuvant therapy for patients with potentially curable metastatic colorectal cancer. J Clin Oncol. 2008;26:1830–5.
5. Van Cutsem E, Kohne CH, Hitre E, et al. Cetuximab and chemotherapy as initial treatment for metastatic colorectal cancer. N Engl J Med. 2009;360:1408–17.
6. Jia SQ, Niu ZJ, Zhang LH, et al. Identification of prognosis-related proteins in advanced gastric cancer by mass spectrometry-based comparative proteomics. J Cancer Res Clin Oncol. 2009;135:403–11.
7. Hildebrandt MA, Yang H, Hung MC, et al. Genetic variations in the PI3K/PTEN/AKT/mTOR pathway are associated with clinical outcomes in esophageal cancer patients treated with chemoradiotherapy. J Clin Oncol. 2009;27:857–71.
8. Biomarkers Definitions Working Group. Biomarkers and surrogate endpoints: preferred definitions and conceptual framework. Clin Pharmacol Ther. 2001;69:89–95.
9. Parkin DM, Bray F, Ferlay J, Pisani P. Global cancer statistics, 2002. CA Cancer J Clin. 2005;55:74–108.
10. Kamangar F, Dores GM, Anderson WF. Patterns of cancer incidence, mortality, and prevalence across five continents: defining priorities to reduce cancer disparities in different geographic regions of the world. J Clin Oncol. 2006;24:2137–50.
11. Pera M, Cameron AJ, Trastek VF, Carpenter HA, Zinsmeister AR. Increasing incidence of adenocarcinoma of the esophagus and esophagogastric junction. Gastroenterology. 1993;104:510–3.
12. Van Cutsem E, Van de Velde C, Roth A, et al. Expert opinion on management of gastric and gastro-oesophageal junction adenocarcinoma on behalf of the European Organisation for Research and Treatment of Cancer (EORTC)-gastrointestinal cancer group. Eur J Cancer. 2008;44:182–94.
13. Gunderson LL. Gastric cancer—patterns of relapse after surgical resection. Semin Radiat Oncol. 2002;12:150–61.
14. Gebski V, Burmeister B, Smithers BM, Foo K, Zalcberg J, Simes J. Survival benefits from neoadjuvant chemoradiotherapy or chemotherapy in oesophageal carcinoma: a meta-analysis. Lancet Oncol. 2007;8:226–34.
15. Macdonald JS, Smalley SR, Benedetti J, et al. Chemoradiotherapy after surgery compared with surgery alone for adenocarcinoma of the stomach or gastroesophageal junction. N Engl J Med. 2001;345:725–30.
16. Sakuramoto S, Sasako M, Yamaguchi T, et al. Adjuvant chemotherapy for gastric cancer with S-1, an oral fluoropyrimidine. N Engl J Med. 2007;357:1810–20.
17. Boige V, Pignon J, Saint-Aubert B, et al. Final results of a randomized trial comparing preoperative 5-fluorouracil (F)/cisplatin (P) to surgery alone in adenocarcinoma of stomach and lower esophagus (ASLE): FNLCC ACCORD07-FFCD 9703 trial. American Society of Clinical Oncology; 2007 June 1–5; Chicago, IL, USA.
18. Cunningham D, Allum WH, Stenning SP, et al. Perioperative chemotherapy versus surgery alone for resectable gastroesophageal cancer. N Engl J Med. 2006;355:11–20.
19. Stahl M, Walz MK, Stuschke M, et al. Phase III comparison of preoperative chemotherapy compared with chemoradiotherapy in patients with locally advanced adenocarcinoma of the esophagogastric junction. J Clin Oncol. 2009;27:851–6.
20. Ku GY, Ilson DH. Multimodality therapy for the curative treatment of cancer of the esophagus and gastroesophageal junction. Expert Rev Anticancer Ther. 2008;8:1953–64.
21. Reynolds JV, Muldoon C, Hollywood D, et al. Long-term outcomes following neoadjuvant chemoradiotherapy for esophageal cancer. Ann Surg. 2007;245:707–16.
22. Mitani Y, Oue N, Matsumura S, et al. Reg IV is a serum biomarker for gastric cancer patients and predicts response to 5-fluorouracil-based chemotherapy. Oncogene. 2007; 26:4383–93.

23. Fletcher JW, Djulbegovic B, Soares HP, et al. Recommendations on the use of 18F-FDG PET in oncology. J Nucl Med. 2008;49:480–508.
24. Shreve PD, Anzai Y, Wahl RL. Pitfalls in oncologic diagnosis with FDG PET imaging: physiologic and benign variants. Radiographics. 1999;19:61–77. quiz 150–151.
25. Antoch G, Stattaus J, Nemat AT, et al. Non-small cell lung cancer: dual-modality PET/CT in preoperative staging. Radiology. 2003;229:526–33.
26. Jayson GC, Zweit J, Jackson A, et al. Molecular imaging and biological evaluation of HuMV833 anti-VEGF antibody: implications for trial design of antiangiogenic antibodies. J Natl Cancer Inst. 2002;94:1484–93.
27. Dehdashti F, Picus J, Michalski JM, et al. Positron tomographic assessment of androgen receptors in prostatic carcinoma. Eur J Nucl Med Mol Imaging. 2005;32:344–50.
28. Kwekkeboom DJ, Teunissen JJ, Bakker WH, et al. Radiolabeled somatostatin analog [177Lu-DOTA0, Tyr3]octreotate in patients with endocrine gastroenteropancreatic tumors. J Clin Oncol. 2005;23:2754–62.
29. Mortimer JE, Dehdashti F, Siegel BA, Trinkaus K, Katzenellenbogen JA, Welch MJ. Metabolic flare: indicator of hormone responsiveness in advanced breast cancer. J Clin Oncol. 2001;19:2797–803.
30. Grosu AL, Weber WA, Franz M, et al. Reirradiation of recurrent high-grade gliomas using amino acid PET (SPECT)/CT/MRI image fusion to determine gross tumor volume for stereotactic fractionated radiotherapy. Int J Radiat Oncol Biol Phys. 2005;63:511–9.
31. Weber WA. Positron emission tomography as an imaging biomarker. J Clin Oncol. 2006;24:3282–92.
32. Beer AJ, Wieder HA, Lordick F, et al. Adenocarcinomas of esophagogastric junction: multidetector row CT to evaluate early response to neoadjuvant chemotherapy. Radiology. 2006;239:472–80.
33. Wieder HA, Beer AJ, Lordick F, et al. Comparison of changes in tumor metabolic activity and tumor size during chemotherapy of adenocarcinomas of the esophagogastric junction. J Nucl Med. 2005;46:2029–34.
34. Lordick F, Ruers T, Aust DE, et al. European Organisation of Research and Treatment of Cancer (EORTC) Gastrointestinal Group: workshop on the role of metabolic imaging in the neoadjuvant treatment of gastrointestinal cancer. Eur J Cancer. 2008;44:1807–19.
35. Weber WA, Ziegler SI, Thodtmann R, Hanauske AR, Schwaiger M. Reproducibility of metabolic measurements in malignant tumors using FDG PET. J Nucl Med. 1999;40:1771–7.
36. Souvatzoglou M, Ziegler SI, Martinez MJ, et al. Standardised uptake values from PET/CT images: comparison with conventional attenuation-corrected PET. Eur J Nucl Med Mol Imaging. 2007;34:405–12.
37. Stahl A, Ott K, Schwaiger M, Weber WA. Comparison of different SUV-based methods for monitoring cytotoxic therapy with FDG PET. Eur J Nucl Med Mol Imaging. 2004;31:1471–8.
38. Arslan N, Miller TR, Dehdashti F, Battafarano RJ, Siegel BA. Evaluation of response to neoadjuvant therapy by quantitative 2-deoxy-2-[18F]fluoro-D-glucose with positron emission tomography in patients with esophageal cancer. Mol Imaging Biol. 2002;4:301–10.
39. Brink I, Hentschel M, Bley TA, et al. Effects of neoadjuvant radio-chemotherapy on 18F-FDG-PET in esophageal carcinoma. Eur J Surg Oncol. 2004;30:544–50.
40. Brucher BL, Weber W, Bauer M, et al. Neoadjuvant therapy of esophageal squamous cell carcinoma: response evaluation by positron emission tomography. Ann Surg. 2001;233:300–9.
41. Cerfolio RJ, Bryant AS, Ohja B, Bartolucci AA, Eloubeidi MA. The accuracy of endoscopic ultrasonography with fine-needle aspiration, integrated positron emission tomography with computed tomography, and computed tomography in restaging patients with esophageal cancer after neoadjuvant chemoradiotherapy. J Thorac Cardiovasc Surg. 2005;129:1232–41.
42. Downey RJ, Akhurst T, Ilson D, et al. Whole body 18FDG-PET and the response of esophageal cancer to induction therapy: results of a prospective trial. J Clin Oncol. 2003;21:428–32.
43. Duong CP, Hicks RJ, Weih L, et al. FDG-PET status following chemoradiotherapy provides high management impact and powerful prognostic stratification in oesophageal cancer. Eur J Nucl Med Mol Imaging. 2006;33:770–8.

44. Flamen P, Van Cutsem E, Lerut A, et al. Positron emission tomography for assessment of the response to induction radiochemotherapy in locally advanced oesophageal cancer. Ann Oncol. 2002;13:361–8.
45. Kato H, Kuwano H, Nakajima M, et al. Usefulness of positron emission tomography for assessing the response of neoadjuvant chemoradiotherapy in patients with esophageal cancer. Am J Surg. 2002;184:279–83.
46. Kim MK, Ryu JS, Kim SB, et al. Value of complete metabolic response by (18) F-fluorodeoxyglucose-positron emission tomography in oesophageal cancer for prediction of pathologic response and survival after preoperative chemoradiotherapy. Eur J Cancer. 2007;43:1385–91.
47. Mamede M, Abreu ELP, Oliva MR, Nose V, Mamon H, Gerbaudo VH. FDG-PET/CT tumor segmentation-derived indices of metabolic activity to assess response to neoadjuvant therapy and progression-free survival in esophageal cancer: correlation with histopathology results. Am J Clin Oncol. 2007;30:377–88.
48. McLoughlin JM, Melis M, Siegel EM, et al. Are patients with esophageal cancer who become PET negative after neoadjuvant chemoradiation free of cancer? J Am Coll Surg. 2008;206:879–86. discussion 86–87.
49. Melcher L, Wong W, Sanghera B, et al. Sequential FDG-PET scanning in the assessment of response to neoadjuvant chemotherapy in operable esophageal cancer. Amercan Society of Clinical Oncology, Annual Proceedings; 2004. Abstract #4056.
50. Port JL, Lee PC, Korst RJ, et al. Positron emission tomographic scanning predicts survival after induction chemotherapy for esophageal carcinoma. Ann Thorac Surg. 2007; 84:393–400.
51. Schmidt M, Bollschweiler E, Dietlein M, et al. Mean and maximum standardized uptake values in [18F]FDG-PET for assessment of histopathological response in oesophageal squamous cell carcinoma or adenocarcinoma after radiochemotherapy. Eur J Nucl Med Mol Imaging. 2009;36:735–44.
52. Smithers BM, Couper GC, Thomas JM, et al. Positron emission tomography and pathological evidence of response to neoadjuvant therapy in adenocarcinoma of the esophagus. Dis Esophagus. 2008;21:151–8.
53. Song SY, Kim JH, Ryu JS, et al. FDG-PET in the prediction of pathologic response after neoadjuvant chemoradiotherapy in locally advanced, resectable esophageal cancer. Int J Radiat Oncol Biol Phys. 2005;63:1053–9.
54. Swisher SG, Maish M, Erasmus JJ, et al. Utility of PET, CT, and EUS to identify pathologic responders in esophageal cancer. Ann Thorac Surg. 2004;78:1152–60.
55. Javeri H, Xiao L, Rohren E, et al. The higher the decrease in the standardized uptake value of positron emission tomography after chemoradiation, the better the survival of patients with gastroesophageal adenocarcinoma. Cancer. 2009;14:14.
56. Konski AA, Cheng JD, Goldberg M, et al. Correlation of molecular response as measured by 18-FDG positron emission tomography with outcome after chemoradiotherapy in patients with esophageal carcinoma. Int J Radiat Oncol Biol Phys. 2007;69:358–63.
57. Kroep JR, Van Groeningen CJ, Cuesta MA, et al. Positron emission tomography using 2-deoxy-2-[18F]-fluoro-D-glucose for response monitoring in locally advanced gastroesophageal cancer; a comparison of different analytical methods. Mol Imaging Biol. 2003;5:337–46.
58. Levine EA, Farmer MR, Clark P, et al. Predictive value of 18-fluoro-deoxy-glucose-positron emission tomography (18F-FDG-PET) in the identification of responders to chemoradiation therapy for the treatment of locally advanced esophageal cancer. Ann Surg. 2006;243:472–8.
59. Gillham CM, Lucey JA, Keogan M, et al. (18)FDG uptake during induction chemoradiation for oesophageal cancer fails to predict histomorphological tumour response. Br J Cancer. 2006;95:1174–9.
60. Lordick F, Ott K, Krause BJ, et al. PET to assess early metabolic response and to guide treatment of adenocarcinoma of the oesophagogastric junction: the MUNICON phase II trial. Lancet Oncol. 2007;8:797–805.

61. Ott K, Herrmann K, Lordick F, et al. Early metabolic response evaluation by fluorine-18 fluorodeoxyglucose positron emission tomography allows in vivo testing of chemosensitivity in gastric cancer: long-term results of a prospective study. Clin Cancer Res. 2008;14:2012–8.
62. Ott K, Weber WA, Lordick F, et al. Metabolic imaging predicts response, survival, and recurrence in adenocarcinomas of the esophagogastric junction. J Clin Oncol. 2006;24:4692–8.
63. Ribi K, Nitzsche E, Schuller J, et al. PET scanning and patient reported dysphagia before and after chemotherapy (CT) for prediction of pathological response after CT and chemoradiotherapy (CRT) in patients with locally advanced esophageal cancer (EC): a multicenter phase II trial of the Swiss. American Society of Clinical Oncology, Annual Proceedings; 2007; Orlando, FL. Abstract #4587.
64. Weber WA, Ott K, Becker K, et al. Prediction of response to preoperative chemotherapy in adenocarcinomas of the esophagogastric junction by metabolic imaging. J Clin Oncol. 2001;19:3058–65.
65. Wieder HA, Brucher BL, Zimmermann F, et al. Time course of tumor metabolic activity during chemoradiotherapy of esophageal squamous cell carcinoma and response to treatment. J Clin Oncol. 2004;22:900–8.
66. Lordick F, Ott K, Krause BJ, et al. Salvage radiochemotherapy in locally advanced gastroesophageal junction tumors that are metabolically resistant to induction chemotherapy: The MUNICON-2 trial. Gastrointestinal Cancers Symposium; 2008; Orlando, FL. Abstract #104.
67. Ku GY, Bains M, Rizk N, et al. Phase II trial of pre-operative cisplatin/irinotecan and radiotherapy for locally advanced esophageal cancer: PET scan after induction therapy may identify early treatment failure. Gastrointestinal Cancer Symposium; 2007 Jan 25–25; Orlando, FL, USA. Abstract #9.
68. Sarkaria IS, Rizk NP, Bains MS, et al. Post-treatment endoscopic biopsy is a poor-predictor of pathologic response in patients undergoing chemoradiation therapy for esophageal cancer. Ann Surg. 2009;249:764–7.
69. Cascini GL, Avallone A, Delrio P, et al. 18F-FDG PET is an early predictor of pathologic tumor response to preoperative radiochemotherapy in locally advanced rectal cancer. J Nucl Med. 2006;47:1241–8.
70. Rizk N, Downey RJ, Akhurst T, et al. Preoperative 18[F]-fluorodeoxyglucose positron emission tomography standardized uptake values predict survival after esophageal adenocarcinoma resection. Ann Thorac Surg. 2006;81:1076–81.
71. Rizk NP, Tang L, Adusumilli PS, et al. Predictive value of initial PET-SUVmax in patients with locally advanced esophageal and gastroesophageal junction adenocarcinoma. J Thorac Oncol. 2009;4:875–9.
72. Kato H, Nakajima M, Sohda M, et al. The clinical application of (18)F-fluorodeoxyglucose positron emission tomography to predict survival in patients with operable esophageal cancer. Cancer. 2009;26:26.
73. Hong D, Lunagomez S, Kim EE, et al. Value of baseline positron emission tomography for predicting overall survival in patient with nonmetastatic esophageal or gastroesophageal junction carcinoma. Cancer. 2005;104:1620–6.
74. van Westreenen HL, Cobben DC, Jager PL, et al. Comparison of 18F-FLT PET and 18F-FDG PET in esophageal cancer. J Nucl Med. 2005;46:400–4.
75. Westerterp M, Sloof GW, Hoekstra OS, et al. 18FDG uptake in oesophageal adenocarcinoma: linking biology and outcome. J Cancer Res Clin Oncol. 2008;134:227–36.
76. Di Fabio F, Pinto C. Rojas Llimpe FL, et al. The predictive value of 18F-FDG-PET early evaluation in patients with metastatic gastric adenocarcinoma treated with chemotherapy plus cetuximab. Gastric Cancer. 2007;10:221–7.
77. Ilson DH, Bains M, Rizk N, et al. Phase II trial of preoperative bevacizumab (Bev), irinotecan (I), cisplatin (C), and radiation (RT) in esophageal adenocarcinoma: Preliminary safety analysis. American Society of Clinial Oncology, Annual Proceedings; 2009; Orlando, FL, USA. Abstract 4573.
78. Van den Abbeele AD. The lessons of GIST—PET and PET/CT: a new paradigm for imaging. Oncologist. 2008;13 Suppl 2:8–13.

79. Ott K, Herrmann K, Krause BJ, Lordick F. The value of PET imaging in patients with localized gastroesophageal cancer. Gastrointest Cancer Res. 2008;2:287–94.
80. Shah MA, Yeung H, Coit D, et al. A phase II study of preoperative chemotherapy with irinotecan(CPT) and cisplatin(CIS) for gastric cancer(NCI 5917): FDG-PET/CT predicts patient outcome. Amercan Society of Clinical Oncology, Annual Proceedings; 2007; Orlando, FL. Abstract #4502.
81. Shah MA, Yeung H, Trocola R, et al. The characteristics and utility of FDG-PET/CT scans in patients with localized gastric cancer (GC). Gastrointestinal Cancers Symposium; 2007; Orlando, FL. Abstract #2.
82. Ott K, Fink U, Becker K, et al. Prediction of response to preoperative chemotherapy in gastric carcinoma by metabolic imaging: results of a prospective trial. J Clin Oncol. 2003; 21:4604–10.
83. Herrmann K, Ott K, Buck AK, et al. Imaging gastric cancer with PET and the radiotracers 18F-FLT and 18F-FDG: a comparative analysis. J Nucl Med. 2007;48:1945–50.

Chapter 12
Circulating Tumor Cells as Biomarkers

Stephen V. Liu, Tong Xu, and Amir Goldkorn

Introduction

When a tumor disseminates beyond the primary site, the negative impact on survival is profound. The pathophysiology underlying this process has naturally been of great interest and has led to a search for the tumor cell in-transit. With recent technical advancements, detection and capture of tumor cells in peripheral blood is now possible. These circulating tumor cells (CTC) have quickly been established as viable biomarkers and promise to greatly expand our understanding of tumor biology and impact our approach to treating cancer. The presence of CTC in the blood has important clinical significance for patients with various types of cancer, and serial measurements have shown that CTC are a dynamic variable that may reflect the complicated clinical course of cancer. Therefore, CTC constitute an invaluable clinical resource for planning and modifying therapeutic maneuvers, because they offer a real-time, readily accessible window into the developing disease process. Furthermore, studies of CTC biology may help to elucidate the basic mechanisms governing cancer dissemination and metastasis.

For the purpose of this discussion, it is important to draw a distinction between CTC and disseminated tumor cells (DTC). Prior to the emergence of more recent technologies, the search for early evidence of disseminated cancer focused on the bone marrow, where these cells are particularly abundant. Cells found in this niche were termed DTC, and studying this reservoir site [1–3] has provided valuable clinical information, particularly in breast cancer [4]. However, the invasive nature of DTC sampling makes serial monitoring impractical. With the advent of new technologies

S.V. Liu, M.D. • T. Xu, Ph.D. • A. Goldkorn, M.D. (✉)
Division of Medical Oncology, Department of Internal Medicine, Norris Comprehensive Cancer Center, Keck School of Medicine, University of Southern California, 1441 Eastlake Avenue, Suite 3440, Los Angeles, CA 90033, USA
e-mail: agoldkor@usc.edu

H.-J. Lenz (ed.), *Biomarkers in Oncology: Prediction and Prognosis*,
DOI 10.1007/978-1-4419-9755-5_12,

to isolate tumor cells from circulating blood, the preponderance of recent studies has focused on CTC monitoring and analysis. DTC have been reviewed elsewhere [5] and a comparison between the two is beyond the scope of this discussion. Instead, this chapter will review the capture and analysis of CTC as well as their clinical utility.

Capture of Circulating Tumor Cells

The absolute number of CTC in circulation at a given time is quite variable and depends on multiple factors such as the underlying biology of the tumor and host, any ongoing treatments, and the method of measurement. It is generally accepted that in relative terms CTC are quite rare, comprising at most only a few cells for every 10^8 leukocytes and 10^{10}–10^{11} erythrocytes. It is only with sophisticated enrichment and identification techniques that CTC can be detected with any regularity. CTC enrichment can be approached using any of several strategies, described in detail below (Fig. 12.1). The strategies can be grouped into four general categories: (1) density gradient centrifugation, which enriches CTC by separating blood into fractions based on relative density, (2) membrane microfiltration, which separates CTC based on their large relative size, (3) immunomagnetic separation, which isolates CTC by binding specific antigens on their cell surface, and (4) whole blood polymerase chain reaction (PCR), which detects DNA mutations or the expression

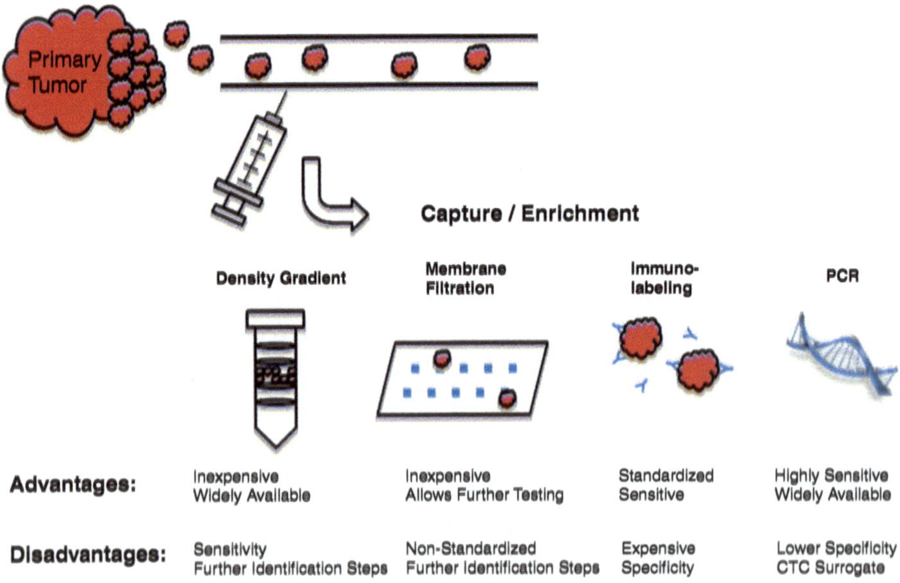

Fig. 12.1 General strategies for CTC capture include density gradient enrichment, membrane filtration, immunomagnetic separation and whole blood PCR

of genes common in CTC. Any combination of the available enrichment and detection modalities can be used to identify and quantify CTC, but each strategy has its own unique advantages and limitations. While each may be effective, the available techniques are inherently different and comparing results must be done cautiously. The methods used for enrichment and identification in any CTC study are central to interpretation of its results and a discussion of these methods needs to frame all further dialogue.

Density Gradient Centrifugation

This CTC enrichment strategy takes advantage of the fact that whole blood can be reliably separated into fractions containing different cell types based on their relative densities. Using this approach, CTC predictably settle into a small fraction of blood that can be carefully removed, reducing the testing volume and greatly increasing the concentration of any CTC. Several density gradient liquids are commercially available, including Ficoll (Amersham Biosciences, Pittsburgh, PA) and Lymphoprep (Axis-Shield, Norton, MA). The density gradient liquid is combined with whole blood and subject to centrifugation, layering groups of cells based on their density. Erythrocytes have the highest density and will collect at the bottom of the centrifugation tube. Neutrophils will collect above the erythrocytes, followed by the standardized density gradient liquid. Above this liquid, the mononuclear cells will collect and plasma, which has the lowest density, will accumulate at the top. The mononuclear cell layer is the fraction of interest and will include monocytes, lymphocytes, epithelial cells, and any CTC, now present in a much higher concentration and accessible to identification assays.

The density gradient enrichment process was used with great frequency, due to its early refinement and relative accessibility. Unlike other assays, it does not require highly specialized equipment or techniques. However, its major limitation is loss of sensitivity due to intermixing of blood layers, especially if separation is not immediate. CTC often migrate into the lower density plasma fraction, excluding themselves from subsequent identification assays; alternatively, CTC may cluster with erythrocytes or leukocytes and are then lost in the higher density fractions. One remedy is a membrane placed above the density gradient, which is commercially available as OncoQuick (Greiner Bio One, Monroe, NC). Nevertheless, comparison with other assays has shown an inferior sensitivity with the density enrichment approach, though it is still frequently encountered today [6].

Membrane Microfiltration

A completely different strategy enriches whole blood via filtration, exploiting the larger relative size of CTC. While blood cells have a size of 5–10 μm, CTC are typically >15 μm and often much larger, with one group showing a mean CTC size of 29.8–33.9 μm [7]. Polycarbonate membranes are laced with 8 μm pores that permit erythrocytes and the vast majority of leukocytes to pass through while trapping CTC on the filter surface. A more recent improvement upon the polycarbonate membranes is the microelectromechanical system (MEMS), a membrane that is micromachined from parylene-C rather than polycarbonate, allowing pore size, shape and spacing to be dictated on a micron level, thus "customizing" the microfilter for optimal cell capture. MEMS has the additional benefit of allowing "on-membrane" electrical lysis of captured cells for molecular analysis of DNA, RNA, or protein [8]. After the cells are captured on a microfilter, additional assays such as immunolabeling or RT-PCR can then be performed on the captured cells. The sensitivity of this approach has been validated by Zabaglo et al. who noted retention of nearly 100% of spiked breast cancer cells [9]. Occasional leukocytes will be trapped on the membrane as well but these are easily excluded based on their different morphology or expression of CD45, a leukocyte antigen absent on CTC and other epithelium-derived cells. A newer MEMS microfilter designed with slots instead of pores is capable of efficiently capturing viable CTC which can be further assayed for live-cell phenotypes (e.g., enzymatic reactions) and potentially expanded in culture [10]. The Isolation by Size of Epithelial Tumor cells (ISET) method applies the same principles but uses a commercially available buffer (for fixation) and a Metablock device for vacuum filtration. Cells are still retained on the membrane for further analysis. Validation studies by Vona et al. demonstrated the ability of ISET to isolate a single tumor cell transferred to 1 ml of whole blood [11]

As with the density gradient approach, filtration simply enriches for a population of cells that includes CTC but still requires a subsequent assay to identify which of the captured cells are actually CTC. The most common approach is fixation on filter followed by immunolabeling using antibodies that target epithelial surface antigens. The antigens of choice are typically cytokeratins, which are cytoskeletal proteins specifically expressed in epithelial cells. When these antibodies are conjugated to fluorescent dyes, automated digital microscopy systems can excite the labeled cells. Fiber-optic array scanning technology (FAST) and laser scanning cytometry (LSC) are systems that quantify the labeled cells and detect their position, allowing subsequent relocation and direct visualization of the cells for cytopathologic confirmation. Automated scanning microscopes now offer rapid and reliable identification of CTC and are much more practical than manual identification [12].

The filtration approach has several advantages over other enrichment strategies. It is relatively inexpensive and largely due to its simplicity, is fairly easy to perform. Filtration offers a high sensitivity, attributable to the few steps involved, which means fewer CTC are lost in processing; moreover, it allows further characterization of captured cells, by various subsequent assays. However, there is a striking lack of standardization. Questions regarding the specifics of the equipment and the protocol persist, including the ideal features of the filter itself and the proper quantity of blood to be subject to filtration. And while the process itself is straightforward, it still requires a subsequent identification step as described above.

Immunomagnetic Separation

This enrichment strategy employs magnetically labeled antibodies to bind epithelial antigens on the cell membrane of CTC. The cells are then exposed to a magnetic field that retains the magnetically immunolabeled cells, while all other cells are washed away. Isolated cells consist of a mixed population of CTC, noncancerous epithelial cells and inadvertently captured leukocytes. Therefore, as with microfiltration, immunomagnetic enrichment necessitates a second "identification" step using additional immunofluorescent (IF) staining with antibodies that allow more specific identification of CTC. Cells expressing CD45, a common leukocyte antigen, are negatively selected while the epithelial markers CK8, CK18 and CK19 are used for positive selection. One study by Witzig et al. used an antibody directed toward epithelial adhesion molecule (EpCAM), which is expressed on the surface of epithelial cells [13]. The EpCAM antibody was conjugated to immunomagnetic beads to capture the targeted cells. Blood from 75 breast cancer patients was subjected to analysis: 25 had no lymph node involvement, 25 had lymph node involvement, and 25 had metastatic breast cancer. In addition, 25 samples from healthy individuals served as negative controls and 15 samples were spiked with carcinoma cells to serve as positive controls. None of the negative controls produced any CTC, while all of the positive controls did. Of the 75 patients with breast cancer, 21 (28%) demonstrated CTC, and all of these were within the node positive or metastatic disease groups. Several other protocols demonstrated efficient identification of CTC with immunomagnetic separation [14, 15].

The CellSearch assay (Veridex, USA) is a standardized, FDA-approved commercial assay that employs EpCAM antibodies coupled to magnetic ferrofluids to bind and magnetically separate CTC, followed by further positive and negative selection with IF. Analysis is semiautomated and requires specialized, standardized equipment. The CellSearch assay offers superior sensitivity to the density gradient enrichment approach and its standardization facilitates translation to the clinical setting [6]. However, the equipment can be cost-prohibitive and its use is time-intense and operator-dependent for cell by cell "judging" of CTC positivity based on stains. In addition, the cells themselves, which are fixed in cuvettes, are not amenable to further molecular analysis.

Perhaps the most important limitation of CellSearch, like all immunolabeling techniques, is its reliance on antigen expression. Antibodies used in this process should ideally target an antigen overexpressed on the surface of tumor cells and not expressed on any other circulating cell. Unfortunately, such specific antigens have yet to be defined. Currently, epithelial cell surface antigens such as EpCam and CKs are targeted. While these are frequently expressed on carcinoma cells, which are epithelium-derived, it is important to acknowledge that these assays detect epithelial cells and not necessarily CTC. Benign epithelial cells can circulate and will be labeled by these assays as CTC, constituting false positive results. Since CTC exist in such small numbers, any false positive results can have a significant impact.

Perhaps more concerning is the possibility of false negative results: as tumor cells enter the circulation, presumably as precursors to metastatic disease, they are observed to undergo several important biologic changes [16, 17]. This can include a change in phenotype termed epithelial to mesenchymal transition (EMT) accompanied by a loss of adhesion molecules and other epithelial cell surface antigens to permit cell migration [18–20]. Depending on which antigens are lost in the transition (and which are targeted by immunolabeling), a significant portion of CTC may not express typical epithelial markers and thus escape detection by any immunolabeling assay. This is particularly troubling since these are potentially the most critical cells to detect and may offer the most potent glimpse into the metastatic process.

Whole Blood PCR

This strategy employs PCR or reverse transcription PCR (RT-PCR) to detect specific DNA mutations or specific gene expression, respectively. Higher levels of circulating DNA had been described in cancer patients as early as 1977, and tumor related DNA was more frequently seen in patients with disseminated disease than in patients with local disease [21]. Use of circulating DNA as a biomarker was limited, however, as it was not possible to distinguish DNA of a dying cell from that of a viable tumor cell. This led to the use of tumor RNA detection, and while free RNA analysis is an area of ongoing research, targeting RNA from CTC by RT-PCR has emerged as a practical and highly sensitive assay which more accurately reflects the presence of live CTC in the blood. Enrichment of whole blood can be performed prior to RT-PCR using modalities such as microfiltration described earlier, and spiking studies using MEMS confirm efficient CTC recovery [8, 22], however RT-PCR can be performed on whole blood without prior enrichment. Blood cells are lysed, either chemically or electrically. Once the cells are lysed, RNA is isolated and used as a template for complementary DNA synthesis. Selected primers are then used to amplify specific genes, and the product can then be analyzed by gel electrophoresis. RT-PCR offers the highest sensitivity of any CTC quantification assay, and it circumvents the technical challenge of actually capturing the CTC; therefore, RT-PCR has been the most widely used CTC detection method to date.

While sensitivity is high, there are several drawbacks to the RT-PCR approach. The most striking disadvantage to RT-PCR is the uncertainty regarding target gene and primer selection. As with immunolabeling, the gene to be amplified should be overexpressed in tumor cells and not in any other cells present. Again, perfectly "tumor-specific" genes have not been described. For example, the use of genes for epithelial markers such as CK19 is commonly described. Unfortunately, these genes are expressed in normal cells as well and have been detected in samples from healthy donors. On occasion, cells will transcribe low levels of genes in a nonspecific manner, referred to as "illegitimate transcription." RT-PCR is so highly sensitive that it can detect illegitimate transcription, which detracts from the specificity of the assay. Combinations of genes can improve the specificity [23, 24], but the optimal combination is still being explored. Some groups have used organ specific marker genes in lieu of the epithelial markers such as prostate specific antigen (PSA) [25] or prostate specific membrane antigen (PSMA) [26] in the setting of prostate cancer, and alpha fetoprotein (AFP) [27] for hepatocellular cancer.

Nevertheless, false positive results were still seen, as benign tissue expressed these markers and transcripts were subsequently identified in the circulation. To address the false positive signal generated by benign tissue, more recent studies have increasingly relied on quantitative real-time PCR, which allows measurement of absolute transcript amounts in cancer versus normal patient samples, thus establishing a cutoff value that distinguishes CTC transcripts from benign transcripts. Last but not least, it is important to remember what RT-PCR actually measures. The CTC themselves are neither visualized nor counted, and the assay only quantifies gene expression, which is essentially a surrogate for CTC. For example, an increase in a particular RT-PCR transcript could signify increase in CTC number, but it could also be the result of elevated gene expression per cell. RT-PCR would not easily distinguish between the two scenarios.

Analysis of Circulating Tumor Cells

The methodologies described above allow capture, enrichment and/or quantification of CTC in some manner and each method provides unique information. Useful data include the presence or absence of CTC, the absolute number of CTC, and the increase or decrease in CTC burden over time (Fig. 12.2). While such measures may

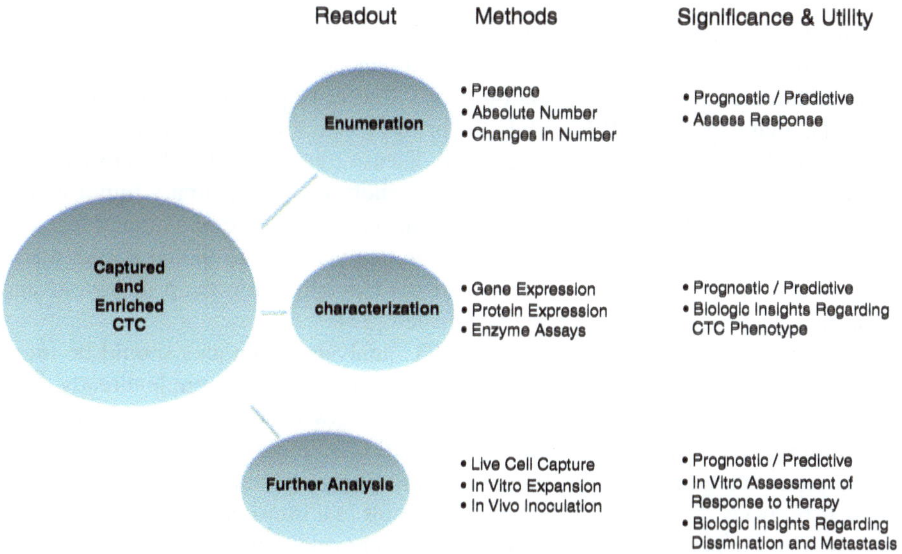

Fig. 12.2 Analysis of CTC after capture and identification can include variables as simple as the presence or absence of a CTC to quantitative analysis of gene expression of the captured cell

seem simplistic, they provide a real-time reflection of changes occurring at the cellular level of the cancer. This is a vast improvement over current radiographic imaging, which documents gross changes in tumor size that necessarily lag far behind any molecular or cellular disease changes. Such improved prognostic and predictive power is particularly relevant with the increasing use of biologic therapies, where disease response may manifest as tumor stabilization or necrosis which can be difficult to assess radiographically. Monitoring CTC numbers may also supplant various chemical serum tumor markers in use today, such as CEA and CA-125, which lack sensitivity and specificity, are often not predictive, or simply do not exist for many tumors [28, 29].

In addition to quantification of CTC and the trends of those values over times, capture of CTC also provides an opportunity for specific molecular characterization. Historically, immunohistochemical (IHC) or IF analysis of antigens on the surface of tumors has provided vital information about a malignancy's identity, outcome, and potential response to therapeutic intervention. However, tissue from primary tumors, tumor recurrences, or metastases often is not accessibly for biopsy, and repeating such biopsies over time is even more impractical due to technical limitations, cost, and patient safety and comfort. Study of captured CTC with IHC or IF provides an immensely powerful alternative which can be obtained cheaply, safely, and repeatedly throughout the course of disease and treatment. One expects that the profile of these cells may differ from that of the original tumor, perhaps reflecting phenotypic changes such as EMT discussed earlier, additional mutations that lead to dissemination, or changes induced by selective pressure from systemic therapy. Such highly informative "real-time" tumor biopsies in the form of CTC identification and molecular analysis are already being performed: Shaffer et al. successfully analyzed CellSearch-captured CTC from patients with prostate cancer for epidermal growth factor receptor (EGFR) expression, chromosome ploidy, and androgen receptor (AR) gene amplification [30]. Wulfing et al. analyzed HER2 expression on CTC from patients with breast cancer after density gradient enrichment and immunomagnetic separation [31]. Of note, 12 patients in this small study had CTC that expressed HER2 when the primary tumor did not. The expression of HER2 on CTC correlated with a decreased disease free survival and a shorter overall survival. Yen et al. compared the KRAS genotype of the primary tumor and of CTC in patients with metastatic colorectal cancer [32]. Of the 33 patients that harbored KRAS mutations in the primary tumor, analysis of CTC noted KRAS mutations in only 28 patients and a potential discordance between the primary site and metastatic lesions has already been established [33].

As with CTC enrichment strategies, CTC analysis techniques should be interpreted cautiously in light of their technical limitations. One example already cited is the difficulty when using RT-PCR in determining whether elevation of a particular transcript is caused by an increase in overall CTC number or increased per-cell expression of the gene. Another factor is the timing of sample collection. Interventions such as biopsies or surgical procedures can result in a transient release of epithelial cells into the circulation. This was described by Pachmann et al. who noted a 1,000-fold increase in circulating epithelial cells during the first 3 days after surgery for breast cancer that resolved after 2–4 days [34]. Depending on the assay and when it was performed, these transient epithelial cells could give the impression of a rise in CTC, underscoring the complexity of these assays and our still-evolving understanding of the information they provide.

Clinical Application of Circulating Tumor Cells

Although various methods of CTC quantification are still evolving and competing for mainstream use, there is already a sizable body of evidence supporting the clinical relevance of each modality (Table 12.1).

Density Gradient Centrifugation

Many studies have successfully employed the density gradient enrichment approach prior to CTC identification [35–37]. Early efforts that employed a density gradient alone proved too cumbersome and the advent of porous membrane enhancement improved outcomes and ease of use. A comparison between standard Ficoll density gradient separation and the OncoQuick membrane centrifugation method showed a higher sensitivity with OncoQuick in spiking assays (87% yield vs. 84%) with significantly fewer non-CTC mononuclear cells coenriched by the process (9.5×10^4 vs. 1.6×10^7) [38].

A study using the OncoQuick membrane density gradient system was applied to 60 women with resected breast cancer and 63 women with metastatic breast cancer [39]. Following density gradient enrichment, cells underwent positive selection with an anti-cytokeratin monoclonal antibody and negative selection with the leukocyte antigen CD45. Using this method, CTC were detected in 38.7% of women with metastatic breast cancer, compared to 8.3% of women with operable breast cancer who did not have overt metastases. In the latter group, there was a correlation between detectable CTC and the presence of DTC in the bone marrow. Serial CTC measurements were obtained in a subset of 25 women with metastatic disease after initiation of systemic therapy. CTC were found more frequently in patients with progressive disease than in those with stable disease or remission (87.5% vs. 43.8%).

Membrane Microfiltration

Vona et al. used ISET to analyze blood samples from 44 patients with newly diagnosed, untreated primary liver cancer but no overt metastases, as well as 30 patients

Table 12.1 Selected clinically significant studies using various CTC capture and enrichment technique

Method	Study	Clinical setting	Study design	Findings
Density gradient centrifugation	Muller et al. [41]	60 women with resected breast cancer and 63 women with metastatic breast cancer.	OncoQuick density gradient system followed by immunolabeling. CTC capture before systemic therapy; subgroup of 25 women with metastatic disease had serial CTC measurements after initiation of therapy.	CTC were more prevalent in patients with metastatic breast cancer than operable breast cancer (38.7% vs. 8.3%). In patients with metastatic disease, CTC more prevalent in poorly controlled cancer than in cases of stable disease or remission (87.5% vs. 43.8%).
Membrane microfiltration	Vona et al. [42]	44 patients with primary liver cancer and no metastases.	ISET device used for CTC capture and identity confirmed pathologically. CTC capture at diagnosis before treatment.	CTC were detected in 52.3% of patients with liver cancer and in none of the control group. Their presence correlated with a shorter overall survival.
	Wong et al. [43]	43 women with metastatic breast cancer.	Density gradient enrichment followed by filtration through a polycarbonate filter. CTC capture while systemic treatment was ongoing.	CTC present prior to therapy correlated with a shorter overall survival and a high level (≥13) was associated with a shorter time to progression.
Immunomagnetic separation	Cristofanilli et al. [48]	177 women with metastatic breast cancer.	CellSearch assay with high burden defined as ≥5 CTC per 7.5 ml of blood. CTC capture prior to starting a new systemic treatment.	High CTC correlated with a shorter progression free survival (2.7 months vs. 7.0 months) and a shorter overall survival (10.1 months vs. over 18 months).
	Cohen et al. [49]	430 patients with metastatic colorectal cancer.	CellSearch assay with high burden defined as ≥3 CTC per 7.5 ml of blood. CTC capture prior to starting a new systemic treatment and at various points during therapy.	High CTC correlated with a shorter progression free survival (4.5 months vs. 7.9 months) and a shorter overall survival (9.4 months vs. 18.5 months). A reduction in CTC from high burden to low burden during therapy was associated with better outcomes compared to patients whose CTC burden remained high.

	de Bono et al. [50]	231 men with metastatic castration-resistant prostate cancer.	CellSearch assay with high burden defined as ≥5 CTC per 7.5 ml of blood. CTC capture prior to starting a new systemic treatment and at various points during therapy.	High CTC correlated with a shorter progression overall survival (11.5 months vs. 21.7 months). A reduction in CTC from high burden to low burden during therapy was associated with better outcomes compared to patients whose CTC burden remained high.
Whole blood polymerase chain reaction	Stathopoulou et al. [53]	148 women with resected breast cancer.	PCR targeting CK19. CTC capture at least 2 weeks after surgery and before any systemic treatment.	Detection of CK19 mRNA prior to adjuvant therapy was an independent poor prognostic factor.
	Ross et al. [54]	104 men with castration-resistant prostate cancer.	PCR targeting PSA. CTC capture prior to starting initial chemotherapy regimen.	PSA mRNA is an independent prognostic factor for time to progression and overall survival.
	Wang et al. [56]	72 patients with resectable colorectal cancer.	PCR targeting CEA. CTC capture immediately prior to resection of primary tumor.	CEA mRNA correlates with depth of invasion, TNM stage, and postoperative metastases.

with hepatitis, 39 with cirrhosis, and 38 healthy individuals [40]. CTC were detected in 23 of the 44 patients with liver cancer and none of the other cohorts analyzed. In this study, the presence of CTC was associated with a shorter overall survival. Wong et al. studied 43 patients with metastatic breast cancer and initially used density gradient enrichment, then passed the isolated fraction of blood through a polycarbonate filter to capture CTC [41]. This study found that the presence of CTC prior to therapy was associated with a shorter overall survival, and an absolute value of ≥13 CTC was associated with a shorter time to progression.

Immunomagnetic Labeling

Immunomagnetic separation has been successfully applied to various clinical settings. Gaforio et al. captured CTC using the immunomagnetic strategy and correlated their presence with progression-free survival (PFS) and overall survival (OS) [42]. Peripheral blood was obtained from 92 patients with breast cancer in various stages prior to initiation of chemotherapy. Blood from 16 healthy patients served as negative controls and no CTC were isolated from these patients, however CTC were detected in 62% of the breast cancer patients. The presence of CTC correlated with expression of estrogen receptors and the presence of lymph node metastases. In addition, detection of CTC correlated with shorter median OS and PFS. CTC were detected in all 11 of the patients who died. Immunomagnetic enrichment was used by Chen et al. to capture CTC from 84 patients with advanced prostate cancer, 69 of whom had metastatic disease [43]. A group of 39 healthy donors served as negative controls. CTC were detected in 62% of the samples and none of the controls. CTC correlated well with PSA and were more prevalent in patients receiving chemotherapy than in those receiving hormonal therapy. Soria et al. used immunomagnetic beads coated with an epithelial-specific antibody (BerEP4) to capture CTC from women with metastatic breast cancer with healthy patients serving as negative controls [44]. The captured cells were then used to assay telomerase activity, in an attempt to establish a molecular marker for cancer. Of the 25 samples, 21 demonstrated telomerase activity (84%) while none of the controls were positive.

An alternative enrichment-free immunolabeling approach has been employed as well. Luttgen et al. isolated CTC from patients with non-small-cell lung cancer by lysing erythrocytes and labeling CTC using antibodies directed against nine cytokeratins [45]. FAST was employed to detect the position of the labeled cells. In their prospective analysis, changes in CTC were correlated with response to chemotherapy. Of the 20 patients with data at time 0, 3, 6, and 9 months, 95% demonstrated a direct correlation between change in CTC count and clinical response to chemotherapy.

The CellSearch assay has been validated and FDA approved in breast, colon, and prostates cancers, and as such has recently become the de facto gold standard for CTC quantification in the clinical setting. A prospective study in breast cancer by

Cristofanilli et al. led to the first FDA approval for the CellSearch system [46]. In this study, 177 women with metastatic breast cancer underwent CTC testing using the CellSearch assay. High CTC burden was defined as five or more CTC per 7.5 ml of peripheral blood while low CTC burden included women with less than five CTC, a cutoff based on a training set analysis that was subsequently confirmed with a validation set. High CTC was associated with a shorter median progression-free survival (2.7 months vs. 7.0 months, $p<0.001$) and a shorter overall survival (10.1 months vs. >18 months, $p<0.001$). Several years later, this assay was validated in patients with colon cancer. In a large, prospective, multicenter study, Cohen et al. measured CTC in 430 patients with metastatic colorectal cancer and in this case, high CTC burden was defined as three or more CTC per 7.5 ml of peripheral blood based on training and validation set analyses [47]. Patients with high CTC at baseline had a shorter median progression-free survival (4.5 months vs. 7.9 months, $p=0.0002$) and overall survival (9.4 months vs. 18.5 months, $p=0.0001$). Conversion from a high CTC to a low CTC was associated with better outcomes when compared to patients whose CTC remained high. More recently, the CellSearch assay has been tested in men with prostate cancer. Using the same definition of high CTC burden as the breast study (five or more CTC per 7.5 ml of peripheral blood), de Bono et al. prospectively studied 231 men with metastatic castration-resistant prostate cancer (CRPC) [48]. Men with high CTC prior to initiating therapy had a shorter median overall survival than men with low CTC (11.5 months vs. 21.7 months). This correlation held true for posttreatment CTC as well. Men who started with high CTC but converted to low CTC with treatment had a longer survival than men whose CTC remained elevated. The converse held true as well; men whose CTC started low but rose during treatment fared worse than those whose CTC remained low (Fig. 12.3). Thus, because of its greater sensitivity and specificity as well as technical feasibility, such serial CTC measurement has the potential to augment or even replace other biologic markers, such as PSA measurements in prostate cancer [49]. It is important to note that CTC are not necessarily indicative of disease burden. CTC studies reported to date have not cited any direct correlation between CTC number and tumor burden. For example, in one study of patients with prostate cancer, CTC number had only a modest association with baseline PSA and correlated more with sites of metastasis and prior treatment, suggesting that the presence of CTC depends more on the biology of the cancer (e.g., pattern of spread) than the burden of disease [50].

Whole Blood PCR

Numerous small studies using RT-PCR have demonstrated clinical significance with this indirect CTC assessment. Stathopoulou et al. used RT-PCR to detect CK19 mRNA in women with stage I and II breast cancer. Detection of CK19 mRNA before initiation of adjuvant therapy was an independent poor prognostic factor

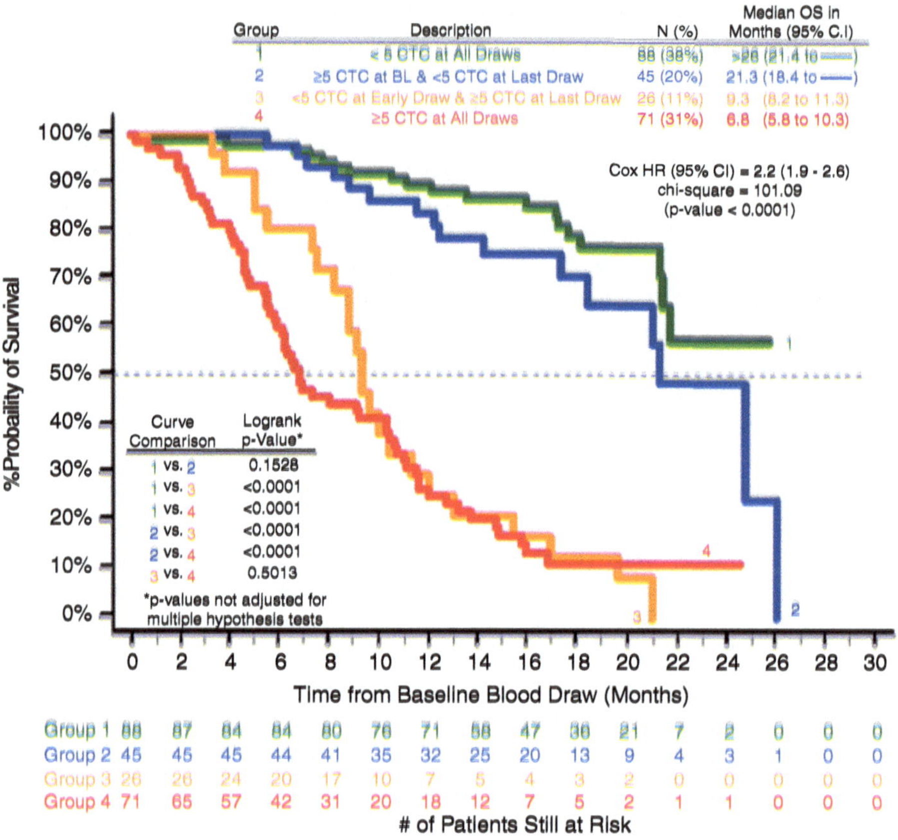

Fig. 12.3 Kaplan-Meier estimates of probability of overall survival (OS) of patients with castration-resistant prostate cancer based on the presence of favorable (<5) or unfavorable (>5) CTC prior to treatment and over the course of treatment. Patients whose CTC were always favorable had the longest OS and those whose CTC were always unfavorable had the shortest OS. Patients whose CTC converted from the unfavorable to the favorable group had a longer survival than those who converted from the favorable to the unfavorable (Reprinted from de Bono JS, Scher HI, Montgomery RB, et al. Circulating tumor cells predict survival benefit from treatment in metastatic castration-resistant prostate cancer. Clin Cancer Res. 2008;14(19):6302–6309. With permission from the American Association for Cancer Research)

[51]. In men with prostate cancer, Ross et al. [52] and Ghossein et al. [37] independently quantified mRNA transcripts for PSA. These groups found PSA mRNA to be an independent prognostic factor for time to progression and overall survival, respectively. CEA mRNA was detected in patients with colorectal cancer undergoing curative resection. CEA mRNA detection correlated with stage at diagnosis and was found to be an independent predictor of postoperative metastasis [53]. RT-PCR continues to be employed in CTC quantification studies, using various target genes (Table 12.1).

Biology of Circulating Tumor Cells

While the clinical utility of CTC measurement has been demonstrated in a multitude of studies, the precise role of CTC in cancer biology is less clear. Many have speculated that CTC represent the critical dissemination step from a primary tumor to distant metastasis. Dramatic changes in phenotype are necessary as cancer cells transition from the environment of the primary tumor, to circulation, to possible "sanctuary niches." and finally to new metastatic sites. For example, the primary tumor environment favors cellular adhesion and angiogenesis in order to promote growth through access to nutrients and oxygen. In contrast, dissemination requires loss of cellular adhesion to facilitate migration into and through the circulation as well as evasion of immune surveillance [54, 55]. It is not clear what triggers this change, in part described as EMT, though some factor such as the transcription factor Twist, have been identified [56]. Once disseminated tumor cells establish metastatic sites, they may need to change yet again, reverting back to their epithelial state (MET) which favors growth and proliferation (Fig. 12.4).

Preliminary findings in these areas have raised more questions than they have answered: Multiple studies have documented the presence of CTC and DTC in the bone marrow of early stage cancers, including breast [57] and prostate [25]. Others have shown that DTC possess a cell surface antigen profile similar to that of so-called cancer stem cells (CSC), a highly tumorigenic and therapy resistant subset of tumor cell thought to promote cancer recurrence and metastasis [58]; still others have shown that CTC have a low Ki67 proliferative index, another characteristic in common with CSC [59].

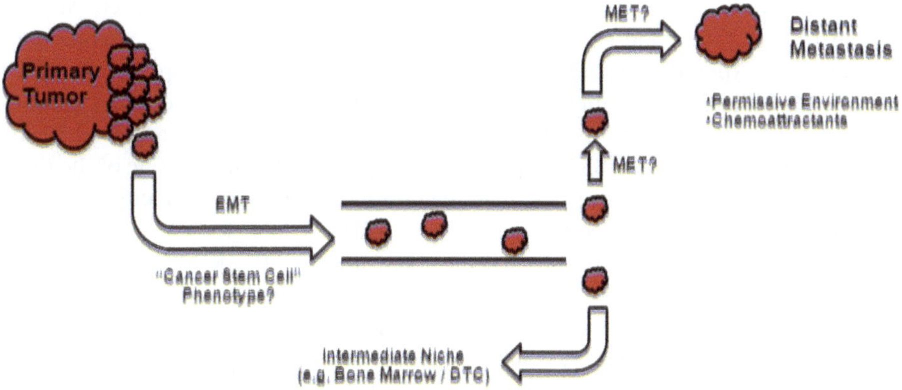

Fig. 12.4 Hypothetical CTC model based on preliminary biologic data. The epithelial to mesenchymal transition (EMT) is induced by the transcriptional factor Twist and this phenotypic change necessary for migration of tumor cells may be more likely to occur in cells with a certain progenitor or "cancer stem cell" phenotype. From the periphery, CTC may seek an intermediary niche such as the bone marrow, or may establish distant metastases, which may require a mesenchymal to epithelial transition (MET) to regain a phenotype necessary for implantation and/or growth

These preliminary findings offer tantalizing glimpses of a complex biology which has yet to be deciphered; does the presence of CTC necessarily portend metastatic disease, or are CTC a common epiphenomenon of primary tumors, and are additional steps necessary for those CTC to become clinical metastases? If so, what are those steps, and are they dependent on changes within the CTC themselves or a subset of CTC (those with a CSC phenotype), or perhaps on signals from the primary tumor or from an enabling niche such as the bone marrow, or maybe alterations in the metastatic target site (the so-called seed versus soil dilemma), or some combination of these factors? It is likely that cells enter the periphery without developing overt metastases and this transition may be necessary but not sufficient. The signals responsible for these multiple steps are largely unknown, and the study of CTC may shed light on the process.

Future Directions

The Technology of CTC Quantification

The most pressing question in regards to CTC analysis involves the best method by which to quantify these cells. Cross-comparison of clinical data obtained from studies employing different methods is imprudent because of the very different pros and cons of these methods already described. A comparison between the OncoQuick and CellSearch assays has been described [6]. In healthy patients, neither assay detected any CTC but in patients with metastatic carcinoma, OncoQuick revealed CTC in 23% of patients compared to 54% detected by the CellSearch assay. The absolute number of CTC detected was also greater with the CellSearch approach. A different study compared immunomagnetic separation (followed by laser scanning cytometry), filtration and RT-PCR in samples from patients with metastatic breast cancer [60]. Apparent sensitivity was lowest in the filtration approach, which revealed CTC in 30% of patients tested, compared to 48% identified with immunomagnetic separation. The highest sensitivity was with multimarker real-time RT-PCR, which found that 83% of patients were positive for at least one of the three PCR markers used (cytokeratin 19, mammaglobin, and prolactin-inducible peptide). The filtration strategy was compared to direct RT-PCR in a study by Pinzani et al. [61] who obtained peripheral blood from 44 women with operable breast cancer prior to curative resection (19 stage I, 20 stage II, 5 stage III) and from 40 healthy women, who served as controls. Peripheral blood was analyzed with ISET and blood from the same sample was also subject to RT-PCR targeting CK19. Neither method detected CTC in the control samples. Both ISET and RT-PCR detected CTC in 12 of the 44 samples from patients with breast cancer. There was concordance between ten of the samples but two samples were only positive by ISET and another two were only positive by RT-PCR. The authors concluded that the two methods could be considered equivalent. Additional studies comparing the different methodologies are warranted, but at this time, all of the available methods continue

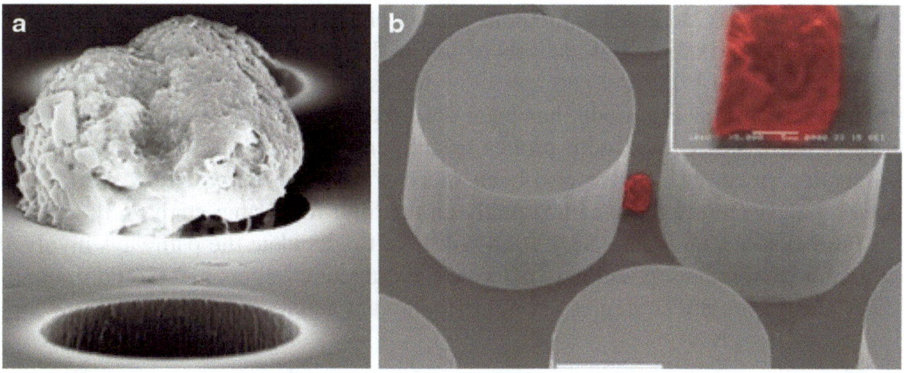

Fig. 12.5 Development of membrane filters used in CTC capture. (**a**) Electron micrograph of CTC captured on a parylene-C pore microfilter (MEMS); (**b**) Scanning electron micrograph of CTC captured with microfluidic device (Reprinted from Nagrath S, Sequist LV, Maheswaran S, et al. Isolation of rare circulating tumour cells in cancer patients by microchip technology. Nature. 2007;450:1235–1238. With permission from Nature Publishing Group)

to be used and each has its own niche and utility. The burden of selecting a method lies with each investigator, and the study results should be interpreted with an understanding of the advantages and limitations of the techniques used.

Newer techniques hold the potential to increase the sensitivity and specificity of CTC detection. Microfluidic devices have been developed and show early promise. The "CTC-chip" was first described by Nagrath et al. and consists of an array of EpCAM antibody-coated microposts exposed to a patient's peripheral blood under precisely defined laminar flow conditions (Fig. 12.5) [62]. The system ensures maximum interaction between any CTC and the labeled microposts and allows quantification without any prelabeling. This system was efficacious in spiking assays and in 116 peripheral blood samples, most of which were from patients with metastatic disease, 115 samples (>99%) demonstrated some degree of CTC. These data were highly reproducible and in a smaller subgroup, the changes in CTC correlated well with clinical course. New equipment and technological advances promise improvement in existing strategies as well. In another approach, a parylene-C membrane slot microfilter has been developed in combination with a constant pressure driving fluid delivery system. This system has demonstrated high efficiency for live cell capture, thus eliminating the need for fixation and permitting extensive analysis of the captured cells [63].

The Biology of CTC

As described earlier, many questions remain about the role of CTC in cancer dissemination, and emerging capture technologies may provide improved opportunities to study these cells. One area of active investigation is the expansion in culture of live captured CTC in order to facilitate further characterization. Current techniques necessitate cell fixation, but analysis of live cells would expand our understanding of the biology of CTC and perhaps allow for as says testing sensitivity to various therapies. A promising model has been described by Talasaz et al. involving activated micropores coated with probes to antigens such as EpCAM [64]. The slot filters described above have also been successfully used to capture live cells and subsequently culture these cells directly on the filter for further study [63].

Further molecular characterization will help to elucidate the pathways involved in tumor dissemination and may offer new therapeutic targets that would dramatically alter treatment strategies in both the adjuvant and metastatic settings.

Clinical Applications of CTC

The majority of clinical data exists in patients with metastatic disease, but there may be even greater utility to CTC analysis in early stage cancer. Many cancer patients who undergo curative therapy for so-called localized tumors eventually suffer disease recurrence and metastasis, caused by early microscopic dissemination of their primary tumor which was not clinically detectable at the time of primary therapy. Such dissemination may be mediated by CTC, and our increasing ability to detect these cells may lead to more accurate prognostic guidelines and better directed therapeutic maneuvers. Specifically, the presence of CTC may indicate which patients with early stage cancer will suffer distant recurrence, allowing administration of aggressive adjuvant therapy to the population most likely to benefit. CTC may also allow early assessment of response to therapy and may expedite changes in ineffective regimens. After completion of indicated therapy, CTC may serve a prominent role in cancer surveillance.

CTC studies in early disease are ongoing and preliminary results are promising. In one study of 70 patients with local breast cancer receiving primary systemic therapy, peripheral blood was tested for CTC at the start of every cycle of neoadjuvant chemotherapy and before and after surgery [65]. Nearly all patients had detectable CTC and the number of CTC correlated with primary tumor size. Of the patients whose CTC burden improved significantly (at least tenfold) with adjuvant therapy, none had experienced a relapse of disease with a posttherapy observation period of 4.5 years. Patients that suffered an increase in CTC burden during therapy had an 11–16-fold hazard ratio for relapse. The larger SUCCESS trial ongoing in Germany seeks to validate these data [66]. In this study, 1,767 patients with node-positive or high risk node-negative breast cancer submitted blood for CTC analysis (using the CellSearch system) after resection but before any systemic treatment. Nearly half of the participants submitted blood at the completion of chemotherapy for further analysis. This study noted CTC in 10% of all patients before the start of systemic treatment. The presence of CTC correlated with the presence of lymph node metastases at the time of surgery. Outcome analysis is not yet mature, but this study may guide the future role of CTC in early cancer therapy.

In advanced disease, one ongoing trial sponsored by the Southwest Oncology Group (SWOG S0421), CTC are collected from men with metastatic castration resistant prostate cancer before and during treatment in a Phase III multi-center therapeutic trial. Specimens in this correlative study are analyzed for CTC number as well as expression of several markers associated with aggressive disease and therapy response [67]. Another ongoing SWOG trial (SWOG S0500) is investigating whether CTC data can be used to guide therapy in real time [68]. Breast cancer patients receiving treatment will undergo CTC analysis using the CellSearch assay in order to quickly identify nonresponders. Patients with elevated CTC prior to therapy will undergo a second analysis after 21 days of therapy. Should CTC fall, therapy will continue, but if CTC rise or remain elevated, patients will be randomized to change therapy, based on CTC alone, or to continue therapy until clinical progression is noted. The results of this study may impact our assessment of ongoing therapy. It could decrease the need for serial imaging and prevent ongoing use of ineffective regimens, preventing unnecessary adverse effects and facilitating initiation of a regimen with proper antitumor activity.

Yet another exciting application of CTC with enormous clinical potential would be in the early diagnosis of cancers. With improvements in capture and analysis, CTC may ultimately replace many less effective screening tests currently available. Though there is scant data to support its current use in that arena, CTC technology is rapidly evolving and may yet prove invaluable for early detection and eradication of occult malignancy.

References

1. Lindemann F, Schlimok G, Dirschedl P, Witte J, Riethmuller G. Prognostic significance of micrometastatic tumour cells in bone marrow of colorectal cancer patients. Lancet. 1992; 340:685–9.
2. Cote RJ, Beattie EJ, Chaiwun B, et al. Detection of occult bone marrow micrometastases in patients with operable lung carcinoma. Ann Surg. 1995;222:415–23.
3. Kollermann J, Weikert S, Schostak M, et al. Prognostic significance of disseminated tumor cells in the bone marrow of prostate cancer patients submitted to neoadjuvant hormonal therapy. J Clin Oncol. 2008;26(30):4928–33.
4. Braun S, Vogl FD, Naume B, et al. A pooled analysis of bone marrow micrometastasis in breast cancer. N Engl J Med. 2005;353(8):793–802.
5. Riethdorf S, Wikman H, Pantel K. Biological relevance of disseminated tumor cells in cancer patients. Int J Cancer. 2008;123:1991–2006.
6. Balic M, Dandachi N, Hofmann G, et al. Comparison of two methods for enumerating circulating tumor cells in carcinoma patients. Cytometry B Clin Cytom. 2005;68(1):25–30.
7. Meng S, Tripathy D, Frenkel EP, et al. Circulating tumor cells in patients with breast cancer dormancy. Clin Cancer Res. 2004;10:8152–62.
8. Zheng S, Lin H, Liu JQ, et al. Membrane microfilter device for selective capture, electrolysis and genomic analysis of human circulating tumor cells. J Chromatogr A. 2007;1162(2):154–61.
9. Zabaglo L, Ormerod MG, Parton M, Ring A, Smith IE, Dowsett M. Cell filtration-laser scanning cytometry for the characterisation of circulating breast cancer cells. Cytometry A. 2003;55A:102–8.

10. Xu T, Lu B, Tai YC, Goldkorn A. A cancer detection platform which measures telomerase activity from live circulating tumor cells captured on a microfilter. Cancer Res. 2010;70(16): 6420–6.
11. Vona G, Sabile A, Louha M, et al. Isolation by size of epithelial tumor cells: a new method for the immunomorphological and molecular characterization of circulating tumor cells. Am J Pathol. 2000;156:57–63.
12. Ntouroupi TG, Ashraf SQ, Seppo A, Kilpatrick MW, Tsipouras P, Tafas T, Bodmer WF. Detection of circulating tumor cells in peripheral blood with an automated scanning fluorescence microscope. Proc ASCO Molecular Markers; 2008. Abstract 8.
13. Witzig TE, Bossy B, Kimlinger T, et al. Detection of circulating cytokeratins-positive cells in the blood of breast cancer patients using immunomagnetic enrichment and digital microscopy. Clin Cancer Res. 2002;8:1085–91.
14. Campos M, Prior C, Warleta F, et al. Phenotypic and genetic characterization of circulating tumor cells by combining immunomagnetic selection and FICTION techniques. J Histochem Cytochem. 2008;56(7):66–75.
15. Bilkenroth U, Taubert H, Riemann D, Rebmann U, Heynemann H, Meye A. Detection and enrichment of disseminated renal carcinoma cells from peripheral blood by immunomagnetic cell separation. Int J Cancer. 2001;92(4):577–82.
16. Comijn J, Berx G, Vermassen P, et al. The two-handed E box binding zinc finger protein SIP1 downregulates E-cadherin and induces invasion. Mol Cell. 2001;7:1267–78.
17. Peinado H, Olmeda D, Cano A. Snail, Zeb and bHLH factors in tumour progression: an alliance against the epithelial phenotype? Nat Rev Cancer. 2007;7:415–28.
18. Mani SA, Guo W, Liao MJ, et al. The epithelial-mesenchymal transition generates cells with properties of stem cells. Cell. 2008;133(4):704–15.
19. Cheng GZ, Chan J, Wang Q, Zhang W, Sun CD, Wang LH. Twist transcriptionally up-regulates AKT2 in breast cancer cells leading to increased migration, invasion, and resistance to paclitaxel. Cancer Res. 2007;67:1979–87.
20. Polyak K, Weinberg RA. Transitions between epithelial and mesenchymal states: acquisition of malignant and stem cell traits. Nat Rev Cancer. 2009;9:265–73.
21. Leon SA, Shapiro B, Sklaroff DM, Yaros MJ. Free DNA in the serum of cancer patients and the effect of therapy. Cancer Res. 1977;37(3):646–50.
22. Lin YG, Merritt WM, Spannuth WA, et al. Efficient recovery of circulating tumor cells (CTC) using novel micro-electro-mechanical system (MEMS)-based platform. Proc Am Assoc Cancer Res; 2008. Abstract LB-298.
23. Hoon DS, Wang Y, Dale PS, et al. Detection of occult melanoma cells in blood with a multiple-marker polymerase chain reaction assay. J Clin Oncol. 1995;13(8):2109–16.
24. Conzelmann M, Linnemann U, Berger MR. Molecular detection of clinical colorectal cancer metastasis: how should multiple markers be put to use? Int J Colorectal Dis. 2005;20:137–46.
25. Katz AE, de Vries GM, Olsson CA, et al. Molecular staging of genitourinary malignancies. Urology. 1996;47(6):948–58.
26. Noguchi M, Miyajima J, Itoh K, Noda S. Detection of circulating tumor cells in patients with prostate cancer using prostate specific membrane-derived primers in the polymerase chain reaction. Int J Urol. 1997;4(4):374–9.
27. Miyamoto A, Nagano H, Sakon M, et al. Clinical application of quantitative analysis for detection of hematogenous spread of hepatocellular carcinoma by real-time PCR. Int J Oncol. 2001;18(3):527–32.
28. Rustin GJ, van der Burg ME. A randomized trial in ovarian cancer (OC) of early treatment of relapse based on CA125 level alone versus delayed treatment based on conventional clinical indicators (MRC OV05/EORTC 55955 trials). JCO. 2009;27 Suppl 18. Abstract 1.
29. Macdonald JS. Carcinoembryonic antigen screening: pros and cons. Semin Oncol. 1999; 26(5):556–60.
30. Shaffer DR, Leversha MA, Danila DC, et al. Circulating tumor cell analysis in patients with progressive castration-resistant prostate cancer. Clin Cancer Res. 2007;13(7):2023–9.

31. Wulfing P, Borchard J, Buerger H, et al. HER2-positive circulating tumor cells indicate poor clinical outcome in stage I to III breast cancer patients. Clin Cancer Res. 2006;12(6):1715–20.
32. Yen LC, Yeh YS, Chen CW, et al. Detection of KRAS oncogene in peripheral blood as a predictor of the response to cetuximab plus chemotherapy in patients with metastatic colorectal cancer. Clin Cancer Res. 2009;15(13):4508–13.
33. Artale S, Sartore-Bianchi A, Veronese SM, et al. Mutations of KRAS and BRAF in primary and matched metastatic sites of colorectal cancer. J Clin Oncol. 2008;26(25):4217–9.
34. Pachmann K. Longtime recirculating tumor cells in breast cancer patients. Clin Cancer Res. 2005;11:5657–8.
35. Pachmann K, Clement JH, Schneider CP, et al. Standardized quantification of circulating peripheral tumor cells from lung and breast cancer. Clin Chem Lab Med. 2005;43(6):617–27.
36. Campos M, Prior C, Warleta F, et al. Phenotypic and genetic characterization of circulating tumor cells by combining immunomagnetic selection and FICTION techniques. J Histochem Cytochem. 2008;56(7):667–75.
37. Ghossein RA, Rosai J, Scher HI, et al. Prognostic significance of detection of prostate-specific antigen transcripts in the peripheral blood of patients with metastatic androgen-independent prostatic carcinoma. Urology. 1997;50:100–5.
38. Rosenberg R, Gertler R, Friederichs J, et al. Comparison of two density gradient centrifugation systems for the enrichment of disseminated tumor cells in blood. Cytometry. 2002;49(4):150–8.
39. Muller V, Stahmann N, Riethdorf S, et al. Circulating tumor cells in breast cancer: correlation to bone marrow micrometastases, heterogeneous response to systemic therapy and low proliferative activity. Clin Cancer Res. 2005;11(10):3678–85.
40. Vona G, Estepa L, Beroud C, et al. Impact of cytomorphological detection of circulating tumor cells in patients with liver cancer. Hepatology. 2004;39:792–7.
41. Wong NS, Kahn HJ, Zhang L, et al. Prognostic significance of circulating tumor cells enumerated after filtration enrichment in early and metastatic breast cancer patients. Breast Cancer Res Treat. 2006;99:63–9.
42. Gaforio JJ, Serrano MJ, Sanchez-Rovira P, et al. Detection of breast cancer cells in the peripheral blood is positively correlated with estrogen-receptor status and predicts for poor prognosis. Int J Cancer. 2003;107:984–90.
43. Chen BT, Loberg RD, Neeley CK, et al. Preliminary study of immunomagnetic quantification of circulating tumor cells in patients with advanced disease. Urology. 2004;65:616–21.
44. Soria JC, Gauthier LR, Raymond E, et al. Molecular detection of telomerase-positive circulating epithelial cells in metastatic breast cancer patients. Clin Cancer Res. 1999;5:971–5.
45. Luttgen MS, Marrinucci D, Lazar D, et al. Circulating tumor cells monitored over time in lung cancer patients. JCO. 2009;27 Suppl 15, abstract 11025.
46. Cristofanilli M, Budd GT, Ellis MJ, et al. Circulating tumor cells, disease progression, and survival in metastatic breast cancer. N Engl J Med. 2004;351:781–91.
47. Cohen SJ, Punt CJ, Iannotti N, et al. Relationship of circulating tumor cells to tumor response, progression-free survival, and overall survival in patients with metastatic colorectal cancer. J Clin Oncol. 2008;26(19):3213–21.
48. de Bono JS, Scher HI, Montgomery RB, et al. Circulating tumor cells predict survival benefit from treatment in metastatic castration-resistant prostate cancer. Clin Cancer Res. 2008;14(19):6302–9.
49. Goodman OB, Fink LM, Symanowski JT, et al. Longitudinal analysis of circulating tumor cell (CTC) counts in prostate cancer patients: assessment of treatment efficacy. JCO. 2008;26 Suppl, abstract 5169.
50. Danila DC, Heller G, Gignac GA, et al. Circulating tumor cell number and prognosis in progressive castration-resistant prostate cancer. Clin Cancer Res. 2007;13(23):7053–8.
51. Stathopoulou A, Vlachonikolis I, Mavroudis D, et al. Molecular detection of cytokeratin-19-positive cells in the peripheral blood of patients with operable breast cancer: evaluation of their prognostic significance. J Clin Oncol. 2002;20:3404–12.

52. Ross RW, Manola J, Hennessy K, et al. Prognostic significance of baseline reverse transcriptase-PCR for prostate-specific antigen in men with hormone-refractory prostate cancer treated with chemotherapy. Clin Cancer Res. 2005;11:5295–8.
53. Wang JY, Wu CH, Lu CY, et al. Molecular detection of circulating tumor cells in the peripheral blood of patients with colorectal cancer using RT-PCR: significance of the prediction of postoperative metastasis. World J Surg. 2006;3:1007–13.
54. Marches R, Scheuermann R, Uhr J. Cancer dormancy: from mice to man. Cell Cycle. 2006;5(16):1772–8.
55. Rossi DJ, Jamieson CH, Weissman IL. Stem cells and the pathways to aging and cancer. Cell. 2008;132:681–96.
56. Yang J, Mani SA, Weinberg RA. Exploring a new twist on tumor metastasis. Cancer Res. 2006;66:4549–52.
57. Pachmann K, Camara O, Hammer U, et al. The impact of systemic chemotherapy on circulating epithelial tumor cells (CETC) in breast cancer. JCO. 2008;26 Suppl, abstract 11001.
58. Balic M, Lin H, Young L, et al. Most early disseminated cancer cells detected in bone marrow of breast cancer patients have a putative breast cancer stem cell phenotype. Clin Cancer Res. 2006;12(19):5615–21.
59. Schindlbeck C, Kampik T, Janni W, et al. Prognostic relevance of disseminated tumor cells in the bone marrow and biological factors of 265 primary breast carcinomas. Breast Cancer Res. 2005;7(6):1174–85.
60. Ring AE, Zabaglo L, Ormerod MG, Smith IE, Dowsett M. Detection of circulating epithelial cells in the blood of patients with breast cancer: comparison of three techniques. Br J Cancer. 2005;92:906–12.
61. Pinzani P, Salvadori B, Simi L, et al. Isolation by size of epithelial tumor cells in peripheral blood of patients with breast cancer: correlation with real-time reverse transcriptase-polymerase chain reaction results and feasibility of molecular analysis by laser microdissection. Hum Pathol. 2006;37(6):711–8.
62. Nagrath S, Sequist LV, Maheswaran S, et al. Isolation of rare circulating tumour cells in cancer patients by microchip technology. Nature. 2007;450:1235–8.
63. Lu B. A novel parylene membrane slot filter for capture, analysis and culture of viable circulating tumor cells from human whole blood. IEEE international conference on micro-electro-mechanical systems; 2010; Hong Kong, China.
64. Talasaz AH, Powell AA, Stahl P, et al. Cell trapping in activated micropores for functional analysis. Conf Proc IEEE Eng Med Biol Soc. 2006;1:1838–41.
65. Pachmann K, Camara O, Hammer U, Joerke C, Krauspe S, Rabenstein C, Runnebaum I, Hoeffken K. The impact of systemic chemotherapy on circulating epithelial tumor cells (CETC) in breast cancer. JCO. 2008;26 Suppl, abstract 11001.
66. Rack BK, Schindlbeck C, Hofmann S, et al. Circulating tumor cells (CTCs) in peripheral blood of primary breast cancer patients. JCO. 2007;25 Suppl 18, abstract 10595.
67. Goldkorn A, Xu T, Lu B, et al. Circulating tumor cell capture and analysis in a multicenter SWOG-coordinated prostate cancer trial. JCO. 2010;28 Suppl 15, A-TPS342.
68. Smerage J, Hayes D, Winer E. Using circulating tumor cells to guide treatment. Http://www.cancer.gov/clinicaltrials/ft-SWOG-S0500. Accessed 29 Sept 2010.

Chapter 13
Focus on Personalized Molecular Based Medicine

Lex H.T. Van der Ploeg, Bud Mishra, Casimir P. Eitner, Jon Burrows, Thomas Wray Tombler Jr., Vladimir Poponin, Daniel J. Knauer, Ilia Ichetovkin, Richard M. Pinnola, Gregory A. Endress, and Patrick Soon-Shiong

L.H.T. Van der Ploeg, Ph.D. (✉)
Rhythm Pharmaceuticals, Managing Director VDP, LLC,
Rhythm, 855 Boylston Street, Boston, MA 02116, USA
e-mail: lex.vanderploeg@gmail.com

B. Mishra, Ph.D.
Department of Computer Science and Mathematics, Courant Institute of Mathematical Sciences, New York University, New York, NY, USA

C.P. Eitner, B.Sc.
OncoPlex Diagnostics, Rockville, MS, USA

J. Burrows, Ph.D.
OncoPlex Diagnostics, Rockville, MD, USA

T.W. Tombler Jr., Ph.D.
ADD Biosensors, Somerset, NJ, USA

V. Poponin, Ph.D.
Nant Holdings, LLC, Costa Mesa, CA, USA

D.J. Knauer, Ph.D.
Manager, Oncology R&D, Vela Diagnostics, 353C Rt. 46 West, Fairfield, NJ 07004, USA

I. Ichetovkin, Ph.D.
Head of Oncology, Vela Diagnostics, 353C Rt. 46 West, Fairfield, NJ 07004, USA

R.M. Pinnola, B.S. • G.A. Endress
NeoDiagnostix, Inc., Rockville, MD, USA

P. Soon-Shiong, M.D.
Departments of Microbiology, Immunology, and Molecular Genetics, Bioengineering, University of California at Los Angeles, Los Angeles, CA, USA

H.-J. Lenz (ed.), *Biomarkers in Oncology: Prediction and Prognosis*,
DOI 10.1007/978-1-4419-9755-5_13, © Springer Science+Business Media New York 2013

Abbreviations

BCC	Basal cell carcinoma
BRCA	Breast cancer susceptibility protein
BRAF	A raf family kinase
cfBRAF	Cell free BRAF
Cone biopsy	Conization
C-Kit	Oncogene
CGH	Comparative genomic hybridization
Cox2	Cyclooxygenase 2
FISH	Fluorescent in situ hybridization
Her2	Human epidermal growth factor receptor 2
KRAS	Kirsten ras
LEEP	Loop electrosurgical excision procedure
miRNA	microRNA
PDAC	Pancreatic duct adenocarcinoma
PARP	Poly ADP ribose polymerase
PDGFR	Platelet derived growth factor receptor
PI3K	Phosphoinositol 3 kinase
SKY	Spectral karyotyping
TCGA	The cancer genome atlas
TGF-B	Transforming growth factor Beta
VEGF	Vascular endothelial growth factor
SCC	Cutaneous squamous cell carcinoma
siRNA	Small interfering RNA
SRM/MRM triple quad mass spectrometry	Selected reaction monitoring triple quad mass spectrometry, multiple reaction monitoring triple quad mass spectrometry

Introduction

While diverse 'Omics capabilities have been applied in academic and industry settings for target identification, target validation, and systems biology advances, their impact to health care delivery has trailed their promise. As is often the case, access to new tools leads believers to pronounce that their ultimate wonders will change the world. These promised technology revolutions often end up as slow technology evolutions that are anticipated to pay off, eventually. We now enter a period of change, where these diverse 'Omics technologies may be applied to improve delivery of health care. Specifically, molecular diagnostic biomarker technologies are gaining stronger inroads in guiding the treatment of cancer. Several success stories apply where prognostic and predictive outcomes allow a calculation of the likelihood of progression to metastatic breast cancer allowing clinicians to modify a given therapeutic approach to alter the disease course [1–4]. Excellent examples include molecular diagnostic markers that predict risk for breast cancer (BRCA1, 2) [5] or those that have power to indicate a suitable treatment based on companion diagnostics (e.g., PARP, BRAF, Her2, Cisplatin in CRC, KRAS mutations) [6]. Markers of toxicity and metabolism, such as CYP enzymes isoforms, have also been identified and are being applied in guiding treatment decisions. These initial successes are supported by a rapidly expanding set of clinical and 'Omics basic research databases (SAGE, BROAD Inst, Karolinska, TCGA, etc.) that—it is hoped—will provide novel, critical insights into disease pathways and networks thereby leading to the development and application of pathway/network-specific treatment decisions individualized for each patient's specific condition. The first clinical applications of these newly gained insights will likely include predictions for the development of improved prognostic and predictive diagnostic tests. The promise of these high content databases is that causal analysis of coordinately regulated genes, other cellular parameters, and clinical traits will herald a reclassification of disease, through its molecular definition, and the discovery of novel clinical trait associations with disease mechanisms. We project that the field of molecular diagnostics in cancer and other indications will eventually lead to a close alliance between the clinical oncologist, pathologist, molecular diagnostic specialist and patient, through which personalized treatment guidance reports will be created. Based on these reports, clinical oncologists and pathologists will be enabled with precise disease classifications and associated treatment regimens.

To accomplish these goals, we are developing a unique biomarker and genomics infrastructure through which we will perform patient stratification by measurement of diverse analytes, including protein analytes and genomics information. Our personalized medicine approach has the following strategic components:

1. Standardize, assemble, interpret patient 'Omics and clinical data and build comprehensive standardized clinical and basic databases.
2. Integrate patient data with data from basic- and drug-discovery research to enhance our systems biology understanding of disease.
3. Pursue discovery and development of diagnostic platform technologies.
4. Apply genetics, proteomics, and high-content patient data capture platforms developed, to inform the clinical databases.
5. Mature and prioritize these data through the application of diagnostic tests to create an integrated, patient-specific treatment guidance report.

The ultimate product will include delivery of a comprehensive report to the physician, aimed at patient-specific diagnostic and prognostic guidance and treatment predictions. In parallel with these efforts, commercially available primary diagnostic platforms will create a menu of diagnostic tests that must be applied to optimally implement patient treatment guidance. Validation and clinical application of next-generation diagnostics and therapeutics, tailored to specific molecular profiling of patient blood and other tissues, will offer safer and more effective treatments for critical illnesses, with an initial focus to oncology. Changing current classification methods of critical illnesses, such as cancer, to a more heavily molecular classification will result in improved patient treatment decisions. In the first section of this chapter, we will discuss examples of our genetics and platform technology developments. The last section of this chapter provides examples of diagnostic tests we developed, aimed at optimal patient guidance for selected cancers. Our initial focus has been in cervical cancer, melanoma and colorectal cancer.

Health Economics

The application of biomarkers can have a positive impact for both patients and payers, due to the converging action on patient-health and health-economics. While many molecular diagnostic tests are developed in a manner that allows one to quantitatively measure sensitivity and specificity, the large numbers of new molecular diagnostic tests that are being developed are creating a challenge for appropriate judicious regulatory approval processes of tests [7].

Numerous risks and concerns regarding development and adoption of biomarkers in medicine have been raised. These include the overall less favorable economics of biomarker products when method classifications (Current Procedural Terminology [CPT code]) are applied to determine reimbursement value, rather than the impact of the test on overall patient health and health economics. This arrangement may hinder development investments in suitable trials, whether retrospective or prospective and can hamper progress. As a result, biomarkers are often developed based on retrospective trial designs, with only a small proportion having the benefit of being an integral part of Phase II and III clinical trials or being supported by insightful health economic data. The advantages of prospective design during Phase II and III of a clinical trial are significant, as the combination of therapeutic and companion diagnostics eventually represents a product that cannot easily be rivaled by second-generation compound and biomarker pairs. While the economic benefits of providing treatment to those that are best matched with a therapeutic is recognized from a payer's perspective, it has taken time for those that develop therapeutics to recognize the inevitable wisdom of this approach.

Numerous regulatory challenges lie ahead, including the need to redefine regulatory oversight for clinical biomarker applications. In this regard, it seems critical to recognize the clinical utility of biomarkers and the value this represents to patients and payers. Making clinical utility the driver will lead clinical and basic researchers to focus on those areas where clinical impact is most profound. Like many European countries, even the US population will eventually be held accountable for the cost of its healthcare system; at that point, the financial justification of biomarker applications will become inescapable.

Personal Genomics and Cancer

Personal individualized genomics is an emerging branch of genomics, where individual genomes are genotyped/haplotyped and deployed to provide the context for analysis of phenotypes, classification of diseases, discovery of disease biomarkers, and interpretation of electronic health records. Naturally, the tools and techniques in this field are intimately related to traditional population genetics, as they strive to uncover how genotypes are associated with phenotypes, building upon the statistical theories of association studies. Several recent developments have now brought this field to the forefront of biomedical and information technology research, as genotype and phenotype data are about to undergo a quantum leap, both in quality and quantity. In addition, the infrastructure needed to manage and interpret the data is being developed.

With the underlying genomics sequencing platforms and software pipelines continuing to improve along a biotechnological Moore's Law, it seems imminent that one will be able to haplotypically sequence (along with their epigenomic annotations) any single-cell in a heterogeneous cell-population. Such a technology, for instance, could be easily devised using single-molecule optical-mapping and a short-read next-generation sequencing platform, integrated with the help of sophisticated map- and sequence-assembly algorithms, e.g., SUTTA [8, 9]. A biomedical tipping point is expected as soon as approximately 10,000 globally sampled, haplotypic reference genomes become available (possibly assimilated with detailed electronic medical records) and ubiquitously accessible via fast hardware that is capable of calling well-interpreted genetic variants in real time. The opportunities created by personalization of translational biomedicine appear limitless; however, the challenges for this emerging field are also countless, even when considered for instance in the narrow context of personal oncogenomics.

Personalized Genomics in Oncology

Personal genomic and bioinformatic analyses have a critical role in the study of tumorigenesis, and in shaping cancer diagnosis, prognosis, and therapies. These analyses build on our assumptions that cancer is a disease of the genome (and epigenome), driven by an un-programmed somatic evolution, which leads to the abnormal activation or inhibition of pathways and networks in the transformed cell and its neighboring tissues. However, cancer progression also exhibits many broad, heterogeneous and nuanced variations that remain poorly modeled and largely unpredictable. A failure to appreciate these variations has been a major hurdle for cancer research, as it single-mindedly pursued its goals with an emphatic, unshakable faith in the underlying singularity of cancer more than its pluralities: Oncologists of the 60s were on a quest for a universal cure. That assumption—that a monolithic hammer would eventually demolish a monolithic disease has, however, been futile. During the last three decades, different models of cancer have been proposed, and pursued: cancer has been variously categorized as viral disease, disease of the genome, disease of the somatic evolution, disease of the aberrant signaling, response to multicellularity (controlled by proliferation, apoptosis, repair, and autophagy), price of repair/regeneration (stem cells), disease of metabolism (Warburg-effect), response to external stress and microenvironment. However, none of the approaches based upon any single characterization seems to have led to uniformly effective therapeutics.

A personalized data-driven and phenomenological-model-based approach [10] may come to the rescue. This approach promises to select diagnostic tests and therapeutic interventions without getting bogged down by the variability, heterogeneity and complexity of the disease and its progression. Crudely speaking, the approach may be thought of as based on the following premises: (1) Carcinogenesis is triggered by "stress" conditions and requires the tumor cells to acquire specific characteristics, denoted by "cancer hallmarks (see below)." (2) Although initiation and progression of cancer is largely stochastic, the carcinogenesis process exhibits well-orchestrated state-transitions, each state roughly corresponding to a "hallmark." (3) Transition from state-to-state is coordinated by perturbation to pathways, networks and complex signaling processes (that control cellular proliferation, motility, apoptosis or anoikis) among cells, which can be interfered with by small-molecules such as kinase inhibitors. (4) The hallmarks of a cancer cell can be characterized directly (chemically) by genomics and transcriptomic assays (e.g., copy-number and mutational profiles) and biomarkers, or indirectly by a state-observer algorithm, which can inform a "supervisory controller" on how to make suitable therapeutic choices (constrained by certain "cost functions" related to toxicity, discomfort to the patient, etc.) by using ideas from mathematical game theory (e.g., "games against nature"). For instance, one wishing to address a "sustained angiogenesis hallmark" may target a receptor for a related growth factor (e.g., TGF-beta through an antisense oligo such as AP 12009 or VEGF through an antibody such as Bevacizumab), a kinase (e.g., a multiple kinase inhibitor for VEGFR, RAF, PDGFR, c-Kit through Sorafenib or Sunitinib), a pathway or network (e.g., PI3K pathway controlling angiogenesis through a small molecule such as BEZ235), and/or the immune system (e.g., a COX2 inhibitor such as Celecoxib).

The targets of this algorithm are cancer phenotypes, often described in terms of "cancer hallmarks": (1) limitless replicative potential, (2) insensitivity to anti-growth signals, (3) self-sufficiency in growth signals, (4) evading apoptosis, (5) tissue invasion and metastasis, (6) sustained angiogenesis, (7) evading immune surveillance, and (8) influencing the microenvironment to sustain the cancer phenotype.

The discrete dynamics that describe the evolution of cancer are often depicted by cancer biologists using "cancer subway maps," in which various states ("subway stations") are labeled by a particular hallmark: a loss-of-function (mutation to a tumor suppressor gene), or a gain-of-function (mutation to an oncogene), and these states are deterministically connected by labeled edges ("colored subway lines"). Thus, a good abstract representation of such a subway map can be provided as a disjoint union of ("colored") Kripke models whose states are labeled by an extended ontology.

Computational Efforts in Cancer Genomics

The computational work leading to informative personalized genomics in cancer must then focus on: (1) characterization, classification, and discovery of hallmarks from tumor-progression data and their description via stable genomic signatures and a list of related diagnostic tests; (2) extraction of the underlying model that describes the discrete dynamics of a particular cancer (which may also depend on the patient's genomics as well as site and stage of the tumor); (3) a database of small-molecules, oligos, or peptides acting as signaling-pathway- or kinase-inhibitor that can control state-dynamics; (4) design of monitors and supervisory controllers such that the modified system satisfies appropriate temporal logic properties. The resulting complete scheme is rather ambitious and not immediately technologically feasible; however, it can be simplified significantly to an initial scheme using biomarker based cancer classification, from which it can further progress.

A simpler approach, as described below, can be used immediately and will not require inference of a more data-intensive temporal dynamic model. It will start with a straightforward static model of the statistical distribution of various tumor-related—'Omics data, constrained by patient's genotype, history and demographics (derived from electronic medical records), and known theories of DNA-protein or protein-protein interactions, and regulatory, metabolic and signaling pathways. A representation of the statistical model could be in the form of a graphical model (a factoring of the joint distributions in terms of conditional probabilities representing the edges of a graph), which could then be used for cancer classification, discovery of biomarkers, or causal structures to identify pathways and genes involved in the tumor [11]. The results of the static model can then be optimally matched to diagnostic tests and therapies and recommended to an oncologist. However, as the results of these tests and therapies accumulate over the lifetime of many cancer patients, the resulting data will be a source of information leading to a phenomenological temporal model with states representing various hallmarks and transitions among them. For a more detailed perspective, we return to the discussion of currently available genomics and transcriptomic profiling for cancer.

Genomics and Transcriptome Data

Cancer, modeled as a genetic disease, involves point mutations, translocations, segmental amplifications, and deletions in the genome that alter specific vulnerable molecular points in cellular regulatory pathways, and thus confer particular cancer-phenotypes (or hallmarks) to the tumor cells. As disease progresses, the tumor cells can acquire further mutations, proliferate or commit apoptosis, thus changing the population-wide genomic profile of a tumor and its cancer-hallmark. Analysis of chromosomal changes by fluorescent in situ hybridization (FISH)-based cytogenetic approaches including comparative genomic hybridization (CGH), spectral karyotyping (SKY), and multiplex-FISH (M-FISH) have mapped various chromosomal regions involved in various cancers [12–16]. Recently, microarray techniques (e.g., array-CGH or matrix-CGH), and next-generation sequencing technologies (e.g., Illumina, 454, ABI-Solid) have become widely available, hastening the speed and improving the resolution at which an oncologist can map regions of DNA sequence from the cancer tissue that are amplified or reduced compared to normal tissue. In addition, genome-wide measurements of single nucleotide polymorphisms (SNPs) [8, 9] can provide detailed diagnostic, prognostic or predictive tumor information. With the advent of single-molecule technologies, which will be able to analyze the base-pair content (at various resolutions) of any individual genomic DNA from a single normal or tumor cell and work with minute amounts of material (e.g., single cell), it will be possible to understand the genetic and epigenetic [10] heterogeneity of a tumor. Epigenetic changes such as DNA methylation, histone modification, and RNA silencing can be involved in regulating many cellular processes, including development, via gene silencing (chromatin structure and transcriptional regulation) and genetic imprinting [17].

Global gene expression profiling with DNA microarrays have been used for over a decade for cancer phenotyping/classification [18–23]. It has furthered our knowledge and state of the art of the regulation of biological processes and has become a tool in the study and classification of human tumors. Semi-quantitative profiles of gene expression have been measured for many cancer types and subtypes and can relate to various cancer classifications and hallmarks [22, 24]. Through unbiased comparative analysis of these profiles, a subset of genes can be found that correlate with tumor phenotype and can serve as diagnostic and prognostic markers of disease, which can be incorporated into cancer pathway analysis or cancer hallmark models. Disease-specific regulatory programs have been studied and combined using techniques such as chromatin immunoprecipitation (ChIP) of tumor biopsies [25].

Nonetheless, for several reasons, the analysis of the cancer genomic data, in isolation, is rather challenging: as cancer progresses, the tumor accumulates many noncausal bystander mutations, thus making the genomic data noisy; amplifications and deletions affect many genes in synteny, which introduce many spurious correlations; clonal amplifications and collapses in a heterogeneous tumor population introducing difficult-to-handle nonstationarity; heterogeneity and variability within the tumor and among the cancer patients; variability due to subjectivity in many current diagnostic tools, tests and pathology review outcomes; all make the analysis very susceptible to Yule-Simpson effects; and finally, for certain groups of cancer (e.g., pancreatic cancer), lack of sufficient patient data and well-preserved biosamples (collected at different stages of the disease progression) weakens the power of statistical inference, since the complexity, dimensionality and multiplicity of hypotheses testing in a typical oncogenomic analysis are huge.

A typical approach to enhance the power of statistical analysis and tame the false discovery rate, involves a Bayesian scheme that combines the genomic data with other 'Omics data, pathway models and patient-specific information, although the issues related to small-sample, heterogeneity and nonstationarity are left to other independent treatments. For this purpose, epigenomic and transcriptomic profiling have received intense attention, though small-RNA, proteomics, and metabolomics are also thought to be no less important. As mentioned earlier, pathway information can be important for understanding biological processes and how they can be disrupted or reprogrammed in disease. However, collecting complex pathway information in a usable form from diverse and heterogeneous sources, including more than 220 pathway databases (http://pathguide.org), can be a major challenge. Thus, a major computational systems biology effort will be a fundamental ingredient needed to improve our personalized analyses of cancers.

Multiplexed Tissue Protein Analysis by Mass Spectrometry

One of the next steps in technology evolution to improve personalized medicine diagnostics is the analysis of functional proteins, pathways and networks. Systematic sequencing studies performed on gene families involved in signal transduction have been extended to include the majority of protein-coding genes in cancer. These analyses have identified many genes and pathways that are linked to human cancer, and mutation analysis has enabled the development of a handful of important diagnostic tests such as the BRCA, KRAS, BRAF, and EGFR mutation assays. As outlined above, while these advances are useful they are not sufficient to fully exploit personalized medicine opportunities for the future. As much as these genomic studies provide a window into the genetic landscape of human cancer and help indicate new targets for personalized diagnostic and therapeutic intervention, the link to functional proteins is often missing. Linking the functional proteins involved in the cellular biochemistry that drives cancer, the activation of these proteins, and their interplay is essential if we are to unlock the true potential of this wealth of genetic information. Developing techniques and strategies to deliver multiplexed protein assays in patient tumors will allow us to understand the nuances of the protein networks that drive cancer, sensitize tumors, or result in treatment resistance.

Current diagnostic tests in routine use for the measurement of protein expression in tissue rely on immunohistochemistry (IHC). Because IHC is antibody based it is subject to the idiosyncrasies of antibody specificity and sensitivity. In the best of cases it is semi-quantitative, hard to reproduce, not easily applied to phosphoproteins, and tissue-intensive due to difficulty of multiplexing. AQUA immunofluorescence techniques have overcome some of the limitations of multiplexing and quantitation, but are still based on antibody binding and staining [26]. The challenge has been to build diagnostic panels for protein analysis that are fit for clinical practice. In order to interrogate complex tissues for specific proteins quantitatively, we developed a diagnostic platform that is capable of multiplexing quantitative protein expression and activation analysis from formalin-fixed-paraffin-embedded FFPE tissue based on mass spectrometry. The goal is to fit these in with clinical practice. Currently we are in the process of distilling down the existing wealth of genomic and proteomic information to assemble rationally designed protein and phosphoprotein markers of clinical interest, thus creating a menu of multiplexed protein test panels to achieve this end.

Targeted Selected Reaction Monitoring (SRM) by Mass Spectrometry as a Diagnostic Tool in Fixed Human Tissues

The majority of human clinical tissue biopsies are formalin-fixed and paraffin-embedded (FFPE). It was recently shown that diagnostically relevant proteins and their phosphorylation status can be targeted and accurately quantitated in FFPE tissues [27, 28] by Selected Reaction Monitoring (SRM) triple quadrupole mass spectrometry [29]. The key to this new use of mass spectrometry is the invention of a process, termed Liquid Tissue, which allows FFPE tissue to be completely dissolved and digested into a mixture of tryptic peptides suitable for quantitative mass spectrometry [30, 31]. The major advantages of using a mass spectrometry approach with tissue are that multiple proteins and their phosphorylation status can be detected and measured from the same cells populations. In addition, the multiplex capability of quantitative SRM and the minute amounts of tissue specimen required, make it practical to employ these capabilities in the clinical setting. In order to successfully detect and quantify the target proteins (analytes) and their phosphorylation status, SRM assays for each analyte of interest can be built and validated. This involves a multistep process where the recombinant human protein for each target is formalin fixed and Liquid Tissue processed. The resultant peptide mixture is then analyzed to identify peptides representative of the target protein. Target peptides are selected which ionize well and are reproducibly detected and quantified. Once suitable peptides have been identified for a protein analyte, the corresponding isotopically labeled synthetic peptides are generated. These peptides are substituted for N15 and C13 on one amino acid and hence are biochemically equivalent, but biophysically distinct from the native peptide because they are a few atomic mass units heavier than the endogenous peptides being measured. Since elemental analysis of the synthetic peptides allows their accurate quantification, a spike of a known amount can be added into an unknown sample and simultaneous detection of the endogenous and spiked peptide (their mass-to-charge is slightly different, enabling resolution) allows absolute quantitation of the endogenous peptide. Once this basic assay has been built, it is further refined and validated in cell lines and xenografts that are known to express the target of interest at differential levels, and finally the tests are performed with human clinical tissues. The refinement of the peptide analyte assays through cell lines and into relevant tissue backgrounds is essential to determine that the representative peptides being tracked are robust in the most complex biological milieu where they will be applied. Individual peptide analyte assays can be run simultaneously in a single tissue sample and multiplex information on large panels of proteins can be generated by adding the appropriate cocktail of heavy control peptides into the sample. In addition to heavy peptides for quantitation of the peptides/proteins of interest, heavy peptides that aid in the determination of quality control parameters and dynamic range control for the assays can also be included (analyzed by LC/MS/MS using a nano-HPLC (Waters, NanoAcquity)) coupled to a triple quadrupole mass spectrometer (Thermo, TSQ Vantage).

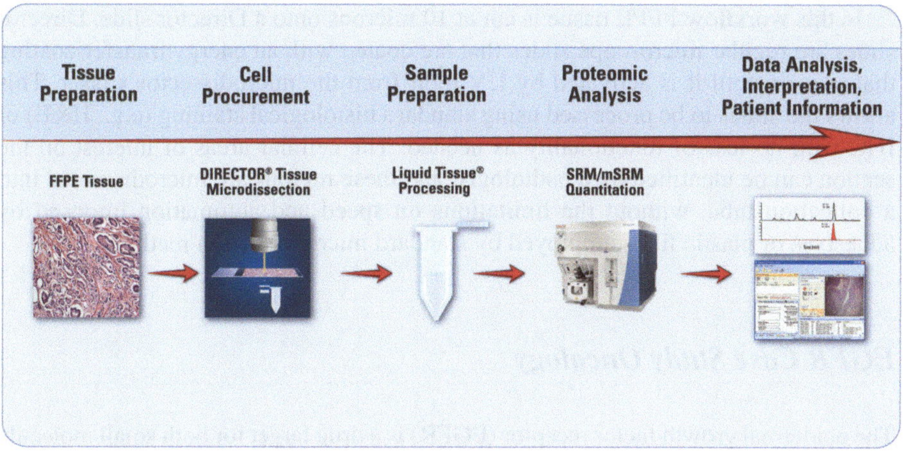

Fig. 13.1 Liquid Tissue®-SRM mass spec workflow

Phosphorylation of target proteins can also be measured using the same techniques; however, a phosphoenrichment step is incorporated. A peptide mixture resulting from the sample preparation is split into two fractions. Ten percent of the fraction is used for analysis of nonphosphorylated protein analytes and the remainder of the fraction is used for phosphoenrichment and analysis of phosphorylated protein analytes. Phosphoenrichment is achieved by capturing the phosphopeptides on TiO_2 beads (Pierce) and eluting only the phosphopeptide fraction for analysis [32]. An expanding menu of robust and specific diagnostic assays for protein analytes of interest in oncology has already been developed, which can be run individually, or in multiplex on a small sample of tumor tissue. Although the current focus is on oncology, this technology is just as applicable to other therapeutic areas. This technology has been successfully reduced to practice as a clinical diagnostic assay for the determination of a panel of plaque proteins to aid in the diagnosis of systemic amyloidosis [33]. In the remaining sections specific examples of the application of SRM technology to targets in oncology are presented.

Expression Pathology's Platform: LMD-Director/ Liquid Tissue/SRM MS and Workflow

A Liquid Tissue®-SRM technology platform has been developed that makes practical multiplexed protein quantitation by SRM mass spectrometry. This allows minute amounts of FFPE tissue to be laser microdissected using Director® slides, processed using the patented Liquid Tissue® reagents and technology, and analyzed by SRM mass spectrometry (Fig. 13.1).

In this workflow FFPE tissue is cut at 10 microns onto a Director slide. Director slides are regular microscope slides that are coated with an energy transfer coating that is inert until it is activated by UV light from the microdissector's laser. This allows the slides to be processed using standard histological staining (e.g., H&E) or IHC with no loss of functionality as needed. The cellular areas of interest on the section can be identified by a pathologist and these regions are microdissected into a collection tube, without the limitations on speed and automation imposed by adhesives or plastic films employed by standard microdissection methods.

EGFR Case Study Oncology

The epidermal growth factor receptor (EGFR) is a drug target for both small molecule (Gefitinb, Erlotinib) and antibody therapeutics (Cetuximab, Panitumamb); these therapies have been approved in non small-cell lung carcinoma (NSCLC) and colorectal carcinoma (CRC), respectively. The small molecule drugs block receptor signaling though blockade of the tyrosine kinase domain, while the antibody therapies block receptor signaling through inhibition of ligand binding. Unfortunately, direct non-quantitative assessment of the EGFR protein expression level by IHC in tumors has not been shown to correlate with response or outcome in patients. Also current genomic tests are indirect in that they measure receptor amplification, RNA levels, the mutation status of receptor or pathway molecules (EGFR or KRAS mutations) but no current assay can directly and quantitatively measure the EGFR target, resistance markers, and the activation state (phosphorylation) of EGFR or its downstream signaling pathway components. Indeed KRAS mutant positive status rules a patient out of receiving EGFR therapy for colon cancer and is thus a negative predictor. There is currently no diagnostic test to positively predict response in the KRAS wild type population. By comparison, the EGFR mutation positive NSCLC tumors (thought to be constitutively active) do show a high response rate to TKI therapy, though there are many nonresponders, thus demonstrating that this genomic test also has limited utility, highlighting the need for other diagnostic tests that can help direct the therapy decision. Since inhibition of EGFR is necessary for the response to these targeted agents, it is critical to measure what levels of receptor activation and downstream signaling determines tumor responsiveness to EGFR targeted therapies in patients.

The currently described approach enables absolute quantification of proteins and their phosphorylation status directly in FFPE tissue. Based on these test characteristics, we developed a panel of new diagnostic assays which measure in a multiplex manner (in selected cells from a tissue sample) the expression and activation of EGFR, plus other receptors and key downstream signaling proteins through quantitation of the total protein and phosphorylation state of these proteins where appropriate (Fig. 13.2).

Quantitative SRM assays were built to measure the nonphosphorylated EGFR, HER2, HER3, IGF1R, cMET, cSRC, and BIM proteins. This protein target multiplex was initially preclinically validated on the A431 tumor cell line (which harbors

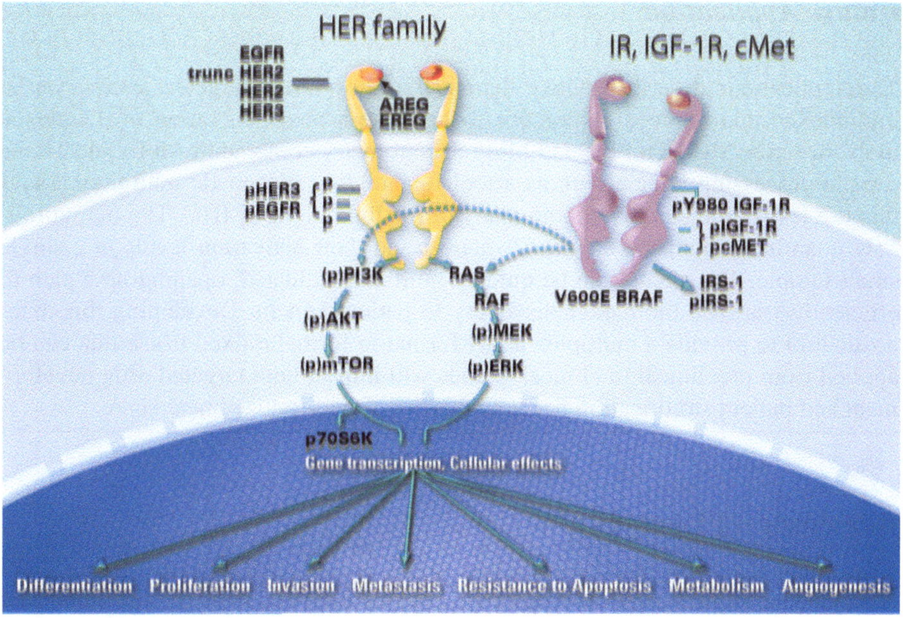

Fig. 13.2 Design of EGFR Rx SRM assay panel

an amplification of the EGFR gene) [34] and HCC827 cells (harboring mutant amplified EGFR, constitutively active cMET and AKT) [35]. In addition, quantitative SRM assays to measure the phosphorylated forms of EGFR, HER3, IGF1R, MET, SRC, ERK, AKT, and p70S6K proteins have been described. This phosphopeptide multiplex assay was initially validated preclinically on the A431 tumor cell line mentioned above. These cells were stimulated with a dose range of EGF (50–200 ng/ml) or in a time course study (EGF 50 ng/ml for 5–30 min). Confluent, EGF stimulated cells were then formalin fixed, subjected to Liquid Tissue® processing, and then phosphoenriched using TiO_2 magnetic beads. The resulting enriched phosphopeptides were then analyzed by mass spectrometry. This method demonstrated the feasibility, and reproducibility of this method for quantitating EGFR pY1197, EGFR pT693, AKT pS473, p-p70S6K pS447, ERK pT202/pY204. In addition to in vitro studies, experiments with phospho-SRM analysis of FFPE NSCLC xenograft explants with extensive independent histopathologic and molecular characterization have been performed, allowing a benchmark to be made for phospho-SRM analysis with standard diagnostic analyses.

Validation studies are currently being extended by using this EGFR Rx panel to measure protein expression and activation in FFPE tissues obtained from relevant human clinical trial cohorts—Gefitinib treated NSCLC and Cetuximab treated CRC. It may be that such studies will correlate EGFR pathway expression, activation and signaling in these tumors with responsiveness to EGFR targeted therapy, and validate this assay for use as a companion diagnostic to guide therapy in both NSCLC and CRC.

Future Application

The applications described above demonstrate how these targeted assays can be multiplexed and reduced to practice to generate a next generation of diagnostic tools for tissue.SRM Triple Quad Mass Spectrometry combined with Liquid Tissue sample processing is emerging as a tool for building diagnostic multiplex assays that use less tissue, and overcome many of the limitations of IHC. The output reliably quantitates both the targets of interest and their activation levels in a single small sample. The assays can be quickly built and validated, opening up a path to efficiently translate biomarker discovery to patient benefit. Developing this diagnostic tool to provide a multiplex assay format in formalin fixed tissue that can be applied from preclinical to clinical studies will impact both targeted drug development and patient stratification needs in this era of personalized healthcare.

BioSensors: Plasmonics

A major goal in biosensor development is the creation and commercialization of a new, molecular, high-data-content diagnostic platform for the detection of biomarkers for individual patient care and personalized disease treatment. The field of plasmonics offers the potential for creating such biosensors. Plasmonic substrate design for specific biomarker applications, relies on nanoscale- precise substrate fabrication creating biosensor devices for the ultra-sensitive detection of target analytes in biological media, e.g., blood, plasma, and other bodily fluids.

The field of plasmonics captures the physics of the interaction of light with plasmonic oscillations of electrons in materials. Raman spectroscopy is a technique based on the inelastic Raman scattering of incident light to give unique frequency shifted fingerprints for molecules and information on their vibrational, rotational, and electronic energies. Raman spectroscopy can take advantage of plasmonic structures and often works over the visible or near IR range of incident light. While standard Raman spectroscopy has a relatively low occurrence of Raman scattering events, substrates can be created that enhance the occurrence of the Raman events many orders of magnitude and result in high levels of sensitivity, down to the single molecule detection regime. Surfaces, and nanosize features therein, play a main role in what is known as Surface Enhanced Raman Spectroscopy (SERS) [36, 37]. In addition to surface features such as surface roughness, it has been shown that several nano- and microengineered architectures have similar or significantly greater Raman enhancement ability. As these substrates utilize plasmonic mechanisms to achieve extreme enhancement abilities, they are often referred to as Plasmonic Enhanced Raman Spectroscopy (PERS) substrates. Examples include plasmonic architectures that have nanometer scale gaps between materials that support plasmons (generally silver and gold) [38], micron or submicron periodicity of features, nanoparticle systems [39], nanorings [40], nanocrescents [41], nanorods [42], and many others.

Extensive simulation capabilities based on plasmonic and material principles can be used to define and optimize designs for PERS nanostructures. The effects of local and/or periodic feature effects can be thoroughly investigated in simulation space over relevant bands of incident light wavelengths. Importantly, this guidance can highlight key parameters relevant during actual fabrication and how to optimize for biomarkers of interest. In the discovery phase of building PERS devices, simulation coupled with experimental results may also be utilized to attain a deep understanding of what needs to be built.

Creation of optimal PERS substrates for reliable biomarker detection requires controlled and reproducible methods for achieving consistently high enhancement of the Raman signal. The interaction of metal features within random or periodic arrays or individually with incident light for the PERS substrates is critical. Individual effects may include feature size, shape, presence of sharp edges, and roughness. The effect of coupled systems of arrays of metal features is determined by type, distance, spacing/gap sizes, and periodicity. It is known that nanogaps, such as gaps less than 100 nm and preferably less than 10 nm [43, 44], have very high local Raman enhancement factors, often referred to as "hot spots," representing localized plasmons. For example, a traditional nanogap is the particle-particle gap seen in silver or gold nanoparticle dimers, trimers and agglomerates. A high local Raman enhancement factor has also been shown in features with sharp edges or points on the nanometer scale, such as diamond, triangle, prism [45], star [46], and similar shapes. Periodic structures utilize the coupling of features to result in enhancement which can often be tuned based on the periodicity, for example, structures can be created that result in efficient absorption of incident light at certain wavelength or wavelength ranges that are generally used in Raman spectroscopy [47].

One example of a controlled PERS substrate that incorporates nanogaps and highly periodic features is a gold coated one-dimensional Nanograting array, shown in Fig. 13.3. The Nanograting array can extend across long distances relative to the grating height and width. The periodicity is shown in a submicron pitch which is approximately 330 nm in the example in Fig. 13.3. The most active areas, referred to as "hot-spots" in enhanced Raman spectroscopy, occurs within the sub-10 nm gaps. Figure 13.3 (top) shows simulation results for the local electric field intensity, which shows the hotspot location in and near the gaps. The pitch of the grating features results in a critical-coupling with the incident light as shown in Fig. 13.4, where the reflectance of the gold coated PERS substrate when the light is correctly polarized relative to the gratings can go to nearly zero. This is impressive as it should be emphasized that gold in the visible range is generally a highly reflective mirror.

A PERS architecture with a two-dimensional array of nanodots is shown in Fig. 13.5. The substrate has gold nanodots of approximately 90 nm in diameter and a square pattern with an X&Y pitch of 330 nm. This structure has controlled periodicity and nanoscale features. The nanodot array can be modified in array layout (e.g., rectangular, hexagonal, or other pattern) and pitches. The duty cycle, which is described by the feature size divided by the pitch, can vary from low duty cycles as in Fig. 13.5 (roughly 27% duty cycle) to nearly touching or touching features. When the features approach touching distances, nanogaps are formed and can result in dramatically increased Raman enhancement.

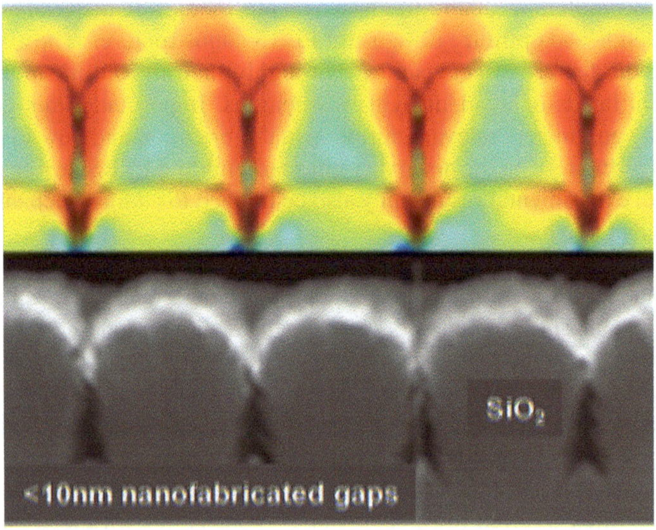

Fig. 13.3 PERS substrate with nanogaps between gold features and submicron periodicity

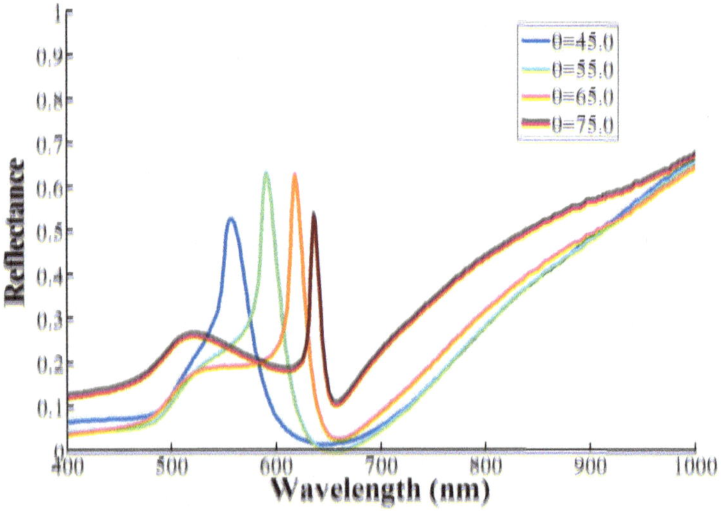

Fig. 13.4 Reflection versus wavelength for the gold coated one-dimensional grating array

Important characteristics of the PERS substrates to be considered in their rational design and fabrication are high enhancement, accessible hot-spots, reproducibility, and consistency. For integration into medical devices for biomarker detection, they will be coupled with analyte delivery systems, electronics, Raman spectroscopy equipment and data analysis software. The target biomarkers will be biological analytes in complex mixtures present in biological fluids such as blood or plasma.

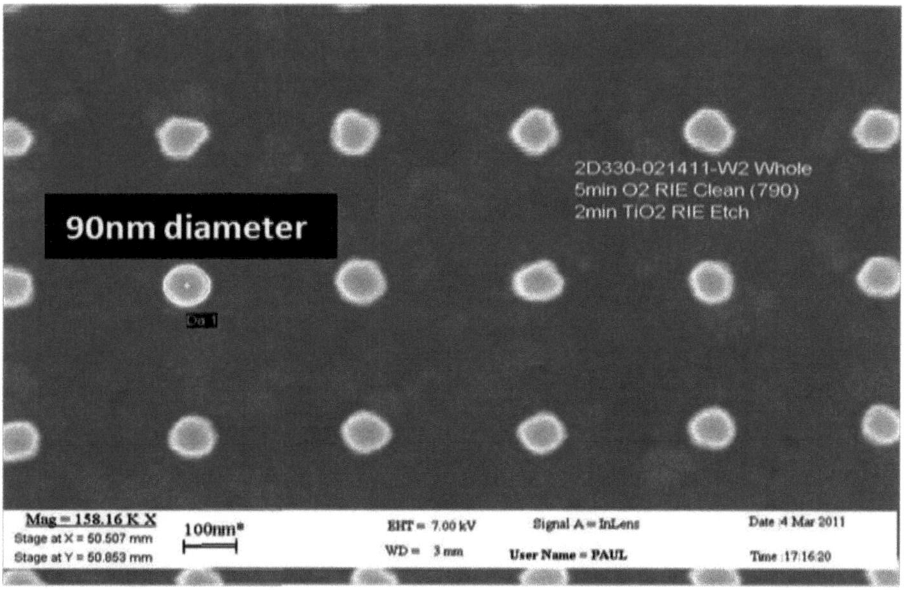

Fig. 13.5 Two-dimensional nanodot array

The biomarkers will need to reach the vicinity of the hotspots in order to be detected, therefore a thorough understanding of the surface chemistry of the substrate and fluid medium will be essential. The data analysis software is required to identify the Raman spectrum of the biomarkers within a matrix of signals from multiple species. A general type of software for this purpose is chemometric software that is used to extract specific signals out of multivariate data using chemical databases. As each biomarker will have a unique Raman signature, the software can be loaded with the biomarker data in order to extract the biomarker signal when present and above the level of detection.

An example of using a PERS substrate for the detection of a controlled substance is presented in Fig. 13.6. In this example, a one-dimensional Nanograting PERS substrate is exposed to a solution of cocaine (concentration of 100 μ(mu)M), briefly rinsed and then dried. The red curve is the optimal operating condition, i.e., incident light polarization state relative to the grating array, and the blue curve is the pure cocaine Raman signal for reference. Comparable results were obtained for measuring cocaine in saliva (not shown).

The rational design and controlled fabrication of highly enhancing PERS substrates can result in the creation of a variety of stable biosensing devices for next generation clinical bio-diagnostics and personalized medicine. Unique biomarker fingerprints can potentially be detected at concentrations as low as few or single molecule levels and extracted from multivariate chemical data in a quantifiable and reliable manner, which can lead to patient-specific diagnostic guidance.

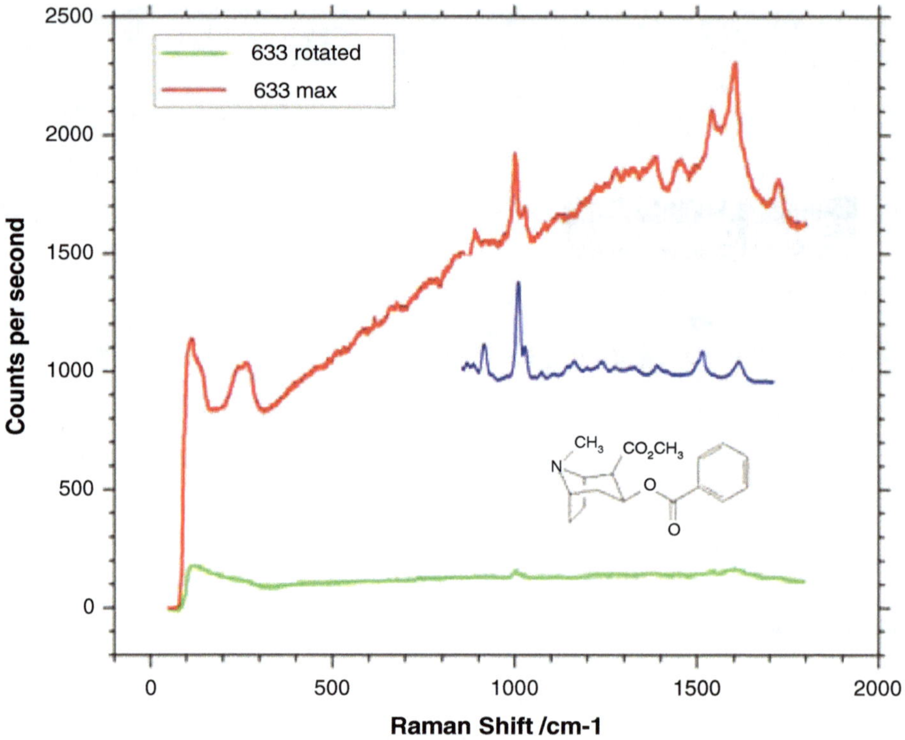

Fig. 13.6 Detection of cocaine with the one-dimensional PERS substrate. Raman measured at 633 nm, 2.8 mW, 1 s integration time

Examples of Companion Diagnostics and Prognostic Markers: BRAF, KRAS, Predictive and Prognostic Biomarkers

The highest value biomarkers in patient management are those that either stratify patients to a particular therapy or predict disease outcome. The classic example is Her2, where overexpression of Her2 determined by either FISH or IHC analysis, selects a subpopulation of patients for anti-Her2 monoclonal antibody therapy (Herceptin) [48]. Recent advances in technology that have led to the development of more selective and more sensitive tests have vastly expanded diagnostic capability and clinical utility. Below are two emerging examples of biomarkers that have recently entered the therapeutic arena.

BRAF V600E Mutant Allele in Melanoma

It is estimated that at least 50% of all stage IV malignant melanoma patients carry a specific somatic mutation in the BRAF gene. This mutation, V600E, which results in

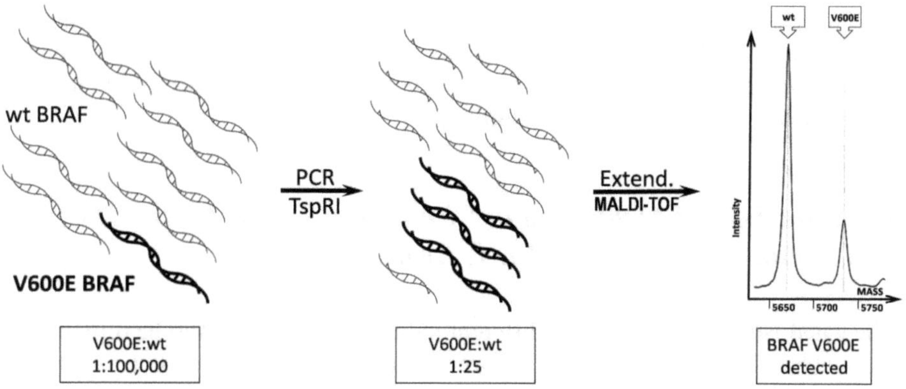

Fig. 13.7 cfBRAF V600E assay

an amino acid change from Valine to Glutamic acid at position 600 in the BRAF kinase, renders the kinase constitutively activated. Phase I/II trial data show more than 80% of late stage melanoma patients who carry this mutation are highly responsive to a specific BRAF inhibitor (RG7204/PLX4032), and go into remission for variable lengths of time [49]. Thus, the presence of BRAF V600E allele is a companion biomarker for BRAF inhibitor therapy. The discovery that this mutation can be detected not only in metastatic tumor biopsies, but as cell-free DNA released from tumors into the circulatory system of these patients [50], has led to the development of a recently available clinical diagnostic assay that uses a MALDI-TOF genotyping platform (MassARRAY Analyzer, Sequenom Inc. San Diego, CA). This test is capable of detecting a few copies of the cfBRAF V600E mutant DNA in 1 ml of plasma or serum. The uniquely high selectivity of this test is in part due to the higher sensitivity of the MALDI-TOF platform, as well as end stage PCR reaction and the inclusion into the reaction mix of a thermostable restriction enzyme specific for the wild type allele of BRAF. In the analytical validation experiments, samples with ratios of wild-type to mutant BRAF alleles up to 100,000:1 were reliably analyzed with just 35 PCR cycles (Fig. 13.7). Specific allelotypes in this approach are determined by single nucleotide extensions of primers designed to interrogate the SNP site. The two peaks, clearly separated by 9 Da on the MALDI-TOF spectrogram corresponding to the A (V600E) or T (wild type), allow reliable detection of the V600E allele when it comprises 5% or more of the sample BRAF DNA. However, the inclusion of the TspRI restriction enzyme allows for the detection of a rare BRAF V600E mutant allele (A), in a background of more than 100,000× excess of wild type BRAF alleles (T).

The high value of this biomarker is several fold: (1) the test immediately identifies a population of melanoma patients that would benefit most from BRAF inhibitor therapy, (2) requires only a blood sample and is thus relatively noninvasive and economical compared to costly and invasive biopsies, (3) the test is analytically very selective and sensitive. The pilot study of plasma from 31 stage IV melanoma patients revealed 78% sensitivity and 100% specificity. This test is currently undergoing intensive development in both retrospective and prospective melanoma clinical trials to mature its clinical utility.

RNA Markers of Melanoma in Circulating Tumor Cells (CTC) and Sentinel Lymph Node(SLN) Evaluation

The gated isolation of CTC's in different indications has proven to be difficult and unreliable. This lack of reliability is largely due to apparently very low numbers of CTC's (<10 per 8 cm^3 of blood) in some cases and or poor performing identification markers. In the case of melanoma, this problem has been overcome by the ability to detect melanoma CTC's without intact cell isolation on a platform such as CellSearch (Veridex LLC, Raritan, NJ). Using four highly specific melanoma RNA cell markers: melanoma antigen recognized by T-cells(MART-1), melanoma antigen gene-A3 family member (MAGE-A3), beta1,4-*N*-acetylgalactosaminyl-transferase (GalNAc-T), and paired box homeotic gene transcription factor 3 (PAX-3), feasibility of accurately detecting melanoma CTC's has been clearly demonstrated in melanoma patients. Using RNA isolated from the PBMC's derived from 5 cm^3 of whole blood, changes in the levels of these markers detected by qRT-PCR have been shown to directly correlate with patient response to biochemotherapy [51]. The potential for these markers to be used to follow treatment response, and as early indicators of relapse, is currently under investigation in multiple prospective clinical trials.

Sentinel lymph node (SLN) status with respect to the presence of metastatic lesions is a pivotal point in the care of early stage melanoma patients. Using FFPE specimens, patients scored negative by standard H&E staining and immunohistochemistry (IHC) using HMB-45 and S-100 as markers, are currently followed by watchful waiting without aggressive follow-up treatment. However, approximately 20% of the patients scored as SLN negative relapse within the first 10 years. A retrospective study of 215 patients was undertaken to evaluate the potential clinical utility of the molecular SLN evaluation utilizing the same four melanoma RNA markers as in the case of CTC detection. Out of 215 patients, 54 were scored positive using a combination of H&E staining and the HMB-45 and S-100 IHC biomarkers. Of the remaining 162 patients that were scored SLN negative by H&E and IHC, 39 progressed to metastatic disease, and were found to carry one or more of the four melanoma RNA markers. The detection of more than one marker correlated with shortened survival time [52, 53]. These statistics indicate that in fact 39 of the patients had occult micrometastases in the SLN that were not detected using H&E and the IHC markers. Another large retrospective trial with 250–500 patients is in progress where the node sampling method is also being evaluated. In the study cited above, sections for IHC evaluation and for qRT-PCR came from a very small and spatially close sampling of the SLN's. It may be that a more comprehensive sampling scheme, where multiple node regions are included, will improve the sensitivity of the 4-marker assay.

KRAS in PDAC Surgical Margins

Our ability to detect exceedingly rare somatic mutant alleles within the background of prevalent wild-type DNA allows for genotyping of the tumor using nontraditional sources of DNA, such as plasma circulating cell-free DNA in case of BRAF V600E. Furthermore, if such a technique is applied to the cancers with well defined somatic mutation widely represented among patients, it may lead to development of sensitive and highly specific assays for detection of occult tumor cells. Unlike RNA or protein markers, where baseline expression level plays a pivotal role, most of the disease-driving somatic mutations (SNP, translocation, deletion, or amplification) are binary (i.e., discrete) by nature and unaffected cells contain no such change. That leaves only technical limitations of the methodology in use as a challenge in detecting of the affected cell.

An excellent example where this approach worked well is the molecular analysis of surgical margins in Pancreatic Duct Adenocarcinoma (PDAC). Pancreatic adenocarcinoma is one of the most aggressive diseases, being the tenth most frequent cancer, and the fourth most common cause of cancer death, with 5-year survival rates well below 10%. Compounding the aggressive nature of this disease, nonspecific and late presentation of symptoms makes less than 20% of diagnosed individuals fit for surgical resection [54]. Margins of surgical resection have long been graded by pathologists microscopically in order to evaluate success of the surgery and provide oncologists with a prognostic marker. However, the subjective nature of the analysis, inherently low sensitivity of microscopic approach and often distorted shape of the tissue specimen result in a relatively weak prognostic value. A 2003 analysis by Lim et al. of 396 patients with resectable pancreatic adenocarcinoma indicates only a mild increase in median survival from 12 months to 19 months for a patient with negative margins [55]. A comparative review by Verbeke and Manon of 13 published data sets [56] show an incongruent relationship between microscopic margin status and clinical outcomes. Lack of standardization of pathological assessment leads to a seemingly counterintuitive observation: two studies with highest proportion of R1 margins also have the best clinical outcomes after resection (Table 13.1) [56].

One of the hallmarks of pancreatic cancer is extremely high involvement of somatic KRAS mutations. Recent search of the COSMIC database indicates that out of 3,760 recorded pancreatic carcinoma cases where KRAS was analyzed, nearly 70% contain one or more mutated RAS alleles More than 99% of those alleles are represented by just three key activating mutations within codon 12 (G12D, G12R, and G12V) [57]. Most of the pancreatic samples in the database did not undergo complete sequencing of the KRAS gene, and as a result there is a possibility of additional mutations outside of codon 12 that was not detected by the methods in use.

The methodology of preferential amplification of mutant KRAS alleles was developed and applied to pancreatic margin analysis by Dr. Hoon's group at the John Wayne Cancer Institute. First, PCR amplification is clamped with a PNA oligomer complementary to the wtKRAS sequence as developed by Thiede et al. [58],

Table 13.1 Survival and margin involvement in pancreatic cancer

Study	Number of patients	Percentage of patients with R1	Median survival (months)	
			R1/R2 patients	R0 patients
Menon et al. [56]	27	82	14	>55
Westgaard et al. [99]	40	45	11	16
Raut et al. [100]	360	17	22	28
Verbeke et al. [101]	26	85	11	37
Neoptolemos et al. [59]	541	19	11	17
Benassai et al. [102]	75	20	9	17
Sohn et al. [103]	616	30	12	19
Millikan et al. [104]	84	29	8	17
Nishimura et al. [105]	157	45	6	12
Sperti et al. [106]	113	17	7	14
Nitecki et al. [107]	174	16	9	–
Yeo et al. [108]	201	29	10	18
Willett et al. [109]	72	51	12	20

[Based on data from Verbeke CS, Menon KV. Redefining resection margin status in pancreatic cancer. *HPB*. 2009;11(4):282–89]

and then the product is detected utilizing RT-PCR. Results from a representative set of samples were also confirmed using a nested PCR approach with bidirectional sequencing. 70 patients with PDAC in two cohorts underwent surgery with intent to cure pancreatic cancer (68 pancreaticoduodenectomy and 2 distal pancreatomy). Pancreatic transection and retroperitoneal margins were identified by ink, suture or in relation to the location of the primary tumor. Paraffin embedded sections included the tumor and margin as a single block. Slides prepared from the block were subjected to H&E staining and microscopic examination by a pathologist to ensure no traces of cancer cells present in the margins submitted for molecular investigation. Primary tumors were typed for KRAS mutations and 81% were found to contain an allele of KRAS with a mutation in codon 12, which is within the statistically expected range. Mutant KRAS alleles were detected in pancreatic transection (17 patients), in retroperitoneal margins (27 patients) and for seven patients—in both. Comparison of overall survival between margin positive and margin negative groups produced significant difference (median 15 months versus 55 months), with a hazard ratio of 2.8 and $p=0.004$. These results would rank KRAS presence in the margins as one of the most significant prognostic markers for PDAC, on par with tumor grade and more robust than KRAS status in primary tumor or perineural invasion.

However, the aggressive nature of the PDAC may lead to questions of clinical utility of such a marker—with metastatic disease recurring in the vast majority of patients within 2 years after resection. Physicians would not likely make a decision on withholding the chemotherapeutic treatment solely based on the predicted statistically significant increase in expected survival time. At the present time the only therapeutic modality that may be driven by such a result is the use of follow-up radiotherapy. The results of a large prospective study of the 541 resections (ESPAC-1) indicate that for the subgroup with microscopically positive margins (R1) chemoradiotherapy did not provide additional benefit. The same study confirmed that margin status ceased to have independent prognostic significance in the presence of tumor grade and nodal status [59], indicating that other parameters may have comparable prognostic value.

Utilization of molecular margin analysis by Dr. Hoon's laboratory appears to perform better than traditional microscopy at stratifying patients into the group with less biologically aggressive cancer. It is only logical to envision that molecular approaches with superior performance may lead to the robust selection of the patients with less aggressive disease who will benefit from chemoradiotherapy. The higher sensitivity KRAS assay developed at the Nant Networks, LLC, combines PNA clamping of wild type allele, end stage PCR and mass spectrometry based product detection. That allows for approximately 100-fold increase in assay selectivity as compared to the original approach employed by Kim et al. [60]. Ongoing retrospective analysis of the samples from several clinical studies will clarify the potential role of the molecular detection of occult tumor cells in the selection of candidates for neoadjuvant or postoperative radiotherapy.

The Application of Genomics to Cervical Cancer: Dtex a Case Study

Cervical cancer is the third most commonly diagnosed cancer and the fourth leading cause of cancer death in females worldwide, accounting for 9% (529,800) of the total new cancer cases and 8% (275,100) of the total cancer deaths among females in 2008. More than 85% of these cases and deaths occur in developing countries. India, the second most populous country in the world, accounts for 27% (77,100) of the total cervical cancer deaths each year. Worldwide, the highest incidence rates are in Eastern, Western, and Southern Africa, as well as South-Central Asia and South America [61].

In countries where adequate resources exist to implement screening programs the incidence of cervical cancer deaths has been greatly reduced, primarily through the widespread availability and use of the Papanicolaou (Pap) test. However, robust cervical cancer screening programs are costly and can be very complex. Cytologic screening alone has reduced the burden of cervical cancer in the US by an estimated 70%, albeit at a cost of $6 billion per annum for screening and intervention [62]. A substantial portion of this cost is attributable to the estimated 10% of women with abnormal test results that require additional follow-up and management [63]. Despite the relatively low incidence of cervical carcinogenesis in this group, these women are subjected to repeated diagnostic testing, invasive procedures, and, when appropriate, surgical treatment [64, 65].

The discovery of the human papillomavirus (HPV) and the incorporation of testing for high-risk, oncogenic HPV types into the management of women with cytological abnormalities have been moderately beneficial. An infection from an oncogenic HPV subtype is required for the development of cervical cancer [66, 67]. Many women with mild cytologic abnormalities do not have HPV infections and, therefore, may be spared needless follow up and invasive procedures because their risk of cervical cancer is considered no greater than those in the general population. The clinical use of HPV testing, however, has its limitations. Studies have shown the vast majority of women (an estimated 80%) will have at least one HPV infection in their lifetime [68]. In addition, the HPV infection rate in young women is very high, i.e., an estimated 45% of women aged 20–24 have been shown to harbor the infection [69]. The high prevalence of HPV infection limits the impact of such testing which is why the use of HPV screening has been confined only to women aged 30 years or older [70]. However, care and follow-up of younger women is particularly critical since their surgical treatment is known to have significant negative consequences and harm [63, 71, 72].

Despite these limitations, the development of high risk HPV testing is considered an improvement over Pap testing alone. Infection with a high risk HPV subtype is widely considered to be a necessary condition for the development of virtually all squamous cell cervical carcinomas. Testing for HPV was initially incorporated into patient management as a triage test for women with Atypical Squamous Cells of Undetermined Significance (ASCUS) Pap results to determine which women should go to colposcopy (direct inspection of the cervix). Its utility in populations with more severe cytologic abnormalities, like Low-grade Squamous Intraepithelial Lesions (LSIL) and High-grade Squamous Intraepithelial Lesions (HSIL), is limited by the high prevalence of HPV infections in these populations. Simply, HPV testing is not able to distinguish women whose abnormalities would progress from those that would regress. Within the last 5 years, the guidelines have been modified to provide practicing physicians with an option to screen older women for high-risk HPV in conjunction with the Pap test. Due to the high prevalence of HPV infection, especially in younger women, screening recommendations have been limited to those women >30 years of age. Whereas a small percentage of HPV positive women may be diagnosed with disease earlier, many more undergo needless follow up testing until carcinogenesis can be ruled out.

The biological complexity of cervical disease development plus the large number of women with either cytological abnormalities and/or oncogenic HPV infections require comprehensive guidelines for clinical management. Both The American College of Obstetricians and Gynecologists (ACOG) and The American Society for Colposcopy and Cervical Pathology (ASCCP) have developed consensus practice recommendations for cytology screening and management of women with abnormal cervical cytology [63, 73–77]. These guidelines were developed to enable clinicians to better distinguish true cervical precancers from benign abnormalities [64]. The recommendations indicate the use of Pap testing, HPV testing, colposcopy, and surgical intervention in various combinations and frequencies depending on the severity of the abnormalities identified by the screening tests. The practice guidelines identify a number of areas for improvement to address unmet medical needs. Most of these opportunities focus on addressing the poor specificity of PAP and HPV testing as a measure of cervical lesions with oncogenic potential.

Histology results from colposcopy-directed biopsy are considered the gold standard in the assessment of cervical cancer development. A histology result of Within

Normal Limits (WNL) confirms the absence of dysplasia. Cervical Intraepithelial Neoplasia grade 1 (CIN-1) lesions indicate only slightly greater risk over normal histology and are therefore not treated. CIN-3 lesions are considered "high grade" and carry a significant risk of cancer development. CIN-2 designations are highly subjective and are the least reproducible. Many physicians find CIN-2 to be the most difficult to manage since such lesions have a higher risk of carcinogenesis, yet a significant proportion have been shown to regress without intervention. Complicating the matter even further is the variability of CIN scoring among the pathology community.

Colposcopy with directed biopsy is used to detect disease and make treatment decisions, but its utility is limited because it has also been shown to have sensitivity challenges [75]. The sensitivity of these tools (Pap, HPV, and colposcopy) enables a larger pool of at-risk women to be identified, but create a situation where the risk of disease development for any specific patient within the pool cannot be determined. Therefore, the guidelines outline an effective method to manage patients based on population disease risks and high frequency testing. The introduction of new techniques could provide greater accuracy and efficiency in the identification of early stage disease development. Utilization of diagnostic tools that provide greater specificity in detecting early cervical carcinogenesis would enable a shift away from population-based management tools to more individualized patient care.

The detection of abnormalities in chromosomal DNA has been shown to be an effective tool for the detection and diagnosis of cancers [78]. Identification of specific DNA amplifications, deletions, translocations, and rearrangements are used to diagnose and guide treatment of a range of hematologic cancers [79]. The complexity of genetic abnormalities in epithelial cell cancers is much greater and has only been utilized for disease detection more recently. The introduction of Fluorescence In Situ Hybridization (FISH) testing for the diagnosis of bladder cancer, or its recurrence, by aneuploidy (abnormal chromosomal number) represents the first major clinical application of cytogenetic abnormalities within epithelial cancers [80, 81]. The potential to employ FISH-based diagnostic tests exists for a wide range of epithelial cancers, including cervical cancer. Molecular and cytogenetic research studies have identified a number of chromosomal abnormalities that are associated with cervical carcinogenesis [82–86]. Both cervical squamous cell carcinomas and adenocarcinomas have representative chromosomal aberrations, including amplification of 1q, 3q, 5p, 8q, 9p, 11q, and 20q along with deletions of 2q, 6p, 8q, 9p, 10q, and 13q among others [87–89]. A small number of these abnormalities, predominantly the amplification of 3q26 and 5p15, have been shown to be involved in the progression of the carcinogenic process and the transition from dysplasia to invasive disease [90–92]. The incorporation of a FISH-based test into current practice to identify these critical events during cervical carcinogenesis would provide clinicians the opportunity for more cost-effective utilization of costly healthcare resources for patients with early disease development as determined by their chromosomal profile.

The role of chromosomal abnormalities in the development of cervical cancer is not surprising. Carcinogenesis is driven by HPV infection. The expression of the viral oncoproteins E6 and E7 results in deregulation of the p53 and Rb tumor

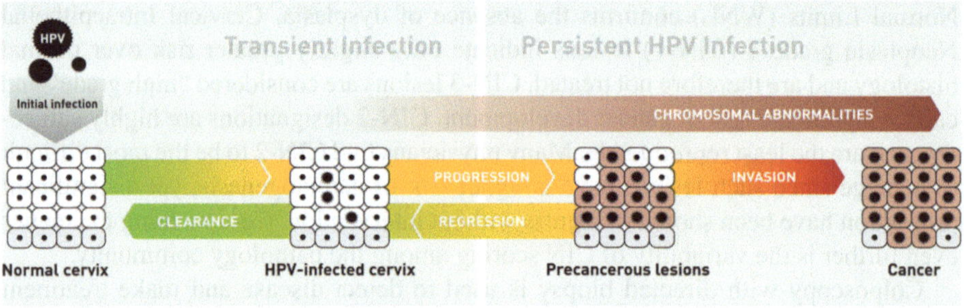

Fig. 13.8 Cervical carcinogenesis processes

suppression pathways and leads to genomic instability [93, 94]. The subsequent development of multiple DNA abnormalities occurs within the unstable cervical cell genome, some of which drive the development of a tumor [87, 89]. The following diagram (Fig. 13.8) illustrates the cervical carcinogenic process.

The ability to detect the damage to the DNA caused by the HPV oncoproteins E6 and E7 complements current practice and would enable the identification of early stage carcinogenesis within specific patients. The Cervical DNA Dtex™ test was developed to address this unmet need. The Cervical DNA Dtex test is designed to identify and enumerate chromosomes 3, 5, and 7 via FISH in cervical specimens from women with mild cytologic abnormalities or high–risk HPV infections. Abnormalities in these chromosomes are associated with high–grade dysplasia and/or cervical cancer. The test results, together with the physician's assessment of the patient's history, other risk factors, and professional guidelines, may be used to guide patient management. Since the Cervical DNA Dtex test is performed using liquid-based cytology it is run out of the same vial from which the Pap and HPV tests are performed. The primary target population for the Cervical DNA Dtex test are patients identified with mild cytological abnormalities and/or high-risk HPV infections that have elevated, but low, risk of developing cervical precancers or cancers that require surgical treatment. This group includes two patient types (a) ASCUS/HPV+ or (b) LSIL. More than 50% of patients treated today present with these clinical indications. Medical research shows these two patient subgroups have identical risk of developing disease (~11%) and are, therefore, clinically equivalent. This means, however, that 8 of every 9 women in these subgroups are overtreated due to the lack of a specific disease marker.

The utility of the Cervical DNA Dtex test was recently confirmed in a clinical study performed at The University of Florida Shands Medical Center [95]. This IRB-approved study was designed to evaluate the use of the Cervical DNA Dtex test to detect cervical cancer within current clinical practice. Within the 26 enrolled subjects, the Cervical DNA Dtex was shown to have 100% sensitivity and 100% specificity for the detection of invasive cervical cancer, outperforming Pap testing, HPV testing, and directed biopsy.

In a recent case study, the clinical benefit of the Cervical DNA Dtex test to detect DNA damage and early cervical carcinogenesis was demonstrated by a clinician in Tennessee earlier this year. A new patient, age 42, visited the clinician's office for a

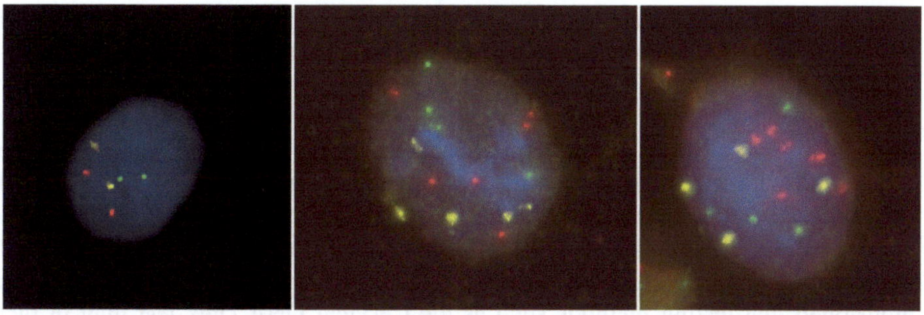

Fig. 13.9 Damaged DNA identified using FISH by Cervical DNA Dtex test. Normal diploid cells would have two copies of each 3q26 (*red*), 5p15 (*green*) and CEN7 (*yellow*) (*left panel*). Aneuploid cells have extra copies of these loci (*middle* and *right panel*)

routine exam. The Pap result was reported as ASCUS/HPV+. The clinician scheduled a 6-month follow-up visit for repeat cytology screening at which time the Pap test showed Atypical Endocervical Cells; the patient retested as positive for high-risk HPV. At the physician's request the residual cytology specimen was sent for Cervical DNA Dtex testing which revealed extensive DNA damage. The clinician then performed a colposcopic exam with directed biopsy and endocervical curettage (ECC). The histology diagnosis was mild dysplasia and the ECC was negative suggesting that the patient was disease-free. The clinician requested the patient return for follow up testing within 3 months at which time another Cervical DNA Dtex test was ordered. Results showed extensive DNA damage (see images below). The clinician performed a conization based upon the recurrent cytological abnormalities, confirmed persistent high-risk HPV infection, and the identification of chromosomal abnormalities associated with carcinogenesis. The histological diagnosis of the cone biopsy specimen revealed cervical adenocarcinoma. The patient subsequently had a hysterectomy performed. Fortunately for this patient, the clinician's diligence uncovered a potentially life-threatening condition at a stage where it could be effectively treated (Fig. 13.9).

While screening test results of ASCUS/HPV+ are common (about 6% of patients) and more than two-thirds of them do not require treatment, these patients represent a difficult population to manage for clinicians [64, 96, 97]. The prevalence of HPV infection, the frequent regression of mild abnormalities, and imperfections with colposcopy make it difficult to assess disease risk patient-by-patient and make individualized management plans. The use of Cervical DNA Dtex to provide a snapshot of disease development at the DNA level is complementary to standard techniques that provide cellular and tissue morphological information.

As the scientific and medical communities advance, the creation of tools and techniques to assess a patient's risk of disease development will lead to more accurate and efficient healthcare. Individualized risk profiling is critical to the early detection and diagnosis of cancer. Risk assessment has been proposed previously for the prevention of cervical cancer but has limited adoption due to the complexity of clinical practice guidelines [98]. The incorporation of Cervical DNA Dtex testing into clinical practice would provide practicing clinicians with valuable insight into the underlying carcinogenesis process and guide clinical practice toward risk-appropriate patient management. In those women presenting with HPV infection and/or a cytologic abnormality, an independent, noninvasive, specific marker of disease from the same sample used for both the Pap and HPV testing has specific implications regarding the likelihood of progression. The ability to detect the same biomarkers within tissue also offers the promise of confirming that the target lesion(s) are excised. In addition, patients without the requisite DNA damage—and therefore at lesser risk—can be spared needless follow up testing and interventions based upon the reliance on nonspecific and highly subjective methodologies. In fact, it is envisioned that testing methods such as the Cervical DNA Dtex test may in fact supplant traditional histology assessment as the gold standard in the diagnosis and classification of disease. It is our belief that only in understanding and measuring the underlying biological mechanisms of disease can one truly realize the promise of personalized medicine leading to more cost-effective healthcare management.

Conclusions

High content patient data capture, whether through genomics, transcriptomics, protein-based methods or other routes, will result in association studies that tie these data to clinical outcomes and result in effective, personalized patient management tools. Managing these large data sets in a controlled manner and developing the algorithms for their in-depth clinical epidemiological evaluations will form the foundation of our efforts to move molecular diagnostics to the forefront in the prevention and management of disease. The outcome of these efforts will result in rational methods for the cost effective individualized treatment and management of diseases in large populations. Their implementation will heavily depend on the development of an array of molecular diagnostic tests employed in conjunction with detailed patient data from centralized data centers. In the US this will require strong support from patient advocacy groups, to help bring this about.

Acknowledgements We thank Michael Carter and Allison Peak for their efforts in helping to finalize the manuscript.

References

1. van't Veer LJ, Dai H, van de Vijver MJ, et al. Gene expression profiling predicts clinical outcome of breast cancer. Nature. 2002;415(6871):530–6.
2. Mittempergher L, de Ronde JJ, Nieuwland M, et al. Gene expression profiles from formalin fixed paraffin embedded breast cancer tissue are largely comparable to fresh frozen matched tissue. PLoS One. 2011;6(2):e17163.
3. Dowsett M, Cuzick J, Wale C, et al. Prediction of risk of distant recurrence using the 21-gene recurrence score in node-negative and node-positive postmenopausal breast cancer patients treated with anastrozole or tamoxifen: a transATAC study. J ClinOncol. 2010;28(11):1829–34.

4. Jänicke F, Schmitt M, Pache L, et al. Urokinase (uPA) and its inhibitor PAI-1 are strong and independent prognostic factors in node-negative breast cancer. Breast Cancer Res Treat. 1993;24(3):195–208.
5. Trainer AH, Lewis CR, Tucker K, Meiser B, Friedlander M, Ward RL. The role of BRCA mutation testing in determining breast cancer therapy. Nat Rev Clin Oncol. 2010;7(12): 708–17.
6. Smith J, Tho LM, Xu N, Gillespie DA. The ATM-Chk2 and ATR-Chk1 pathways in DNA damage signaling and cancer. Adv Cancer Res. 2010;108:73–112.
7. Parker D. PMC, Personalized medicine coalition. The adverse impact of the US reimbursement system on the development and adoption of personalized medicine diagnostics. Boston Healthcare. 2010. www.bostonhealthcare.com/objects/PDFs/ReimbursementIssueBrief.pdf. Accessed 18 May 2011.
8. Narzisi G, Mishra B. Comparing de novo genome assembly: the long and short of it. PLoS One. 2011;6(4):e19175.
9. Narzisi G, Mishra B. Scoring-and-unfolding trimmed tree assembler: concepts, constructs and comparisons. Bioinformatics. 2011;27(2):153–60.
10. Ramakrishnan N, Tadepalli S, Watson LT, Helm RF, Antoniotti M, Mishra B. Reverse engineering dynamic temporal models of biological processes and their relationships. Proc Natl Acad Sci USA. 2010;107(28):12511–6.
11. Ramakrishnan N, Mishra B. Reverse engineering dynamic temporal models of biological processes and their relationships. Proc Natl Acad Sci USA. 2010;107(28):12511–6.
12. Vaske CJ, Benz SC, Sanborn JZ, et al. Inference of patient-specific pathway activities from multi-dimensional cancer genomics data using PARADIGM. Bioinformatics. 2010;26(12): i237–45.
13. McNeil N, Ried T. Novel molecular cytogenetic techniques for identifying complex chromosomal rearrangements: technology and applications in molecular medicine. Expert Rev Mol Med. 2000;2000:1–14.
14. Ionita I, Daruwala R, Mishra B. Mapping tumor suppressor genes using multipoint statistics from copy-number variation data. Am J Human Genet. 2006;79(1):13–22.
15. Daruwala R-S, Rudra A, Ostrer H, Lucito R, Wigler M, Mishra B. A versatile statistical analysis algorithm to detect genome copy number variation. Proc Natl Acad Sci USA. 2004;101(46):16292–7.
16. Mathew JP, Chinnaiyan A, Bader G, et al. From bytes to bedside: computational biology for biomedical translational research. PLoS Computational Biol. 2007;3(2):1–12.
17. Rauch A, Ruschendorf F, Huang J, et al. Molecular karyotyping using an SNP array for genomewide genotyping. J Med Genet. 2004;41:916–22.
18. Robertson KD. DNA methylation and human disease. Nat Rev Genet. 2005;6:597–610.
19. Schena M, Shalon D, Davis RW, Brown PO. Quantitative monitoring of gene expression patterns with a complementary DNA microarray. Science. 1995;270:467–70.
20. Lockhart DJ, Dong H, Byrne MC, et al. Expression monitoring by hybridization to high-density oligonucleotide arrays. Nat Biotechnol. 1996;14:1675–80.
21. Brenner S, Johnson M, Bridgham J, et al. Gene expression analysis by massively parallel signature sequencing (MPSS) on microbead arrays. Nat Biotechnol. 2000;18:630–4.
22. Golub TR, Slonim DK, Tamayo P, et al. Molecular classification of cancer: class discovery and class prediction by gene expression monitoring. Science. 1999;286:531–7.
23. Reed J, Pittenger B, Magonov S, et al. Single molecule transcription profiling with AFM. Nanotechnology. 2007;18:1–15.
24. Dhanasekaran SM, Barrette TR, Ghosh D, et al. Delineation of prognostic biomarkers in prostate cancer. Nature. 2001;412:822–6.
25. Blais A, Dynlacht BD. Constructing transcriptional regulatory networks. Genes Dev. 2005; 19:1499–511.
26. Rubin MA, Zerkowski MP, Camp RL, et al. Quantitative determination of expression of the prostate cancer protein alpha-methylacyl-CoA racemase using automated quantitative analysis (AQUA): a novel paradigm for automated and continuous biomarker measurements. Am J Pathol. 2004;164(3):831–40.

27. Nishimura T, Nomura M, Tojo H, et al. Proteomic analysis of laser-microdissected paraffin-embedded tissues: (2) MRM assay for stage-related proteins upon non-metastatic lung adenocarcinoma. J Proteomics. 2010;73(6):1100–10.
28. Güzel C, Ursem NT, Dekker LJ, et al. Multiple reaction monitoring assay for pre-eclampsia related calcyclin peptides in formalin fixed paraffin embedded placenta. J Proteome Res. 2011;10(7):3274–82.
29. Gallien S, Duriez E, Domon B. Selected reaction monitoring applied to proteomics. J Mass Spectrom. 2011;46:298–312.
30. Hood BL, Darfler MM, Guiel TG, et al. Proteomic analysis of formalin fixed prostate cancer tissue. Mol Cell Proteomics. 2005;4(11):1741–53.
31. Bateman NW, Sun M, Bhargava R, et al. Differential proteomic analysis of late-stage and recurrent breast cancer from formalin-fixed paraffin-embedded tissues. J Proteome Res. 2011;10(3):1323–32.
32. Tong J, Taylor P, Peterman SM, Prakash A, Moran MF. Epidermal growth factor receptor phosphorylation sites Ser991 and Tyr998 are implicated in the regulation of receptor endocytosis and phosphorylations at Ser1039 and Thr1041. Mol Cell Proteomics. 2009;8(9):2131–44.
33. Sethi S, Theis JD, Leung N, et al. Mass spectrometry-based proteomic diagnosis of renal immunoglobulin heavy chain amyloidosis. Clin J Am SocNephrol. 2010;5(12):2180–7.
34. Yamasaki F, Johansen MJ, Zhang D, et al. Acquired resistance to erlotinib in A-431 epidermoid cancer cells requires down-regulation of MMAC1/PTEN and up-regulation of phosphorylated akt. Cancer Res. 2007;67:5779.
35. Engelman JA, Zejnullahu K, Mitsudomi T, et al. MET amplification leads to gefitinib resistance in lung cancer by activating ERBB3 signaling. Science. 2007;316:1039–43.
36. Moskovits M. Surface enhanced spectroscopy. Rev Modern Physics. 1985;57:783–826.
37. Stiles PL, Dieringer JA, Shah NC, Van Duyne RP. Surface-enhanced raman spectroscopy. Annl Rev Analytical Chem. 2008;1:601–26.
38. Gunnarsson L, Bjerneld EJ, Xu H, Petronis S, Kasemo B, Kall M. Interparticle coupling effects in nanofabricated substrates for surface-enhanced raman scattering. Applied Phyics Letters. 2001;78:802–4.
39. McFarland AD, Van Duyne RP. Single silver nanoparticles as real-time optical sensors with zeptomole sensitivity. Nano Lett. 2003;3:1057–62.
40. Clark AW, Glidle A, Cumming DRS, Cooper JM. Plasmonic split-ring resonators as dichroic nanophotonic DNA biosensors. J Am Chem Soc. 2009;131:17615–9.
41. Shumaker-Parry JS, Rochholz H, Kreiter M. Fabrication of crescent-shaped optical antennas. Adv Mater. 2005;17:2131–4.
42. Sau TK, Murphy CJ. Seeded high yield synthesis of short au nanorods in aqueous solution. Langmuir. 2004;20:6414–20.
43. Wang H, Levin CS, Halas NJ. Nanosphere arrays with controlled sub-10 nm gaps as surface-enhanced raman spectroscopy substrates. J Am Chem Soc. 2005;127:14992–3.
44. Im H, Bantz KC, Lindquist NC, Haynes CL, Oh SH. Vertically oriented sub-10 nm plasmonic nanogap arrays. Nano Lett. 2010;10:2231–6.
45. Pastoriza-Santos I, Liz-Marzan LM. Synthesis of silver nanoprisms in DMF. Nano Lett. 2002;2:903–5.
46. Nehl CL, Liao HW, Hafner JH. Optical properties of star-shaped gold nanoparticles. Nano Lett. 2006;6:683–8.
47. Deng X, Braun GB, Liu S, et al. Single-order, subwavelength resonant nanograting as a uniformly hot substrate for surface-enhanced raman spectroscopy. Nano Lett. 2010;10:1780–6.
48. Ross JS. Breast cancer biomarkers and HER2 testing after 10 years of anti-HER2 therapy. Drug News Perspect. 2009;22(2):93–106.
49. Bollag G, Hirth P, Tsai J, et al. Clinical efficacy of a RAF inhibitor needs broad target blockade in BRAF-mutant melanoma. Nature. 2010;467(7315):596–9.

50. Shinozaki M, O'Day SJ, Kitago M, et al. Utility of circulating B-RAF DNA mutation in serum for monitoring melanoma patients receiving biochemotherapy. Clin Cancer Res. 2007;13(7):2068–74.
51. Koyanagi K, O'Day SJ, Gonzalez R, et al. Serial monitoring of circulating melanoma cells during neoadjuvant biochemotherapy for stage III melanoma: outcome prediction in a multicenter trial. J Clin Oncol. 2005;23(31):8057–64.
52. Takeuchi H, Morton DL, Kuo C, et al. Prognostic significance of molecular upstaging of paraffin-embedded sentinel lymph nodes in melanoma patients. J Clin Oncol. 2004; 22(13):2671–80.
53. Nicholl MB, Elashoff D, Takeuchi H, Morton DL, Hoon DS. Molecular upstaging based on paraffin-embedded sentinel lymph nodes: ten-year follow-up confirms prognostic utility in melanoma patients. Ann Surg. 2011;253(1):116–22.
54. Landis SH, Murray T, Bolden S, Wingo PA. Cancer statistics, 1999. CA: A Cancer Journal for Clinicians. 1999;49(1):8–31.
55. Lim JE, Chien MW, Earle CC. Prognostic factors following curative resection for pancreatic adenocarcinoma: a population-based, linked database analysis of 396 patients. Ann Surg. 2003;237(1):74–85.
56. Verbeke CS, Menon KV. Redefining resection margin status in pancreatic cancer. HPB. 2009;11(4):282–9.
57. Catalogue of somatic mutations in cancer. http://www.sanger.ac.uk/genetics/CGP/cosmic/. Accessed 22 Aug 2011.
58. Thiede C, Bayerdörffer E, Blasczyk R, Wittig B, Neubauer A. Simple and sensitive detection of mutations in the ras proto-oncogenes using PNA-mediated PCR clamping. Nucleic Acids Res. 1996;24(5):983–4.
59. Neoptolemos JP, Stocken DD, Dunn JA, European Study Group for Pancreatic Cancer, et al. Influence of resection margins on survival for patients with pancreatic cancer treated by adjuvant chemoradiation and/or chemotherapy in the ESPAC-1 randomized controlled trial. Ann Surg. 2001;234(6):758–68.
60. Kim J, Reber HA, Dry SM, et al. Unfavourable prognosis associated with K-ras gene mutation in pancreatic cancer surgical margins. Gut. 2006;55(11):1598–605.
61. Ferlay J, Shin HR, Bray F, Forman D, Mathers C, Parkin DM. GLOBOCAN 2008, Cancer incidence and mortality worldwide: IARC CancerBase No. 10. Lyon, France: International agency for research on cancer. 2010. http://globocan.iarc.fr. Accessed 18 May 2011.
62. Davidson, Nancy. Cervical Cancer SPORE Program. Cervical Cancer SPORE Program Description. The Johns Hopkins University. 2004. Web. http://pathology2.jhu.edu/ccspore/introduction.html. Accessed 18 May 2011.
63. Wright Jr TC, Massad LS, Dunton CJ, Spitzer M, Wilkinson EJ, Solomon D. 2006 Consensus guidelines for the management of women with cervical intraepithelial neoplasia or adenocarcinoma in situ. 2006 American society for colposcopy and cervical pathology-sponsored consensus conference. Am J Obstet Gynecol. 2007;197:340–5.
64. American College of Obstetricians and Gynecologists. ACOG practice bulletin No. 99: management of abnormal cervical cytology and histology. Obstet Gynecol. 2008;112:1419–44.
65. American College of Obstetricians and Gynecologists. ACOG practice bulletin No. 109: cervical cytology screening. Obstet Gynecol. 2009;114:1409–20.
66. zur Hausen H. Condylomata acuminata and human genital cancer. Cancer Res. 1976;36(2 pt 2):794.
67. Walboomer JM, Jacobs MV, Manos MM, et al. Human papillomavirus is a necessary cause of invasive cervical cancer worldwide. J Pathol. 1999;189(1):12–9.
68. Herrero R, Munoz N. Human papillomavirus and cancer. Cancer Surv. 1999;33:75–98.
69. Dunne EF, Unger ER, Sternberg M, et al. Prevalence of HPV infection among females in the United States. JAMA. 2007;297:813–9.
70. Schiffman M, Castle PE, Jeronimo J, Rodriguez AC, Wacholder S. Human papillomavirus and cervical cancer. Lancet. 2007;370(9590):890–907.

71. Jakobsson M, Gissler M, Sainio S, Paavonen J, Tapper AM. Preterm delivery after surgical treatment for cervical intraepithelial neoplasia. Obstet Gynecol. 2007;109:309–13.
72. Crane JM. Pregnancy outcome after loop electrosurgical excision procedure: a systematic review. Obstet Gynecol. 2003;102:1058–62.
73. ASCUS-LSIL Triage Study (ALTS) Group. Results of a randomized trial on the management of cytology interpretations of atypical squamous cells of undetermined significance. Am J Obstet Gynecol. 2003;188:1383–92.
74. ASCUS-LSIL Triage Study (ALTS) Group. A randomized trial on the management of low-grade squamous intraepithelial lesion cytology interpretations. Am J Obstet Gynecol. 2003;188:1393–400.
75. ASCUS-LSIL Triage Study (ALTS) Group. Post-colposcopy management strategies for patients with low-grade squamous intraepithelial lesions or human papillomavirus DNA-positive atypical squamous cells of undetermined significance: two-year prospective study. Am J Obstet Gynecol. 2003;188:1401–5.
76. ASCUS-LSIL Triage Study (ALTS) Group. Prospective follow-up suggests similar risk of subsequent cervical intraepithelial neoplasia grade 2 or 3 among women with cervical intraepithelial neoplasia grade 1 or negative colposcopy and directed biopsy. Am J Obstet Gynecol. 2003;188:1406–12.
77. Wright TC, Massad LS, Dunton CJ, Spitzer M, Wilkinson EJ, Solomon D. For the 2006 ASCCP-sponsored consensus conference. 2006 Consensus guidelines for the management of women with abnormal cervical cancer screening tests. Am J Obstet Gynecol. 2007;197:346–55.
78. Sandberg AA, Meloni-Ehrig AM. Cytogenetics and genetics of human cancer: methods and accomplishments. Cancer Genet Cytogenet. 2010;203:102–26.
79. Bernheim A. Cytogenomics of cancers: from chromosome to sequence. Mol Oncol. 2010;4:309–22.
80. Sarosdy MF, Schellhammer P, Bokinsky G, et al. Clinical evaluation of a multi-target fluorescent in situ hybridization assay for detection of bladder cancer. J Urol. 2002; 168:1950–4.
81. Skacel M, Fahmy M, Brainard JA, et al. Multitarget fluorescence in situ hybridization assay detects transitional cell carcinoma in the majority of patients with bladder cancer and atypical or negative urine cytology. J Urol. 2003;169:2101–5.
82. Heselmeyer K, Macville M, Schröck E, et al. Advanced-stage cervical carcinomas are defined by a recurrent pattern of chromosomal aberrations revealing high genetic instability and a consistent gain of chromosome arm 3q. Genes Chromosomes Cancer. 1997;19:233–40.
83. Soder AI, Hoare SF, Muir S, Going JJ, Parkinson EK, Keith WN. Amplification, increased dosage and in situ expression of the telomerase RNA gene in human cancer. Oncogene. 1997;14:1013–21.
84. Thein AT, Han X, Heyderman E, Fox M, Steele SJ, Parrington JM. Molecular cytogenetic analysis of five newly established cervical cancer cell lines using G banding and fluorescence in situ hybridization. Cancer Genet Cytogenet. 1996;91:28–36.
85. Heselmeyer K, Schröck E, du Manoir S, et al. Gain of chromosome 3q defines the transition from severe dysplasia to invasive carcinoma of the uterine cervix. Proc Natl Acad Sci USA. 1996;93:479–84.
86. Kirchhoff M, Rose H, Petersen BL, et al. Comparative genomic hybridization reveals a recurrent pattern of chromosomal aberrations in severe dysplasia/carcinoma in situ of the cervix and in advanced-stage cervical carcinoma. Genes Chromosomes Cancer. 1999;24:144–50.
87. Allen DG, White DJ, Hutchins AM, et al. Progressive genetic aberrations detected by comparative genomic hybridization in squamous cell cervical cancer. Br J Cancer. 2000;83:1659–63.
88. Baudis M. Genomic imbalances in 5918 malignant epithelial tumors: an explorative meta-analysis of chromosomal CGH data. BMC Cancer. 2007;7:226.

89. Lando M, Holden M, Bergersen LC, et al. Gene dosage, expression, and ontology analysis identifies driver genes in the carcinogenesis and chemoradioresistance of cervical cancer. PLoS Genet. 2009;5:e1000719.
90. Heselmeyer-Haddad K, Janz V, Castle PE, et al. Detection of genomic amplification of the human telomerase gene (TERC) in cytologic specimens as a genetic test for the diagnosis of cervical dysplasia. Am J Pathol. 2003;163:1405–16.
91. Heselmeyer-Haddad K, Sommerfeld K, White NM, et al. Genomic amplification of the human telomerase gene (TERC) in pap smears predicts the development of cervical cancer. Am J Pathol. 2005;166:1229–38.
92. Fitzpatrick MA, Funk MC, Gius D, et al. Identification of chromosomal alterations important in the development of cervical intraepithelial neoplasia and invasive carcinoma using alignment of DNA microarray data. Gynecol Oncol. 2006;103:458–62.
93. Dyson N, Howley PM, Munger K, Harlow E. The human papilloma virus-16 E7 oncoprotein is able to bind to the retinoblastoma gene product. Science. 1989;243:934–7.
94. Band V, De Caprio JA, Delmolino L, Kulesa V, Sager R. Loss of p53 protein in human papillomavirus type 16 E6-immortalized human mammary epithelial cells. J Virol. 1991;65: 6671–6.
95. Smith K. Balanky E. (Study) Evaluate the performance of Cervical DNA Dtex testing to detect invasive cancer within current clinical practices. Conducted February 9, 2010 to December 20, 2010. Personal Communication: April 15th, 2011.
96. Wang SS, Walker JL, Schiffman M, Solomon D. Evaluating the risk of cervical precancer with a combination of cytologic, virologic, and visual methods. Cancer Epidemiol Biomarkers Prev. 2005;14:2665–8.
97. Walker JL, Wang SS, Schiffman M, Solomon D. Predicting absolute risk of CIN3 during post-colposcopic follow-up: results from the ASCUS-LSIL Triage Study (ALTS). Am J Obstet Gynecol. 2006;195:341–8.
98. Castle PE, Sideri M, Jeronimo J, Solomon D, Schiffman M. Risk assessment to guide the prevention of cervical cancer. Am J Obstet Gynecol. 2007;197:356.e1–6.
99. Westgaard A, Tafjord S, Farstad IN, Cvancarova M, Eide TJ, Mathisen O, Clausen OP, Gladhaug IP. Resectable adenocarcinomas in the pancreatic head: the retroperitoneal resection margin is an independent prognostic factor. BMC Cancer. 2008 Jan 14;8:5.
100. Raut CP, Tseng JF, Sun CC, Wang H, Wolff RA, Crane CH, Hwang R, Vauthey JN, Abdalla EK, Lee JE, Pisters PW, Evans DB. Impact of resection status on pattern of failure and survival after pancreaticoduodenectomy for pancreatic adenocarcinoma. Ann Surg. 2007 Jul;246(1):52–60.
101. Verbeke CS, Leitch D, Menon KV, McMahon MJ, Guillou PJ, Anthoney A. Redefining the R1 resection in pancreatic cancer. Br J Surg. 2006 Oct;93(10):1232–7.
102. Benassai G, Mastrorilli M, Quarto G, Cappiello A, Giani U, Mosella G. Survival after pancreaticoduodenectomy for ductal adenocarcinoma of the head of the pancreas. Chir Ital. 2000 May–Jun;52(3):263–70.
103. Sohn TA, Yeo CJ, Cameron JL, Koniaris L, Kaushal S, Abrams RA, Sauter PK, Coleman J, Hruban RH, Lillemoe KD. Resected adenocarcinoma of the pancreas-616 patients: results, outcomes, and prognostic indicators. J Gastrointest Surg. 2000 Nov–Dec;4(6):567–79.
104. Millikan KW, Deziel DJ, Silverstein JC, Kanjo TM, Christein JD, Doolas A, Prinz RA. Prognostic factors associated with resectable adenocarcinoma of the head of the pancreas. Am Surg. 1999 Jul;65(7):618–23.
105. Nishimura Y, Hosotani R, Shibamoto Y, Kokubo M, Kanamori S, Sasai K, Hiraoka M, Ohshio G, Imamura M, Takahashi M, Abe M. External and intraoperative radiotherapy for resectable and unresectable pancreatic cancer: analysis of survival rates and complications. Int J Radiat Oncol Biol Phys. 1997 Aug 1;39(1):39–49.
106. Sperti C, Pasquali C, Piccoli A, Pedrazzoli S. Survival after resection for ductal adenocarcinoma of the pancreas. Br J Surg. 1996 May;83(5):625–31.

107. Nitecki SS, Sarr MG, Colby TV, van Heerden JA. Long-term survival after resection for ductal adenocarcinoma of the pancreas. Is it really improving? Ann Surg. 1995 Jan;221(1):59–66.
108. Yeo CJ, Cameron JL, Lillemoe KD, Sitzmann JV, Hruban RH, Goodman SN, Dooley WC, Coleman J, Pitt HA. Pancreaticoduodenectomy for cancer of the head of the pancreas. 201 patients. Ann Surg. 1995 Jun;221(6):721–31; discussion 731–3.
109. Willett CG, Lewandrowski K, Warshaw AL, Efird J, Compton CC. Resection margins in carcinoma of the head of the pancreas. Implications for radiation therapy. Ann Surg. 1993 Feb;217(2):144–8.

Chapter 14
Clinical Validation of Biomarkers

Sumithra J. Mandrekar and Daniel J. Sargent

Introduction

Medical treatment for patients is driven by the combination of the expected outcome for the patient (prognosis), and the ability for treatment to improve the expected outcome (prediction). Traditionally, anatomic staging systems have been used to provide predictions of individual patient's outcome, and to a lesser extent, guide the choice of treatment by defining a set of patients who may benefit from therapy. With the introduction of novel agents and "targeted" therapies, biomarkers have the potential to supplement existing anatomic and/or pathologic information in patient stratification (risk assessment), treatment response identification (surrogate markers), and/or in differential diagnosis (identifying which patient is likely to respond to which drug[s]). There are several challenges in the translation of biomarker information from preliminary, hypothesis generating studies into well-controlled clinical studies, which are critical for determining their clinical utility. This is evident from the multitude of reports of promising biomarker activity from early studies in various disease settings; however, reports of the successful validation of these markers in prospective large-scale randomized clinical trials are far less frequent.

Biomarkers have been (and are being) developed for various diseases to estimate disease-related patient trajectories (i.e., prognostic signatures) and to predict patient-specific outcome to different treatments (i.e., predictive tools) [1–10]. A prognostic marker is a single trait or signature of traits that separates a population with respect to the outcome of interest in the absence of treatment, or despite nontargeted "standard" treatment. Prognostic marker validation is relatively straightforward, as it is

S.J. Mandrekar, Ph.D. (✉) • D.J. Sargent, Ph.D.
Department of Health Sciences Research, Mayo Clinic, 200 First St SW, Harwick 8, Rochester, MN 55905, USA
e-mail: mandrekar.sumithra@mayo.edu

H.-J. Lenz (ed.), *Biomarkers in Oncology: Prediction and Prognosis*,
DOI 10.1007/978-1-4419-9755-5_14,

associated with the disease or the patient, and not with a specific therapy. Therefore, it can be established (at least in theory) using the marker and outcome data from a series of patients (with adequate follow-up) treated uniformly with placebo or with standard treatment [10–12]. A predictive marker, on the other hand, is a single trait or signature of traits that separates a population with respect to the outcome of interest in response to a particular (targeted) treatment. Designs for predictive marker validation are therefore inherently more complex and require at a fundamental level data from a randomized study [12].

Two critical issues in the clinical validation of biomarkers are the choice of the clinical trial design and logistical issues surrounding the biomarker assays. In this chapter we first discuss the technical feasibility, assay performance metrics and the logistics of specimen collection for biomarker assays. Next, we review the various trial designs for predictive marker validation and discuss the relative merits and limitations of each design based on the strength of the preclinical evidence, and the prevalence of a marker. These designs rest on the assumption that the technical feasibility, assay performance metrics and the logistics of specimen collection are well established and that initial results demonstrate promise with regard to the predictive ability of the marker(s). A careful consideration of the design and logistics is essential in the determination of the clinical utility of a biomarker, and its successful integration into routine clinical practice.

Biomarker Assays

The clinical validation of biomarkers is challenging given the multitude of marker assessment methods and the possibility that one drug can impact several molecular pathways. The accessibility of the marker status using the specimens obtained/available from a patient versus the specimens that are needed in theory (i.e., the concept of what you need versus what you get) poses another important but real challenge. The cost and feasibility of obtaining the specimens in a real world setting also needs careful consideration in determining the clinical utility and viability of testing the biomarker in clinical practice. Two trials, I-SPY (investigation of serial studies to predict therapeutic response with imaging and molecular analysis) and BATTLE (biomarker integrated approaches of targeted therapy of lung cancer elimination trial), have attempted to address these issues by using diverse data types, in the case of I-SPY to identify biomarkers predictive of response to therapy, and in BATTLE, by randomizing patients to treatment choices based on multiple biomarker profiles [13, 14]. In this section, we provide a broad overview of the specimen collection logistics, and the assay performance criteria for biomarker assessment.

Procedures for specimen collection including the time points of collection, processing, shipment, and storage (taking into account the longevity) of specimens for future research must be clearly outlined prior to launching a marker validation trial. The type of specimen, tissue versus serum for example, required for the biomarker assessment is an important component in assessing the logistics issues. While this is biologically and scientifically driven, serum based biomarkers are usually preferred for their simplicity, lesser cost, better feasibility in a clinical setting (if validated) and fewer ethical issues in case of multiple blood draws from a patient. The assay performance, which influences the association between the biomarker status and therapeutic activity, is impacted by all of these factors.

The technical protocol for the assay has to be well developed and validated prior to launching a marker validation trial. This includes the performance characteristics of the assay, such as the optimal assay methodology, the assay reproducibility and validity, assay failure rates, and local versus central testing. Whether a local laboratory (an on-site laboratory where the patient is treated) or a central laboratory (where all testing is done in one central facility determined at the start of the study) is required for testing of a biomarker depends on many factors, with the intended ultimate clinical use of the biomarker and the assay methodology being the two key components. For example, is the biomarker status determined based on immunohistochemistry (IHC), fluorescent in situ hybridization (FISH), or other microarray based high dimensional classifiers? The sophistication of some of these techniques makes a local assessment of the marker status infeasible, expensive, and/or unreliable. The use of commercially available kits might be a solution, but again the acceptance of this for routine clinical use is dependent on the simplicity of the kit, timeliness of the results, and the cost to the patient.

The determination of whether within the conduct of a prospective clinical trial, local or central testing of a possible predictive biomarker should be allowed depends on many factors as noted above. A key driver of the decision is intended ultimate clinical use of the biomarker. If it is envisioned that central testing of the marker will always be required, then the choice is clear. Similarly, if the assay technique is well established, the results unambiguous (such as presence or absence of a specific mutation), and biospecimens readily suitable for assay without significant preprocessing, then local biomarker determination for trial eligibility is likely preferred. In many cases the situation is usually less clear: the assay may be most optimally centrally performed at the present time, but with the intention of local testing if the biomarker is validated. In this case, when feasible, local testing may be acceptable to allow patients to enter the trial, with central confirmation required for the patient to be included in the trial's primary analysis. In this way, data can be generated on the concordance rate between local and central testing, which may help guide the future use of the biomarker. An example of where the central testing was done after the fact, and was discordant in a high proportion of cases compared to the local testing results is described below.

Trastuzumab (Herceptin), a human monoclonal antibody, is approved for treatment of human epidermal growth factor receptor 2 (HER2)-positive breast cancer patients in the advanced as well as the adjuvant setting [15]. Subsequent analyses, however, have raised the possibility of a beneficial effect of Herceptin in a more broadly defined patient population than that defined in the two trials. Specifically, post-hoc central testing for HER2 expression from the available tumor tissue blocks has demonstrated that patients with tumors that were negative for FISH and had less than immunohistochemical (IHC) 3+ staining by central testing also derived benefit from Herceptin, thus suggesting that the definition for HER2 positivity based on FISH or IHC for the adjuvant disease setting may need to be refined [16–19]. Additionally, questions regarding the reproducibility and the validity of the assay due to a high degree of discordance (approximately 25%) in the HER2 results between central and local testing remain relevant [18]. Since patients deemed HER2 negative based on the local evaluation were not enrolled onto the trials, the validity of HER2 as a predictive marker could not be fully established, and the question remains open whether Herceptin therapy may benefit a potentially larger group than the approximately 20% of patients defined as HER2 positive by central testing in these two trials. This raises two important questions: (1) choice of using a central facility versus local laboratories for patient selection for therapeutic intervention trials, which clearly depends on the reliability and reproducibility of the assay and the complexity of the assay; and (2) a potential need for a repeat assessment of the patient's marker status on a second sample, when feasible and ethically appropriate, if the first assessment deems the patient as ineligible for the trial in question.

Clinical Trial Designs for Predictive Marker Validation

The ultimate goal of developing and validating a predictive marker is that the marker will be useful in clinical practice to dictate the choice of therapy for an individual patient. Thus, the same level of rigor required for the validation of a new therapy is appropriate for a predictive marker validation, which is to conduct a prospectively designed randomized controlled trial (RCT) to test for a differential effect of treatment depending on the marker status i.e., a marker by treatment interaction. In some instances, where a prospective RCT is not possible due to ethical and/or logistical (large trial and long time to complete) considerations, a well conducted, prospectively specified retrospective validation can also aid in bringing forward effective treatments to marker defined patient subgroups in a timely manner [10].

Data from an RCT and availability of specimens from a large number of patients are both essential for a sound retrospective validation, as otherwise it would be impossible to isolate any causal effect of the marker on therapeutic efficacy from the multitude of other factors arising from a nonrandomized design and/or selected samples. For example, the marker of tumor microsatellite instability has been proposed to be a predictive marker for the efficacy of 5-fluorouracil (5-FU) based chemotherapy in colon cancer. Data from cohorts of patients treated and untreated with 5-FU, but not randomized between the treatments, have been used for this analysis [20, 21]. Specifically, data came from a cohort of nonrandomized patients where the median age of the treated patients was 13 years younger than those of the nontreated patients was utilized, thus rendering any meaningful statements about the predictive value of the marker impossibly confounded [20, 21].

Several designs have been proposed and utilized in the field of biomarkers for validation of predictive markers. Broadly speaking, these designs can be either retrospective or prospective, where prospective designs can be further classified into the following:

- Enrichment or targeted designs
- Unselected or all-comers designs
  - Sequential testing strategy
  - Marker based designs
- Hybrid designs
- Adaptive designs

We discuss the salient features of these designs, along with pertinent examples below.

Retrospective Designs

In this approach, patient specimens from two or more arms of a previously conducted randomized clinical trial are assessed. The treatment effect (comparing one treatment to another) is then tested separately within the two (or more) marker-defined groups. Ideally, this approach also includes a test for a marker by treatment interaction effect, which if significant, implies that the effect of treatment differs between patients with different marker values. This approach of testing for the predictive effect of a marker through the use of data collected from a previously conducted randomized controlled trial (RCT) comparing therapies for which a marker is proposed to be predictive is particularly effective in settings where a prospective RCT might be impossible due to ethical and logistical considerations. A summary of the essential elements for a successful retrospective validation utilizing data from a previously well conducted RCT is provided below [10, 12]:

- Availability of samples on a large majority of patients to avoid selection bias in the patients who have/do not have the samples
- Precisely stated algorithm for assay techniques and scoring system
- Prospectively stated hypothesis, analysis techniques, and patient population
- Upfront sample size and power justification for all subgroup analyses

An example of a marker that has been successfully validated using data collected from previous RCTs is KRAS as a predictor of efficacy of panitumumab and cetuximab in advanced colorectal cancer, where it was demonstrated that the benefit is restricted to patients with wild type KRAS status [22–28]. In a prospectively specified analysis of data from a previously conducted randomized Phase III trial of panitumumab versus best supportive care (BSC), KRAS status was assessed on 92% (427/463) of the patients enrolled, with 43% having the KRAS mutation [22]. The hazard ratio for treatment effect comparing panitumumab versus BSC on progression free survival (PFS) in the wild type and mutant subgroups was 0.45 and

0.99 respectively, with a significant treatment by *KRAS* status interaction ($p < 0.0001$). Similarly, retrospective data on KRAS status and cetuximab from Phase III and Phase II trials have demonstrated a statistically significant advantage in the progression-free and/or overall survival for patients with wild type KRAS, with no survival benefit in patients with *KRAS* mutant status [24–28]. Based on these data, all ongoing clinical trials sponsored by the US National Cancer Institute (NCI) with these agents in colorectal cancer have been or are being modified to only include KRAS wild type patients and the label for panitumumab monotherapy has been restricted to KRAS wild type patients.

In summary, this prospective-retrospective strategy maybe a reasonable alternative to a prospective trial when (1) a prospective RCT is ethically impossible based on results from previous trials, and/or (2) a prospective RCT is not logistically feasible (large trial and long time to complete). If two or more findings from large well designed retrospective analyses (that meet all of the above mentioned criteria) of data from prospective RCT trials demonstrate consistent findings regarding the predictive validity of a marker, this may be sufficient to establish the predictive utility of the marker and possibly move it into routine clinical practice [12].

Prospective Designs

While prospectively specified analyses from retrospective cohorts (i.e., using banked biospecimens from a previously conducted RCT) may provide strong evidence for a predictive marker effect in some cases, there remains no substitute for a well-conducted prospective RCT. One key issue that drives the design of a marker validation trial is the hypothesized effectiveness of the new treatment regimen: is it effective in all patients regardless of the marker status, or only within certain marker-defined subgroups? A comparison of the performance of the targeted versus the all-comers designs demonstrated that the targeted design required fewer randomized (and screened) patients compared to the all-comers design in cases where there is an underlying true predictive marker and the cut-point for determining the marker status is well established [29–31]. The strength of the preliminary evidence, accuracy of the assay and the prevalence of the marker under consideration are important factors in the trial design determination. In this section, we discuss the different trial designs using specific clinical trials as examples where possible.

Enrichment or Targeted Designs

An enrichment design screens patients for the presence or absence of a marker or a panel of markers, and then only includes patients in the clinical trial who either have or do not have a certain marker characteristic or profile. The enrichment design results in a stratification of the study population, with a goal of understanding the safety, tolerability, and clinical benefit of a treatment in the subgroup of the patient population defined by a specific marker status. This design is based on the paradigm that not all patients will benefit from the study treatment under consideration, but rather that the benefit will be restricted to a subgroup of patients who either express or do not express a specific molecular feature.

An enrichment design strategy of enrolling only HER2 positive patients was used in two national intergroup adjuvant breast cancer trials: the National Surgical Adjuvant Breast and Bowel Project trial (NSABP B-31) comparing doxorubicin and cyclophosphamide followed by paclitaxel every 3 weeks with the same regimen plus 52 weeks of trastuzumab beginning with the first dose of paclitaxel, and the North Central Cancer Treatment Group trial (NCCTG N9831) comparing three regimens: doxorubicin and cyclophosphamide followed by weekly paclitaxel, the same regimen followed by 52 weeks of trastuzumab after paclitaxel, and the same regimen plus 52 weeks of trastuzumab initiated concomitantly with paclitaxel. A combined analysis of these two trials demonstrated that Trastuzumab combined with paclitaxel after doxorubicin and cyclophosphamide significantly improves disease free survival among women with surgically removed HER2-positive breast cancer [15]. In this case, the enrichment strategy seems to have been successful: only approximately 20% of women are HER2 positive, and if there truly were no benefit from Herceptin in 80% of women that are deemed HER2 negative, a much larger sample size would have been required to establish statistically significant results in an unselected study. Subsequent analyses of the data, however, have raised the possibility of a beneficial effect of Herceptin in a more broadly defined patient population, details of which were discussed in the previous section on biomarker assays pertaining to the trade-offs relating to local versus central testing [16–19]. Thus, while the enrichment strategy did clearly and quickly define an effective treatment for a subset of patients, several other questions regarding the predictive utility of HER2 were left unanswered due to the issues of assay reproducibility and inclusion of only biomarker defined subgroups. An unselected design, allowing for both HER2 positive and negative patients, may have helped provide these answers in a definitive and ultimately timelier manner.

In general, an enrichment design is appropriate when (1) therapies have modest absolute benefit in the unselected population, but cause significant toxicity, (2) in the absence of selection, therapeutic results are similar whereby a selection design (even if incorrect) would not hurt, (3) an unselected design is ethically impossible based on previous studies, (4) there is compelling preliminary evidence to suggest that patients with or without that marker profile do not benefit from the treatments in question, and (5) assay reproducibility and accuracy is well-established. In summary, unless there is compelling preliminary evidence that not all patients will benefit from the study treatment under consideration (such as the case with KRAS gene status in colorectal cancer) [22, 25], it is prudent to include and collect specimens and follow-up information from all patients (since all patients are screened anyway) in the trial to allow for future testing for other potential prognostic markers in this population, as well as other marker assessment techniques [10, 12, 32, 33].

Unselected or All-Comers Designs

In the all-comers design strategy, all patients meeting the eligibility criteria are entered into the trial. The ability to provide adequate tissue may be an eligibility criterion for these designs, but not the specific biomarker result or the status of a biomarker characteristic. These designs are differentiated from each other by the protocol specified approach to the prespecified type I and type II error rates (influencing sample size), analysis plans (including a single hypothesis test, multiple tests, or sequential tests), and randomization schema.

Sequential Testing Strategy Designs

These designs utilize a single primary hypothesis that is either tested in the overall population first and then in a prospectively planned subset or in the marker-defined subgroup first, and then tested in the entire population if the subgroup analysis is statistically significant [34, 35]. The first is recommended in cases where the experimental treatment is hypothesized to be broadly effective, and the subset analysis is ancillary. The latter (also known as the closed testing procedure) is recommended when there is strong preliminary data to support that the treatment effect is strongest in the marker-defined subgroup, and that the marker has sufficient prevalence that the power for testing the treatment effect in the subgroup is adequate. Both these approaches appropriately control for the type I error rates associated with multiple testing. A modification to this approach, taking into account potential correlation arising from testing the overall treatment effect and the treatment effect within the marker defined subgroup has also been proposed [36].

Marker Based Designs

The marker by treatment interaction design uses the marker status as a stratification factor (i.e., assumes that the overall population can be split into marker defined subgroups) and randomizes patients to treatments within each marker subgroup (see Fig. 14.1) [12, 37–39]. The fundamental difference between this design and a single large RCT is that the marker by treatment interaction design is clearly a prospective (and a definitive) markers validation trial, where (1) only patients with a valid markers result are allowed to be randomized, (2) the sample size is prospectively specified separately within each marker-based subgroup, and (3) the randomization is stratified by marker status [12].

In contrast, the marker based strategy design randomizes patients to have their treatment either based on or independent of the marker status (see Figs. 14.2 and 14.3) [12, 37–39]. A limitation of the design presented in Fig. 14.2 is that it cannot examine the true interaction between a treatment regimen and marker status as

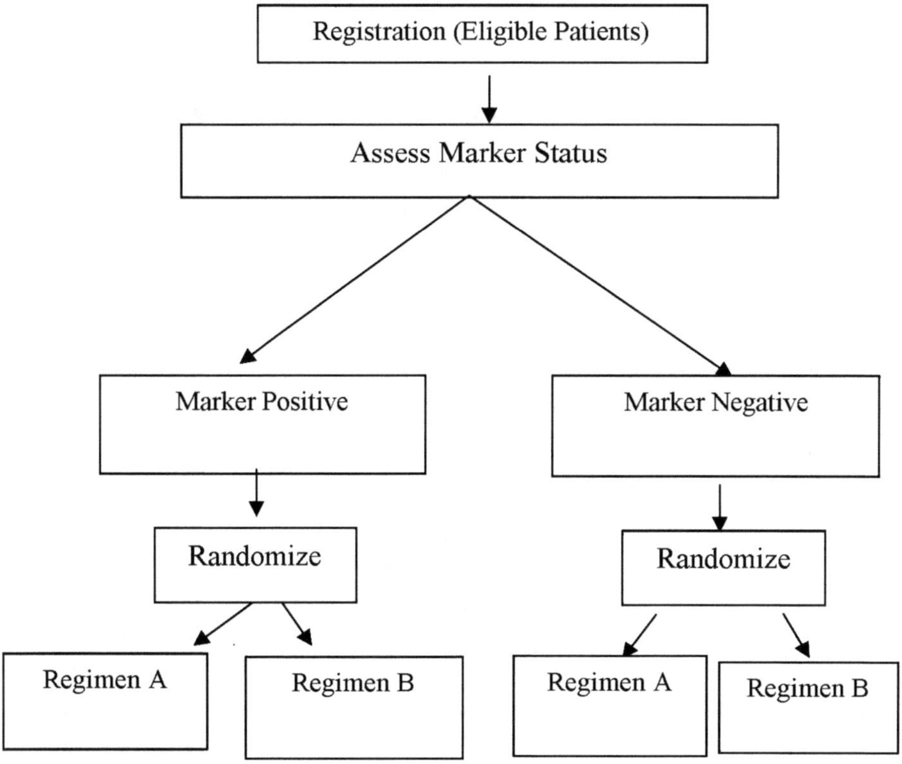

Fig. 14.1 Marker by Treatment Interaction Design (upfront stratification by marker status)

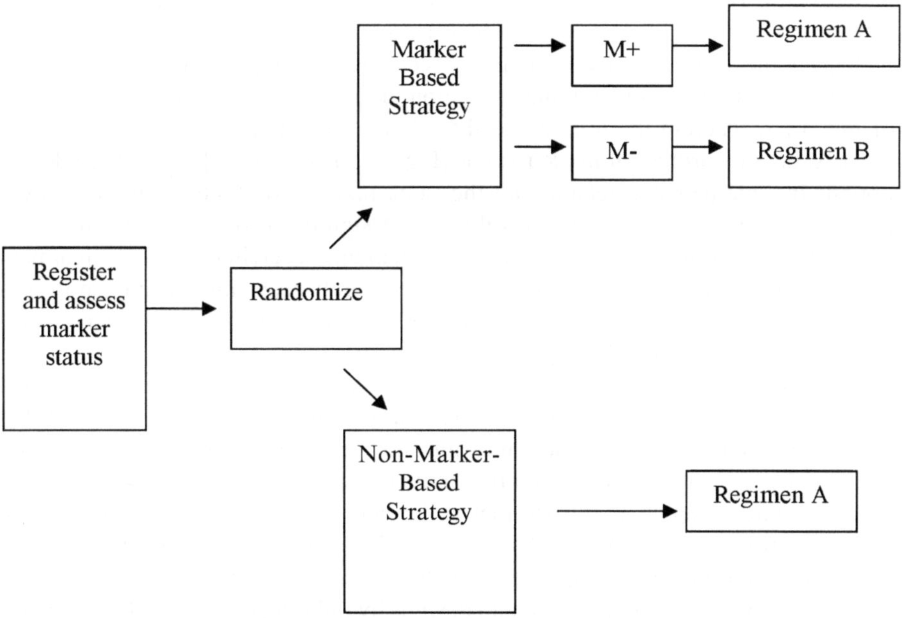

Fig. 14.2 Marker Based Strategy Design (no randomization in the non-marker-based strategy arm; *M+* marker positive, *M−* marker negative)

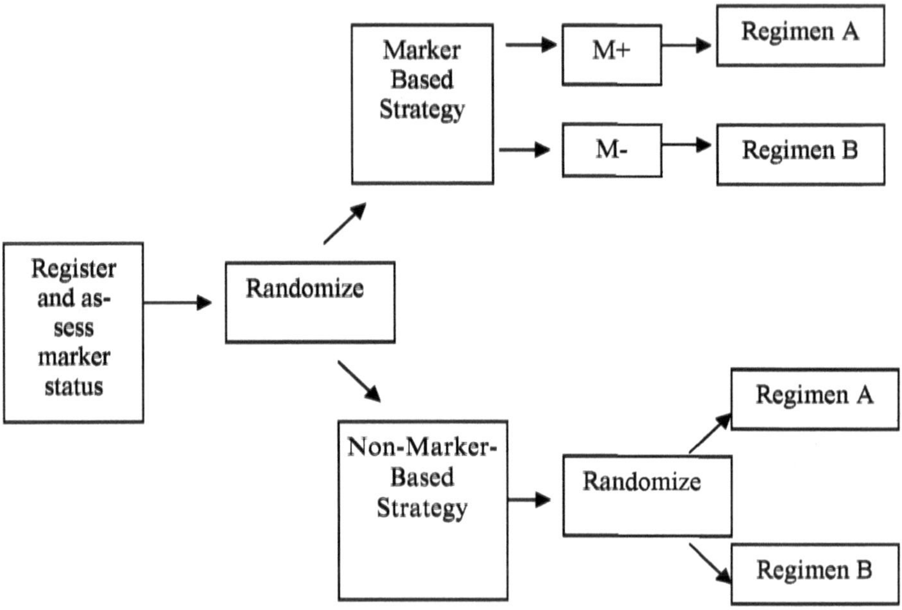

Fig. 14.3 Marker Based Strategy Design (second randomization in the non-marker-based strategy arm; *M+* marker positive, *M−* marker negative)

patients with a certain marker status never receive the alternative treatment. A design to evaluate the true interaction between a treatment and marker status requires patients in the different marker groups to receive both therapies. This can be accomplished by including a second randomization in the non-marker-based strategy arm of Fig. 14.2, wherein the non-marker-based arm patients are randomized to regimens A, or B regardless of marker status (Fig. 14.3) [12, 27–29]. Both these design options include patients treated with the same regimen on both the marker based and the non-marker-based arms resulting in a significant overlap (driven by the prevalence of the marker) in the number of patients receiving the same treatment regimen in both arms. As a consequence, the overall detectable difference in outcomes between the arms is reduced (depending on the marker prevalence), thus resulting in a comparatively larger trial [12, 37–39].

A head-to-head comparison of the marker based designs (in the setting of a marker or markers that can be distilled to a single binary measure) suggested that the marker by treatment interaction design may be superior to the marker based strategy design in terms of the number of events (and hence the total sample size) required (while keeping all the parameters the same for both designs) under specific clinical settings [12, 37]. While the impact of the error in measurement of the biomarker on the efficiency of these designs needs to be explored further, it is likely that it will have a similar effect on both designs by inflating the required sample size due to patient misclassification [12].

Hybrid Designs

In this design, only a certain marker defined subgroup of patients is randomized to have their treatment based on their marker status, whereas patients in the other marker defined subgroups are assigned the standard of care treatment(s) [12] (see Fig. 14.4 for an illustration). This design is an appropriate choice when there is compelling prior evidence demonstrating the efficacy of a certain treatment(s) for a marker defined subgroup, thereby making it unethical to randomize patients with that particular marker status to other treatment options. This design is powered to detect differences in outcomes only in the marker defined subgroup that is randomized to treatment choices based on the marker status (marker positive subgroup in Fig. 14.4), similar to an enrichment design strategy. However, unlike the enrichment design, the hybrid design provides additional value: since all patients are screened for marker status to determine whether they are randomized or assigned the standard of care treatment(s), it seems prudent to include and collect specimens and follow-up

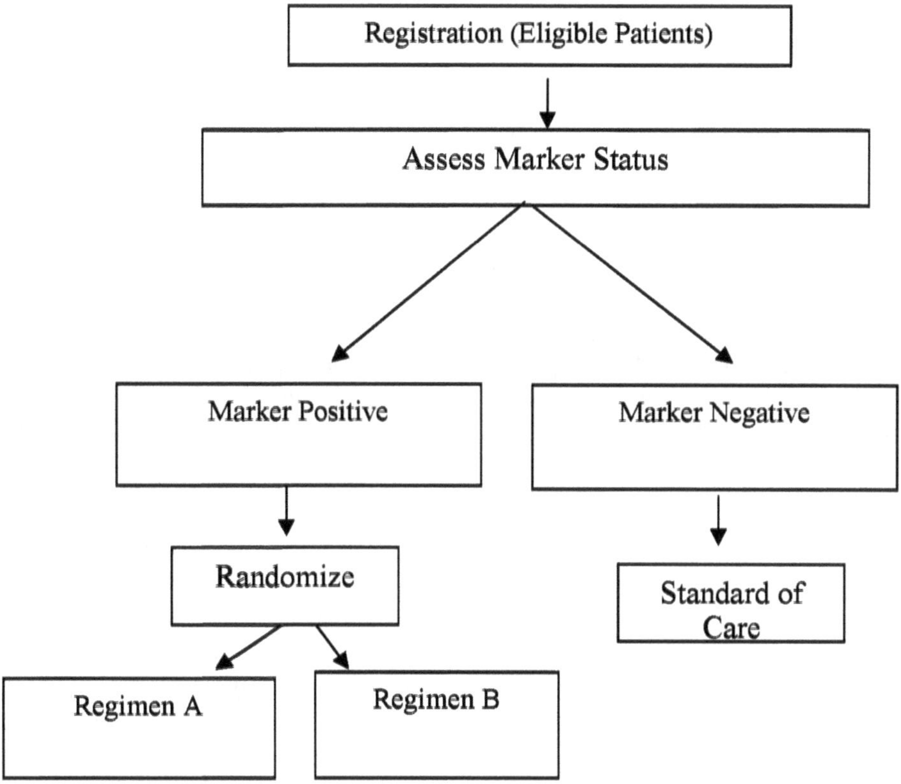

Fig. 14.4 Hybrid Design

from "all" patients in the trial to allow for future testing for other potential prognostic markers in this population.

Adaptive Designs

A number of innovative designs have been proposed recently that use an adaptive strategy for analysis. They differ on the type and degree of adaptation allowed. The biomarker adaptive threshold design is similar to the sequential testing strategy designs discussed earlier and can be implemented one of two ways: (1) the new treatment is compared to the control in all patients at a prespecified significance level, and if not significant, a second stage analysis involving finding an "optimal" cut-point for the predictive marker is performed using the remaining alpha; or (2) under the assumption that the treatment is effective only for a marker driven subset, no overall treatment to control comparisons are made, instead, the analysis focuses on the identification of optimal cut-points [40]. Both these approaches were concluded to be superior (in terms of the power and number of events required to detect an effect at a prespecified overall type I error rate) to the classic nonadaptive design approaches in the simulation studies. Two issues need further consideration: (1) the added cost of a somewhat larger sample size and/or redundant power dictated by the strategy of partitioning the overall type I error rate and (2) use of data from the same trial to both define and validate a marker cut-point.

The adaptive accrual design outlines a strategy to adaptively modify accrual to two predefined marker defined subgroups based on an interim futility analysis [41]. Specifically, the trial follows the following scheme: (1) begin with accrual to both marker defined subgroups; (2) if the treatment effect in one of the subgroups fails to satisfy a futility boundary at the interim analysis, terminate accrual to that subgroup, and (3) continue accrual to the other subgroup until the planned total sample size is reached, including accruing subjects that had planned to be included from the terminated subgroup. This design demonstrated greater power than a nonadaptive trial in simulation settings; however, this strategy might lead to a substantial increase in the accrual duration depending on the prevalence of the marker. In addition, the futility boundary is somewhat conservative and less than optimal as it is set to be in the region where the observed efficacy is greater for the control arm than the experimental regimen.

The outcome based adaptive randomization design uses a Bayesian hierarchical framework to adaptively (based on outcome from the accumulated data in the trial) randomize patients to treatments based on the biomarker status [13]. The design is extensively described in the context of the phase II BATTLE (biomarker-integrated approaches of targeted therapy of lung cancer elimination trial) trial in advanced non-small-cell lung cancer. Patients are classified into five biomarker subgroups based on their biomarker profile, and subsequently adaptively randomized. The adaptive accrual and adaptive randomization designs require a rapid and reliable endpoint, which is somewhat challenging as most oncology trials use time to event endpoints as the gold standard for validation trials.

Conclusion

Biomarkers are becoming increasingly common in cancer treatment to provide a patient-specific prediction of outcome to different treatments. The goal of a predictive biomarker is to select the optimal therapy from among multiple treatment options, and deliver individualized treatment regimens to patients, thereby increasing the potential for a favorable clinical outcome such as improved survival and/or decreased toxicity. The ultimate clinical utility of a biomarker depends on the following:

1. What is the added value of marker assessment in every patient in relation to the prevalence of the marker?
2. Is the incremental benefit of treatment selection based on the marker worthwhile when considering the added costs and complexity induced by the marker measurement?
3. Is the new treatment option effective in all patients regardless of the marker status (the magnitude of benefit may differ within the marker-defined subgroups) or just within the marker-defined subgroup(s)?

A careful consideration of the issues outlined in this chapter is essential to determine the clinical utility of a biomarker, and its routine integration into clinical practice to guide treatment selection and inform patient management.

Acknowledgments Supported in part by the National Cancer Institute Grants: Mayo Clinic Cancer Center (CA-15083), and the North Central Cancer Treatment Group (CA-25224).

References

1. Taube SE, Jacobson JW, Lively TG. Cancer diagnostics: decision criteria for marker utilization in the clinic. Am J Pharmacogenomics. 2005;5(6):357–64.
2. Bonomi PD, Buckingham L, Coon J. Selecting patients for treatment with epidermal growth factor tyrosine kinase inhibitors. Clin Cancer Res. 2007;13(15 Pt 2):s4606–12.
3. Paik S. Clinical trial methods to discover and validate predictive markers for treatment response in cancer. Biotechnol Annu Rev. 2003;9:259–67.
4. Augustine CK, Yoo JS, Potti A, et al. Genomic and molecular profiling predicts response to temozolomide in melanoma. Clin Cancer Res. 2009;15(2):502–10.
5. Riedel RF, Porrello A, Pontzer E, et al. A genomic approach to identify molecular pathways associated with chemotherapy resistance. Mol Cancer Ther. 2008;7(10):3141–9.
6. Garman KS, Acharya CR, Edelman E, et al. A genomic approach to colon cancer risk stratification yields biologic insights into therapeutic opportunities. Proc Natl Acad Sci USA. 2008;105(49):19432–7.
7. Anguiano A, Nevins JR, Potti A. Toward the individualization of lung cancer therapy. Cancer. 2008;113 Suppl 7:1760–7.
8. Salter KH, Acharya CR, Walters KS, et al. An integrated approach to the prediction of chemotherapeutic response in patients with breast cancer. PLoS One. 2008;3(4):e1908.
9. Garman KS, Nevins JR, Potti A. Genomic strategies for personalized cancer therapy. Hum Mol Genet. 2007;16(Spec No.2):R226–32.
10. Simon RM, Paik S, Hayes DF. Use of archived specimens in evaluation of prognostic and predictive biomarkers. J Natl Cancer Inst (Commentary). 2009;101:1–7.

11. Mandrekar SJ, Sargent DJ. Genomic advances and their impact on clinical trial design. Genome Med (Commentary). 2009;1(7):69.
12. Mandrekar SJ, Sargent DJ. Clinical trial designs for predictive biomarker validation: theoretical considerations and practical challenges. J Clin Oncol. 2009;27(24):4027–34.
13. Zhou X, Liu S, Kim ES, Herbst RS, Lee JJ. Bayesian adaptive design for targeted therapy development in lung cancer—a step towards personalized medicine. Clin Trials. 2008;5: 181–93.
14. Esserman J, Perou C, Cheang M, et al. Breast cancer molecular profiles and tumor response of neoadjuvant doxorubicin and paclitaxel: the I-SPY TRIAL (CALGB 150007/150012, ACRIN 6657). J Clin Oncol. 2009;27:LBA515 [abstract].
15. Romond EH, Perez EA, Bryant J, et al. Trastuzumab plus adjuvant chemotherapy for operable HER2-positive breast cancer. N Engl J Med. 2005;353(16):1673–84.
16. Paik S, Kim C, Jeong J, Geyer CE, et al. 2007 ASCO annual meeting proceedings: benefit from adjuvant trastuzumab may not be confined to patients with IHC 3+ and/or FISH-positive tumors: central testing results from NSABP B-31, Part I. J Clin Oncol. 2007;25(18S):511.
17. Perez EA, Romond EH, Suman VJ, et al. ASCO annual meeting proceedings: updated results of the combined analysis of NCCTG N9831 and NSABP B-31 adjuvant chemotherapy with/without trastuzumab in patients with HER2-positive breast cancer, Part I. J Clin Oncol. 2007;25(18):512.
18. Perez EA, Suman VJ, Davidson NE, et al. HER2 Testing by local, central, and reference laboratories in specimens from the North Central Cancer Treatment Group N9831 intergroup adjuvant trial. J Clin Oncol. 2006;24(19):3032–8.
19. Paik S, Kim C, Wolmark N. HER2 status and benefit from adjuvant trastuzumab in breast cancer. N Engl J Med. 2008;358(13):1409–11.
20. Elsaleh H, Joseph D, Grieu F, et al. Association of tumour site and sex with survival benefit from adjuvant chemotherapy in colorectal cancer. Lancet. 2000;355:1745–50.
21. Elsaleh H, Powell B, McCaul K, Grieu F, et al. p53 alteration and microsatellite instability have predictive value for survival benefit from chemotherapy in stage III colorectal carcinoma. Clin Cancer Res. 2001;7:1343–9.
22. Amado RG, Wolf M, Peeters M, et al. Wild-type KRAS is required for panitumumab efficacy in patients with metastatic colorectal cancer. J Clin Oncol. 2008;26(10):1626–34.
23. Freeman D, Juan T, Meropol NJ, et al. Association of somatic KRAS gene mutations and clinical outcome in patients with metastatic colorectal cancer receiving panitumumab monotherapy. Eur J Cancer. 2007;5(Suppl):239 (abstr O3014).
24. Jonker DJ, O'Callaghan CJ, Karapetis CS, et al. Cetuximab for the treatment of colorectal cancer. N Engl J Med. 2007;357:2040–8.
25. Karapetis CS, Khambata-Ford S, Jonker DJ, et al. K-ras mutations and benefit from cetuximab in advanced colorectal cancer. N Engl J Med. 2008;359(17):1757–65.
26. Van Cutsem E, Lang I, D'haens G, et al. KRAS status and efficacy in the first-line treatment of patients with metastatic colorectal cancer (mCRC) treated with FOLFIRI with or without cetuximab: the CRYSTAL experience. J Clin Oncol. 2008;26(15):2.
27. Bokemeyer C, Bondarenko I, Hartmann JT, et al. KRAS status and efficacy of first-line treatment of patients with metastatic colorectal cancer (mCRC) with FOLFOX with or without cetuximab: the OPUS experience. J Clin Oncol. 2008;26(15):4000.
28. Van Cutsem E, Lang I, D'haens G et al. The CRYSTAL study: assessment of the predictive value of KRAS status on clinical outcome in patients with mCRC receiving first-line treatment with cetuximab or cetuximab plus FOLFIRI. 10th World Congress on Gastrointestinal Cancer 2008, Abstract O-031.
29. Hoering A, Leblanc M, Crowley JJ. Randomized phase III clinical trial designs for targeted agents. Clin Cancer Res. 2008;14(14):4358–67.
30. Simon R, Maitournam A. Evaluating the efficiency of targeted designs for randomized clinical trials. Clin Cancer Res. 2004;10(20):6759–63.
31. Maitournam A, Simon R. On the efficiency of targeted clinical trials. Stat Med. 2005;24(3): 329–39.

32. Sparano JA, Paik S. Development of the 21-gene assay and its application in clinical practice and clinical trials. J Clin Oncol. 2008;26:721–8.
33. Cardoso F, Van't Veer L, Rutgers E, Loi S, Mook S, Piccart-Gebhart MJ. Clinical application of the 70-gene profile: the MINDACT trial. J Clin Oncol. 2008;26:729–35.
34. Simon R, Wang SJ. Use of genomic signatures in therapeutics development. Pharmacogenomics J. 2006;6:166–73.
35. Bauer P. Multiple testing in clinical trials. Stat Med. 1991;10:871–90.
36. Song Y, Chi GYH. A method for testing a prespecified subgroup in clinical trials. Stat Med. 2007;26:3535–49.
37. Mandrekar SJ, Sargent DJ. Clinical trial designs for predictive biomarker validation: one size does not fit all. J Biopharm Stat. 2009;19(3):530–42.
38. Mandrekar SJ, Grothey A, Goetz MP, et al. Clinical trial designs for prospective validation of biomarkers. Am J Pharmacogenomics. 2005;5(5):317–25.
39. Sargent DJ, Conley BA, Allegra C, et al. Clinical trial designs for predictive marker validation in cancer treatment trials. J Clin Oncol. 2005;23(9):2020–7.
40. Wang SJ, O'Neill RT, Hung HMJ. Approaches to evaluation of treatment effect in randomized clinical trials with genomic subset. Pharm Stat. 2007;6:227–44.
41. Jiang W, Freidlin B, Simon R. Biomarker-adaptive threshold design: a procedure for evaluating treatment with possible biomarker-defined subset effect. J Natl Cancer Inst. 2007;99(13):1036–43.

Chapter 15
Regulatory Issues

Maxwell T. Vergo and Al B. Benson III

Introduction

It is critical that biomarker tests are held to certain standards of safety and efficacy prior to widespread use in the medical community. This regulation process consists of thorough examination of the biomarker test's full history including its analytical performance, its manufacturing under accepted standards, its adequate preclinical and clinical data for efficacy and safety, its ability to add to current medical decision making, and finally its post-approval monitoring all as pertains to the intended use of the biomarker test. The Food and Drug Administration (FDA) is the government body that regulates and approves biomarkers tests and therefore this section will focus on the process needed for a biomarker test to move from development to clinical use. In the FDA, laboratory test systems sold by a manufacturer or developed by a lab for commercial use are known as "in vitro diagnostic" (IVD) devices. The laboratory test systems developed to detect important biomarkers would fit under this category.

For example, the gene chip and analytes needed to look at tumor gene expression in stage II colon cancer or the reagents needed in order to stain for HER2 expression on breast cancer cells would both be classified as IVD devices and are subject to FDA regulation. The Office of In Vitro Diagnostic Device Evaluation and Safety (OIVD) is the specific office within the FDA which handles these matters. This chapter aims to explain how the FDA accomplishes its task so that medical developers will be better equipped to develop biomarker tests without unnecessary delays

M.T. Vergo, B.S., M.D. (✉)
Division of Hematology and Oncology, Department of Medicine, Feinberg School of Medicine, Robert H. Lurie Comprehensive Cancer Center, Northwestern Memorial Hospital, 676 N. St. Clair Street, Suite 850, Chicago, IL 60611, USA
e-mail: mvergo@nmff.org

Al B. Benson III, M.D., F.A.C.O.
Division of Hematology and Oncology, Department of Medicine, Feinberg School of Medicine, Robert H. Lurie Comprehensive Cancer Center, Northwestern Memorial Hospital, Chicago, IL, USA

H.-J. Lenz (ed.), *Biomarkers in Oncology: Prediction and Prognosis*,
DOI 10.1007/978-1-4419-9755-5_15,

and with proper safety and efficacy standards in mind. In this terminology, safety requires that the probable benefit from its intended use outweighs any probable risk and efficacy requires that a significant portion of the target population will derive clinically significant results.

Much of the information contained in this chapter is taken from the FDA OIVD website [1] as well as a review article [2]. Other sources will be specifically referenced. Examples were added by the authors to solidify concepts for the readers.

IVD Device Risk Profiles

One of the most important initial considerations is the risk classification of an IVD device. There are three categories including Class I (lowest risk), Class II (moderate risk), and Class III (greatest risk). The decisions to place an IVD device into one of these three categories derives from both the intended use of the device and the indication for use of the device. Intended use refers to what is being tested (i.e., HER2 immunohistochemistry on tumor cells) while indication for use refers to why the patient is being tested (to determine candidacy for trastuzumab as therapy). The intended use combined with the indications for use will determine the class of the device and subsequently the process it must undergo for premarket authorization. In the context of IVD tests, risk can be conceptualized as the severity or likelihood of harm to the patient if the test gave an undetected incorrect result.

Class I devices are those which present low risk to the patient both as defined by its intended use and its indication for use. In terms of biomarker tests, since they usually require only a peripheral blood measurement or tumor sample processing the testing process would pose minimal risk by itself to the patient. On the other hand, biomarker tests would only be classified as Class I if their indication for use was low risk, meaning that the risk to the patient of an incorrect result would be minimal. Biomarker tests which are used to determine therapy or even prognosis would not generally be Class I devices since erroneous results in these categories could be quite harmful to the patient. An example of a Class I device may be an immunohistochemistry test system to detect a marker which is used adjunctively with other information for diagnosis of colorectal cancer. In this case, an incorrect result would most likely be detected in conjunction with other adjunctive clinical or biomarker information. In addition, analyte-specific reagents (ASRs) which are single reagents used for the purpose of quantifying or identifying a specific substance, ligand, or biologic target are in this risk classification as long as they are not indicated for screening blood bank samples (Class II) or donor screening (Class III).

Class II devices are those which present moderate risk to the patient. These biomarker tests may be used in order to determine prognosis or monitor a patient already diagnosed with cancer but would not be indicated for making treatment decisions, which would put the patient at high risk. For example, a testing system for measuring loss of heterogeneity at 18q (18qLOH) in stage II and III colon cancer which portends a worse prognosis but does not predict response to adjuvant chemotherapy may be considered a class II IVD device. Since retrospective data have been inconsistent on 18qLOH its role is under investigation in a current large prospective study.

Class III devices are those which pose the highest risk to the patient and most biomarker tests used in oncology fall under this category due to their indication of use which tend to be focused around diagnosis, use of therapy, choice of appropriate therapy, and response to therapy. In addition, any device testing for a new analyte (i.e., novel tumor surface marker) or for any existing analyte being considered for an intended use for which no other submission has previously been cleared for (i.e., same device used to measure thymidylate synthase expression in colon cancer now being considered in breast cancer to assess tumor sensitivity to chemotherapy), then this device becomes Class III regardless of its indication of use. The risk profile may, however, allow down-classification to class II or I under certain circumstances.

We will see in the sections to come how the risk profile of the IVD device impacts its approval process.

Investigational Device Exemption

In order to accumulate enough preclinical (Class II and Class III) and clinical data (Class III mostly) on a device for approval by the FDA, a laboratory or manufacturer may need to apply for an IDE. It is critically important to emphasize that the FDA offers a pre-IDE service which it likens to a "free FDA consulting service." The purpose is to allow the manufacturer a chance to plan ahead by anticipating what the FDA will likely require in terms of a submission mechanism and subsequent approval in an informal and nonbinding agreement. This allows the manufacturer to better hone their preclinical and clinical data collection.

The FDA distinguishes "research" from "investigational" use of IVD devices. Research use is defined as basic science or animal based studies. IVD devices used for this purpose are not required to comply with most device regulations but must carry the label "For Research Use Only. Not for use in diagnostic procedures." On the other hand, investigational use is for clinical investigation in humans and its regulation by the FDA is determined by whether it is determined to have "nonsignificant risk" as opposed to "significant risk." An investigational use only (IUO), IDE exempt IVD device must be judged to have a nonsignificant risk, which would include being noninvasive, requiring noninvasive sampling (phlebotomy acceptable risk), not introducing a source of energy into the subject, and having an accepted gold standard for which to compare to. Nonsignificant risk IUO IVD device uses are monitored by local institutional review boards (IRBs) but generally are not reviewed by the FDA. An example would be assessing a new hepatocellular carcinoma (HCC) marker in patients with this disease and comparing this with the traditional AFP marker. Of note, an IVD device may be appropriate for IUO (nonsignificant risk) if the results are not returned for patient care or decision making. If there is a significant risk, such as a novel HCC marker that will be used to determine progression of disease while on sorafenib therapy, then this requires compliance with FDA's Investigational Device Exemption (IDE) regulations and IDE approval is required prior to initiating the clinical investigation with the device. Of course, in the case of an IDE the local IRB continues to monitor the device's use in addition to the FDA. An IDE should describe the nature of the proposed study, how the risks associated with participation of the study will be clearly communicated to individuals, and details of informed consent [3].

We will briefly review some of the important measures the FDA requires in preclinical data in the next section.

Analytical Performance Measures

Biomarker tests require some specific rigors in their preclinical studies in order to assure the FDA approval process is as expedited as possible without unnecessary delays. This section summarizes some important points to take into account during the preapproval process from a publication by Dr. Mansfield et al. in 2007 [4].

Measurement of the accuracy and trueness of the device is important. The trueness is how close the average value is to the "true" value and measures the bias of the device. Accuracy is how close each measurement is to the "true" value and measures bias as well as imprecision of the device. The "true" value is usually some comparison test or standard appropriate as a reference and ideally should be the same specimen type as being used in the device's measurement as well as the same type of data (qualitative, semiqualitative, or quantitative).

Precision and reproducibility deal with the closeness of agreement between measurements under stipulated controlled conditions. This can yield a standard deviation or coefficient of variation. Repeatability is measured within a given run and reproducibility is measured between different laboratories/manufacturing plants. The precision around medical decision points is most important to include.

Linearity and the reportable range are other important analytic measures to include. This has to do with assuring over what range the response is linear, or monotonic. Especially important is assuring this linearity is tested at the highest and lowest ranges and at medical decision points.

Traceability involves assuring there is adequate calibration and controls for the device as well as a measurement of how stable the testing materials are over time (i.e., expiration dates, calibration intervals, etc.).

For quantitative tests, it is important to establish the limits of detection and limits of quantification. These are critical to report so that medical professionals using the device can understand how to assess a low quantitative value and what a negative result means.

Analytical specificity is used to report potential interfering substances, which could cause false positives or negatives, or to detect cross reacting substances in the patient sample. This involves measuring the specific quantity of substance the device is testing and then assessing the magnitude of potential interference or cross reactivity from substances that may be present in the sample.

Assay cutoffs are critical to determine and further assure the cutoffs represent clinically valuable information. Qualitative cutoffs are usually designated at a value above or below which the chance of a false result approaches that of a true result. In a quantitative cutoff, three standard deviations are frequently used (or 95–99% for non-Gaussian curves).

Lastly, quality control samples must be developed so the device is able to be challenged at regular intervals to assure it is still operating as intended.

An extensive literature search was performed on appropriate conduct and reporting of diagnostic tests and was synthesized into the Standards for Reporting of Diagnostic Accuracy (STARD) initiative [5]. The result was a checklist and flow diagram which can be used by journals, researchers, and authors alike to assure all relevant information is included when reporting on diagnostic tests. A similar review from the UK on REporting on tumour MARKer prognostic studies (REMARK) resulted in a summary table creating a rigorous reporting standard for both prognostic and predictive tumor marker studies [6].

Approval Processes

As stated earlier, the approval process the FDA uses depends on the risk profile of the IVD device. In general, most class I devices are exempt from premarket review. Class II devices are reviewed relatively rapidly (given that all data needed are provided). On the other hand, Class III IVD devices can take the longest to receive approval and involve the most comprehensive review. We aim to summarize the pathways possible for each class of IVD device in this section.

Class I IVD devices can either achieve an exempt status or a reserved status. Most devices in this class will be exempt from submission to the FDA. Exempt Class I IVD devices must still comply with "general controls," which includes being manufactured according to Quality System Regulation (QSR), labeling requirements, manufacturer and device registration with the FDA, post-marketing regulation, notification of the FDA with changes to the device, and record keeping. Reserved Class I IVD devices generally have a substantially important intended use for preventing human illness or a potential unreasonable risk and must undergo a process referred to as Premarket Notification [510(k)], which will be described in more detail shortly.

Class II IVD devices in the moderate risk category undergo a clearance process based on if there is a predicate (previously cleared) device for the same intended use to compare with the new device. If the FDA decides that the new Class II IVD device is "substantially equivalent" to the predicate device, then the appropriate review process is called Premarket Notification [510(k)]. The 510(k) process involves evaluation of the preclinical data as well as assuring substantial equivalence and often also "special controls" are met. Special controls are controls set up by the FDA to assure safety and efficacy are met by the given device including performance specifications, labeling recommendations, mandatory performance standards, and postmarket surveillance. The 510(k) may or may not require clinical data to support the application depending on the intended use. This process usually takes approximately 3 months to complete.

If the Class II IVD device is not considered substantially equivalent, then it technically is considered a Class III IVD device. In this case, it may be possible to undergo a De Novo Review which is more comprehensive then a 510(k) but less administratively burdensome then the process for other Class III devices.

Class III IVD devices (other than Class I or II devices without a predicate analyte or intended use) are approved by a process called Premarket Approval (PMA). This process is the most comprehensive and labor intensive in order to match the high risk of the device. As opposed to the 510(k) process which allows comparison of one device to another as part of the approval process, the PMA mechanism requires a complete review of the device design, manufacturing, and both preclinical and clinical studies as well as inspection of the laboratory or manufacturing process physically. Often times the FDA statisticians will process the raw data on their own to assure accuracy of reporting and summarize potential biases affecting the data. The FDA examines the preclinical data looking for accuracy and reproducibility of the measured analyte under controlled conditions as well as clinical data looking at the performance at outside laboratories/institutions. The clinical data must also add value to decision making in some way in order to gain approval. The PMA process on average takes about 8.5 months for approval.

Figure 15.1 summarizes this approval process based on the risk profile of the IVD device.

Of note, there is an expedited review for 501(k) or PMA submissions that exists for devices which help diagnose or treat a life-threatening or irreversibly debilitating condition and which fill an unmet medical need in one of the following ways: breakthrough technology, no approved alternative, significantly clinically meaningful advantage, or in the best interest of patients. The manufacturer must request this review and approval will put the submission to the head of the line in its respective approval process.

For example, a new technology for measuring her2 gene amplification using chromogenicity instead of fluorescence, called SPOT-Light® HER2 CISH™, was submitted for a PMA review on March 11, 2005 and was approved on January 7, 2008. This required the highest level of review due to the fact that it would be used for important decision making (i.e., use of trastuzumab in breast cancer) and did not have a predicate device with which to compare. The approval required data collected in regards to the analytical performance of the device as well as satisfactory agreement rates with current standards such as FISH and immunohistochemistry staining for her2 expression. On the other hand, Ikoniscope® oncoFISH™ her2 Test System was simply using a new automated system for enumerating FISH signals with use of already approved her2 FISH DNA probes, which allowed them to apply through the 510(k) process. This required they prove their new automated system performed substantially equivalent with an already approved automated her2 FISH system (BioView Duet™ System) and was approved in a mere 6.5 months.

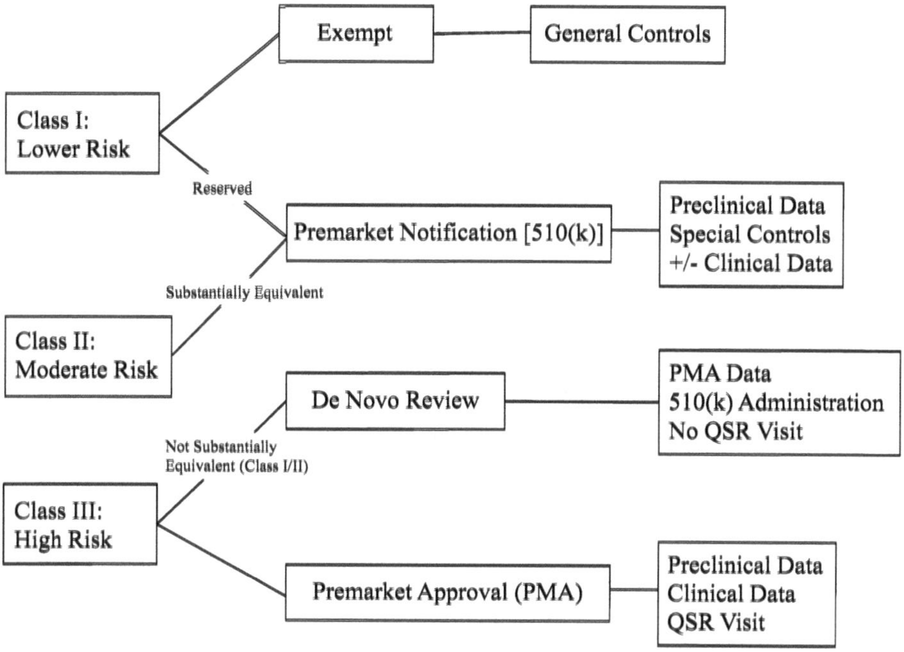

Fig. 15.1 FDA approval process based on risk profile of IVD device

Combination Products

A combination product involves the combination of two or more single-entity products. In the emerging age of personalized oncology care, these tend to be drug-device, biologic-device, or biologic-drug-device combinations. These accompanying devices could be as simple as a delivery system for a drug or biologic, but can be biomarker tests which help determine who is a potential candidate (or not a potential candidate) for the drug or biologic.

The FDA Office of Combination Products (OCP) is charged with assigning a primary mode of action (PMOA) to combination products. The PMOA is determined by which entity of the combination provides the most important therapeutic action or greatest overall contribution to the overall intended effect. With this determination made, which is not always straight forward, the request for FDA approval is triaged to the most appropriate branch including the Center for Biologic Evaluation & Research (CBER), the Center for Drug Evaluation & Research (CDER), or the Center for Devices and Radiologic Health (CDRH) [7].

The future of oncology care is the co-development of companion devices which help select patients who would benefit most (or exclusively) from a therapeutic drug option. The other possibility is to have identified a known biomarker which significantly effects prognosis and then design a therapeutic drug option, which would target the biomarker. In either of these settings, it is essential that the IVD device be appropriately analytically validated prior to being used in a large therapeutic drug trial.

A caution should be taken if the IVD device has not undergone rigorous validation prior to use in a large therapeutic clinical trial with the potential for achieving a combination product. For example, the TOGA trial found the addition of trastuzumab to chemotherapy in HER2 positive (HER2 immunohistochemistry [IHC] with 3+ staining or fluorescence in situ hybridization [FISH] positivity) metastatic gastric carcinoma improved overall survival [8]. Although an initial validation study showed a 93.5% concordance between FISH positivity by PharmDx kit (Dako Denmark A/S) and IHC 3+ staining by HercepTest (Dako) [9], analysis of the TOGA data revealed a 23–26% rate of FISH positivity with patients who were IHC 0/1+ or 2+ staining (negative) which is a significantly higher false negative rate then as determined in breast cancer patients for which the HercepTest was FDA approved [10]. Further evaluation will need to be undertaken to assure the proper biomarker device is approved for use in combination with trastuzumab in advanced gastric cancer patients.

These combination products are not always synchronous though. For example, in 2004 the FDA approved the use of cetuximab in metastatic EGFR expressing colorectal cancer patients as monotherapy in patients refractory to oxaliplatin-based or irinotecan-based regimens as well as in combination with irinotecan for patients refractory to irinotecan-based regimens. The combination IVD device approved at the same time was a qualitative immunohistochemical kit system called Dakocytomation EGFR PharmDx®, which measures the relative expression of EGFR on neoplastic cells compared to normal cells. With the identification of KRAS mutations in codons 12 and 13 leading to a downstream resistance to anti-EGFR monoclonal antibody antagonism [11], the FDA reviewed retrospective data available for KRAS mutant versus wild-type patients from seven large prospective randomized controlled trials utilizing an anti-EGFR monoclonal antibody with or without chemotherapy. Based on these retrospective data, the FDA approved a drug label change to add the recommendation that cetuximab not be used in patients with KRAS mutations in codons 12 or 13. Despite this, currently the FDA has not approved an IVD device for diagnosing KRAS mutations in codon 12 or 13. This highlights the challenges of regulating combination products. Ideally, a prospective study randomized by KRAS mutational status (measured by an FDA approved IVD device) would have been undertaken to accomplish the approval by the FDA but clearly this is not always possible and feasible as it may delay implementation of emerging clinical data, which has an important critical impact on patient care. Use of retrospective data to gain test marketing authorization can be acceptable, but requires careful attention to sample bias, analyte stability in stored samples, and assuring informed consent issues have been addressed [12]. This also emphasizes the utility of building tissue banks with well-annotated samples linked to high quality clinical data, such as the National Cancer Institute and the Cooperative Group repositories, so that future retrospective studies may be feasible.

More information is available at the website [13].

Multivariate Index Assays

These are a subset of IVD devices that are emerging on the market which are unique and are being classified as multivariate index assays (IVDMIAs) [14]. These devices are defined as combining values of multiple variables using an interpretation function to yield a single, patient-specific result and provide a result whose derivation is nontransparent and cannot be independently derived or verified by the end user. For example, calculating creatinine clearance by the Cockcroft method by inputting the patient's sex, age, height, weight, and serum creatinine results in a single, patient-specific result but the process is verifiable and transparent since the equation is given. On the other hand, consider gene expression profiling devices, which measure expression of a large number of genes and then calculate a patient score via an algorithm with no transparency or reproducibility for the general oncologist to double check the device. In addition to this difficulty, IVDMIAs are often times being used for calculating recurrence risk or predicting response to therapeutic agents making them moderate to high risk devices. The first IVDMIA approved by the FDA for breast cancer was MammaPrint® which is a gene expression profiling device to assess the risk of recurrence. Other gene expression profile systems are being investigated actively in stage II colon cancer patients to help with selecting a population who may benefit more robustly from chemotherapy. Kato recently published an explanation of the preferred diagnostic algorithm, called linear classifier, for IVDMIAs with the hope of creating an accepted standard for this new class of devices [15].

Postmarket Interventions

There are two mechanisms for assuring safety after an IVD device is approved by the FDA. The first is the Quality System regulation. This regulation requires the manufacturer or laboratory to have incorporated appropriate design, manufacturing, and change control processes, as well as a number of other controls. Second, there is a requirement that manufacturers or laboratories report adverse events to the FDA (see ref. [16] for the website). These reports are monitored by the FDA technical analysts. This assures corrective actions can be taken in a timely fashion when problems are identified and has the advantage to be able to identify rare adverse events since it is a centralized reporting mechanism.

Conclusion

As the development of biomarker tests for oncologic care accelerates, it is critical to balance scientific advancement with scientific prudence by assuring a standardized comprehensive review of efficacy and safety for these biomarker tests by the

FDA prior to commercial availability. In order to assure these standards are met and biomarker tests are able to be approved without delay, pre-IDE consultation is encouraged to help guide the preclinical and clinical studies that will be needed to support an application. Researchers, manufacturers, and laboratories should become familiar with published standards for reporting specific results, such as diagnostic accuracy or prognostic and predictive biomarkers. Emphasis is placed on the quality and solid validation of an IVD device especially if it may be used as a combination product for selecting appropriate populations of patients for therapeutic management. Increasingly complicated devices, IVDMIAs, are becoming more common but require special attention prior to being approved for commercial use. Since innovative biologically driven clinical trial designs are becoming a cornerstone in oncology with the advent of targeted therapies, new biomarkers, and emerging technologies it is also critical that the FDA remains flexible and open to accepting data from varied novel clinical study designs for commercial use without significantly delaying use in patient care. Large tumor repositories linked to high quality randomized clinical trials are critical to advancing personalized oncology care and assuring there is robust safety and efficacy data available readily as new therapies or biomarkers emerge. Lastly, the postmarket interventions are just as important as the preclinical and clinical data collected prior to approval for an IVD device and must be planned prior to approval.

References

1. In vitro diagnostics. http://www.fda.gov/cdrh/oivd/. Accessed 16 Oct 2010.
2. Mansfield E, O'Leary TJ, Gutman SI. Food and drug administration regulation of in vitro diagnostic devices. J Mol Diagn. 2005;7:2–7.
3. Gutman S, Kessler LG. The US food and drug administration perspective on cancer biomarker development. Nat Rev Cancer. 2006;6:565–71.
4. Mansfield E, Tezak Z, Altaie S, et al. Biomarkers for pharmacogenetic and pharmacogenomic studies: locking down analytical performance. Drug Discov Today: Technol. 2007;4:17–20. doi:10.1016/j.ddtec.October.
5. STARD Group. Towards complete and accurate reporting of studies of diagnostic accuracy: the STARD initiative. Clin Chem. 2003;49:1–6.
6. McShane LM, Altman DG, Sauerbrei W, et al. Reporting recommendations for tumour MARKer prognostic studies (REMARK). Br J Cancer. 2005;93:387–91.
7. Lauritsen KJ, Nguyen T. Combination products regulation at the FDA. Clin Pharmacol Ther. 2009;85:468–70.
8. Van Cutsem E, Kang Y, Chung H, et al. Efficacy results from the ToGA trial: A phase III study of trastuzumab added to standard chemotherapy (CT) in first-line human epidermal growth factor receptor 2 (HER2)-positive advanced gastric cancer (GC). J Clin Oncol. 2009;27:18s (Suppl; abstr LBA4509).
9. Hofmann M, Stoss O, Shi D, et al. Assessment of HER2 scoring system for gastric cancer: results from a validation study. Histopathology. 2008;52:797–805.
10. Bang Y, Chung H, Xu J, et al. Pathologic features of advanced gastric cancer (GC): relationship to human epidermal growth factor receptor 2 (HER2) positivity in the global screening programme of the TOGA trial. J Clin Oncol. 2009;27:15s (Suppl; abstr 4556).

11. Lievre A, Bachet JB, Boige V, et al. KRAS mutations as an independent prognostic factor in patients with advanced colorectal cancer treated with cetuximab. J Clin Oncol. 2008;26:374–9.
12. US Food and Drugs Administration. Guidance on informed consent for in vitro diagnostic device studies using leftover human specimens that are not individually identifiable- guidance for sponsors, institutional review boards, clinical investigators and FDA staff. US Food and Drugs Administration [online]. http://www.fda.gov/cdrh/oivd/guidance/1588.html (2006). Accessed 12 Mar 2010.
13. Combination products. http://www.fda.gov/OC/combination/. Accessed 20 Mar 2010.
14. US Food and Drugs Administration. Draft guidance for industry, clinical laboratories, and FDA staff: in vitro diagnostic multivariate index assays. US Food and Drugs Administration [online], http://www.fda.gov/cdrh/ode/guidance/1584.pdf (2007). Accessed 10 Mar 2010.
15. Kato K. Algorithm for in vitro diagnostic multivariate index assay. Breast Cancer. 2009;16:248–51.
16. MedWatch: The FDA Safety Information and Adverse Event Reporting Program. http://www.fda.gov/medwatch/. Accessed 18 Mar 2010.

Chapter 16
Biomarkers for Safety Assessment and Clinical Pharmacology

Stan Louie and Jared Russell

Background

The drug development landscape has changed dramatically in the last few decades. New methods for the identification of novel targets have lead to the development of new and unique classes of anticancer compounds. Recent advances have been sparked by the deployment of computerized modeling and in silico screening, where "hit" candidates are quickly validated using high throughput screening (HTS) greatly accelerating the advancement of lead candidates. As a result, a more rapid development cycle from bench top to bedside is being realized.

Despite these advances, the cost for developing new pharmaceutical agents is rapidly approaching $900 million per drug. A large proportion of this cost is attributed to drugs that fail to reach the market, which accounts for approximately 75% of all drugs tested. One strategy to reduce drug development cost is to improve the ability to predict for potential failure. This includes identifying suboptimal agents while in early stages of development. Equally important is the ability to detect, manage or mitigate potential toxicities. A major drawback of current strategies is that preclinical animals models are heavily relied on for toxicokinetic studies, however, these animal models are not completely reflective of human specific metabolism. In addition, the types of animal models used are often genetically homogeneous

S. Louie, Ph.D. (✉)
Clinical Pharmacy and Pharmaceutical Economics and Policies,
University of Southern California, 1985 Zonal Avenue, Los Angeles, CA 90033, USA
e-mail: slouie@usc.edu

J. Russell, B.S.
Pharmacology and Pharmaceutical Sciences, University of Southern California,
Los Angeles, CA, USA

H.-J. Lenz (ed.), *Biomarkers in Oncology: Prediction and Prognosis*,
DOI 10.1007/978-1-4419-9755-5_16,

and thus restrict the types of toxicities that may be observed. Currently, most safety biomarkers or biomarkers of toxicity are only effective when significant toxicities are either present or the injury has already occurred.

Despite technological advances, drug failures continue to occur in the late stages of clinical trials, where promising agents with targeted pharmacologic activity were found to have significant and even potentially lethal adverse events. A number of these agents are found to have life-threatening adverse events after they have already received FDA approval and been on market. Examples include nonsedating antihistamines and cyclooxygenase-2 (COX-2) inhibitors, where both cases were found to cause an increased risk for life-threatening cardiac events in otherwise healthy individuals [1]. Despite increased pharmacovigilance efforts, it is still very difficult to develop methods and models that can comprehensively predict for all potential drug toxicities. An important consideration is the low incidence of these types of events in toxicologic studies, where acute toxicity is more often the emphasis. Compounding the problem, clinical trials are often designed to restrict patient ages and limit the types of comorbid conditions that may increase the risk for drug-related toxicities. These exclusionary criteria contribute to the problem of early toxicity detection. A restrictive strategy permits agents to progress further into clinical trials without detection. This is one of the reasons why the FDA mandates postmarketing surveillance studies.

A number of methods have been employed to determine pharmacokinetics and pharmacodynamics (PK/PD) in relation to pharmacologic and toxicologic responses. In these types of assessments, the premise is that there is correlation between pharmacologic exposure and the manifestation of drug toxicity. To establish this type of relationship, dose escalations are necessary to identify and characterize potential adverse events. This can be accomplished by administering a dose that is ten times higher than the targeted dosing. A more important factor is the length of observation periods, where long-term exposure may reveal a different adverse event profile than those seen in acute dose escalation studies.

These issues put into question the reliability and capability of present strategies to project safety margins. Other issues include developing strategies to accurately identify at risk populations, such as elderly or pediatric patients, who often have significantly different clearance as compared to adults.

Biomarker development to determine pharmacodynamics and safety have been deployed to predict disease response to drug therapy and safety profile in both animals and humans. Drug failure is often associated with lower drug exposure, whereas toxicities are attributed to higher intensity of exposure. Despite new technologies and increased vigilance, the ability to comprehensively define disease response to drug therapy still requires years to optimize. However, if a specific drug utilizes a particular pathway, it stands to reason that previous experience can be use to model or even predict for drug responses. In addition, the identification of potential toxicities continues to be a challenge since comprehensive insights into the mechanism(s) dictating the desired effect and toxicity have not often been fully elucidated. Without a comprehensive understanding, it is difficult to develop a strategy for using biomarkers to predict efficacy and toxicity. This chapter will review the various methods used to identify a reliable biomarker and examples showing how they have been employed.

Biomarkers

The strategy of using biomarkers in drug development dramatically changed following Food and Drug Administration (FDA) endorsement of employing these measures to screen, diagnosis, and monitor disease responses. To put things into perspective, it is necessary to define terms. Previously, the term "biomarkers" referred to the analysis of tissues and body fluids for chemicals, metabolites of chemicals, enzymes, and other biochemical substances. More recently, biomarker has been more precisely defined as an objective measure or indicator of normal biological properties, pathogenic processes, or pharmacologic responses in reaction to therapeutic intervention [2]. Biomarkers can be circulating endogenous proteins (e.g., cytokines, peptides), genes, RNA, carbohydrates, chemicals, or metabolites.

Identifying biomarkers capable of predicting pharmacologic responses or anticipating toxic manifestation either in animal or earlier in human trials continues to be a high priority. Unlike clinical end points, which can be defined as how a patient may feel, function, response or survive, biomarkers cannot be subjective indicators. Rather these objective measures must correlate closely with the amount of toxic metabolites interacting with macromolecules where the level of reactive metabolites correlates with the emergence of toxic manifestations. Similarly, biomarkers can be employed as surrogate endpoints in determining pharmacologic responses.

When assessing potential risks towards drug-related toxicities, biomarkers can be useful in identifying hazards, quantifying exposure and the associated response with the probability of drug-induced injury. There are three classes of biomarkers, which include biomarkers of exposure, effect, and susceptibility. When discussing exposure biomarkers, it is often referring to exogenous substances or metabolites that are found within an organism where changes in biomarker levels correlate with toxic exposure. Biomarkers of effect often are referring to a measurable biochemical, physiological, or behavioral change within the organism. In contrast, biomarkers of susceptibility are an indicator of inherent or acquired ability of an organism to respond to xenobiotic challenges. These types of biomarkers are used to identify at risk populations who may be more susceptible to encounter adverse events.

When assessing risks in relation to chemical exposure, it is necessary to take a multifaceted approach to adequately incorporate the following components: identification of toxic component(s) and confirmation of the incriminating chemical causing an adverse effect. Following this assessment, a dose–response relationship should be established for whether drug exposure correlates with pharmacologic effect or the emergence of toxicity. Although more difficult, it may be necessary to determine whether reactive drugs or their metabolites can produce protein adducts that can serve as haptens or immunogens, which can promote immune-mediated toxicities.

Safety Biomarkers

The successful implementation of a safety biomarker must able to detect the presence or absence of clinical toxicity. This has been the "Holy Grail" of drug toxicity. One key characteristic of a predictive safety biomarker includes the ability to predict for individual toxicity or identifying at risk populations. Such is the case in using HLA B5701 for genetic testing, where the absence of this gene will indicate that an HIV patient can safely receive abacavir without encountering serious hypersensitivity reactions. Alternatively, patients with a polymorphism along the uridine diphosphate glucuronosyltransferase (UGT) gene may have an increased risk for developing irinotecan-induced toxicities.

The ability to identify drug safety early in the development cycle will provide important input as to whether the particular agent should be advanced along the development process. This plays an important role in the Go/No Go decision analysis. These types of technology can also be used for risk assessment and the mitigation of potential risks. How these biomarkers will be employed will depend largely on the sensitivity and specificity of the particular test.

The right type of safety biomarkers should have a balance between sensitivity and specificity. When the sensitivity of the test is set too high, this may compromise the specificity, where frequent high false positives may arise. These types of results can reject an otherwise safe and potentially useful drug. Conversely when the sensitivity is set lower to increase specificity; it may lead to a higher number of false negatives. In this situation, agents that may be unsafe can advance deeper into the development process, wasting time and resources that could be spent on the development of other drugs.

Attributes of Ideal Safety Biomarkers

The features of an ideal biomarker for detecting drug-induced toxicities should include the following: (1) the ability to detect injury prior to clinical manifestation or exhausting compensatory reserves, (2) reproducible results across various species of animals, (3) quantifiable to determine the degree or intensity of injury, and (4) uses a sample source that is easily procured (e.g., blood or fluids). As one of the criteria of an ideal biomarker, the ability to translate results from animals over to humans is a critical feature. Having this ability will allow rigorous testing and standardization to establish well-defined relationships between the level of a biomarker and the degree of tissue injury consistent with histological findings within the tested animals.

When the mechanism leading to toxicity is known, the ability to predict toxicity and determine the threshold where risk of toxicity will be increased greatly. Key insights into these mechanism(s) will enhance decision-making to either stop drug development or redesign the compound to circumvent the generation of toxic metabolites. Oftentimes, the parent drug is not the incriminating agent responsible for drug toxicity; rather it is often a reactive metabolite that is the causal agent.

In these types of situation, it may be very difficult to dissect the mechanism leading to toxicity. When the underlying mechanism for how toxicities occur is known, "positive array" data is often used to initiate biomarker development.

Currently, safety profiling monitors the emergence of toxicity manifestations or aberrations found in laboratory values. Available biochemical markers can only detect the presence of ongoing toxicologic process or a toxicologic injury that has already occurred. Presently there are no good predictors for toxicities except for genetic biomarkers to predict for potential toxicities or identify individuals at risk for drug-related toxicities. To address some of these issues, new technology is being employed in biomarker development. This includes using methods such as proteomics, metabolomics, and lipidomics to identify and evaluate subtle changes that may indicate the emergence of toxicities.

Since high drug concentration or rapid formation of toxic metabolites are often good determinants for adverse events potential, it is not surprising that individuals who are unable to eliminate the specific agents are more likely to encounter adverse events. Most genetic biomarkers evaluate the polymorphism along metabolic gene enzymes, where carriers of the variant gene often have a lower capacity to eliminate the specific compound or metabolite.

Technology Integration in Biomarker Development

Prior to addressing the elements of biomarker assay development, it is important to recognize that a number of new technologic platforms are currently available. In addition, there are a number of techniques where biomarker development will evolve in the next few years. Once the platform is chosen, the biomarker target must be verified in terms of its ability to predict drug exposure in relation to the degree of tissue injury.

Proteomic

Tumor Detection

The ability to detect the presence of a disease infers that the condition have specific characteristics that distinguish it from normal cellular proliferation. This biochemical alteration is often the consequence of disease, which can be compared to profiles of samples from healthy individuals. It is critical to note that early detection is not synonymous with disease diagnosis. Disease diagnosis is often accompanied by symptoms and presence of tumor mass that is later confirmed to be malignancy. In contrast, early detection can occur in individuals who are asymptomatic, where screening assays are able to identify individuals who have evolving diseases.

The ability to identify patients who are in early stages of disease can dramatically improve treatment success, often resulting in complete remission.

In the case of malignancies, it is surmised that the tumor produces a significantly different protein pattern as compared to normal cells. This supposition is derived from the finding that tumor tissues have aberrant gene(s) leading to the production of specific aberrant protein(s) that are found only in the tumor proteome. Therefore, tumor tissues are thought to be a rich source for cancer proteins where these differences could serve as biomarkers. This can be analyzed by detecting for one specific protein, or an array of proteins, where pattern changes may infer the presence of malignancies. Profiling the tumor tissue proteome can lead to the identification of proteomic signatures corresponding to clinicopathological features. When a distinctive signature is identified and the results are reproducible, these are characteristics of a good biomarker candidate.

Proteins expressed in an individual with tumors may have subtle differences when compared with a healthy individual. This may include difference in protein expression levels and/or difference in the level of posttranslational processing of the proteins. To distinguish these subtle differences will require sensitive and robust instrumentation such as liquid chromatography mass spectrometry (LC-MS). More specifically, the type of mass spectrometry (MS) that is most used in proteomic biomarker development is an ion trap or matrix-assisted laser desorption ionization time of flight MS (MALDI-TOF). The major advantages of using LC-MS are that only a small sample size is required to distinguish differences, with high precision and low variability.

Samples obtained from a suspected tumor mass often require a technologically challenging procedure to accurately procure the sample. The advantage of using samples procured from the mass is that only a small amount of tissue is required to definitively determine whether it is malignant or not. At first glance, this approach does not appear to be advantageous over the currently employed method of determining malignancies using histological analyses. However, using proteomic profiling, this method may allow for definitive diagnosis by profiling protein(s) found in the tissue.

As stated earlier the acquisition of sample is challenging and thus alternative sampling strategies using circulating peptides found in the blood (e.g., whole blood, plasma, or serum) or biological fluids are easier to obtain. However, the level of protein expression found in the circulation must be high enough for detection, even when using sensitive instrumentation such as LC-MS. In addition, samples from the blood may be susceptible to degradation and thus positive detection may only occur in subjects with a more advanced disease state.

Toxicity Detection

Proteomic analysis has also been used to detect potential toxicity. The principal premise is that reactive species can interact with proteins, therefore, detecting protein adducts may be a good surrogate marker of chemical exposure. Quantifying protein adducts has been employed as biomarker for increased risk of toxicities or carcinogenesis.

Similarly, drug metabolism often produces reactive metabolites that can react nonspecifically to proteins. These protein-metabolite adducts can be used to determine the level of exposure. When adducts react with critical enzymes, they can inactivate enzymes and reduce the clearance of xenobiotics or toxic endobiotics. Alternatively, protein adducts that are not eliminated in a timely fashion may promote hapten formation, and possibly initiate immunological-mediated or hypersensitivity reactions.

Although the detection of protein adducts is not a new concept to evaluate potential carcinogenesis, new methods to determine the abundance of these adducts are dramatically enhanced when using LC-MS. In the past, adducts were detected in either hemoglobin or albumin using gas chromatography mass spectrometry (GC-MS). This method often required chemical derivatization to volatilize the sample for GC-MS analysis. However, the chemical modification can also potentially alter the target protein during the sample processing. In contrast, no chemical derivation is often necessary for proteomic analysis using LC-MS. A major drawback of using ion trap LC-MS is that this method cannot easily quantify the signature protein. Using ion trap LC-MS can only provide information as to the presence or absence of the targeted protein. However, the level of protein adducts may be quantified when using tandem triple quadrupole MS. Using this technique, it is possible to quantify the level of protein adducts found in a sample. However, this approach is more often referred as metabolomic analyses.

Metabolomics

Metabolomics is a biological systems approach that complements genomic, transcriptomic, and proteomic investigation. Since metabolites represent the byproducts of the genome and proteome, metabolomics analysis is physiological phenotyping where measuring metabolites can establish the wellness or disease evolution in an individual. Metabolomic analysis can detect the accumulation of metabolites, which may indicate a defect in the enzyme that catalyzes the production of the next metabolite. This technology utilizes triple quadrupole LC-MS, which is able to quantify multiple analytes simultaneously or what is more commonly referred to as multiplexing.

To validate the presence of mechanistic defects, the use of RNA or protein arrays may be used for confirmation. This is an example as how metabolomic analysis can provide insights into the metabolic pathways and networks downstream of gene expression and enzymatic pathways. When metabolites found in a particular pathway can be quantified reproducibly, they may indicate a good metabolomic candidate has been found.

Metabolomics is ideally suited for diagnostic development, especially since biochemical substances are proven effective biomarkers for disease. Moreover, metabolomics can be employed in a wide array of diseases. This technology can profile endogenous metabolites in a myriad of biomatrices to characterize the various metabolites. More importantly, this technology allows multianalyte determination simultaneously, and thus, the output is a profile and not just a single signal. Presently, two analytic platforms are intensely being developed, which is based on nuclear magnetic resonance (NMR) spectroscopy and the combination of LC-MS. Currently NMR has a lower sensitivity when compared to LC-MS, but it has the advantage that analysis is more rapid and requires less sample preparation. In contrast, LC-MS, the current standard instrumentation for metabolomic analysis, is reproducible and has high sensitivity; however, the sample preparation can be complex.

Metabolomic analysis is powerful in that it will allow investigators to compare the normal metabolism of endogenous substrates and the rate by which these anabolites or catabolites are formed. Alterations in the levels of the metabolites may indicate aberration from normal physiological function. A change in this normal profile can indicate a change in enzyme expression and thus allow for accumulation of metabolites. Metabolite accumulation may utilize alternative pathways or mechanisms for systemic clearance, which can lead to the formation of toxic metabolites and thus the evolution of disease or drug-related toxicities.

Currently metabolomic analysis is limited by the lack of comprehensive metabolite databases to distinguish between wellness and disease. Another drawback is validating the sample processing procedures, which can oftentimes be complex and technically challenging. This is due to the number of components that are found in a specific pathway, where extraction efficiency may not be equal across all metabolites, and thus there are many complications to consider for the analyses. When metabolomic analysis is combined with either transcriptomics or genomics data, this technology can provide a comprehensive analysis of the proximity of an aberration that leads to disease etiology.

Genetic Biomarkers for Efficacy and Drug Safety

Genetic biomarkers can be used to identify individuals at risk for drug-related adverse effects. Examples include the ability to identify patients at risk for irinotecan (CPT-11) or 6-mercaptopurine (6MP) related drug toxicities; two prime examples of predictive biomarkers. To successfully develop predictive biomarkers, it is necessary to comprehensively understand the disposition and elimination pathways. In addition, these tests must be verified using large cohorts to test their ability to predict and discriminate patients at risk. In both cases described, specific polymorphisms have identify individuals who may have a compromised capacity to eliminate either the parental or active metabolite, and thus an increased risk for drug-related toxicities. These genetic biomarkers are surrogate markers correlating drug disposition with genetic polymorphism, where reduced ability to eliminate a specific compound will their increase their risk for drug-related toxicities. A number of polymorphic enzymes have been determined, where the predominant enzymes that have been identified include intracellular enzymes, such as the cytochrome P450 enzymes and UDP-glucuronosyl transferase.

Uridine Diphosphate Glucuronosyltransferase (UGT) Polymorphism

Irinotecan (CPT-11) is a topoisomerase inhibitor used for the treatment of colon and lung cancer. Both severe diarrhea and myelosuppression are toxicities that have been associated with CPT-11. Pharmacokinetic analysis has demonstrated that subjects who are unable to adequately eliminate SN-38, the active metabolite of CPT-11, are most likely to encounter CPT-11-mediated toxicities. CPT-11 is predominantly metabolized to form SN-38 through biotransformation mediated by hepatic carboxylesterase I and II (Fig. 16.1). CPT-11 can also be inactivated through metabolism mediated by CYP3A4 to form inactive metabolites 7-ethyl-10-[4-*N*-(5-aminopentanoic acid)-1-piperidino]carbonyloxycamptothecin (APC) and 7-ethyl-10-(4-amino-1-piperidino) carbonyloxycamptothecin (NPC) [3].

SN-38 is an active metabolite with topoisomerase inhibitory activity that is 100- to 1,000-fold more potent than its parent compound. Not only is SN-38 toxic towards tumor cells but cytotoxic towards susceptible cells found in the bone marrow and the intestinal tract. SN-38 is primarily eliminated through metabolism catalyzed by uridine diphosphate glucuronosyltransferase (UGT) 1A1 to form SN-38 glucuronide (SN-38G), an inactive metabolite that is excreted in the urine and bile. SN-38G excreted in the bile and into the intestines can be hydrolyzed by intestinal microflora to liberate SN-38 [4].

UGT 1A1 is a highly polymorphic enzyme that is predominantly expressed in the liver. CPT-11 toxicity was found to be inversely related to the rate of glucuronidating SN-38, where patients expressing low levels of UGT 1A1 experience severe toxicity [5]. Initially this was found in Japanese subjects who were either heterozygous or homozygous for UGT 1A1*28. These individuals were at significantly higher risk for developing severe CPT-11-related toxicities. It was later found that individuals, regardless of ethnicity, who are homozygous UGT1A1*28 are less able to form the SN-38G and thus are at increased risk for hematologic toxicity such as neutropenia [5]. An accumulation of SN-38 in the gut can also increase the risk for intractable diarrhea events as well as myelosuppression; however, no biomarker is commercially available to predict this adverse event.

Thiopurine Methyl Transferase (TPMT) Polymorphism

Pharmacogenetic tests have also been developed and are commercially available to identify patients who may be at increased risk for developing thiopurine-induced

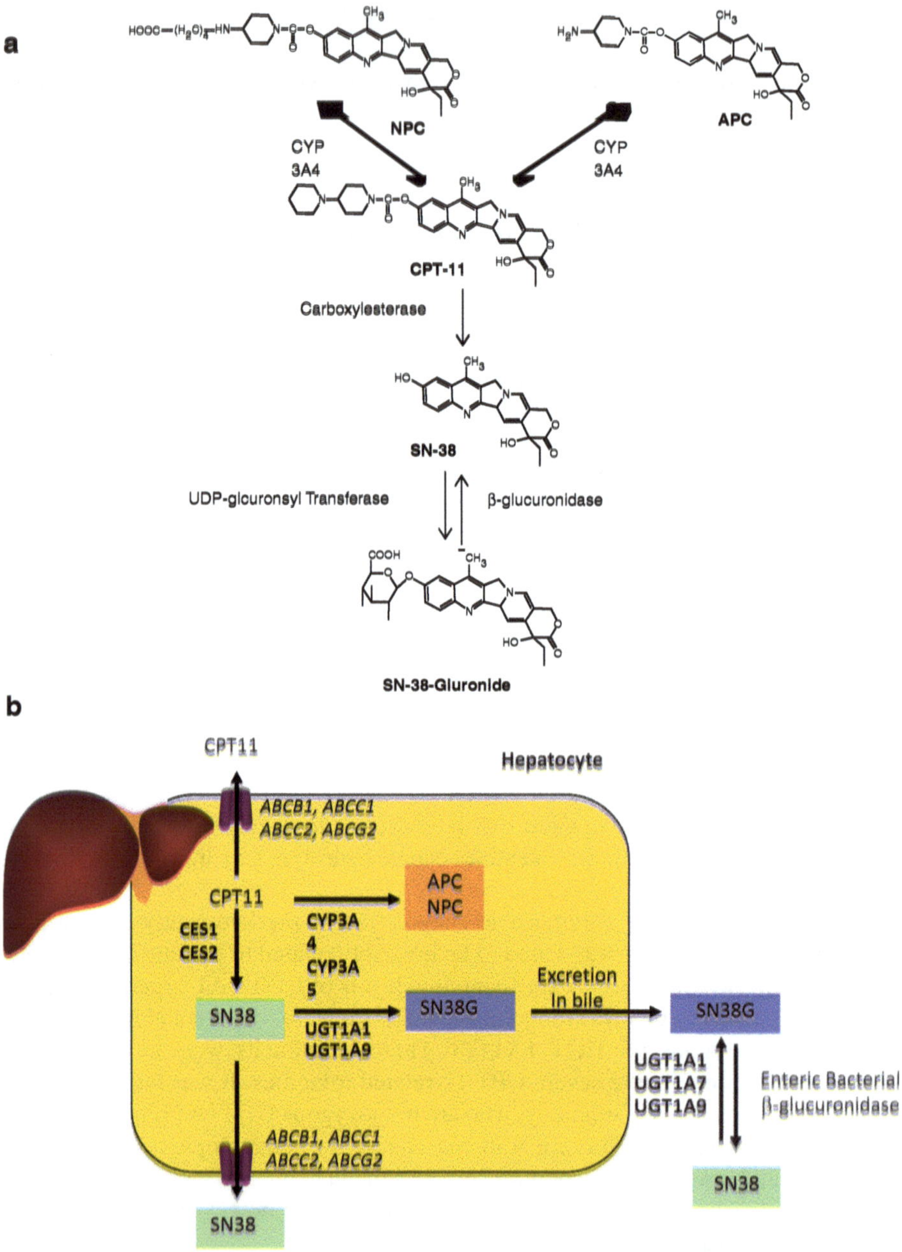

Fig. 16.1 Irinotecan (CPT11) is metabolized either by cytochrome p450 3A4 (CYP3A4) or carboxylesterase. CYP3A4 mediated metabolism forms two inactive metabolites 7-ethyl-10-[4-*N*-(5-aminopentanoicacid)-1-piperidino]carbonyloxycamptothecin(APC)and7-ethyl-10-(4-amino-1-piperidino) carbonyloxycamptothecin (NPC). In contrast carboxylesterase mediated metabolism forms SN38, a biologically active metabolite that is more cytotoxic as compare to CPT11. SN38 can be further biotransformed to SN38-glucuronidate (SN38G), an in active metabolite, where the reaction is catalyzed by UDP-glucuronyl transferase (Panel (**a**)). In Panel (**b**), the hepatic biotransformation of CPT11 is overviewed, where the SN38 and SN38G are cleared from the hepatocytes through export mediated by ATP binding cassettes (ABCs)

toxicities. Thiopurine is a class of drugs that includes 6-mercaptopurine (6MP), 6-thioguanine, and azathiopurine, which is used to treat acute lymphoblastic leukemia, autoimmune disorders, inflammatory bowel disease, and in the prevention of organ transplant rejections. Although they have a broad spectrum of pharmacologic activity, thiopurines have a relatively narrow therapeutic index where individuals who are unable to eliminate these agents may be at increased risk for developing life-threatening myelosuppression.

Thiopurine-induced toxicity has been associated with a polymorphism along the gene coding for thiopurine methyl transferase (TPMT). TPMT is a critical enzyme catalyzing the s-methylation of 6MP to form 6-methylmercaptopurine (MeMP), an inactive metabolite (Fig. 16.2). In this reaction, the methyl group is donated by s-adenosyl-methioine (SAMe), where MeMP can be further metabolized by xanthine oxidase to form 2,8-dihydroxy-6-methylmercatopurine. Alternative metabolism of 6MP can be initially metabolized by xanithine oxidase, where the s-methylation is the second step, where both xanthine oxidase and TPMT will lead to the formation of 2,8-dihydroxy-6-methylmercatopurine [6].

The clearance of thiopurines is dependent on TPMT activity, which correlates with intracellular 6-thiopurine triphosphate concentrations in red blood cells. Polymorphisms along TPMT have been shown to reduce expression of the enzyme and/or have reduce the capacity to eliminate thiopurines. Low TPMT activity correlated with increased potential for thiopurine-induced toxicities. In contrast, high levels of TPMT correlate with decreased therapeutic effectiveness.

A number of variants have been identified along the TPMT gene, and are designated as *1 (wild type), *2, *3A and *3C. In patients who are carriers of the variant, intracellular thiopurines are less likely to undergo S-methylation and thus have reduced clearance. Decreased metabolism will allow the thiopurine to be anabolized to form 6-thioguanine triphosphate, the active moiety, where increased levels can potentially lead to profound myelosuppression.

Approximately 89% of a Caucasian population that was studied was found to be homozygous for the wild-type gene and have high TPMT enzymatic activity. Eleven percent (11%) of the study subjects were found to be heterozygous with intermediate TPMT enzymatic activity. However, 1 out of 300 subjects were found to be homozygous for low TPMT enzymatic activity and were at high risk for developing severe myelosuppression [7–9]. In patients with low TPMT activity, dosage attenuation was able to maintain clinical outcomes with reduced severity and incidence of thiopurine-induced toxicities as comparable to subjects with normal TPMT activity receiving normal dosages.

Dihyrdropyrimidien Dehydrogenase and Thymidylate Synthetase Polymorphism

5-Fluorouracil (5FU) is fluoropyrimidine that has been the cornerstone for the treatment of gastroesophageal, colorectal, and breast cancers. Unfortunately, severe

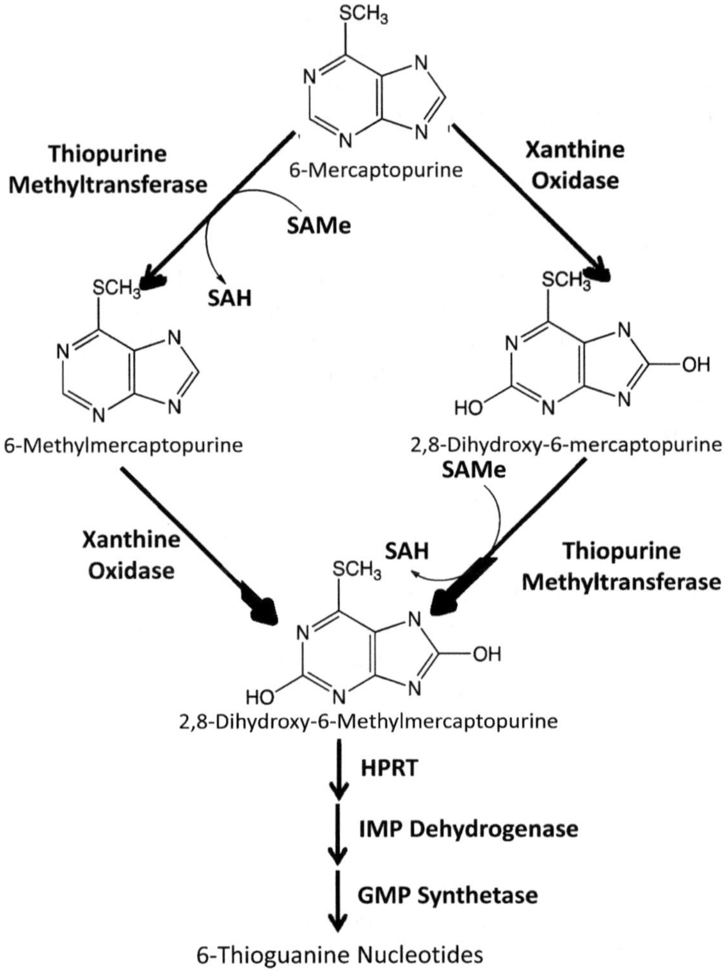

Fig. 16.2 Biotransformation of 6-mercaptopurine (6MP) is summarized, where thiopurine methyltransferase (TPMT) methylates the conversion of 6MP to 6-methylmercaptopurine (MeMP), an inactive metabolite. In this reaction, the methyl group is donated by s-adenosyl-methioine (SAMe). MeMP can be further metabolized by xanthine oxidase to form 2,8-dihydroxy-6-methylmercatopurine. Alternative metabolism of 6MP can be mediated by xanithine oxidase, where the s-methylation is the second step. The combination of xanthine oxidase- and TPMT-mediated metabolism will lead to the formation of 2,8-dihydroxy-6-methylmercatopurine, inactive metabolite

toxicity occurs in approximately 30% of patients treated with 5FU-based regimens. 5FU has a narrow therapeutic window, where the drug concentration required for tumor response is within the general range where toxicity may also occur. Inherited genetic variability in a number of key metabolic enzymes involved in the 5FU metabolic pathway has been associated with drug-related toxicities [9].

5FU is a prodrug that requires biotransformation into its active moieties, which include several active metabolites able to inhibit thymidylate synthase (TS),

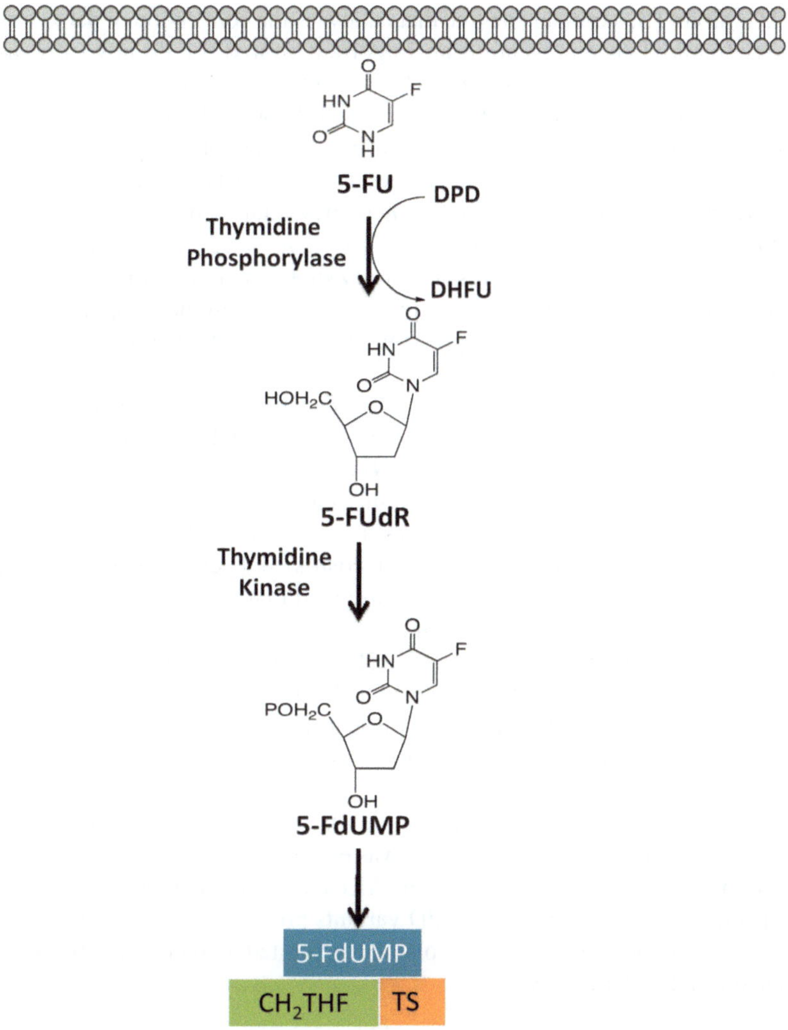

Fig. 16.3 5FU is a prodrug that requires intracellular biotransformation to form the active moieties, 5-FdUMP. Initially 5FU is initially converted FUDr, which is catalyzed by thymidine phosphorylase (TP). FUDR is then converted to 5-FdUMP, one of the active moieties, where this reaction is catalyzed by thymidine kinase. 5-FdUMP inhibits thymidylate synthase (TS), a critical enzyme in normal and tumor DNA synthesis. Both, 5FU and its anabolite, 5-fluorodeoxyuridylate (5FdUMP), can bind tightly onto TS to form a stable ternary complex resulting in enzymatic inhibition. Alternatively, 5FU can also under metabolism mediated by dihydropyrimidine dehydrogenase (DPD), which biotransforms 5FU into DHFU, an inactive metabolite

a critical enzyme in normal and tumor DNA synthesis. In the catabolic pathway, dihydropyrimidine dehydrogenase (DPD) is a rate-limiting catabolic enzyme important to inactivate 5FU (Fig. 16.3). Genetic polymorphisms in TS and DPD may predict for clinical response and accumulation of 5FU and its anabolic products, respectively.

5FU inhibits TS, a critical enzyme that catalyzes the conversion of deoxyuridylate to deoxythymidylate representing an important source for de novo thymidylate synthesis, which is required for DNA synthesis. 5FU and its anabolite, 5-fluorodeoxyuridylate (5FdUMP), can bind tightly onto TS to form a stable ternary complex resulting in enzymatic inhibition [9–11]. One polymorphism involves the 5′ regulatory region of the TS gene promoter and consists of either double (2R) or triple (3R) repeats of a 28 bp sequence, where these mutations influenced TS expression. Studies have shown that 3R had activity that was 2.6 times higher than 2R, where elevated levels of TS expression or enzymatic activity correlated with resistance towards 5FU. The role of TS in predicting for antitumor response was clinically verified where the mRNA expression level was predictive for tumor response and overall survival [11].

In contrast to TS, DPD is responsible for deactivating more than 80% of 5FU that is administered, where 5–20% is excreted unchanged in the urine. Structurally DPD has two FAD, two FMN and eight [4Fe-4S] clusters that are arranged in two electron transfer chains. Impairment of this catabolic pathway can lead to 5FU accumulation resulting in severe toxicities. Patients with DPD deficiency encounter intense 5FU-related toxicities including mucositis, alopecia, diarrhea, neutropenia, skin rash and neurologic toxicities. It is estimated that 3–5% of the population has partial DPD deficiency, where the detection of this genetic variation may prevent severe drug related adverse events [12]. 5FU-induced toxicity has led to almost 100% mortality in patients with complete DPD deficiency, even cases where topical 5FU exposure has resulted in fatality. This test would also be an important test for patients receiving capecitabine, an oral prodrug of 5FU, where the active moiety will utilize the same pathways.

There are rapid genetic tests that can identify individuals with DPD deficiency. The incidence of partial DPD deficiency was estimated to be 3–5% in the Caucasian population. However, the incidence in the African American population is estimated to be as high as 8% [13]. Specific DPD variants produce a truncated protein; however, these mutations have only explained a limited number of adverse effects attributed to DPD deficiency.

Cytochrome P450 Polymorphism as Biomarkers

Cytochrome P450 (CYP) is a superfamily of enzymes critical in metabolizing a wide spectrum of xenobiotics and endobiotics with varying physicochemical properties. CYP enzymes involved in the metabolism of anticancer agents have been reported in 2C8, 2C9, 2C19, 2D6, and 3A4. The predominant isotype found in the liver is CYP3A4 which metabolizes hydrophobic substance including cancer therapeutic drugs, accounting for approximately 60% of all cytochrome P450 enzymatic activity found in the human liver and about 70% of the activity in enterocytes [14]. However, other isotypes are also important as alternative, primary or secondary metabolic pathways for numerous anticancer agents.

CYP3A4 Polymorphism

CYP3A4 metabolizes a wide array of therapeutic agents and endogenous substrates. This may explain why agents utilizing this metabolic pathway are associated with a number of drug–drug interactions. One example of this is a two-way drug–drug interaction between paclitaxel and doxorubicin. Drug–drug interactions can lead to altered metabolism and disposition of a drug when coadministered. Since both paclitaxel and doxorubicin are critical components in breast cancer regimens, coadministering these two agents together is a strong possibility. Paclitaxel is metabolized by CYP3A4 and CYP2C8, both with known polymorphisms, to form 6α-hydroxypaclitaxel and 3′p-hydroxypaclitaxel, respectively [15–17]. When doxorubicin was administered in combination with paclitaxel, response rates in breast cancer patients significantly increased. However, this combination was also associated with higher rate of congestive heart failure. Both clinical responses and cardiotoxicity were attributed to paclitaxel-mediated inhibition of doxorubicin metabolism, allowing for doxorubicin accumulation and increasing the incidence in cardiotoxicity. When docetaxel is substituted for paclitaxel, similar interaction with doxorubicin was found, further supporting the concept of drug–drug interaction. [15]. As has been previously mentioned, paclitaxel and doxorubicin have a two-way interaction, where doxorubicin can also inhibit the formation of 3′p-hydroxypaclitaxel, indicating that it can inhibit CYP2C8. More recently, polymorphisms along CYP2B8 have demonstrated a reduced conversion of paclitaxel to 3′-p-hydroxypaclitaxel; however, there is no data confirming whether this polymorphism impacts clinical outcome [15–18].

CYP2B6 Polymorphism

Genetic polymorphisms along the CYP2B6 gene have been shown to influence the pharmacokinetics for substrates metabolized by this enzyme. Unlike other polymorphisms where the variants were found to have decreased metabolism as compared to the wild-type enzyme, this polymorphism is associated with increased drug clearance. Normally, polymorphisms associated with increased drug clearance are accompanied by a decreased risk of toxicities. However, subjects carrying these types of variants are more likely to encounter disease relapse due to decreased drug exposures. Patients with the variant CYP2B6*6 (Q172H and K262R) were found to eliminate cyclophosphamide faster which corresponded with a shorter plasma cyclophosphamide half-life when compared to either homozygous or heterozygous CYP2B6*1 (wild-type). As expected, subjects with the polymorphism CYP2B6*6 were less lightly to develop leukocytopenia as compared to carriers of CYP2B6*1 [19].

However, other CYP2B6 polymorphism (G516T) was shown to have the opposite effect, where TT carriers were found to be poor metabolizers of CYP2B6 substrates. Patients with this polymorphism had increased plasma concentrations of efavirenz and nevirapine, nonnucleoside reverse transcriptase inhibitors (NNRTI) used for HIV, with the TT genotype as compared to patients who are homozygous for GG. Drug level corresponded to the increased incidence of toxicities. For NVP, altered pharmacokinetics and immunologic response to NVP containing regimens were observed [20]. For patients receiving EFV, patients with G516T were more likely to experience CNS toxicities, which included headaches, hallucination, and vivid dreams [21].

CYP2D6 Polymorphism

Tamoxifen is an antagonist of estrogen receptor (ER) and is employed in treating patients with early and advanced breast cancers that are positive for ER. Other uses for tamoxifen include in situ ductal carcinoma and as primary chemoprevention in women who are identified as high-risk for the development of breast cancer. Although the dosage of tamoxifen is standardized, there is considerable interindividual variation for tamoxifen and its metabolites.

Tamoxifen is eliminated by CYP-mediated metabolism to form several primary and secondary metabolites. When using CYP3A4/5, *N*-desmethyl-tamoxifen is the primary metabolite accounting for approximately 90% metabolites. Alternatively, tamoxifen can undergo CYP2D6 mediated metabolism forming 4-hydroxy-tamoxifen. However, both *N*-desmethyl-tamoxifen (via CYP2D6) and 4-hydroxy-tamoxifen (via CYP3A4/5) are further metabolized to form 4-hydroxy-*N*-desmethyl-tamoxifen (endoxifen), where both 4-hydroxy-tamoxifen and endoxifen are important active metabolites exhibiting similar potencies [9]. The plasma level of endoxifen can be up to 14-fold higher than 4-hydroxyl-tamoxifen. Currently there are more than 80 allelic variants found in CYP2D6 where a large number are associated with increased, decreased, or an absence of enzymatic activity.

The FDA has approved a microarray-based pharmacogenetic CYP2D6 test (AmpliChip CYP450 Test) that can evaluate 27 variants of CYP2D6. This include identifying variants with lower enzymatic capacity such as those found in CYP2D6*3, *4, *5, and *6 variants. These types of variants are most commonly seen in subjects who are of Asian or African descent [9]. In contrast, ultrarapid variants have also been identified, CYP2D6 2XN, which can also be identified using this microarray system. Individuals of Middle Eastern and Ethiopian descent are most commonly associated with CYP2D6 2XN. Despite these findings, there is currently no recommendation for individuals who are found to be either intermediate or poor metabolizers with regards to tamoxifen dosing. This may be due to the role of CYP3A4/5 and other as yet unidentified mediated pathways, which metabolites can use for systemic clearance. In addition, the role of efflux transporters has not been definitively characterized, which may play a role in biliary excretion of tamoxifen and its metabolites. When all of the elimination pathways are integrated into this model, these types of testing will be able to guide in the optimal dosing of individuals.

Genetic Test to Identify Drug-Related Hypersensitivity Reactions

Very recently, a genetic test has been developed that is able to predict for subjects who are at risk for developing hypersensitivity reactions towards abacavir. Approximately 3–8% of patients receiving abacavir will develop hypersensitivity towards this antiretroviral agent. This is dependent on the ethnicity, where 8% of Caucasians encounter hypersensitivity reactions, and only 2% of Africans will encounter hypersensitivity reactions. The incidence in African Americans is approximately 4%.

This potentially severe allergic reaction is characterized by skin rash, gastrointestinal, and respiratory symptoms, where the reactions become more intense with subsequent dosing. When the reaction is encountered, it normally occurs in the first 6 weeks of therapy. When a patient with suspected hypersensitivity reaction is rechallenged, fatal events have been reported. To eliminate this adverse reaction, a genetic test has been developed and is now commercially available to identify individuals who may at risk for drug-related hypersensitivity reactions. It was found that patients who are positive for HLA B5701 were found to have an increased risk for abacavir-mediated hypersensitive reaction. In contrast, patients who test negative for this polymorphism were found to have no risk for the developing this immunologically related reaction [22]. In the PREDICT study, patients testing negative for HLA B5701 had no reported incidence of hypersensitivity reactions, which was confirmed by skin patch testing.

ABC Polymorphism in Relations to Toxicities

Currently, cellular transporter polymorphisms are being investigated as potential biomarkers to predict for drug-related toxicities. Since a number of these transporters are key factors in regulating intracellular levels of drugs, it is understandable that polymorphisms along ATP binding cassettes (ABCs) such as ABCB1 (P-glycoprotein), ABCC1 (MRP1), ABCC2 (MRP2), ABCC4 (MRP4), and ABCG2 (BCRP) will play a role in clinical response and toxicity. All of these transporters are efflux transporters that pump their substrates into the extracellular space.

Polymorphisms and Clinical Outcomes to EGFR Antibodies

ATP binding cassette G2 (ABCG2) or breast cancer resistance protein (BCRP) is a cellular efflux transporter. This is a highly polymorphic cellular efflux transporter protein that is expressed at high levels in the blood brain barrier, kidneys, intestines and liver. Increased expression of ABCG2 on cancer cells was associated with resistance to anthracycline and camptothecin analogs. Interestingly, polymorphisms in ABCG2 were also found to be associated with adverse effects in relations with the EGFR inhibitor, gefitinib [23]. An association between allelic variants found along EGFR, ABCG2, and ABCB1 correlating with an increased incidence of diarrhea and skin toxicity were found in gefitinib-treated patients. One single-nucleotide polymorphism (SNP) in the ABCG2 gene was found to be associated with diarrhea in 124 patients receiving oral gefitinib. Forty-four percent (44%) of patients who are heterozygous ABCG2 421C>A (Q141K) developed diarrhea, compared to only 12% of wild-type patients reporting diarrhea. Patients carrying the 421C>A variant have been shown to have significantly higher drug accumulation, which may be attributed to low ABCG2 protein expression and an increased risk for diarrhea [24–26]. More interestingly is that this SNP was not associated with skin toxicity suggesting that an alternative drug action may be the cause of this adverse effect.

Polymorphism in EGFR was associated with responsiveness to EGFR inhibitor therapy in lung cancer. A variant along exon 13 in EGFR (R421K) was associated with increased progression free survival and overall survival in colorectal cancer patients receiving cetuximab and CPT-11-based therapy [27]. Another polymorphism along EGFR showed short allele carriers were more prone to have grade 2–3 skin toxicity compared with those who carried the long alleles. In the same study a polymorphism in EGFR 61G/G genotypes was associated with improved overall survival [27].

A prospective trial was undertaken to investigate pharmacogenomic and pharmacokinetic determinants of skin rash and diarrhea in 80 patients treated with erlotinib [28]. The polymorphisms along ABCG2, EGFR, CYP3A4 and 3A5 were all interrogated to assess for association with erlotinib toxicity. Skin toxicity was associated with trough erlotinib concentration, which was associated with a polymorphism in the EGFR intron 1. Diarrhea was linked to two polymorphisms in the EGFR promoter, -216G/T and -191C/A. The newly identified ABCG2 polymorphisms, 1143C/T and -15622C/T, are associated with differential erlotinib concentrations, but there has not been a definitive association with toxicity.

Conclusion

Although the ultimate goal is to develop biomarkers that can predict both outcomes and potential toxicities for drug development, it is obvious that the development of biomarkers will trail drug development. This is particularly the case for the development of safety biomarkers where comprehensive pharmacologic understanding of how the specific drug is metabolized and eliminated is compulsory. Currently there are predictive biomarkers that are able to identify subjects who may be at risk for the development of toxicities. In the future, it is very conceivable that biomarkers using different technologies will complement each other. This is certainly the case when using genetics or microarrays with biomarkers that employ metabolomic technology. With the advances in technology, the types of data will not come from a single source but will be a comprehensive evaluation, or more simply a systemic approach.

References

1. Monahan BP, Ferguson CL, Killeavy ES, Lloyd BK, Troy J, Cantilena Jr LR. Torsades de pointes occurring in association with terfenadine use. JAMA. 1990;21:2788–90.
2. Biomarkers Definitions Working Group. Biomarkers and surrogate endpoints: preferred definitions and conceptual framework. Clin Pharmacol Ther. 2001;69:89–95.
3. Santos A, Zanetta S, Crestell T, et al. Metabolism of irinotecan (CPT-11) by CYP3A4 and CYP3A5 in humans. Clin Cancer Res. 2000;6:2012–20.
4. Kaneda N, Nagata H, Furuta T, Yokokura T. Metabolism and pharmacokinetics of camptothecin analogue CPT-11 in the mouse. Cancer Res. 1990;50:1715–20.
5. Cote J-F, Kirzin S, Kramar A, et al. UGT1A1 Polymorphism can predict hematologic toxiticity in patients treated with irinotecan. Clin Cancer Res. 2007;13:3269–75.
6. Weinshilboum R. Thiopurine pharmacogenetics: clinical and molecular studies of thiopurine methyltransferase. Drug Metab Dispos. 2001;29:601–5.
7. Cheok MH, Evans WE. Acute lymphoblastic leukaemia: a model for the pharmacogenomics of cancer therapy. Nat Rev Cancer. 2006;6:117–29.
8. Relling MV, Hancock ML, Rivera GK, et al. Mercaptopurine therapy intolerance and heterozygosity at the thiopurine S-methyltransferase gene locus. J Natl Cancer Inst. 2008;91:2001–8.
9. Tan S-H, Lee S-C, Goh B-C, Wong J. Pharmacogenetics in breast cancer therapy. Clin Cancer Res. 2008;14:8027–41.
10. Mercier C, Ciccolini J. Profiling dihydropyrimidine dehydrogenase deficiency in patients with cancer undergoing 5-fluorouracil/capecitabine therapy. Clin Colorectal Cancer. 2006;6:288–96.
11. Lenz HJ, Danenberg KD, Leichman CG, et al. p53 and thymidylate synthase expression in untreated stage II colon cancer: associations with recurrence, survival, and site. Clin Cancer Res. 1998;4:1227–34.
12. Ezzeldin H, Diasio R. Dihydropyrimidine dehydrogenase deficiency, a pharmacogenetic syndrome associated with potentially life-threatening toxicity following 5-fluorouracil administration. Clin Colorectal Cancer. 2004;4:181–9.
13. Mattison LK, Fourie J, Desmond RA, Modak A, Saif MW, Diasio RB. Increased prevalence of dihydropyrimidine dehydrogenase deficiency in African-Americans compared with Caucasians. Clin Cancer Res. 2006;12(18):5491–5.
14. Linder MW, Prough RA, Valdes Jr R. Pharmacogenetics: a laboratory tool for optimizing therapeutic efficiency. Clin Chem. 1997;43(2):254–66.
15. Kumar GN, Walle UK, Walle T. Cytochrome P450 3A-mediated human liver microsomal taxol 6 alpha-hydroxylation. J Pharmacol Exp Ther. 1994;268(3):1160–5.
16. Cresteil T, Monsarrat B, Alvinerie P, Treluyer JM, Vieira I, Wright M. Taxol metabolism by human liver microsomes: identification of cytochrome P450 isozymes involved in its biotransformation. Cancer Res. 1994;54(2):386–92.
17. Sonnichsen DS, Liu Q, Schuetz EG, Schuetz JD, Pappo A, Relling MV. Variability in human cytochrome P450 paclitaxel metabolism. J Pharmacol Exp Ther. 1995;275(2):566–75.
18. Sparano JA. Compilation of phase I and II trial data of docetaxel and doxorubicin in the treatment of advanced breast cancer and other malignancies. Semin Oncol. 1998;25(6 Suppl 13): 10–5.
19. Nakajima M, Komagata S, Fujiki Y, et al. Genetic polymorphisms of CYP2B6 affect the pharmacokinetics/pharmacodynamics of cyclophosphamide in Japanese cancer patients. Pharmacogenet Genomics. 2007;17:431–45.
20. Haas DW, Ribaudo HJ, Kim RB, et al. Pharmacogenetics of efavirenz and central nervous system side effects: an adult AIDS clinical trials group study. AIDS. 2004;3:2391–400.
21. Saitoh A, Sarles E, Capparelli E, et al. GYP2B6 genetic variants are associated with nevirapine pharmacokinetics and clinical response in HIV infected Children. AIDS. 2007;21:2191–9.
22. Mallal S, Phillips E, Carosi G, (PREDICT-1 Study Team), et al. HLA-B*5701 screening for hypersensitivity to abacavir. N Engl J Med. 2008;358(6):568–79.
23. Cusatis G, Gregorc V, Li J, et al. Pharmacogenetics of ABCG2 and adverse reactions to gefitinib. J Natl Cancer Inst. 2006;98(23):1739–42.

24. Mizurai S, Aozasa N, Kotani H. Single nucleotide polymorphisms result in impaired membrane localization and reduced ATPase activity in multidrug transporter ABCG2. Int J Cancer. 2004;109:238–46.
25. Imai Y, Nakane M, Kage K, et al. C421A polymorphism in the human breast cancer resistance protein gene is associated with low expression of Q141K protein and low-level drug resistance. Mol Cancer Ther. 2002;1:611–6.
26. Goncalves A, Esteyries S, Taylor-Smedra B, et al. A polymorphism in the EGFR extracellular domain is associated with progression-free survival in metastatic colorectal cancer patients receiving cetuximab-based treatment. BMC Cancer. 2008;8:169.
27. Graziano F, Ruzzo A, Loupakis F, et al. Pharmacogenetic profiling for cetuximab plus irinotecan therapy in patients with refractory advanced colorectal cancer. J Clin Oncol. 2008;26(9): 1427–34.
28. Rudin CM, Liu W, Desai A, et al. Pharmacogenomic and pharmacokinetic determinants of erlotinib toxicity. J Clin Oncol. 2008;26:1119–27.

Chapter 17
Biomarker Discovery Strategies: DNA, RNA, and Protein

Eduardo Vilar and Josep Tabernero

Abbreviations

NGS	Next-generation sequencing
PCR	Polymerase chain reaction
ddNTPs	Dideoxynucleotides
FRET	Fluorescent energy software resonance transfer
bp	Base pair
SNP	Single nucleotide polymorphism
CNV	Copy number variation
LOH	Loss of heterozygosity
CGH	Comparative genomic hybridization
FFPE	Formalin-fixed paraffin-embedded
SAGE	Serial analysis of gene expression
PCR qRT-PCR	Quantitative reverse transcriptase
MM	Mismatch
PM	Perfect match
FDR	False discovery rate
2D-PAGE	Polyacrylamide gel electrophoresis
MS	Mass spectrometry
DIGE	Differential in-gel electrophoresis
MALDI	Matrix-assisted laser desorption ionization

E. Vilar, M.D., Ph.D. (✉)
Department of Internal Medicine, University of Michigan Comprehensive Cancer Center,
1858 BSRB 109 Zina Pitcher, Ann Arbor, MI 48109, USA
e-mail: evilar@umich.edu

J. Tabernero, M.D.
Department of Medical Oncology Service, Vall d'Hebron University Hospital,
Ps. Vall d'Hebron 119-129, Barcelona 08035, Spain
e-mail: jtabernero@vhio.net

H.-J. Lenz (ed.), *Biomarkers in Oncology: Prediction and Prognosis*,
DOI 10.1007/978-1-4419-9755-5_17, © Springer Science+Business Media New York 2013

TOF Time-of-flight
SELDI Surface-enhanced laser desorption and ionization
TMA Tissue microarray
CMA Cell line microarray
XMA Xenograft microarrays
GSEA Gene set enrichment analysis

The Long and Winding Road of Biomarker Discovery

During the last two decades the medical community has steadily increased its interest in the field of biomarkers. This may be explained by to the outburst of the application of molecular biology techniques to medical sciences and the ability for translating faster these discoveries into the clinical setting. As the number of basic and clinical investigators involved in this common effort grows, there is a necessity to clearly establish concepts and basic definitions regarding the process of biomarker development and validation. The Biomarkers Definition Working Group has helped to improve the terminological accuracy in this field and has defined unequivocally the terms *clinical endpoint, biomarker, and surrogate endpoint* [1]. Following its recommendations a *clinical endpoint* would be defined as a "*characteristic or a variable that reflects how a patient feels, functions or survives.*" Then a *biological marker* would be a "*characteristic that is objectively measured and evaluated as an indicator of normal biological process, pathogenic process or pharmacologic responses to a therapeutic intervention.*" Therefore, a biomarker may be implemented for diagnosis, staging, prognosis, prediction of response to treatment, or final monitoring of clinical response. But it is obvious that the final goal would be to establish a *surrogate endpoint*, which is a "*biomarker intended to substitute for a clinical endpoint.*" Therefore, a surrogate endpoint is expected to predict clinical benefit based on epidemiologic, therapeutic, pathophysiologic, or other scientific evidence. It is important to understand that only a subset of biomarkers will finally qualify as surrogate markers, although all surrogate endpoints are technically biomarkers.

Furthermore, definition of a pipeline for biomarker studies is needed if we want to improve the standardization of biomarker validation. Due to the fact that many clinical investigators have already started to conduct biomarker studies a parallel model that resembles the steps of drug development process is being incorporated in this scenario. This pathway has been stratified in six sequential steps: (1) discovery, (2) qualification, (3) verification, (4) research assay optimization, (5) clinical validation, and (6) commercialization. The terms such as *validation, qualification*, and *evaluation* have introduced a high degree of confusion in the literature as they have been used interchangeably. Therefore, we think that the term *qualification* should make reference to the process of linking a biomarker to a biologic entity and then establishing a surrogate endpoint when this association is demonstrated; this specific process would include the final part of the discovery, qualification and verification steps [2]. At the same time *validation* is commonly seen as the process to test the performance of an assay and define the most optimal conditions to be applied. In this way a particular analytical procedure to measure a biomarker can be considered precise (the measurements are reproducible) and accurate (a correlation between the measure of the biomarker and the clinical endpoint exists). In general, the steps of research assay optimization and clinical validation integrate into the term of *validation*. Finally, *evaluation* would refer to the process of determining the surrogate endpoint status under a clinical point of view and therefore is also linked to the last phases of the clinical validation.

In the present chapter we focus in the initial step of the biomarker discovery process. As this phase is truly embracing the concept of discovery is conceptually and technologically very far from the final steps meant for clinical validation. In the last years high-throughput analysis have became the mainstay in the discovery process taking advantage of cutting-edge technologies. These techniques generate a large amount of data, but many candidates will not reach the last stages of the biomarker discovery process. Here we describe the biologic principles behind these techniques and provide the principal applications as well as the major advantages and disadvantages of each one. Finally bioinformatics and system biology tools will be discussed.

Strategies for Discovering Cancer Biomarkers

In the current research scenario we are constantly challenged by new techniques and methodological resources that offer data analyzed under very different scopes. Genomics, transcriptomics, proteomics, and epigenetics are now becoming classical fields as new disciplines such as peptidomics, metabolomics, and many others continue emerging. All of them are potential sources of cancer biomarker and probably the future success of this field will be on combining this multilayered information. Here we present the most significant strategies involved in biomarkers discovery by their source of biologic material: (1) DNA, (2) RNA, and (3) protein strategies (Table 17.1). This classification is arbitrary in many aspects but helps to classify these techniques. Although it could be argued that metabolomics or epigenetics can be considered to fall into one of these categories, we have decided to place them apart due to the fact that we are using several techniques at the same time to analyze a specific biological question.

DNA Biomarkers Discovering Strategies

DNA Sequencing

The implementation and designing of DNA sequencing protocols have greatly impacted our knowledge of the molecular biology of cancer and deeply changed the landscape of basic and clinical research in oncology [3]. At the present time molecular characterization of tumors by DNA sequencing is redefining the way that therapies

Table 17.1 Biomarker discovery strategies as developed in this chapter

DNA strategies
DNA sequencing
SNP arrays
CGH arrays
SAGE
RNA strategies
Gene expression profiling
qRT-PCR
Protein strategies
Mass spectrometry (MALDI-TOF, SELDI)
2D-PAGE, DIGE
FISH
Immunohistochemistry
TMA, CMA, XMA
Multiplex ELISA
Multiplex Western Blot
Protein microarrays
Others
Epigenetics
Metabolomics
Integromics
Magnetic resonance spectroscopy
Circulating tumor cells
Pharmacogenomic markers

are implemented in the clinical setting. There are several examples of well-established genetic alterations used to predict response versus resistance to targeted therapies such as *KRAS* and *BRAF* mutations for anti-EGFR therapies in colorectal cancer [4,5], *EGFR* mutations for tyrosine kinase inhibitors in lung cancer, *c-KIT* amplification for the tyrosine kinase inhibitor imatinib in GIST, the fusion protein *BCR-ABL* for imatinib in chronic myeloid leukemia and *ERB-B2* amplification for the antibody against ERB-B2 receptor Trastuzumab in breast cancer [6, 7]. Dideoxy enzymatic sequencing, also known as Sanger protocol, is currently the most extended option for molecular characterization of tumors and continues to be the gold standard for sequencing [8]. However, in the last decade a general perception that there was no more room for improvement of this protocol has been growing. Therefore, different research groups started to developed new methods to characterize sequences in a high-throughput way and at a lower cost. These new techniques have been generally named as *Next Generation Sequencing (NGS)* as all of them shared the common principle of sequencing-by-synthesis, although differences in the methodology to generate sequences and the biochemistry of cycling exist.

Dideoxy sequencing is a polymerase-driven synthesis of DNA strands complementary to the template whose sequence wants to be determined. Template is prepared from an initial polymerase chain reaction (PCR) followed by a cleanup process or from a miniprep of a plasmid vector used to cloned the DNA fragment of interest. Sanger protocols consist in a single primer extension reaction including the four species of dideoxynucleotides (ddNTPs) labeled with fluorescent dyes that have different emission wavelengths. The products of sequencing reactions are analyzed by electrophoresis in a capillary that will separate them by denaturalization allowing a single-base-pair resolution. At the end of the capillary a single wavelength will excite the fluorochromes linked to the ddNTPs and then recognized by fluorescent energy software resonance transfer (FRET). Therefore, the identity of every nucleotide is recognized and computers algorithms will translate these signals to DNA sequences. These techniques have been refined after introducing major advances in the automation of the process by using capillary electrophoresis, in the high-throughput implementation by being able to analyze 96–384 sequencing reactions simultaneously, in template preparation, in development of ddNTP by labeling them with fluorescent dyes, in the use of engineered thermostable polymerases that are highly efficient incorporating ddNTPs thus increasing the amount of template linearly, and finally in the establishment of core facilities at research centers. At the present time Sanger capillary-based sequencers such as ABI3730XL are able to generate 1–2 million base-pair (bp) per 24 h with an average of 550–800 bp of read length and an accuracy of 99.9% [8, 9]. It has been successfully applied for cancer biomarker discovery even in a high-throughput context. A complete genomic landscape of breast, colorectal [10], pancreatic [11], and brain tumors [12] has been published by a research group in a tremendous comprehensive effort to provide us with a complete overlook of the mutational spectrum behind these tumors. However, the application of dideoxy sequencing to mammalian-sized genomes such as those coming from human tumors has been restricted to large genome centers with high levels of technical experience, and sophisticated bioinformatic support available in order to handle this amount of information, so a clear distinction between real genomic signals and noise could be established. It is also important to bear in mind that the cost of these experiments is exceedingly high, so it was only achievable to collaborations among large research groups. Finally, another disadvantage is that the analogic output displayed by the Sanger protocol makes difficult to identify those mutations coming from nonabundant cell populations within tumors. Probably the desire of increasing the high-throughput organization and reducing the cost have been the main triggers for developing a new generation of sequencing tools [13].

Several biotechnology companies have established partnerships with research laboratories that have been the pioneers in the development of NGS. At the present time the principal platforms that are commercially available are 454/Roche, Solexa/Illumina, and SOLiD/Applied. All of them are based on the concept of cyclic array sequencing although important differences among these platforms exist. NGS would be able to decrease the costs of sequencing by analyzing in a physical two-dimensional array millions of distinct sequencing features at the same time. Every one of these features is an unknown sequence of DNA that can share the same well with other features because they are physically immobilized on the surface of the array. This sequencing process is cyclic in nature because in each cycle the identity of a single base position is interrogated for all features in a parallel way. Briefly, an enzymatic reaction is coupled to either light emission or fluorescent incorporation and is

Table 17.2 Sequencing platforms

Platform	Cycle sequencing method	Amplification approach	Read length (bp)	Throughput (million bp/day)	Time/run
3730XL	Polymerase Dye terminators	PCR	>800	1–2	3 h
Roche 454 FLX	Polymerase Pyrosequencing	Emulsion PCR	400	200	10 h
Solexa/Illumina	Polymerase Reversible dye terminators	Bridge PCR	25–35	>200	2.5 day
SOLiD/ABI	Ligase	Emulsion PCR	25–35	200–300	6 day

finally detected by imaging techniques leading a base call for all of the features after every cycle. Although this is the basic principle behind NGS, every platform is remarkably different in the two fundamental aspects: (1) the methodology used to generate the DNA features, and (2) the biochemistry implemented for performing the cyclic sequencing. In Table 17.2 we have summarized these differences between the main platforms and compared their performance to the Sanger method.

In general, the amplification approach for handling and generating the DNA features is based on either emulsion PCR or bridge PCR. Emulsion PCR implies that DNA features are prepared by fragmentation of the genomic DNA and then ligated to adaptor sequences. Multiple PCRs of these DNA features will be performed in a water-in-oil emulsion located in a single PCR compartment facilitating a clonal amplification. Those amplicons generated in the emulsion PCR compartments are captured by 1 μ(mu)m paramagnetic beads bearing one of the two primers (forward or reverse) and then all beads are recovered by immobilization on a glass substrate. In contrast to this in the bridge PCR approach a set of universal primers that have been designed to target universal adaptors are immobilized on a two-dimensional glass slide. So PCR reagents and DNA features are located in the aqueous phase where the PCR will take place and final DNA clones derived from these PCR will be physically retained by primers attached to the surface. The biochemistry of the reactions is also a differential feature between platforms. 454/Roche is taking advantage of the principle of sequencing-by-synthesis based on pyrosequencing reactions, so addition of a single nucleotide species involves the release of a pyrophosphate that is detected in luciferase reaction. Solexa/Illumina use a dye terminator chemistry that requires a reengineered DNA polymerase and modified dye labeled nucleotides as substrates. SOLiD/ABI uses a ligase instead of a polymerase, so labeled nonamers are introduced and the identity of every position within each nonamer is correlated with the identity of the fluorochrome. Finally there is a fourth platform different to the three previous that follows the idea on single-molecule sequencing. Helicos BioSciences is the proprietary of this technology that obviates the initial clonal amplification of the template. Sample DNA is initially fragmented and disperse in single DNA molecules thorough an array. Successive sequence cycles with fluorescent labeled nucleotides will resolve the complete sequence [9, 14].

Genome-Wide Single Nucleotide Polymorphism (SNP) Arrays

SNPs are the most common source of genetic variation in the human genome. A single nucleotide change can be considered as a SNP when the frequency of the minor allele is higher than 1% in a population, otherwise is either a variation or a mutation. The International Haplotype Project (also known as HapMap Project) revealed the presence of limited haplotype diversity within small chromosomal segments and the tendency of all of the SNPs in these segments to be transmitted by blocks [15]. This concept is known as linkage disequilibrium and subsequently the HapMap project defined the patterns of linkage disequilibrium throughout the whole genome [16]. This fact has had tremendous consequences in the way that whole genome-wide molecular epidemiology and biology studies are conducted because the identification of tagging SNPs in this blocks gives the opportunity to perform this massive genotyping projects using only the most informative SNPs.

For those studies focusing in SNP identification the source of DNA (genomic or tumor) is crucial to answer the questions proposed. Therefore, population studies using germ-line DNA of cases and controls from a specific population will inform about genetic variation predisposing for cancer development. This particular design has reported the association of a 8q24 variant in prostate [17] and colorectal cancer [18], and has led to the identification of *MYC* as a putative responsible for this association in colorectal cancer [19]. In addition the combination of SNP arrays studies using germ-line and tumor DNA gives the opportunity to detect copy number variation (CNV) and loss of heterozygosity (LOH) even with more resolution than comparative genomic hybridization (CGH) arrays [15].

There are two main vendors of SNP arrays technology. Although both platforms are involving the use of oligonucleotide probes one is spotting them on gene chips (Affymetrix) and the other absorbing them on beads (Illumina). In addition both platforms need to decrease the complexity of the genome and generate whole genome amplified DNA before starting the genotyping process. In general this is carried through sequential steps that cleave the genomic DNA using restriction enzymes, ligate common adaptor sequences to restriction sites and eventually extend these fragments using single or dual universal PCR primers able to recognize the adaptor sequences (in Affymetrix SNPs) or allele-specific designed primers (in Illumina chips). This process is crucial as it allows the amplification on thousands of DNA fragments simultaneously [16].Another important difference between these platforms strives in the hybridization technologies that they use: Affymetrix arrays are using an allele-specific approach and Illumina a tag-specific array. Affymetrix SNP arrays are manufactured using a photolithographic process and 40 different 25-mer oligonucleotide probes for each SNP locus are tiled, including perfect match and mismatch probes. On the other side Illumina is using specific oligonucleotide tags that are linked to particular SNPs. Therefore, Affymetrix presents a platform with a fixed set of SNPs arrayed and Illumina is more amenable for customization.

These platforms require the use of high-quality DNA that is obtained from fresh or frozen samples. Genotyping of DNA obtained from formalin fixed paraffin embedded (FFPE) tissue has also been reported although fewer chances exist to scale up the number of SNPs at the same level of those experiments performed with fresh material. This is especially relevant for the study of LOH and CNV in tumors samples using SNPs arrays. On the contrary, germ-line DNA is easily extracted from fresh or frozen lymphocytes.

RNA Biomarkers Discovering Strategies

Gene Expression Profiling

Gene expression can be assessed using many different approaches and technologies whose selection may depend on the ultimate goal of the researcher. Those interested on biomarker discovery will certainly decide to consider the use of DNA chips also known as DNA microarrays [20, 21]. However, other technologies are emerging again with renewed forces in the gene expression arena such as serial analysis of gene expression (SAGE) [22, 23], which is especially true after the appearance of a new wave of sequencing methods. Finally, a very popular platform used to interrogate gene expression at a smaller scale is quantitative reverse transcriptase PCR (qRT-PCR) which has gained popularity to validate those biomarkers coming from "fishing expeditions" with DNA microarrays.

DNA microarrays will allow the determination of mRNA levels of thousands of genes simultaneously. The choice of using standard chips from the different commercially available providers or building a custom spotted microarray in house has to be made depending again on scientific goals, availability of resources and budget considerations. This large-scale platform is based on the stable characteristics that are ruling the chemical relations between mRNA and cDNA species. There are two options for designing microarray probes: full-length cDNAs and oligonucleotides. The first is based on our knowledge of the genome sequence that has enabled researchers to design primers and amplify probe sequences by PCR that will be subsequently printed on the array. The advantage of using long PCR products as probes is that they result in stronger signals. This implies an extra effort preparing probes, assuring their quality and also provides a poor distinction among gene families and splice variants. The second option is short single-stranded DNA segments, oligonucleotides, or oligos that can be synthesized and then printed or directly synthesized on a substrate (in situ synthesis). Oligos are probably the most popular option because are standardized, so the majority of commercial platforms are based on them but also researchers building their own custom in-house microarrays can purchase them to be printed. Oligonucleotide probes can be short (25-mer) or long (50 to 70-mer). Although long probes are better in terms of hybridization they offer poorer discrimination than short ones, which is secondary to cross-hybridization. Therefore, multiple independent probes that target different regions of the same RNA have to be incorporated in these arrays to enhance hybridization specificity. This problem has turned into an opportunity because commercial platforms will provide in the same array mismatch (MM) probes which are identical to perfect

Table 17.3 Microarray platforms comparison

Array	Format	Total RNA (μg)	Detection method	Sensitivity	No. human genes
Agilent Human 1A (V2) Human 1B	60-mer	5–50	Two-channel Cy3 and Cy5	1:1,000,000	18,000 19,000
Amersham/Codelink Human whole genome bioarray	30-mer	0.2–2	Single-channel Streptavidin-Alexa Fluor 647	1:900,000	45,000
Affymetrix Human Genome U133 Plus 2.0	25-mer	5	Single-channel Streptavidin-phycoerythrin	1:100,000	39,500
NimbleGen	24-mer	15	Single-channel Streptavidin-Cy3		
Spotted cDNA		5–10	Two-channel Cy3 and Cy5	1:300,000	Customized

match (PM) probes with the exception of a single base located in the middle of the oligonucleotide in order to measure the signal-to-noise ratio, thus controlling the hybridization problems at the same time. Detection systems are optimized to work in a single- or dual-color mode. In single color arrays one sample is hybridized per array and in dual-color (also known as two-channel or two-colors) two mRNA samples will be labeled with two different fluorescent dyes such as Cy3 (green) or Cy5 (red). Then samples labeled with these dyes are competitively hybridized thus comparing transcript abundance between two different biological samples being one a reference sample (normal tissue) and the other an mRNA sample coming from an experimental setting or tumor cells. This method provides with a direct comparison between samples but will require complex normalization algorithms when samples assayed in different arrays needs to be compared.

Different companies are producing microarray platforms as shown in Table 17.3. They have differences regarding probes format, starting amount of RNA, detection method and also number of genes and transcript variants that are able to assess. Selection of a particular platform has to be guided by the nature of the study and the goals. Many academic institutions have established core facilities that provide researchers with the opportunity not only to access these platforms from different companies but also to produce their own customized arrays. Therefore, the option of spotted cDNA is still reasonable for those researchers whose are towards a more restricted number of genes.

There are two major concerns that were raised earlier in the application of DNA microarrays and are still object of debate: the most optimal way to extract meaningful biological conclusions from large amounts of data and how to appropriately establish comparisons between different experiments and laboratories. Soon after microarray experiments started to be a frequent approach in research projects and publications, a working group of experts define guidelines for the submission of microarray data and the minimal amount of information that have to be publicly available before publishing a microarray experiment (MIAME) [24]. In addition it became obvious that statistical thresholds in microarray need to follow the concept of multiple test correction and multiple comparisons. Therefore, researchers involved in expression studies started to became familiar with Bonferroni correction to adapt the level of significance to the actual number of probes tested in every experiment. However, these stringent P-value cutt-offs are increasing the number of false negatives, so Benjamini and Hochberg introduced the concept of False Discovery Rate (FDR) which basically tells us how many of the selected genes from a profile or signature could be false positives [25]. Even applying this methodology the reproducibility of the data from several laboratories analyzing the same biologic context is low and when direct comparison of signatures defining the same biologic state are compared one realized that there is an evident lack of reproducibility [26]. Probably in the following years a consensus will be adopted to establish the rules and optimal approaches to metaanalyze expression data sets.

Protein Biomarkers Discovering Strategies

The cancer proteome refers to a collection of proteins expressed by a given cancer cell and this may be assessed not only by studying directly from the primary tumor but also from plasma and other body fluids such as urine, cerebrospinal fluid, nipple aspirate, pancreatic and bile fluids, saliva and bronchoalveolar lavage and many others. Although at the present time genomics are at the center of the stage of biomarker discovery, the vast majority of biomarkers that have been approved by the US Food and Drug Administration are protein biomarkers such as CA-125, PSA, CA-19–9, CEA, and many others [27]. In addition there is a central argument to claim the importance of protein biomarkers over RNA-based ones related with the fact that some mRNA changes have low correlation with their corresponding proteins. This may be the reflection of cotranslational and posttranscriptional events, protein-protein interactions and differences in the distribution among cellular compartments [28]. There are two main strategies for studying the proteome: targeted and untargeted. In targeted techniques the proteins studied are previously known and experiments are designed for assessing a number of protein analytes determined a priori. Examples of targeted techniques are protein microarrays, tissue microarrays and multiplex western blots. On the contrary untargeted approaches are meant for identifying a relative low number of novel and unknown proteins that exhibit differences in abundance between tumor and normal tissues or different tumor subtypes. Untargeted technologies include two-dimensional polyacrylamide gel electrophoresis (2D-PAGE) and different methods based on mass spectrometry (MS) [29].

The technology involved in proteomic studies has greatly evolved in the last years. 2D-PAGE was the first tool introduced in this field and generates proteins maps based on the use of immobilize pH gel gradients to separate them firstly by isoelectric points, followed by sodium dodecyl sulphate polyacrylamide electrophoresis to perform a second separation by molecular weights. A map of hundreds of spots where everyone represents different proteins, different isoforms of the same protein or posttranscriptional variants help to identify these spots using MS [30]. The drawbacks of this technique are related with the fact that it requires a large amount of starting material, has low sensitivity for less-abundant proteins, has a relatively complex and time-consuming protocol, and finally has difficulties to resolve hydrophobic, very large, and very small proteins [30, 31]. Differential in-gel electrophoresis (DIGE) represents a step further in the development of 2D-PAGE and is essentially based on labeling protein extracts with fluorescent dyes. It is physically resolved in the same way as 2D-PAGE but after scanning the gel a map with dots of different colors corresponding to each labeled protein pool can be compared for assessing differences, thus improving its sensitivity, reproducibility and quantitative resolution. The second wave of proteomic technologies has brought the possibility to implement high-throughput dynamics to the field. Matrix-assisted laser desorption ionization (MALDI) coupled to a time-of-flight (TOF) mass spectrometer and its more refined version named surface-enhanced laser desorption and ionization (SELDI) TOF are the principal techniques. In brief, SELDI-TOF starts with a sample of unfractioned proteins that is applied to the surface of a protein-binding chip. Then the chip is rinsed in order to remove the unbound proteins and subsequently the bound proteins are treated with a chemical compound that absorbs laser energy and transfers it to molecules present in the sample protonating and ionizing them. Then the chip is introduced in a vacuum chamber, irradiated with a laser launching the proteins as charged ions that will be detected by an electrode. Molecular weights are calculated based on their time of flight and the identification of peptides or proteins is based on matches with theoretical spectra obtained from publicly available protein databases. An obvious advantage of this technique is that is high-throughput and the amount of starting material is much more reduced compared to 2D-PAGE. However, it requires extensive upfront fractionation of protein mixtures and purification to obtain absolute protein quantification [30, 31]. DIGE and SELDI-TOF are able to generate a protein profile from a tumor cell or tissue in comparison with normal samples or other tumor subtype counterparts.

The majority of the time subsequent proteomic studies require further detailed analyses of protein to protein interactions and dynamics within a pathway. In this context the most appropriate platforms are targeted proteomic studies such as protein microarrays. Protein microarrays allow combining the quantification of several proteins from the same pathway and also different cellular subsets from the same tissue or different tissues simultaneously. Basically a protein microarray is a miniaturized ligand-binding assay where antibodies are captured and immobilize in a membrane. Then lysates are hybridized to the array providing a way to quantify and interpret signals associated.

Finally, tissue microarrays (TMA) will represent the latest technical step in validating protein biomarkers that have been suggested from mRNA or proteomic profiling. TMA is a technology that displays arrayed histopathology samples coming from tissues or cell lines on a single microscope slide [32]. The most common source of tissue is FFPE samples, but also arrays including panels of well-established cell lines as the panel of the NCI60 (cell line microarray, CMA), xenografts (xenograft microarray, XMA), and fresh frozen samples have been reported previously.

The integration of cell lines in TMAs provides with the possibility to introduce positive and negative controls. XMA is a strong platform to integrate the discovery and validation process of candidate biomarkers earlier in the drug development setting. TMA has been frequently applied to validation studies, especially to assess the expression of candidate biomarkers derived from gene expression arrays. However, it is starting to be implemented in the discovery step as this resource combined with automated quantification instruments are becoming more available

TMA are frequently generated from FFPE. Therefore, large pathologic repositories of tumor samples with high quality clinical annotation and long follow up could be used for validation studies. It is also possible to construct TMAs from frozen samples, although the technical complexity of using a cryostat has limited its application. TMAs are able to combine 40–800 samples in the same slide allowing to multiplex the detection of different biomarkers at the same. This fact also has implications related with standardization of antibody concentrations and processing of samples, so TMA are reducing the variability observed in former large pathologic studies due to batch effects. Initially samples have to be inspected by an expert pathologist to determine which areas of interest from the tissue block will be included in the TMA. Then cores of tissue are extracted from a donor paraffin block and placed in a recipient paraffin block. This block is subsequently sectioned on a microtome generating a tissue slide. Therefore, a complete and correct annotation of the samples arrayed is essential for a successful interpretation. Finally, a major challenge for pathologist has been generating an accurate quantification of a marker from TMA histospots that can be correlated with expression values in a continuous scale. Automated systems recently developed such as the AQUA platform that uses multicolor immunofluorescent histochemistry generates a value for histospot that is being stained. A critical point in the automated reading of TMAs is that antibody titers could have profound effects on the association between the expression of a biomarker and a clinical outcome. This resource will improve the interpretation and the application of immunohistochemistry to larger cohort of samples.

TMA technology has several major advantages [33]. First, TMAs provide a prospective assessment of hundreds of samples at the same time as pathologists select representative tumor areas without an a priori knowledge of the distribution of the staining or antibodies that will be used later. Second, this technology is high-throughput, so a large number of samples can be handled and assayed simultaneously. Third, the reduction of variability and the increase of reproducibility are notorious; all samples are probed against antibodies or other hybridization methods at the same time using the same concentrations and sharing the exact same experimental setting. Likewise, visualization of staining, results and data recording are performed in parallel. Fourth, this process allows multiple validation studies coming from the same TMA, thus saving time and reducing costs compared to the same study performed with conventional whole-sections. This technology obviously has several pitfalls. TMAs depend largely in the quality of the tissue of origin, so factors such as sample processing, storage and retrieval of tissues are important. Other weakness depend on the use of appropriated validated antibodies, the establishment of standard laboratory procedures for handling TMAs and appropriately trained personnel with technical skills required to built the TMAs.

Finally, MALDI-TOF and these related techniques have been mainly applied to the study of peptides or proteins. However, recently it has also been implemented to study nucleic acids. This has been possible due to the improvement in sample preparation procedures that avoid the formation of adducts in the negatively charged backbone structure of nucleic acids. In addition, implementation of these techniques using a high-throughput powerflow has leaded to commercial development and increasing interest among the scientific community, There are commercial platforms based on this principle such as Sequenom that are now enabling researchers to perform SNP genotyping, DNA sequencing, gene expression studies and microsatellite analysis using the same resource [34] (a complete description on the technical aspects behind these platforms can be found in ref. [34]).

Integration of Data Generated from Different Experimental Platforms: The Challenge for Bioinformatics

All of these technological advances would not have impacted so decisively in the molecular biology of cancer without the concurrent development of bioinformatic tools and also without the appearance of a new discipline called integromics. Tumor samples can now be characterized for changes in gene expression and CNVs, the presence of SNP variants, and for comprehensive mutational panel. The future of cancer biology rests on the integration of all these layers of information in an adequate way and the development of tools to mine this vast amount of information.

The first example about how to mine information successfully appeared after the generalization of expression array studies. It was obvious since the beginning that mRNA expression arrays were dealing with a large amount of expression information generated from a relative low number of samples [26]. A part from the challenges behind a correct biostatistical interpretation that we have outlined previously, it is also notorious the fact that simple observation of upregulated and downregulated probes do not provide enough insights about the identification of deregulated pathway in tumor subtypes or phenotypes. Therefore, systems biology tools such as gene set enrichment analysis (GSEA) enable us to cross-match this information with data describing the behavior of protein "actors" in different pathways [35] and also providing a quantification of the level of confidence of these assessment. In addition a huge effort updating the annotation of the pathways deposited in public repositories has been recently accomplished. Therefore, public databases like GO, KEGG, Biocarta, and others have been improved with new entries and documented more solidly to verify the information provided by them. All together has helped to reinforce the process of pathway analysis [36].

There are many other systems biology tools that have appeared on the scene. Here we highlight the "Connectivity Map" because it is a resource that may be important in developmental therapeutics. Briefly it helps to relate the expression data from cell lines treated with more than 1,500 compounds with gene profiles defining a tumor subtype, phenotype, or other query signature using the GSEA [37]. We are now starting to see new studies arising based on this tools that have successfully identified pathways and new drugs to be investigated in new tumor contexts. One example is the development of a clinical trial assessing the effect of Cytarabine in Ewing Sarcoma patients based on the results obtained from the application of the principle of the "Connectivity Map." Cytarabine was found to modulate in vitro the expression patterns of the EWS/FLI1 fusion protein which is present in approximately 95% of Ewing Sarcoma cases [38]. Although the phase I/II based on this finding was negative, it represents the first fast transition of a concept derived from the integration of expression data in silico to in vitro/in vivo and then to clinical investigation [39]. Also it remind us that more work needs to be done before finding the best way to interpret and apply gene expression data stratified by molecular tumor subtype to the field of developmental therapeutics. Other platform that is able to relate gene expression information in order to discover new relations between tumor subtypes and targeted therapies or between tumor subtypes and new mutational events that may be mechanistically related is the Oncomine platform [40]. This systems biology tools has been developed by the group led by Arul Chinnaiyan at the University of Michigan which has also pioneered the discovery of protein fusions in epithelial tumors. Starting from the study of gene outliers in expression data and developing algorithms in silico to find candidate genes to be rearranged, this group identified successfully protein fusions in prostate cancer such as those between *TMPRSS2* and *ERG* or *ETV1* [41]. The initial bioinformatic approach was further validated by using other techniques such as FISH and qPCR. This study has revitalized the search of protein fusions in epithelial cancers and it is a demonstration that chromosomal aberrations could be a major genetic event in solid tumors [42]. In addition this example illustrate how bioinformatic data is useful for hypothesis generation and how validation studies are performed with technologies that are different to the ones used in the discovery step.

Conclusions

Despite of the increasing number of biomarker studies published in the literature in the last years very few of them have been approved by the FDA [27]. This concept has been called the "biomarker paradox" and gives a clear picture of the current situation of research in this field: a highly active research community with poor translation in the clinical arena. Furthermore as we have detailed in Table 17.1 many new molecular biology tools have been developed and may be the source for new biomarker studies such as epigenetics, metabolomics, circulating tumor cells and pharmacogenomic markers. Therefore, a more profound knowledge of discovery techniques by clinical investigators may help to develop new studies to be performed in parallel to drug development initiatives. This fact is especially relevant for clinical investigation in oncology where molecular subclassification is demonstrating everyday that better selection of patients may render improvements in survival for patients. This concept constitutes the "pharmaceutical industry nightmare" which restricts the number of patients that are being treated with a drug to only those that will derive a clear benefit based on new predictive biomarkers [28]. The level of technical complexity of these technologies is substantially high, so clinicians need to collaborate closely with molecular biologists involved in these field and have clear idea of the biology principles behind every of these tools. In addition, large-scale arrays need to be complemented with complex bioinformatics development to distinguish those candidates among thousands of signals. Therefore, an exciting future is now open in the biomarker discovery arena with many challenges but also opportunities in the horizon.

Acknowledgements Eduardo Vilar was supported by a fellowship from "la Caixa," Barcelona, Spain.

References

1. Biomarkers Definitions Working Group. Biomarkers and surrogate endpoints: preferred definitions and conceptual framework. Clin Pharmacol Ther. 2001;69(3):89–95.
2. Chau CH, Rixe O, McLeod H, Figg WD. Validation of analytic methods for biomarkers used in drug development. Clin Cancer Res. 2008;14(19):5967–76.
3. Wood LD, Parsons DW, Jones S, et al. The genomic landscapes of human breast and colorectal cancers. Science. 2007;318(5853):1108–13.
4. Jimeno A, Messersmith WA, Hirsch FR, Franklin WA, Eckhardt SG. KRAS mutations and sensitivity to epidermal growth factor receptor inhibitors in colorectal cancer: practical application of patient selection. J Clin Oncol. 2009;27(7):1130–6.
5. Amado RG, Wolf M, Peeters M, et al. Wild-type KRAS is required for panitumumab efficacy in patients with metastatic colorectal cancer. J Clin Oncol. 2008;26(10):1626–34.
6. Gschwind A, Fischer OM, Ullrich A. The discovery of receptor tyrosine kinases: targets for cancer therapy. Nat Rev Cancer. 2004;4(5):361–70.
7. Strebhardt K, Ullrich A. Paul Ehrlich's magic bullet concept: 100 years of progress. Nat Rev Cancer. 2008;8(6):473–80.
8. Strausberg RL, Levy S, Rogers YH. Emerging DNA sequencing technologies for human genomic medicine. Drug Discov Today. 2008;13(13–14):569–77.
9. Shendure JA, Porreca GJ, Church GM. Overview of DNA sequencing strategies. Curr Protoc Mol Biol. 2008;Chapter 7, Unit 71.
10. Sjoblom T, Jones S, Wood LD, et al. The consensus coding sequences of human breast and colorectal cancers. Science. 2006;314(5797):268–74.
11. Jones S, Zhang X, Parsons DW, et al. Core signaling pathways in human pancreatic cancers revealed by global genomic analyses. Science. 2008;321(5897):1801–6.
12. Parsons DW, Jones S, Zhang X, et al. An integrated genomic analysis of human glioblastoma multiforme. Science. 2008;321(5897):1807–12.
13. Rogers YH, Venter JC. Genomics: massively parallel sequencing. Nature. 2005;437(7057): 326–7.
14. Voelkerding KV, Dames SA, Durtschi JD. Next-generation sequencing: from basic research to diagnostics. Clin Chem. 2009;55(4):641–58.
15. Dutt A, Beroukhim R. Single nucleotide polymorphism array analysis of cancer. Curr Opin Oncol. 2007;19(1):43–9.
16. Syvanen AC. Toward genome-wide SNP genotyping. Nat Genet. 2005;37(Suppl):S5–10.
17. Gudmundsson J, Sulem P, Manolescu A, et al. Genome-wide association study identifies a second prostate cancer susceptibility variant at 8q24. Nat Genet. 2007;39(5):631–7.

18. Tomlinson I, Webb E, Carvajal-Carmona L, et al. A genome-wide association scan of tag SNPs identifies a susceptibility variant for colorectal cancer at 8q24.21. Nat Genet. 2007;39(8): 984–8.
19. Pomerantz MM, Ahmadiyeh N, Jia L, et al. The 8q24 cancer risk variant rs6983267 shows long-range interaction with MYC in colorectal cancer. Nat Genet. 2009;41(8):882–4.
20. Katagiri F, Glazebrook J. Overview of mRNA expression profiling using DNA microarrays. Curr Protoc Mol Biol. 2009;Chapter 22, Unit 22.4.
21. Hardiman G. Microarray platforms—comparisons and contrasts. Pharmacogenomics. 2004;5(5):487–502.
22. Velculescu VE, Vogelstein B, Kinzler KW. Analysing uncharted transcriptomes with SAGE. Trends Genet. 2000;16(10):423–5.
23. Porter D, Yao J, Polyak K. SAGE and related approaches for cancer target identification. Drug Discov Today. 2006;11(3–4):110–8.
24. Brazma A, Hingamp P, Quackenbush J, et al. Minimum information about a microarray experiment (MIAME)—toward standards for microarray data. Nat Genet. 2001;29(4):365–71.
25. Benjamini Y, Hochberg Y. Controlling the false discovery rate: a practical and powerful approach to multiple testing. J Roy Statist Soc Ser B. 1995;57:289–300.
26. Ioannidis JP. Microarrays and molecular research: noise discovery? Lancet. 2005;365(9458): 454–5.
27. Ludwig JA, Weinstein JN. Biomarkers in cancer staging, prognosis and treatment selection. Nat Rev Cancer. 2005;5(11):845–56.
28. Omenn GS. Strategies for plasma proteomic profiling of cancers. Proteomics. 2006;6(20): 5662–73.
29. Sanchez-Carbayo M. Antibody arrays: technical considerations and clinical applications in cancer. Clin Chem. 2006;52(9):1651–9.
30. Alessandro R, Belluco C, Kohn EC. Proteomic approaches in colon cancer: promising tools for new cancer markers and drug target discovery. Clin Colorectal Cancer. 2005;4(6): 396–402.
31. Wulfkuhle JD, Liotta LA, Petricoin EF. Proteomic applications for the early detection of cancer. Nat Rev Cancer. 2003;3(4):267–75.
32. Takikita M, Chung JY, Hewitt SM. Tissue microarrays enabling high-throughput molecular pathology. Curr Opin Biotechnol. 2007;18(4):318–25.
33. Camp RL, Neumeister V, Rimm DL. A decade of tissue microarrays: progress in the discovery and validation of cancer biomarkers. J Clin Oncol. 2008;26(34):5630–7.
34. Jurinke C, Oeth P, van den Boom D. MALDI-TOF mass spectrometry: a versatile tool for high-performance DNA analysis. Mol Biotechnol. 2004;26(2):147–64.
35. Subramanian A, Tamayo P, Mootha VK, et al. Gene set enrichment analysis: a knowledge-based approach for interpreting genome-wide expression profiles. Proc Natl Acad Sci USA. 2005;102(43):15545–50.
36. Adriaens ME, Jaillard M, Waagmeester A, Coort SL, Pico AR, Evelo CT. The public road to high-quality curated biological pathways. Drug Discov Today. 2008;13(19–20):856–62.
37. Lamb J. The connectivity map: a new tool for biomedical research. Nat Rev Cancer. 2007;7(1):54–60.
38. Stegmaier K, Wong JS, Ross KN, et al. Signature-based small molecule screening identifies cytosine arabinoside as an EWS/FLI modulator in Ewing sarcoma. PLoS Med. 2007;4(4):e122.
39. Steven GD, Mark DK, Stephen LL, et al. Phase II study of intermediate-dose cytarabine in patients with relapsed or refractory Ewing sarcoma: a report from the Children's Oncology Group. Pediatr Blood Cancer. 2009;52(3):324–7.
40. Rhodes DR, Kalyana-Sundaram S, Tomlins SA, et al. Molecular concepts analysis links tumors, pathways, mechanisms, and drugs. Neoplasia. 2007;9(5):443–54.
41. Tomlins SA, Rhodes DR, Perner S, et al. Recurrent Fusion of TMPRSS2 and ETS Transcription Factor Genes in Prostate Cancer. Science. 2005;310(5748):644–8.
42. Kumar-Sinha C, Tomlins SA, Chinnaiyan AM. Evidence of recurrent gene fusions in common epithelial tumors. Trends Mol Med. 2006;12(11):529–36.

Chapter 18
Biomarkers for Go/No Go Decisions

Ben Markman and Josep Tabernero

Background

Drug discovery and development in medical oncology is a process that was developed primarily for traditional cytotoxic agents that have formed the backbone of systemic cancer therapies for several decades. It is based on the premise that more is better, at least in terms of antineoplastic effect, and therefore toxicity is the factor setting the ceiling on administrable dose.

The process deserves more detailed explanation because it is still the framework that is used as a standard even though the playing field has shifted somewhat. Drug discovery begins with the identification and assessment of lead compounds from a larger pool of candidates. This laboratory phase is based on physiological and pharmacological parameters. Preclinical evaluation then follows in studies conducted in cell lines and animal models, including toxicity studies, in an attempt to match as closely as possible the conditions to be encountered when the drug enters human trials. Unfortunately, despite best intentions, these models are not a perfect fit and often interspecies differences can lead to unexpected or idiosyncratic reactions.

A compound that ticks all the necessary boxes through the discovery process progresses to clinical evaluation in human subjects. This typically involves three core phases. Phase I trials seek to answer the question "is the drug safe." The primary objectives are to determine the maximum tolerated dose (MTD), the dose limiting

B. Markman, M.B.B.S., F.R.A.C.P.
Monash Institute of Medical Research, Monash University,
27-31 Wright St, Clayton, Victoria, 3168 Australia
e-mail: ben.markman@monash.edu.au

J. Tabernero, M.D. (✉)
Department of Medical Oncology Service, Vall d'Hebron University Hospital,
Ps. Vall d'Hebron 119-129, Barcelona 08035, Spain
e-mail: jtabernero@vhio.net

H.-J. Lenz (ed.), *Biomarkers in Oncology: Prediction and Prognosis*,
DOI 10.1007/978-1-4419-9755-5_18, © Springer Science+Business Media New York 2013

toxicities (DLTs) and the recommended phase II dose (RP2D). Phase II trials seek to answer the question "does the drug work." The primary objective is to show preliminary antitumor activity, together with ongoing safety analyses. Phase III trials seek to answer the question "does the drug perform better than the current standard-of-care." The primary objective is to demonstrate an improvement in a predefined survival parameter when compared to what is considered to be the current gold standard. If this can be objectively shown, then application for drug registration is submitted with the intention of achieving regulatory approval by the relevant government bodies, otherwise known as the approval phase. Postmarketing surveillance, a less stringently defined phase IV, exists to monitor for and report any rare but important toxicities that may have gone undetected during the initial three phases of clinical development.

Flaws in the System

This process of sequential phases is lengthy, costly and inefficient. At the start of this decade, the mean clinical and approval phase length for all small molecule drugs approved in the United States (US) was 82 months (having peaked in the late 1980s at 122 months), with antineoplastic agents amongst the slowest [1]. This is not taking into consideration the discovery and preclinical phases that invariably add many more years to the duration, implying a total requirement of some 8–12 years. Monetary costs are also high. It has been estimated that approximately US$700–1,700 million is required to complete a drug development program [2].

Significant investment of time and resources is readily justified from an industry perspective when returns are adequate and secure. A major difficulty in drug discovery is the inefficiency and hence risk inherent to the process. The US Food and Drug Administration (FDA) estimated that the likelihood of a new compound entering phase I clinical evaluation has only an 8% chance of reaching the market [3]. This compares with 14% in 1985. In other words, despite all our innovations and advances, the success rate for drug approval in no greater now than 25 years ago. Other analyses are similarly disappointing. The success rates for compounds passing from first-in-man studies to registration during 1991–2000 for ten big pharmaceutical companies in the US and Europe was 11% for all therapeutic areas [4]. Attrition rates in oncology were particularly poor with a miserly success rate of 5%. Failure occurred at all stages of development. Attrition of compounds entering phase I and II assessment in oncology is approximately 60% and more than 70%, respectively. Even in the more advanced settings these figures are disturbingly high. Of new compounds entering phase III, 45% overall and 59% in oncology fail. And for drugs successfully completing all three phases of clinical development, a staggering 23% overall and 30% in oncology fail to be registered, despite the investment of the magnitude previously described by the sponsoring companies.

These unsettling figures beg an important question: why are the attrition rates so high? In the early 1990s, the primary causes for drug failure centered on adverse pharmacokinetics (PK) and bioavailability results (~40%). Recognition of these problems allowed effective solutions—by 2000 they accounted for less than 10%. The major causes of the last 10 years have been lack of efficacy (30%) and safety issues (30%) [4]. Another important consideration is the type of agents entering development, which in recent times has reflected the rise of targeted therapies.

Targeted Therapies

Targeted therapies are drugs or other substances that block the growth and spread of cancer by interfering with specific molecules involved in tumor growth and progression. We now have a far more advanced understanding of the complex cellular biology of cancer and the multiple signaling pathways that play a crucial role in the malignant process. This enables the identification of key switches or nodes, potentially druggable, in pathways contributing to traits considered the hallmarks of cancer. Often these are either not present in normal cells or are altered or functioning at a subnormal or supranormal level. By exploiting such differences between malignant and nonmalignant cells, targeted therapies seek to maximize benefits whilst minimizing toxicities. This contrasts with the more traditional cytotoxic chemotherapy that damages DNA and therefore nonspecifically targets all dividing cells, narrows the therapeutic index, and increases the side effect profile.

Though the use of targeted agents is not new, there is an undoubted boom in research and development that has been and continues to be invested in this arena. Categories include tyrosine kinase inhibitors, small molecules, monoclonal antibodies, and antisense oligonucleotides, amongst others. A number of these have now found their place in the therapeutic armamentarium available to the medical oncologist (see Table 18.1).

But despite all their promise, few novel agents have achieved registration to date. One study examined the likelihood of transition through the various stages of development for 137 kinase inhibitors for use in oncology over the period 1995–2007 [5]. The probability rates were 0.80, 0.69 and 0.85 for phase I–II, phase II–III, and phase III-market, indicating a 53% overall attrition rate. This compared favorably to the total cohort of 974 oncology drugs (attrition rate 82%), but clearly leaves considerable room for improvement. This study also demonstrated that kinase inhibitors had improved timelines, reaching the market about 21 months faster. The causes suggested for these improvements with kinase inhibitors related to clinical trial design, patient stratification, representative animal models and the use of biomarkers. However, targeted agents not classified as kinase inhibitors were not included in this analysis. Irrespective, it demonstrates how new classes of drugs with novel mechanisms-of-action can impact the drug development process. The next question is how.

Table 18.1 Targeted therapies approved for clinical use*

Drug	Type of agents	Target/s	Indication
Cetuximab	Monoclonal antibody	EGFR	Metastatic CRC, SCCHN
Panitumumab	Monoclonal antibody	EGFR	Metastatic CRC
Erlotinib	Tyrosine kinase inhibitor	EGFR	Advanced NSCLC, advanced pancreatic cancer
Gefitinib	Tyrosine kinase inhibitor	EGFR	Advanced NSCLC[a]
Trastuzumab	Monoclonal antibody	HER2	Breast cancer
Lapatanib	Tyrosine kinase inhibitor	EGFR, HER2	Advanced breast cancer
Bevacizumab	Monoclonal antibody	VEGF	Metastatic CRC, advanced NSCLC, metastatic breast cancer, metastatic RCC, glioblastoma[b]
Rituximab	Monoclonal antibody	CD20	NHL, CLL[a]
Imatinib	Tyrosine kinase inhibitor	KIT, BCR-ABL, PDGFR	GIST, Ph+CML, Ph+ALL
Sunitinib	Tyrosine kinase inhibitor	VEGFR 1,2,3, PDGFR α(alpha)/β(beta), KIT, FLT-3, RET	GIST, advanced RCC
Sorafenib	Tyrosine kinase inhibitor	CRAF, BRAF, VEGFR 1,2,3, KIT, FLT-3, PDGFRβ(beta), RET	Advanced RCC, unresectable HCC
Temsirolimus	Small molecule	mTOR	Advanced RCC
Everolimus	Small molecule	mTOR	Advanced RCC[b]
Dasatinib	Tyrosine kinase inhibitor	BCR-ABL, SRC family, KIT, PDGFRβ(beta)	Ph+CML, Ph+ALL
Bortezomib	Small molecule	26S Proteasome	Multiple myeloma, mantle cell lymphoma[b]
Alemtuzumab	Monoclonal antibody	CD52	B-CLL

[a]only EMEA
[b]only FDA
CRC - colorectal cancer, SCCHN - squamous cell cancer of the head and neck, NSCLC - non-small cell lung cancer, RCC- renal cell carncimona, NHL - non-Hodgkins lymphoma, CLL - chronic lymphocytic leukemia, GIST - gastrointestinal stromal tumor, Ph+ - Philadelphia chromosome (bcr-abl) positive, HCC - hepatocellular carcinoma
*Approvals as of late 2009

Reducing Attrition

Other than questioning why attrition rates are so high, the other key concern is how to reduce failure rates in oncology drug development. Each step of the process has potential for improvements. But ideally, weeding out the good from the bad earlier rather than later will be of greater benefit.

In the discovery phase focused in the laboratory, we need to demonstrate strong proof-of-concept (PoC). Specifically, the intended target must be demonstrable, shown to be relevant to the signaling pathway of interest, and the tumor needs a degree of dependency upon the target. If pathway crosstalk and feedback exists then pharmacological inhibition of a redundant target is likely to be ineffective. In the transition from the basic science to preclinical phases of development, early attempts to identify potential toxicity are important. This can involve techniques such as gene knockouts and RNA interference to assess to impact on the health of cells, and pre-clinical toxicology studies are imperative prior to human testing. For improved physiologic relevance, the animal models chosen to study tumor biology and drug efficacy need to be as representative as possible. Despite their relative ease, xeno-graft models provide a comparatively artificial platform. Though more time-consuming and technically challenging, genetic animal models (transgenic or knockout animals) are an improvement. Unfortunately, oncology is one of the areas where animal models of efficacy are notoriously unpredictable [6].

In an attempt to overcome some of the limitations of animal models, recently designated phase 0 trials have emerged. Otherwise known as human microdosing studies, these exploratory, first-in-man studies are intended to speed up the development process by establishing very early on whether the new agent behaves in human subjects as was expected from animal studies. Phase 0 studies involve the administration of a single subtherapeutic dose to a limited number of patients. Endpoints include extensive agent characterization, especially PK parameters, and target-assay development, including molecular imaging studies. They give no data on safety or efficacy, being by definition a dose too low to cause therapeutic effect. Such studies may be carried out to rank promising new candidate molecules according to those which have the best PK profiles in humans. They therefore enable go/no-go decisions based on relevant human models instead of relying on inconsistent animal data [7].

Biomarkers are also playing an increasing role as new drugs under investigation enter the early phases of clinical development. Biomarker objectives include assisting in PoC and dosing issues in phase I, and in target population selection in phase I and II (discussed below). The large and costly phase III studies need appropriate designs, including relevant statistical considerations, prior to initiation. And early discontinuation of development for commercial reasons must also be factored into this complex equation. We will now turn our attention to biomarkers.

Biomarkers

The US National Institutes of Health Biomarkers Definitions Working Group defined a biomarker as "a characteristic that is objectively measured and evaluated as an indicator of normal biological processes, pathogenic processes, or pharmacologic responses to a therapeutic intervention" [8]. This broad definition provides a starting point but little framework for practical use. Subtypes of biomarkers are therefore described to improve utility and clarity. These are not mutually exclusive as any given biomarker can serve multiple purposes simultaneously. They can be defined as prognostic, predictive/resistance, pharmacodynamic (PD) and surrogate biomarkers (summarized in Table 18.2).

Prognostic biomarkers are implicated in mechanisms of disease causality or the oncologic process, such as the risk of developing a disease, its spread or aggressiveness, or survival rates. They are usually not modulated or influenced by treatment intervention. Predictive biomarkers predict the efficacy (or lack thereof for the case

Table 18.2 Types of biomarkers and their functions

Type	Function
Pharmacodynamic	Target inhibition, cellular effects
	Evaluate MoA
	PK/PD modelling: schedule/dose
	OBD
Surrogate	Registrational endpoints
Prognostic	Predicts course of disease independent of treatment
Predictive	Identification of patients likely to respond
	Identification of patients likely to suffer adverse events
Resistance	Identification of patients with resistance: primary or acquired

MoA mechanism of action, *PK* pharmacokinetic, *PD* pharmacodynamic, *OBD* optimal biologic dose

of resistance biomarkers) of a particular treatment in a given clinical scenario. They thus can improve patient selection for a treatment based on the likelihood of benefit or alternatively minimize the chance of a patient being exposed to toxicities when there is little chance the therapy will be of value. In addition, the capacity to predict can also refer to toxicities, in which case a drug may either be withheld or administered at a reduced dose (without insinuating that the individual is resistant). Pharmacodynamic (PD) biomarkers are markers of drug effect. They imply assessment prior to and following an intervention to detect a change from baseline. They characterize molecular and functional effects of a drug. A correlation with clinical activity is not implied. Surrogate markers similarly demonstrate treatment modulation but in nontumor tissue. If a strong correlation between PD effects in the tumor and surrogate material can be shown then the latter may serve as an effective alternative to monitor for drug effect. As for PD biomarkers, a relation between surrogate markers and clinical endpoints is not necessarily found but this is the ultimate goal.

Current techniques employed to identify potential biomarkers are enormous and varied. They can assess chromosomes (cytogenetics), DNA (direct sequencing), RNA (gene expression signatures generated using high throughput microarray analyses), and proteins (proteomics, crystallography, immunohistochemistry). Whereas these biomarkers look at specific changes at a cellular or molecular level, imaging techniques can be considered to evaluate a more physiological composite endpoint (positron emission tomography (PET) scans and dynamic magnetic resonance imaging are examples). Finally, clinical endpoints are also potentially useful as biomarkers.

Criteria that make a biomarker valuable include a sound scientific base such that it is mechanistically understood, can be measured reproducibly with high sensitivity and specificity in the desired tissue type, and has a clinically relevant impact on treatment or outcomes. In oncology, there have been a few important wins that serve to illustrate their desired utility and lead to considerable optimism for their use. The earliest example extends back 30 years to the biochemical detection of the estrogen receptor (ER) on breast tumors; assessment of hormone receptor status has long since been an integral part of the pathologic description of this type of cancer as it is the primary determinant for response to tamoxifen and other hormonal treatments. Similarly in breast cancer, measurement of the HER2 status (also known as erbB2) by immunohistochemistry or in situ hybridization techniques is routine, as positivity predicts for response to anti-HER2 therapies such as the monoclonal antibody trastuzumab. In chronic myeloid leukemia, demonstration of the Philadelphia chromosome (cytogenetics) or BCR-ABL (quantitative real time polymerase chain reaction) predicts for response to imatinib mesylate, a potent and specific inhibitor of the bcr-abl tyrosine kinase. PET scans are now employed as a PD biomarker of response in lymphoma, such that a failure to achieve a complete metabolic response can result in a change of therapy. And most recently, determination of KRAS status, in particular codon 12 and 13 mutations, has been recommended prior to initiation of monoclonal antibodies targeting EGFR (cetuximab, panitumumab) in metastatic colorectal cancer, as the presence of mutations predicts for resistance to these therapies.

On face value, these examples afford much reason for optimism and support for the use of biomarkers in drug development. After all, they have had a permanent impact on treatment decisions for these disease entities that ultimately translates into patient benefits. In reality, the road to successful biomarker identification, validation, and implementation is fraught with difficulties and uncertainties.

The Biomarker Hypothesis

The theory is that early investment (phase I–II) in biomarkers will accelerate development time lines and reduce costs for novel agents entering the system. It will increase the probability of registrational success through increased scientific understanding of the drug, target and pathway by demonstrating proof of mechanism-of-action, proof of mechanism-of-resistance (primary and secondary), and by PD exploration to assist in choosing the right schedule and dose. Additionally, it will permit focused clinical studies with higher probability of establishing benefit through adaptive study designs and prospective screening of patients for enrolment. But taking this theory further, it suggests that effective use of biomarkers can assist those involved in drug development to make go/no-go decisions. In other words, biomarkers can lead to early rational choices as to the value of pursuing a drug along its maturation process or admitting defeat where an agent is destined to fail.

So are biomarkers indeed assisting us with such go/no go decisions? Goulart et al. performed a comprehensive assessment of the trends in biomarker usage in phase I trials [9]. Of all phase I abstracts submitted during the period 1991–2002 to the American Society of Clinical Oncology (ASCO), 20% (503 of 2,458) included biomarker studies, a proportion that significantly increased over time. The strongest determinant for inclusion of biomarker studies was drug class, with trials of targeted therapies far more likely to incorporate these elements than those of cytotoxic treatments. Of these abstracts, only the 87 that were subsequently published as peer-reviewed articles were subject to further scrutiny. The authors found that biomarker studies contributed to dose selection and schedule selection for phase II studies in 13 and 8%, respectively. However, in 86 of the 87 trials, endpoints for safety/toxicity (MTDs, DLTs) and efficacy (responses) were the defining factors for dose and schedule selection. Therefore, in only one study was information from biomarkers used directly to reach these goals. Additionally, in 39% of trials the biomarkers provided evidence of mechanism-of-action, in 13% they were used to select a patient population for phase I enrolment and in 19% they were considered to be potentially useful for selecting a patient population for subsequent studies.

Though this study does not include studies beyond 2002, a period in which biomarker usage has continued to rise, and the authors definition of biomarkers is tighter than the standard (where clinical criteria are included), the findings provide some initial insights in that we are not hitting the mark with biomarkers as optimally as desired.

Functions of Biomarker Use

Mechanism of Action

It would appear logical that providing evidence that a drug is performing its intended function on a molecular level is a basic requirement; should it fail to do so, a "no go" decision would be imminent. However, this is based on the assumption that we truly understand the target and the pathway and thus effects that any pharmacological intervention would incur.

Unfortunately, for all our progress, our knowledge is far from complete. In addition, mechanistic proof of drug action can be difficult to convincingly determine. Consider the epidermal growth factor (EGFR), a target rationally selected for use in colorectal cancer based on sound preclinical data relating to its role in tumorigensis and its association with aggressive disease and poor prognosis. Many trials of anti-EGFR antibodies therefore used EGFR positivity by immunohistochemistry (IHC) as a criterion for patient selection. However, it has been consistently reported from clinical studies that EGFR protein expression levels by IHC correlate poorly with response to these antibodies [10, 11]. Others have demonstrated clinical response rates of up to 25% in patients whose tumors do not express EGFR by IHC [12]. Therefore, should signal have been weak in early studies, this may have led to premature and inappropriate curtailment of development. Results were strong enough to achieve registration; however, drugs such as cetuximab are likely being withheld in patients who could still benefit.

Subsequent research points to other biomarkers, such as *KRAS* and *BRAF* gene status as well as the expression levels of some of the naturally occurring EGFR ligands, as genuine predictors of response or resistance [13–15]. To understand this, consider that under normal circumstances, the membrane-bound EGFR is activated by endogenous ligands, signaling sequentially through RAS to RAF, which passes signal to MEK and ultimately to ERK, which enters the nucleus to activated transcription factors, altering the regulation of key genes. The EGFR monoclonal antibodies cetuximab and panitumumab target the extracellular domain of the receptor tyrosine kinase. In the presence of mutations affecting downstream RAS or RAF, these elements become constitutively activated, implying ongoing signal transduction irrespective of pharmacological inhibition of the upstream receptor. This improved understanding has been practice changing.

Targeting EGFR has run into similar uncertainties with the use of tyrosine kinase inhibitors, specifically erlotinib and gefitinib, in non-small-cell lung cancer (NSCLC). EGFR is a critical tumorigenic factor in the development and progression of NSCLC and is overexpressed in a majority of patients with this cancer. However, in studies of unselected patients the overall response rate is only about 10% [16]. Certain characteristics have been associated with higher response rates, in particular female patients, non-smokers, East Asian ethnicity and adenocarcinoma histology. It was subsequently determined that two activating mutations (deletion in exon 19 and L858R substitution) have a striking correlation with EGFR-TKI sensitivity. They are also more commonly detected in patients with the characteristics described above. Prospective phase II studies confirmed clinical benefit rates of about 90% when patients were selected based on the presence of these mutations [17, 18]. More recently, phase III data have demonstrated superior progression free survival with gefitinib over chemotherapy for the first-line treatment of NSCLC when patients entered were nonsmokers or light ex-smokers with adenocarcinoma, with even more striking benefits for those with EGFR activating mutations [19]. This improved understanding of the mechanism of action (MoA) of these agents has led to the European Medical Agency (EMEA) to approve gefitinib for use in locally advanced or metastatic NSCLC with activating mutations of EGFR.

In both of these examples—monoclonal antibodies and TKIs targeting EGFR—ongoing translational research efforts have continued to enlighten us about important mechanistic details. This highly credible work has ultimately led to better patient selection and improved outcomes.

Proof of Concept

Biomarkers can also be used to demonstrate PoC in cases where new drugs or drug classes are administered in new clinical settings to provide evidence of the desired biologic consequence or activity, not only to reassure investigators but also to provide impetus to the development process. It does not imply ascertainment of, but can be associated with, MoA. In common with MoA biomarkers, they principally fall into the PD biomarker category.

Despite preclinical support for targeting the mammalian target of rapamycin (mTOR) as cancer therapy, monotherapy with mTOR inhibitors has not reaped the expected rewards. Based on laboratory work indicating that tumors with functional loss of the tumor suppressor PTEN should be sensitized to mTOR inhibition, a PoC study was designed to demonstrate activity of rapamycin in PTEN null glioblastomas [20]. Paired tumor samples were obtained pre- and post-treatment. They found reduced tumor cell proliferation, the magnitude of which was associated with the degree of mTOR inhibition (measured by levels of activation of the downstream biomarker S6 ribosomal protein) more so than PK parameters. Increased activation of the upstream biomarker Akt (due to the loss of negative feedback) was seen in about half of the patients; this was associated with a significantly shorter time to progression. Thus biomarker studies contributed to demonstrating activity of this agent and to the recommendation that mTOR inhibition could be combined with agents targeting upstream elements to prevent potentially undesirable effects of feedback loops.

A phase I study of AZD0530, an oral potent inhibitor of Src kinase, likewise sought to demonstrate PoC [21]. The PD biomarkers pFAK and p-paxillin were selected because their phosphorylation by Src is critical for the migratory phenotype typically induced by pathway activity and had previously been seen in preclinical models. With the demonstration that these biomarkers were inhibited in tumor tissue following AZD0530 administration, the authors concluded that inhibition of Src activity had been effectively shown in human cancers for the first time.

Dose and Schedule Selection

Dose and schedule selection are typical study objectives from phase I trials. They are traditionally linked to the MTD and safety data as well as PK parameters. Antitumor effects can also contribute although the absence of signal at this early stage does not rule out further development. For cytotoxic agents, the choice is tightly linked with the highest dose that has acceptable toxicity. But targeted therapies have substantially different and unique side effect profiles, which are often milder and with little dose-dependent organ toxicity. Consequent to their good tolerability, an MTD based on DLTs may not be reached. Therefore, targeted, noncytotoxic anticancer agents pose challenges to the current phase I paradigm of dose selection based on toxicity and alternative measures are required. Despite this need, a recent study found that the majority of phase I studies continue to use traditional endpoints of toxicity and PK data for selection of the recommended phase II dose [22]. Novel endpoints were not routinely incorporated into the study design and rarely formed the primary basis for dose selection.

More research is needed to define suitable molecular measures of drug effect and the means to incorporate them in the early drug development process. Researchers in the field now speak of the "optimal biologic dose," which is a dose that reliably achieves a target plasma concentration or inhibits a drug target. PK parameters can shed light on the former, while PD biomarker studies help determine the latter; a combination of both PK and PD data is likely to provide the most robust solution. A phase I study of the mTOR rapalog everolimus (also known as RAD001) provides a pertinent example [23]. The authors collected pre- and on-treatment steady-state tumor and skin biopsies for all patients and evaluated a selection of tissue biomarkers. They reported dose- and schedule-dependent inhibition of the mTOR pathway with near complete and sustained inhibition of the downstream pathway elements pS6K1 and peIF-4G at 10 mg/day and ≥50 mg/week, with good concordance between changes seen in tumor and skin. These doses were also tolerable. With lower doses failing to achieve complete mTOR inhibition, the investigators concluded that these two dose/schedules could be recommended for future study.

Patient Selection

Use of unselected patient populations in the early phases of drug development is common. However, the target of a therapy is often limited to a subset of individuals (which may or may not be linked to a tumor type). Ignoring this is likely to dilute any potential benefits of the agent under investigation. The presence of HER2 overexpression was an entry criterion for trials of trastuzumab in women with breast cancer. Should this not have been requisite, the response rates in an unselected population may not have been sufficiently high to warrant further drug development of an agent that has ultimately impacted enormously on the survival of women with HER2 overexpressing breast cancer.

Despite the clear success of trastuzumab in this selected population, a significant proportion of women fail to respond to the monoclonal antibody. One described mechanism of resistance in a subset of these patients is the presence of a truncated form of the HER2 protein that has lost most of its extracellular domain. Named p95HER2, it is unable to be bound by trastuzumab yet it retains kinase activity and can thus continue to propagate tumor promoting growth signals. On the other hand, lapatinib retains activity against p95HER2 as it targets the intact tyrosine kinase domain of the receptor. In one study of 46 women with metastatic HER2 overexpressing breast cancer treated with trastuzumab, only one of nine patients with p95HER2 achieved a response, whereas 19 of 37 (51%) with the full length protein responded [24]. This demonstrates that greater awareness of resistance mechanisms may help to further improve patient selection.

If we do not understand the target and pathway correctly, limiting treatment to specific subgroups may entirely inappropriate. At present, there is huge interest in the development of inhibitors targeting the PI3K/Akt pathway. This signaling cascade plays a vital role in many aspects of the malignant process, genetic aberration of key pathway elements is frequent in human cancer, and pathway activation leads to resistance to many traditional anticancer agents. Preclinical studies suggest that tumors with constitutive pathway activation—due to genetic changes especially mutations of PI3K and functional loss of PTEN—are most susceptible to PI3K inhibitors. It may therefore appear tempting to limit patient enrolment to only those patients who tumors harbor one of these key aberrations. A number of early phase trials of PI3K inhibitors are presently enrolling many of which have strong biomarker components. To date, clinical responses rates have been disappointing. Interestingly, there is no clear signal that these drugs benefit only those patients with genetic aberration [25, 26]. There are many potential reasons for this—combination therapy may be more effective than the current monotherapy trials, many of the patients are heavily pretreated, the biomarker assays are not validated, not all genetic aberrations are being assessed, and pathway inhibition is incomplete. However, the important point in this context is whether pathway mutations truly predict for response, or conversely, whether the absence of a mutation predicts for resistance. If the former line of thinking is pursued, selection criteria may be refined to improve the likelihood of detecting signal and thus handing investigators the confidence to proceed with development, but at the risk of denying others from a treatment to which they may yet respond. We need to be confident that our understanding of the molecular biology is accurate, but we must also remain vigilant that there may be alternate explanations and that what we encounter in the laboratory may not be reflected in the clinic.

Surrogate Endpoints

Traditional endpoints for anticancer therapies include response rates and survival times. Changes in the anatomical measurement of tumor lesions provide the basis for response criteria. Improved overall survival times are the ultimate goal of anticancer therapy. But survival times are scrutinized more in the later stages of drug development. And because many targeted therapies are cytostatic, response rate is not necessarily the optimal manner to assess success. Investigators are therefore looking for alternate, surrogate endpoints to provide useful measures of drug effect or benefit, and therefore help meet registrational endpoints. Blood, plasma or serum, skin, hair follicles, buccal mucosa, and urine can all provide tissue as a source for surrogate biomarker investigations, as can imaging techniques and clinical measures. These have the advantage that they are relatively easy and noninvasive to acquire. Importantly, if a nontumor tissue or test is going to serve as a surrogate, a strong correlation with intratumoral changes (for drug effect) or with traditional endpoints (for treatment benefit) needs to be demonstrated.

Treatment-induced skin toxicity is common with anti-EGFR antibodies in multiple tumor types, leading to the hypothesis that the presence and severity of skin rash could potentially serve as a surrogate biomarker of treatment efficacy [27, 28]. This was evaluated in the EVEREST trial, a dose-escalation study of cetuximab in mCRC. The investigators found that increasing the treatment dose until rash was at least of moderate severity led to improved outcomes compared to those whose rash was mild or absent [29]. However, it is important to note that even patients without skin toxicity may still achieve clinical benefit.

Agents targeting the vascular endothelial growth factor pathway have been associated with treatment-induced hypertension. Although the precise mechanism leading to an increase in blood pressure is unclear, it has been proposed that the magnitude of the elevation could act as a surrogate of efficacy. This has been investigated in various settings, including with bevacizumab (a VEGF specific blocking monoclonal antibody) in colorectal and breast cancer, and sunitinib (an anti-VEGF receptor TKI, amongst other targets) in metastatic renal cell cancer, and warrants ongoing study [30–32].

Finally, ABT-263 is a novel inhibitor of the antiapoptotic Bcl-2 family proteins. Preclinical toxicities observed decreased circulating platelet survival times that is believed to be mediated by Bcl-XL inhibition. During phase I evaluation, transient and dose-related thrombocytopenia was again documented, consistent with the preclinical models. Because this change was predictable and manageable, the authors concluded that not only was the reduced platelet count providing MoA confirmation, but it was also a PD surrogate of drug effect that could be used to guide adaptive dose-escalation study designs [33].

Answering the Question

Substantial overlap is evident between these various objectives to which biomarker studies can contribute. But what may appear suspicious from the above discussion is that a definite "go" or "no go" decision based on such biomarkers seems lacking. So at present, are biomarkers really answering key questions in the development process?

One difficulty when formulating a response is that the "no go" side of the equation is less transparent in the literature. That is, there is a publication bias towards positive studies (irrespective of biomarker status). If biomarkers have provided some indication that a given drug is not hitting the mark, the wider community may not have the opportunity to learn about why. A negative corollary of this tendency is that due to the inherent competitiveness of the industry, knowledge is frequently not shared. A new biomarker may be under investigation simultaneously at multiple sites. The potentially expensive lesson that it is not of value may need to be learnt many times over due to this secretive nature when time and money could have been redirected to other promising options.

"Go" decisions, on the other hand, may be more reportable, but as discussed, it is rare that a biomarker study is the sole determinant of a drugs fate. They often contribute to important trial objectives. They may have a key role in selecting a dose and schedule in the absence of DLTs and when PK profiles are adequate. Providing evidence of MoA or PoC is reassuring, but is neither necessary nor sufficient. In addition, safety and toxicity will never be ignored in the decision making process. It is true that targeted therapies as a heterogeneous group are considered more tolerable than cytotoxics, but they have brought with them unique side effects that are no less relevant, such as trastuzumab-induced cardiotoxicity or the hypertension, gastrointestinal perforation or thrombotic complications associated with use of bevacizumab. Finally, if a novel compound shows early indications of antitumor activity, ongoing development will ensue irrespective of biomarker data emerging from the trial, even if they are contrary to expectation. They may spur further translational investigations that may ultimately assist in, for example, better selecting a population or help define resistance mechanisms, so they are far from obsolete. But they do not categorically define the "go" decision.

Biomarkers Not Hitting the Mark

Currently, biomarkers are not being extensively developed, though exploration of their use is on the rise. There is, however, substantial potential utility if they are used correctly. It is worth asking why they are underused. The reasons extend beyond questions of "go/no go," as we have seen that they can and do contribute to important decision making, even if more in an ancillary role. Drug development is driven by the pharmaceutical industry. This required enormous investment that needs to be offset by profitability, which in turn depends on drug registration. There is a clear clinical regulatory pathway. A biomarker regulatory pathway is far less certain. Industry is going to continue take the conservative approach and walk the former path simply because it is known and established.

Consider also some of the limitations of early biomarker development. The link between those responsible for drug and biomarker discovery and those in clinical development departments is currently inadequate. Early studies tend to have a much shorter follow up than later phase studies; this in turn caps the information that can be gleaned from biomarker data. The transition through each phase of development through to registration occurs as rapidly as is feasible. Including biomarker studies adds complexity that inevitably slows this process and adds cost. A single institution study conducted over a recent 7 year period showed that the budget cost per subject enrolled onto trials that included biomarkers compared to those that did not was almost double (an additional US$6,675 was required per subject on average) [34]. In addition, early clinical trials are frequently not powered to discover or develop promising biomarkers. Finally, not all drugs necessarily need biomarkers. If a compound has high efficacy, limited resistance and low toxicity, some of the reasons why we might desire a useful biomarker are negated. This is not a negative but may limit further biomarker development.

A key consideration is the lack of standardization and validation of biomarkers. There are multiple agents in various stages of development targeting the insulin-like growth factor receptor (IGF-R) pathway, yet to date strategies to improve patient selection based on biomarker studies have provided confusing data, in part due to the multitude of techniques explored. Perhaps the most promising use for biomarkers with these therapies is the case for Ewing sarcoma. The genetic hallmark of this tumor, present in 85% of patients, is the t(11;22) chromosomal translocation. The resulting EWS-FLI-1 fusion protein is transforming only in the presence of IGF-1R, achieved either by downregulating IGFBP-3, increasing IGF-1 promoter, or both [35]. This dependence on IGF-R pathway elements provides the rationale for treating Ewing sarcoma with this drug class; indeed, multiple responses have been observed in early clinical trials [36]. Despite these encouraging signs of activity, multiple methods are employed to evaluate the presence of the translocation or its resultant protein, including IHC, fluorescence in situ hybridization and polymerase chain reaction techniques.

The case for PTEN assessment is similarly unsatisfactory. It is recognized that mutations of PTEN account for only a proportion of cases leading to functional loss; loss of heterozygozity occurs due to other mechanisms including promoter methylation. Ultimately, researchers need a tool to demonstrate the end result—PTEN functional loss—regardless of the mechanism, for which there is no validated technique. Presently, IHC is widely used to serve this purpose. But cut-offs have not been set for what is considered to be functional loss (complete loss, low level expression?) nor have the choice of antibodies been standardized. Considering PTEN is frequently lost in a broad range of tumor types and that its loss may influence the effectiveness of agents targeting not only PI3K but also HER2 and EGFR, the need for improvement is substantial.

Importantly, acquisition of biological samples restricts biomarker development. Although biomarkers can be sourced from many tissue, drug effects in tumor tissue are of most interest, at least until a genuine surrogate can be found. But tumor biopsies are often technically difficult to obtain and are not without risk. Often, there is a need for two or possibly more biopsies for optimal evaluation of a biomarker of interest. This leaves many patients understandably reluctant to provide consent for what ultimately are exploratory studies.

Others hold a more pessimistic view towards biomarkers. Critical of the paucity of evidence for their utility, they claim the investment of capital and resources is not justified in its current form. Consider for example therapies targeting VEGF, of which there are multiple agents either under evaluation or approved for use. Despite extensive studies to date of a plethora of potential options, there are currently no validated biomarkers for selecting patients who will respond to antiangiogenic therapy. Quoting published studies demonstrating that biomarkers have not contributed to go/no go decisions, some biomarker skeptics believe sponsors of phase I studies should reconsider the value of including any biomarker evaluations. Furthermore, trials that add anything more than minimal risk from biomarker studies, especially invasive tumor biopsies, without a strong scientific basis and a testable hypothesis could be considered unethical [37].

A Way Forward

The limitations to effective biomarker use do not imply a lack of potential. On the contrary, they hold great promise for improving aspects of drug development and ultimately patient care. But these obstacles need to be tackled. The heterogeneity of how biomarkers are employed in development at present is a core problem. Just as a phased drug development process has provided a useful framework for cytotoxic agents for many years, a similar approach should improve efficiency of the development process for biomarkers and in turn targeted therapies.

One group proposed a "pharmacological audit trail" designed to link molecular target status with PK parameters and PD endpoints of drug effects on target, pathway and downstream biological processes in order to answer key questions in preclinical and clinical phases of drug development [2, 38]. As a drug successfully passes the sequential, connected questions proposed in the audit, each with an increasing degree of difficulty, the probability of successful development increases. First, investigators need to assess the expression of the molecular target and/

or determine if the corresponding signaling pathway involved is activated. Next, achievement of active concentrations of drug in plasma, blood and tumor tissue needs to be ascertained. Activity against the desired target must be shown. Then modulation of the pathway needs to be achieved. In turn, achievement of the desired biologic effect is critical. Finally, if this checklist of PK and PD criteria can be successfully completed, the key question is whether or not these findings translate into a clinically relevant response.

A second group put forward a comprehensive set of guidelines for study design for biomarker evaluation [39]. Dividing biomarker development into discovery, evaluation of classification accuracy and impact on clinical outcomes, they focused on the intermediate stage. Their proposal, relevant for biomarkers used for classification and prediction, hinges on prospective specimen collection and retrospective blinded evaluation (labeled PRoBE design). In other words, biologic specimens and clinical data are collected in the absence of knowledge of patient outcome. After outcome is known, randomly selected case and control subjects have their specimens assayed. By doing so, they hope to generate biomarkers with that can discriminate reliably and reproducibly and not due to artifact or bias. This is achieved through five phases asking more than 20 questions about the level of evidence in favor of the biomarker, from weakest to strongest, with the earlier phases generally necessary to design later phases. This design is not without its limitations. For example, this quantity of questions implies a large number of studies. The authors concede it may not be necessary to answer all of them or to perform them in strict order. Also, should the biomarker discovery phase be weak or flawed, the PRoBE study will simply confirm that the discovery did not work. However, the authors are to be commended on their attempts to provide a structure for biomarker evaluation and validation. Future proposals and discussion in time will refine the biomarker development process.

Further to the need for guidelines for biomarker discovery and development, these processes also need to occur at appropriate points in the drug approval timelines (see Fig. 18.1). For PD biomarkers, optimal timing for validation and standardization should take place during the preclinical phase, prior to entry into phase I evaluation. If this is not done, as so often is the case, spurious results can lead to inadequate trial design for subsequent phases in addition to substantial expense. This holds true for predictive biomarkers, though the rigorous scrutiny for this type takes place later, ideally between phases I and II. This is because phase II provides the first opportunity for correlative studies with a sufficient number of patients treated at the recommended dose. Novel markers discovered in late phase II trials would delay entry into phase III. In reality, idealized timelines are not pragmatic in many instances. The nature of translational research implies a clichéd cycle of knowledge from the bench to bedside to bench again that does not adhere to unidirectional development, and nor should it. Investigators at all stages of drug development need to remain open to possibility and to continue to ask questions. Only in this way will progress ensue. It is perhaps indicative of the need for a change to the current paradigm of drug development where the divisions between the traditional phases of development are becoming increasingly blurred. Nevertheless, it should still be concluded that the earlier that biomarker validation and standardization occurs, the more pertinent any findings or decisions based on these biomarkers will become.

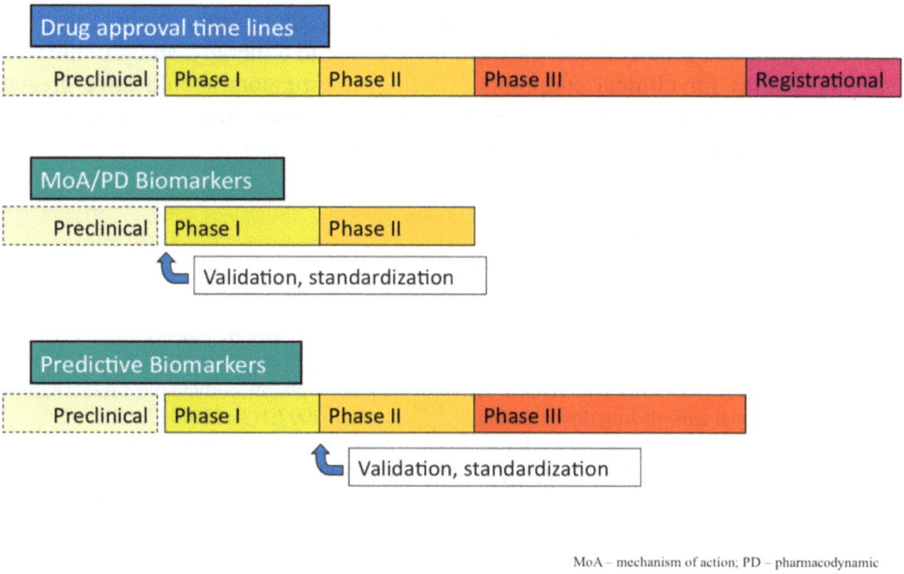

Fig. 18.1 Biomarker development in drug approval timelines

Conclusion

Biomarker development is an expanding area. Its importance parallels the rise of new, targeted therapies with novel mechanisms of action as anticancer treatments. These agents are providing the medical oncologist with an improved armamentarium with which to treat cancer patients.

The drug development process remains lengthy and costly with high attrition rates an ongoing cause for concern. Therefore, one of the objectives of biomarkers is to assist in important "go/no go" decisions for investigators at all stages of this process. Though at times they make a significant and relevant contribution to recommendations if and how a new agent should progress through to the next phase of development, at present this occurs relatively infrequently.

There are several reasons as to why the theoretical benefits of biomarker use not being attained to the full potential. From additional expense, to uncertain regulatory pathways, difficulties in tissue acquisition and doubts over reproducibility and interpretation, there is undeniable room for improvement for how biomarkers can be utilized. Further, drug response is multifactorial and prospective biomarkers are innumerable, and therefore random associations that reach statistical significance will occur, erroneously encouraging more investment.

Despite these shortcomings, biomarkers hold much promise. Validation and standardization will add enormously to the scientific robustness of identified biomarkers. Further, guidelines integrating biomarker with drug development will be advantageous. By doing so, biomarkers will continue providing evidence for PoC and MoA, they will help identify patients at high risk of toxicity, those more likely to respond to a treatment and predict those who will be resistant to a therapy, and provide reliable surrogates for clinical endpoints. In turn, investigators should have greater confidence not only to incorporate biomarker studies into drug development, but also to use biomarker data in key decision-making processes.

References

1. Reichert JM. Trends in development and approval times for new therapeutics in the United States. Nat Rev Drug Discov. 2003;2(9):695–702.
2. Sarker D, Pacey S, Workman P. Use of pharmacokinetic/pharmacodynamic biomarkers to support rational cancer drug development. Biomark Med. 2007;1(3):399–417.
3. Food and Drug Administration. Introduction or stagnation: challenge and opportunity on the critical path to new medical products. http://www.fda.gov/ScienceResearch/SpecialTopics/CriticalPathInitiative/CriticalPathOpportunitiesReports/ucm077262.htm#toolkit. Last accessed 15 June 2009.
4. Kola I, Landis J. Can the pharmaceutical industry reduce attrition rates? Nat Rev Drug Discov. 2004;3(8):711–5.
5. Walker I, Newell H. Do molecularly targeted agents in oncology have reduced attrition rates? Nat Rev Drug Discov. 2009;8(1):15–6.
6. Booth B, Glassman R, Ma P. Oncology's trials. Nat Rev Drug Discov. 2003;2(8):609–10.
7. Kummar S, Kinders R, Rubinstein L, et al. Compressing drug development timelines in oncology using phase '0' trials. Nat Rev Cancer. 2007;7(2):131–9.
8. Biomarkers Definitions Working Group. Biomarkers and surrogate endpoints: preferred definitions and conceptual framework. Clin Pharmacol Ther. 2001;69(3):89–95.
9. Goulart BH, Clark JW, Pien HH, Roberts TG, Finkelstein SN, Chabner BA. Trends in the use and role of biomarkers in phase I oncology trials. Clin Cancer Res. 2007;13(22 Pt 1): 6719–26.
10. Cunningham D, Humblet Y, Siena S, et al. Cetuximab monotherapy and cetuximab plus irinotecan in irinotecan-refractory metastatic colorectal cancer. N Engl J Med. 2004;351(4): 337–45.
11. Saltz LB, Meropol NJ, Loehrer Sr PJ, Needle MN, Kopit J, Mayer RJ. Phase II trial of cetuximab in patients with refractory colorectal cancer that expresses the epidermal growth factor receptor. J Clin Oncol. 2004;22(7):1201–8.
12. Chung KY, Shia J, Kemeny NE, et al. Cetuximab shows activity in colorectal cancer patients with tumors that do not express the epidermal growth factor receptor by immunohistochemistry. J Clin Oncol. 2005;23(9):1803–10.
13. Di Nicolantonio F, Martini M, Molinari F, et al. Wild-type BRAF is required for response to panitumumab or cetuximab in metastatic colorectal cancer. J Clin Oncol. 2008;26(35): 5705–12.
14. Allegra CJ, Jessup JM, Somerfield MR, et al. American Society of Clinical Oncology provisional clinical opinion: testing for KRAS gene mutations in patients with metastatic colorectal carcinoma to predict response to anti-epidermal growth factor receptor monoclonal antibody therapy. J Clin Oncol. 2009;27(12):2091–6.
15. Khambata-Ford S, Garrett CR, Meropol NJ, et al. Expression of epiregulin and amphiregulin and K-ras mutation status predict disease control in metastatic colorectal cancer patients treated with cetuximab. J Clin Oncol. 2007;25(22):3230–7.
16. Kris MG, Natale RB, Herbst RS, et al. Efficacy of gefitinib, an inhibitor of the epidermal growth factor receptor tyrosine kinase, in symptomatic patients with non-small cell lung cancer: a randomized trial. JAMA. 2003;290(16):2149–58.

17. Sequist LV, Martins RG, Spigel D, et al. First-line gefitinib in patients with advanced non-small-cell lung cancer harboring somatic EGFR mutations. J Clin Oncol. 2008;26(15): 2442–9.
18. Sunaga N, Tomizawa Y, Yanagitani N, et al. Phase II prospective study of the efficacy of gefitinib for the treatment of stage III/IV non-small cell lung cancer with EGFR mutations, irrespective of previous chemotherapy. Lung Cancer. 2007;56(3):383–9.
19. Mok TS, Wu YL, Thongprasert S, et al. Gefitinib or carboplatin-paclitaxel in pulmonary adenocarcinoma. N Engl J Med. 2009;361(10):947–57.
20. Cloughesy TF, Yoshimoto K, Nghiemphu P, et al. Antitumor activity of rapamycin in a Phase I trial for patients with recurrent PTEN-deficient glioblastoma. PLoS Med. 2008;5(1):e8.
21. Tabernero J, Cervantes A, Hoekman K, et al. Phase I study of AZD0530, an oral potent inhibitor of Src kinase: First demonstration of inhibition of Src activity in human cancers. J Clin Oncol. 2007;25(18suppl):3520.
22. Kelloff GJ, Bast Jr RC, Coffey DS, et al. Biomarkers, surrogate end points, and the acceleration of drug development for cancer prevention and treatment: an update prologue. Clin Cancer Res. 2004;10(11):3881–4.
23. Tabernero J, Rojo F, Calvo E, et al. Dose- and schedule-dependent inhibition of the mammalian target of rapamycin pathway with everolimus: a phase I tumor pharmacodynamic study in patients with advanced solid tumors. J Clin Oncol. 2008;26(10):1603–10.
24. Scaltriti M, Rojo F, Ocana A, et al. Expression of p95HER2, a truncated form of the HER2 receptor, and response to anti-HER2 therapies in breast cancer. J Natl Cancer Inst. 2007;99(8):628–38.
25. LoRusso P, Markman B, Tabernero J, et al. A phase I dose-escalation study of the safety, pharmacokinetics (PK), and pharmacodynamics of XL765, a PI3K/TORC1/TORC2 inhibitor administered orally to patients (pts) with advanced solid tumors. J Clin Oncol. 2009; 27(15S):3502.
26. Shapiro G, Kwak E, Baselga J, et al. Phase I dose-escalation study of XL147, a PI3K inhibitor administered orally to patients with solid tumors. J Clin Oncol. 2009;27(15S):3500.
27. Saltz L, Kies M, Abbruzzese J, Azarnia N, Needle M. The presence and intensity of the cetuximab-induced acne-like rash predicts increased survival in studies across multiple malignancies. Proc Am Soc Clin Oncol. 2003;22:204 (abstract 817).
28. Peeters M, Siena S, Van Cutsem E, et al. Association of progression-free survival, overall survival, and patient-reported outcomes by skin toxicity and KRAS status in patients receiving panitumumab monotherapy. Cancer. 2009;115(7):1544–54.
29. Tejpar S, Peeters M, Humblet Y, et al. Phase I/II study of cetuximab dose-escalation in patients with metastatic colorectal cancer (mCRC) with no or slight skin reactions on cetuximab standard dose treatment (EVEREST): pharmacokinetic (pk), pharmacodynamic (PD) and efficacy data. J Clin Oncol. 2007;25(18suppl):4037.
30. Scartozzi M, Galizia E, Chiorrini S, et al. Arterial hypertension correlates with clinical outcome in colorectal cancer patients treated with first-line bevacizumab. Ann Oncol. 2009;20(2): 227–30.
31. Rixe O, Billemont B, Izzedine H. Hypertension as a predictive factor of Sunitinib activity. Ann Oncol. 2007;18(6):1117.
32. Schneider BP, Wang M, Radovich M, et al. Association of vascular endothelial growth factor and vascular endothelial growth factor receptor-2 genetic polymorphisms with outcome in a trial of paclitaxel compared with paclitaxel plus bevacizumab in advanced breast cancer: ECOG 2100. J Clin Oncol. 2008;26(28):4672–8.
33. Roberts A, Gandhi L, O'Connor OA, et al. Reduction in platelet counts as a mechanistic biomarker and guide for adaptive dose-escalation in phase I studies of the Bcl-2 family inhibitor ABT-263. J Clin Oncol. 2008;26(15suppl):3542.
34. Goulart BHL, Roberts TG, Clark JW. Utility and costs of surrogate endpoints (SEs) and biomarkers in phase I oncology trials. J Clin Oncol. 2004;22(14suppl):6012.
35. Gualberto A, Pollak M. Emerging role of insulin-like growth factor receptor inhibitors in oncology: early clinical trial results and future directions. Oncogene. 2009;28(34):3009–21.

36. Scotlandi K, Picci P. Targeting insulin-like growth factor 1 receptor in sarcomas. Curr Opin Oncol. 2008;20(4):419–27.
37. Ratain MJ, Glassman RH. Biomarkers in phase I oncology trials: signal, noise, or expensive distraction? Clin Cancer Res. 2007;13(22 Pt 1):6545–8.
38. Workman P. How much gets there and what does it do? The need for better pharmacokinetic and pharmacodynamic endpoints in contemporary drug discovery and development. Curr Pharm Des. 2003;9(11):891–902.
39. Pepe MS, Feng Z, Janes H, Bossuyt PM, Potter JD. Pivotal evaluation of the accuracy of a biomarker used for classification or prediction: standards for study design. J Natl Cancer Inst. 2008;100(20):1432–8.

Index

H.-J. Lenz (ed.), *Biomarkers in Oncology: Prediction and Prognosis*, DOI 10.1007/978-1-4419-9755-5,

Q

MIX
Papier aus verantwortungsvollen Quellen
Paper from responsible sources
FSC® C105338

If you have any concerns about our products,
you can contact us on
ProductSafety@springernature.com

In case Publisher is established outside the EU,
the EU authorized representative is:
Springer Nature Customer Service Center GmbH
Europaplatz 3, 69115 Heidelberg, Germany

Printed by Libri Plureos GmbH
in Hamburg, Germany